Differentiation Antigens in Lymphohemopoietic Tissues

IMMUNOLOGY SERIES

1. Mechanisms in Allergy: Reagin-Mediated Hypersensitivity
   Edited by Lawrence Goodfriend, Alec Sehon and Robert P. Orange
2. Immunopathology: Methods and Techniques
   Edited by Theodore P. Zacharia and Sidney S. Breese, Jr.
3. Immunity and Cancer in Man: An Introduction
   Edited by Arnold E. Reif
4. *Bordetella pertussis:* Immunological and Other Biological Activities
   J.J. Munoz and R.K. Bergman
5. The Lymphocyte: Structure and Function (in two parts)
   Edited by John J. Marchalonis
6. Immunology of Receptors
   Edited by B. Cinader
7. Immediate Hypersensitivity: Modern Concepts and Development
   Edited by Michael K. Bach
8. Theoretical Immunology
   Edited by George I. Bell, Alan S. Perelson, and George H. Pimbley, Jr.
9. Immunodiagnosis of Cancer (in two parts)
   Edited by Ronald B. Herberman and K. Robert McIntire
10. Immunologically Mediated Renal Diseases: Criteria for Diagnosis and Treatment
    Edited by Robert T. McCluskey and Giuseppe A. Andres
11. Clinical Immunotherapy
    Edited by Albert F. LoBuglio
12. Mechanisms of Immunity to Virus-Induced Tumors
    Edited by John W. Blasecki
13. Manual of Macrophage Methodology: Collection, Characterization, and Function
    Edited by Herbert B. Herscowitz, Howard T. Holden, Joseph A. Bellanti, and Abdul Ghaffar
14. Suppressor Cells in Human Disease
    Edited by James S. Goodwin
15. Immunological Aspects of Aging
    Edited by Diego Segre and Lester Smith
16. Cellular and Molecular Mechanisms of Immunologic Tolerance
    Edited by Tomáš Hraba and Milan Hašek

17. Immune Regulation: Evolution and Biological Significance
Edited by Laurens N. Ruben and M. Eric Gershwin

18. Tumor Immunity in Prognosis: The Role of Mononuclear Cell Infiltration
Edited by Stephen Haskill

19. Immunopharmacology and the Regulation of Leukocyte Function
Edited by David R. Webb

20. Pathogenesis and Immunology of Treponemal Infection
Edited by Ronald F. Schell and Daniel M. Musher

21. Macrophage-Mediated Antibody-Dependent Cellular Cytotoxicity
Edited by Hillel S. Koren

22. Molecular Immunology: A Textbook
Edited by M. Zouhair Atassi, Carel J. van Oss, and Darryl R. Absolom

23. Monoclonal Antibodies and Cancer
Edited by George L. Wright, Jr.

24. Stress, Immunity, and Aging
Edited by Edwin L. Cooper

25. Immune Modulation Agents and Their Mechanisms
Edited by Richard L. Fenichel and Michael A. Chirigos

26. Mononuclear Phagocyte Biology
Edited by Alvin Volkman

27. The Lactoperoxidase System: Chemistry and Biological Significance
Edited by Kenneth M. Pruitt and Jorma O. Tenovuo

28. Introduction to Medical Immunology
Edited by Gabriel Virella, Jean-Michel Goust, H. Hugh Fudenberg, and Christian C. Patrick

29. Handbook of Food Allergies
Edited by James C. Breneman

30. Human Hybridomas: Diagnostic and Therapeutic Applications
Edited by Anthony J. Strelkauskas

31. Aging and the Immune Response: Cellular and Humoral Aspects
Edited by Edmond A. Goidl

32. Complications of Organ Transplantation
Edited by Luis H. Toledo-Pereyra

33. Monoclonal Antibody Production Techniques and Applications
Edited by Lawrence B. Schook

34. Fundamentals of Receptor Molecular Biology
Donald F. H. Wallach

35. Recombinant Lymphokines and Their Receptors
Edited by Steven Gillis

36. Immunology of the Male Reproductive Organs
Edited by Pierre Luigi Bigazzi

37. The Lymphocyte: Structure and Function
Edited by John J. Marchalonis
38. Differentiation Antigens in Lymphohemopoietic Tissues
Edited by Masayuki Miyasaka and Zdenek Trnka
39. Cancer Diagnosis In Vitro Using Monoclonal Antibodies
Edited by Herbert Z. Kupchik

Additional Volumes in Preparation

Differentiation Antigens in Lymphohemopoietic Tissues

edited by

MASAYUKI MIYASAKA
The Tokyo Metropolitan Institute of Medical Science
Tokyo, Japan

ZDENEK TRNKA
Basel Institute for Immunology
Basel, Switzerland

MARCEL DEKKER, INC. New York and Basel

Library of Congress Cataloging-in-Publication Data

Differentiation antigens in lymphohemopoietic tissues.

(Immunology series ; v. 38)
Foreword in English and French.
Includes bibliographies and index.
1. Histocompatibility antigens. 2. Tissue specific antigens. 3. Lymphocytes. 4. Leucocytes. 5. Immunology, Comparative. I. Miyasaka, Masayuki. II. Trnka, Z. III. Series. [DNLM: 1. Antigens--immunology. 2. Cell Differentiation. 3. Hematopoietic Stem Cells--physiology. 4. Lymphocytes--physiology.
W1 IM53K v.38 / WH 200 D569]
QR184.3.D54 1988 616.07'92 87-24543
ISBN 0-8247-7805-7

MARCEL DEKKER, INC.
270 Madison Avenue, New York, New York 10016

Current printing (last digit):
10 9 8 7 6 5 4 3 2 1

PRINTED IN THE UNITED STATES OF AMERICA

Series Introduction

It all started with a single, fertilized cell. Mitosis followed by differentiation gives rise to a multicellular animal—a community of cells with different properties and skills cooperating to give a functioning whole being. Of the forces that drive differentiation we still have only limited knowledge, but the consequences are revealed in the several specialized systems that provide the essential elements of life. The system most remarkable in its development is the lymphohemopoietic system, which has the responsibility for such a large number of essential bodily functions, ranging from cellular nutrition to metabolic homeostasis to immunity.

A system with so critical a role in the body's economy is best examined from a phylogenetic point of view. Vertebrates differ in form and function depending on their life-style and stage of evolution, yet the general outline of the lymphohemopoietic system has remained relatively constant. The reason undoubtedly lies in the importance of this system for survival. Even a minor change often leads to disease; a drastic change is incompatible with life.

The present book is the first to deal comprehensively with the distinctive antigens of the lymphohemopoietic system from a comparative point of view. Drs. Miyasaka and Trnka have assembled an outstanding group of experts who have explored this subject thoroughly. The book fills an important niche in the Immunology Series.

Noel R. Rose

Foreword

Scientific research is a lottery in which the scientist gambles that he will discover not only something new, but something that during his lifetime will make a significant contribution to the human condition. Those who have chosen to pursue a scientific career in immunology have placed their bets well.

The dazzling profusion and diversity of new immunological knowledge has given us the details with which we are able today to describe precisely the different aspects of the immune defense system.

The field of immunology, once defined as the science that deals with "the defense against nonself in respect of self," is now an area of research so vast that subdisciplines within immunology have become disciplines of themselves.

I can recall that as recently as the end of World War II, the small lymphocyte was regarded by pathologists as a cell of little interest or significance. Its function was unknown and it was largely ignored. This cell, neglected and even scorned, was destined to become the focal point of immunology. Likewise, the thymus, considered by most pathologists to be some redundant evolutionary relic like the appendix or an extra digit, has now become the new master of "self."

In the decade 1940-1950, the proposition that immunity could be induced against self-antigens was still a heresy. I well remember an epic confrontation at the 1950 International Congress of Hematology in Buffalo between Ernest Witebsky, a pupil and disciple of Ehrlich and a staunch defender of the dogma of "horror autotoxicus," and William Dameshek, who believed in the existence of autoimmune phenomena. Ehrlich's dogma was in fact itself worse than a heresy. It could not be repudiated even though there was the most detailed clinical evidence against it, for to deny its authority would have been sacrilege at that time. Several years later Ernest Witebsky, a gentleman and a great scholar, having himself done the appropriate experiments, became a convert: autoimmunity thus took the proper place that it has in immunology today.

Another subject that perplexed immunologists for many years was the incredible diversity of antibodies. The long controversy between those who believed in a template theory, which held that antibodies were made by being tailored to fit antigens, and those who believed, without really understanding how it came about, in the preexistence of this fabulous molecular diversity has now been decided in favor of the second point of view. But what a long and tortuous path has been negotiated to establish a logical explanation for how this vast repertoire of molecules came into being! Eventually, the new techniques of molecular biology provided the key to the resolution of this question.

But happily for the new generation of scientists there are a multitude of important questions still to be answered, particularly in regard to the mechanisms that allow the distinction of self from nonself. The part played by the histocompatibility antigens in this regard is still obscure. Do these antigens present only foreign antigens or a mixture of auto-, allo-, and xenoantigens, and in what form?

What is the nature of the signal that the histocompatibility antigens transmit to the internal structure of the cell to evoke the enormously complex sequence of events that leads to elimination of the foreign antigen and establishment of the immune state?

There is not much doubt that the discriminatory functions of the histocompatibility antigens are supported and reinforced by other cell-surface molecules, which act as multiple, main, or auxiliary receptors and transmitters of any number of signals.

It is to this task of identifying and describing these multiple "agents of contact and cooperation," which act like sensors on the cell surface, that scientists are now turning their attention. With characteristic egocentricity, the first studies on this subject have been done in the human. The histocompatibility workshops have borne their fruit: extensive collaborative research programs have been undertaken to unearth new molecules described as differentiation antigens, which are more or less specific for certain lines of cells or for certain tissues. The harvest has been rich and the rewards are increasing as the rate of research increases through the systematic use of monoclonal antibodies.

It was natural enough to extend this type of research to study the cells of other animal species. The diversity of the cell populations of animals studied in this way will offer new data with which to contemplate the processes of evolution. In addition, it will be possible through experiment to study and hopefully to uncover the physiological role of new molecular entities.

Masayuki Miyasaka and Zdenek Trnka have been responsible for bringing together in this book certain ideas and data, still as yet incomplete, concerning cell-surface antigens. The volume has the merit of collecting data that are sparse and difficult to find in the literature. The book will thus be of great value for all those who wish to have this information for further research.

If there is one single, crucial, baffling question that confronts scientists, it is that which concerns the regulation of developmental processes in biology. How and by what instructions can such a wonderfully coordinated structure as a living being develop, organize, restrict, and define its perfect internal equilibrium through a genetic program that, in spite of its sophistication, seems completely inappropriate for the prodigious task it has to accomplish—that of making the most successful of all species: a frail human being? Some of the clues to this may lie in the surface antigens of lymphocytes.

Jean Dausset

Foreword

La vie d'un scientifique est un pari. Pari certes de découvrir un fait nouveau mais aussi, par le choix de sa discipline, pari que celle-ci prendra dans les quelques années de sa vie d'homme un essor significatif. Ceux d'entre nous qui ont choisi comme thème d'étude l'Immunologie, ont dans ce sens fait le bon choix.

On ne peut qu'être ébloui par l'extraordinaire éclosion foisonnante de nos connaissances dans ce domaine, de la précision avec laquelle on peut aujourd'hui décrire les différentes étapes de la défense de l'intégrité de l'organisme.

L'Immunologie: science de "la défense contre le non-soi dans le respect du soi" est devenu une discipline tellement vaste qu'on est déjà obligé d'en distinguer des sous-ensembles qui deviennent eux-mêmes progressivement des disciplines à part entière.

Qu'on se souvienne simplement qu'à la fin de la deuxième guerre mondiale la signification des petits leucocytes, les lymphocytes, était totalement ignorée. Cellules presque négligées, méprisées, elles sont désormais au centre de nos préoccupations. Le thymus était considéré par beaucoup comme un reliquat de l'évolution au même titre que l'appendice ou que les restes du sixième orteil. Il est devenu le maître éducateur du soi.

Et la croyance même en une possible auto-immunisation était encore en 1940/1950 une hérésie. Je me souviens encore d'une épique empoignade au cours du Ier Congrès International d'Hématologie tenu à Buffalo en 1950 entre Ernest Witebsky, fidèle élève d'Erlich, lui-même tenant de l'horror autotoxicus et William Dameshek tenant de l'auto-immunité. Le dogme d'Erlich était pire qu'une hérésie et ne pouvait être contradit même par les observations les plus minitieuses d'un clinicien. C'eût été un sacrilège. Quelques années plus tard Ernest Witebsky, en grand gentleman et grand savant ayant expérimenté lui-même, était converti. L'auto-immunité a prenait ainsi la place éminente qui lui revient aujourd'hui.

Un autre sujet de perplexité des immunologistes a été pendant très longtemps l'incroyable diversité des anticorps. La longue querelle entre ceux qui pensaient que l'anticorps "se moulait" sur l'antigène et était ainsi fait sur mesure et ceux qui admettaient, sans la comprendre, la fabulause diversité préfabriquée, s'est enfin résolue en faveur des seconds. (Mais quel long chemin pour arriver à un mécanisme logique de la création d'un immense répertoire.) La biologie moléculaire a été à cet égard le "sésame ouvre toi."

Mais il reste encore, heureusement pour les jeunes chercheurs, bien d'autres mécanismes à déchiffrer, en particulier celui de la reconnaissance spécifique du soi et du non-soi. Le rôle exact de présentation des molécules du complexe majeur d'histocompatibilité est encore obscur. Présentent-elles seulement les antigènes étrangers ou l'ensemble des auto-, des allo- et des hétéro-antigènes et sous quelle forme?

Quelle est la nature du signal qu'elles transmettent aux structures intracellulaires pour promouvoir la cascade impressionnante d'événements qui vont en définitive conduire à l'élimination de l'intrus?

Dans cette mission les molécules du complexe majeur d'histocompatibilité sont sans doute aidées, confortées par d'autres molécules à la surface de la cellule où se trouvent de multiples récepteurs, capteurs principaux ou auxiliaires de nombreux signaux.

C'est à cette tâche de détection puis de description de ces multiples "agents de contact et de coopéeration" qui se trouvent en antenne à la surface des cellules de l'organisme que ce sont plus récemment attachés les chercheurs. Avec l'égocentrisme habituel c'est vers l'Homme que se sont dirigées les premières études. L'exemple des workshops d'histocompatibilité a été suivi avec fruit. D'immenses travaux collaboratifs ont été menés pour dépister de nouvelles molécules dites de différenciation car plus ou moins spécifiques d'une lignée cellulaire donnée ou d'un tissu. La récolte a été riche, la quête se poursuit à un rythme accéléré grâce à la découverte puis à l'usage systématique des anticorps monoclonaux de Milstein et Köhler.

Il était naturel d'étendre ces recherches aux cellules animales, qui par leur diversité apportent de nouveaux éléments de réflexion sur l'évolution et surtout qui vont permettre grâce à l'expérimentation, impossible chez l'Homme, possible chez l'animal, d'étudier et nous l'espérons d'élucider le rôle physiologique et respectif de ces nouvelles entités.

A l'initiative de M. Miyasaka et Z. Trnka ce volume apporte des notions, encore fractionnelles, en ce domaine de l'Immunologie. Il a le mérite de les rassembler alors qu'elles étaient éparses donc difficiles d'accès, dans la littérature scientifique. Ce livre sera donc d'une grande utilité pour tous ceux qui veulent profiter de ces connaissances acquises pour aller plus loin et ouvrir de nouvelles perspectives.

Car s'il y a une question lancinante que le Biologiste se pose c'est bien celle qui concerne le développement. Comment, par quels signaux un tel édifice harmonieux, celui d'un être vivant, peut-il se développer, s'organiser, s'auto-limiter, établir ses équilibres, ses interactions à l'aide d'un programme génétique qui, malgré ses dimensions nous parait encore dérisoire devant l'immense tâche à accomplir: un petit d'Homme.

Jean Dausset

Preface

During the past few years new knowledge on cellular differentiation in lympho-hemopoietic tissue has been acquired with bewildering rapidity. Many technical advances have greatly facilitated the study of differentiation antigens or cell-surface antigens, the expression of which can be correlated with the extent of cellular maturity or differentiation or with cellular derivation. The most important advance has been the introduction of monoclonal antibody technology. Another major technical advance has been the application of molecular biology. These technologies have provided a new dimension to our understanding of various cell-surface molecules in relation to their function and, as a result, have produced in a short time an accumulation of a large amount of information that has not been fully collated.

One aim of the study of cell differentiation is to understand the mechanisms of generation of diversity. Ironically, people engaged in this research have been generators of diversity through the use of various animal species. Although an enormous amount of information on differentiation antigens is becoming available in a wide spectrum of animal species, there has been relatively little effort to create a common thread across the spectrum, which is reflected by the fact that there has been no single up-to-date and comprehensive summary of the entire field, possibly because of such a rapid accumulation of new knowledge and evolution of new thoughts. The same progress has also widened the psychological gap between scientists using different animal species.

The aim of this book is to provide, conveniently within one volume, a comprehensive review of these antigens investigated in various animal species in order to enhance cross-cultural interactions among scientists working on various animal species. The book consists of 15 chapters dealing with various differentiation antigens associated with lymphohemopoietic tissue in a variety of animal species. With humans and mice, which have been most intensively investigated, more space is given to describe in detail cell-surface components defined by monoclonal antibodies, whereas other species are represented by single chapters. The book is designed so that each chapter stands up in its own right, and hence, there is little need to cross-refer when one wants to obtain an overview of antigens in one particular species of animal.

Although we are aware that multiauthored books often suffer from heterogeneity of style, we solicited contributions from various people who have been most actively engaged in each research area in order to assure expertise in each subject. And we are extremely fortunate in having a list of first-class contributors for our book, each of whom has endeavored to provide clear-cut and up-to-date information obtained in individual species. We hope that the outcome of our effort may help to clarify many diverse observations obtained in various animal species. We have attempted to control the size of the book, but not at the expense of thoroughness and scientific merit. We hope that the book will be of value to a diverse group of readers. Although it is primarily directed at people in the field of cellular immunology, we hope that the book will also be of general interest to any persons interested in lymphohemopoietic cell differentiation, be they cell biologists, hematologists, zoologists, clinicians, or veterinarians.

We are indebted to the many colleagues who helped us in compiling this book. We wish to thank all those contributors who generously agreed to give their valuable time and meticulous effort and to share their special knowledge with all who read this book. The stimulating environment generated by the scientists in the Basel Institute for Immunology, where both of us worked for some years, has been extremely important in providing us with the motivation to complete this book, and to these researchers we are very grateful. We wish to express our gratitude to Kerry Doyle and Elaine Grohman for their editorial assistance with the manuscript and to other staff members at Marcel Dekker, Inc., especially the Vice President, Graham Garratt, who shepherded the book through editing and production. Finally, we express our sincere appreciation of the understanding and warm support of our families.

Masayuki Miyasaka
Zdenek Trnka

Contributors

Joseph A. Aprile Department of Medical Oncology, Fred Hutchinson Cancer Research Center, Seattle, Washington

Cynthia L. Baldwin International Laboratory for Research on Animal Diseases, Nairobi, Kenya

Atul K. Bhan Department of Pathology, Harvard Medical School, and Department of Pathology, Massachusetts General Hospital, Boston, Massachusetts

Ina Bhan Department of Pathology, Tufts University School of Medicine, and Department of Pathology, New England Medical Center, Boston, Massachusetts

Reinhard Burger Institute for Immunology, University of Heidelberg, Heidelberg, Federal Republic of Germany

H. Joachim Deeg* Fred Hutchinson Cancer Research Center, Seattle, Washington

Louis Du Pasquier Basel Institute for Immunology, Basel, Switzerland

Martin F. Flajnik Basel Institute for Immunology, Basel, Switzerland

---

**Present affiliation*: Lombardi Cancer Research Center, Georgetown University, Washington, D.C.

Douglas G. Gilmour* Department of Microbiology, New York University School of Medicine, New York, New York

Wayne R. Hein Basel Institute for Immunology, Basel, Switzerland

Thierry Hercend Départment de Biologie Clinique, Institut Gustave Roussy, Villejuif, France

Ellen Hsu† Basel Institute for Immunology, Basel, Switzerland

Wilfred A. Jefferies†† Division of Immunology, Swiss Institute for Experimental Cancer Research, Lausanne, Switzerland

James F. Kaufman Basel Institute for Immunology, Basel, Switzerland

Yukio Koide Department of Microbiology and Immunology, Hamamatsu University School of Medicine, Hamamatsu, Japan

Warren C. Ladiges Transplantation Biology Program, Fred Hutchinson Cancer Research Center, and Division of Animal Medicine, University of Washington, Seattle, Washington

Joan K. Lunney Animal Parasitology Institute, Agricultural Research Service, U.S. Department of Agriculture, Beltsville, Maryland

Bonnie J. Mathieson Laboratory of Experimental Immunology, Biological Response Modifiers Program, Division of Cancer Treatment, National Cancer Institute–Frederick Cancer Research Center, Frederick, Maryland

Susan McClure Basel Institute for Immunology, Basel, Switzerland

John P. McKearn§ Medical Products Department, E. I. duPont de Nemours and Co., Glenolden, Pennsylvania

---

**Present address*: London, England.
Present affiliations:
†Department of Biochemistry, Columbia University College of Physicians and Surgeons, New York, New York.
††Ludwig Institute for Cancer Research, Stockholm, Sweden.
§Searle Research and Development, Monsanto Co., St. Louis, Missouri.

Stefan C. Meuer Division of Applied Immunology, German Cancer Research Center, Heidelberg, Federal Republic of Germany

Masayuki Miyasaka* Basel Institute for Immunology, Basel, Switzerland

W. Ivan Morrison International Laboratory for Research on Animal Diseases, Nairobi, Kenya

Jan Naessens International Laboratory for Research on Animal Diseases, Nairobi, Kenya

Mark D. Pescovitz† Immunology Branch, National Cancer Institute, National Institutes of Health, Bethesda, Maryland

J. Richard L. Pink Central Research Unit, F. Hoffmann-La Roche & Co., Basel, Switzerland

Robert F. Raff Department of Transplantation Biology, Division of Oncology, Fred Hutchinson Cancer Research Center, Seattle, Washington

Hubert Schaefer Institute for Immunology, University of Heidelberg, Heidelberg, Federal Republic of Germany

Friedrich Schuening Department of Transplantation Biology, Fred Hutchinson Cancer Research Center, Seattle, Washington

Susan O. Sharrow Immunology Branch, National Cancer Institute, National Institutes of Health, Bethesda, Maryland

Joan Stein-Streilein Departments of Medicine and Microbiology/Immunology, University of Miami School of Medicine, Miami, Florida

Rainer Storb Department of Transplantation Biology, Fred Hutchinson Cancer Research Center, Seattle, Washington

Zdenek Trnka Basel Institute for Immunology, Basel, Switzerland

---

Present affiliations:
*Department of Immunology, Tokyo Metropolitan Institute of Medical Science, Tokyo, Japan.
†Department of Surgery, University of Minnesota, Minneapolis, Minnesota.

J. Michael Wilkinson Department of Biochemistry, The Hunterian Institute, Royal College of Surgeons of England, London, England

Pamela L. Witte Department of Pathology, University of Texas Health Science Center, Dallas, Texas

Takato O. Yoshida Department of Microbiology and Immunology, Hamamatsu University School of Medicine, Hamamatsu, Japan

Contents

1
Functional Significance of Human T-Lymphocyte-Associated Antigens

STEFAN C. MEUER
German Cancer Research Center, Heidelberg, Federal Republic of Germany

THIERRY HERCEND
Institut Gustave Roussy, Villejuif, France

I. INTRODUCTION

A high degree of functional heterogeneity exists within the T-cell population. In this regard, human T lymphocytes recognize antigens in a very specific fashion, perform immunoregulatory activities, and execute unique effector functions. T lymphocytes proliferate to soluble and cell-surface antigens as well as polyclonal activators, are responsible for cytotoxic killer activity in cell-mediated lympholysis, and produce soluble mediators. Perhaps more important, T lymphocytes regulate the function of many other cells in an inductive or suppressive fashion (1-7).

The development of monoclonal antibodies restricted in their reactivity to cells of the human T lineage provides the basis for an advanced understanding of T-cell differentiation and unique functional programs that individual mature T-cell subpopulations perform. Moreover, these reagents have greatly improved in vitro techniques for the isolation of highly pure subsets of human T lymphocytes. Thus, it is now possible to correlate some normal and abnormal functional properties of T-lymphocyte subpopulations in vitro with in vivo disorders of the immune response. Most recently, the combination of monoclonal antibodies with cell cloning techniques has been successfully employed to delineate the functional significance of T-cell surface molecules.

The rapidly increasing number of monoclonal antibodies already produced and an expected acceleration of future production required the organization of a forum in which the abundant data available from many investigators could be compared by means of biochemistry, surface binding, and functional activities. International workshops on human leucocyte differentiation antigens took place in Paris (1981) and Boston (1984). As a result of these workshops, clusters of differentiation were defined. In this chapter we shall, therefore, describe the various lymphoid differentiation antigens according to this cluster definition (8,9).

II. CD2-T11. A GLYCOPROTEIN INVOLVED IN T-CELL ACTIVATION

Human T lymphocytes were first identified when it was observed that all thymus-derived cells spontaneously form rosettes with sheep erythrocytes (10-13). The E-rosetting capacity, which is acquired early in thymic ontogeny, is then maintained on all peripheral T lymphocytes. This phenomenon provided means by which to enumerate cells in the T lineage at a time when no specific antisera were available. Subsequently, with the development of monoclonal antibodies, the sheep-erythrocyte receptor has been identified as a 50 Kd glycoprotein. This 50 Kd structure demonstrates considerable structural conservation on T cells of such phylogenetically distinct species as lemur and man (14-20).

A series of monoclonal antibodies which were produced against the T11 surface protein define three distinct epitopes of this molecule (21). Two of these, $T11_1$ and $T11_2$ are expressed on resting T lymphocytes and thymocytes, whereas a third, $T11_3$, is found only on activated T cells. Monoclonal antibodies specific for the $T11_1$ epitope are unique in their capacity to inhibit E-rosette formation, indicating that $T11_1$ represents the human T-lymphocyte E-rosette receptor. More important, anti-$T11_2$ and anti-$T11_3$ in concert activate human T cells to express their individual functional programs in the absence of antigen and/or antigen-presenting cells. This activation results in proliferation and release of regulatory mediators. Since the T11 structure is not physically linked to T3-Ti (see below), which is the receptor complex for specific antigen, T-cell activation through CD2 appears to represent an antigen-independent "alternative pathway" of T-cell triggering (21).

The physiological significance of this alternative pathway has yet to be identified, since a natural ligand that could engage this pathway remains unknown. Nevertheless, the identification of an antigen-independent mode of T-cell triggering has prompted speculations regarding the involvement of the T11-mediated activation processes in T-cell differentiation. Most recently, a T helper cell-derived novel lymphokine, termed IL4a, has been proposed to bind to T11 with the consequence of inducing proliferation of resting human T lymphocytes in the absence of accessory cells (22).

Moreover, a 45 Kd cell-surface molecule (T11TS) detected on sheep erythrocytes by a monoclonal antibody was recently shown to bind directly to CD2 (23). It is not known at present whether the interaction between CD2 and T11TS produces functional effects. Nevertheless, the fact that some antibodies directed at the T11 glycoprotein have been reported to inhibit the immune response is not surprising (24).

III. CD3-T3. THE T3 MOLECULAR COMPLEX IS INVOLVED IN ANTIGEN RECOGNITION

The T3 molecular complex consists of at least three individual sets of molecules, namely, the 25 Kd glycosilated T3 γ chain, the 20 Kd glycosilated T3 δ chain, and the 20 Kd nonglycosilated T3 ϵ chain (25). Both the appearance of the T3 molecular complex in late intrathymic ontogeny at the time that immunologic competence is acquired and its known critical role in T-lymphocyte function suggested that T3 was closely linked to an important recognition receptor or cell-cell interaction molecule (26,27). Antibodies directed against T3 were unique in their capacity to block the induction phase as well as the effector phase of cell-mediated lympholysis, to inhibit T-lymphocyte proliferative responses to soluble antigen, and to be mitogenic for resting T cells in the presence of accessory cells. In the latter case, activation was accompanied by a release of T-cell lymphokines, including interleukin 2 and γ interferon (27-31). Incubation of T cells with anti-T3 induces modulation of the T3 complex (27). It is not known at present whether modulation occurs as a consequence of internalization of the T3 complex or, alternatively, by external shedding from the membrane. In fact, both possibilities have been suggested (27,32). It seems likely that these discrepancies are due to the isotype of monoclonal antibodies which have been employed to induce modulation (internalization in the case of IgG antibodies and external shedding in the case of IgM antibodies).

As mentioned above, anti-T3 antibodies possess potent mitgenic activity for resting T cells, provided accessory cells are present (33-35). This mode of activation is in marked contrast to the T11-mediated mode of T-cell triggering which occurs independent of metabolic activities in accessory cells (21). In the process of T-cell triggering by anti-T3, accessory cells apparently serve two purposes. First, antibody oligomerization via Fc receptors has been shown to represent a critical requirement for the initiation of T-cell activation. Anti-T3 antibodies in soluble form inhibit T-cell function (28). Oligomerization can also be artificially induced by multimeric surface binding of anti-T3 monoclonal antibodies, e.g., to Sepharose beads (36). Second, monocytes contribute in the process of primary T-cell activation through soluble mediators, such as interleukin 1, which is critically required by human T lymphocytes for the production of interleukin 2. In contrast, the expression of receptors for interleukin 2 appears to be independent of monocyte-secreted interleukin 1 (35).

IV. Ti. THE ANTIGEN RECOGNITION STRUCTURE

In the membrane of mature T lymphocytes, the T3 complex is noncovalently associated with a heterodimer of approximately 90 Kd clonotypic determinants (37-39). This molecule represents an antigen-recognition structure on the majority of human T cells, independent of subset derivation, specificity, or regulatory function (40). This heterodimer was termed Ti, for T-cell idiotype. The close functional linkage of T3 and Ti is demonstrated by a number of findings. Thus, modulation of T3 induced by anti-T3 antibodies leads to comodulation of Ti, and vice versa (36). Moreover, with respect to the quantitative surface expression, T3 and Ti exist at a 1:1 ratio, suggesting that each Ti molecule is linked to one T3 complex in the membrane (37). Finally, activities of anti-T3 and anti-Ti monoclonal antibodies are indistinguishable from each other. Thus, in soluble form, these antibodies inhibit T-cell function, whereas, following multimerization, the same antibodies can individually trigger T lymphocytes in a fashion identical to that induced by the natural ligand of Ti, namely antigen itself (40). A linkage between the T-cell receptor, Ti and T3 does not exist only for human T lymphocytes, but was recently found to exist for murine T cells as well (41). Although monoclonal antibodies to murine T3 are not available, molecular cloning and surface cross-linking experiments in immunochemical studies proved that the T3-Ti relationship represents a general fact.

Peptide map analysis of isolated α and β chains from individual T-cell clones with distinct specificities indicated that both chains contain variable (V) and constant (C) regions and are unrelated to each other (42,43). Moreover, both chains are glycosilated. These findings have been confirmed by molecular cloning of the genes that are encoding Ti α and β (44,45). In the human, these genes are localized on chromosome 7 (β gene) and chromosome 14 (α gene). The corresponding protein chains are generated following rearrangement of V, D, J, and C genes, similarly to those occurring in the case of immunoglobulins (46). Finally, both Ti α and β chains belong to the family of molecules that includes immunoglobulins and the MHC gene products (47).

A third rearranged gene, located on chromosome 7 like the Ti β genes, has been cloned and sequenced (48,49). Only very recently has a corresponding gene product been identified. However, its biological function remains unclear at present. Studies, particularly from the murine system, indicated that a Ti γ chain may be expressed at very early stages of T-cell ontogeny during thymic development (50). In the peripheral compartment, it has been suggested that mature cytolytic mouse T lymphocytes, but not helper T lymphocytes, express Ti γ (49). Very recent studies in the human system, however, demonstrate that, independent of biological activity (cytotoxic/noncytotoxic), Ti γ is not surface expressed by the majority of mature T lymphocytes (51,52). Therefore, one must conclude that a Ti α/β structure serves as a receptor which allows for MHC-restricted antigen recognition by human T lymphocytes (53). However, it has been shown that minor populations of cytotoxic T lymphocytes exist which recognize target cells (particular tumor cells) in an MHC-independent fashion (54,55). This subset can be delineated through surface expression of a 220 Kd molecule, NKH1 (56,57), whose function is presently unknown. It has been demonstrated that a α/β Ti heterodimer is expressed on these "unconventional" T lymphocytes as well (54) and employed for MHC-unrestricted antigen recognition.

V. CD4-T4. A SUBSET-RESTRICTED GLYCOPROTEIN

Profound changes in cell surface antigens mark the various stages of T-cell ontogeny (17). In man the earliest lymphoid cells within the thymus lack mature T-cell antigens such as T3, but express antigens carried by bone marrow cells of several lineages. This population accounts for approximately 10% of thymic lymphocytes and is reactive with two monoclonal antibodies, anti-T9 and anti-T10. Although these two antibodies are not specific for T cells, since they react with normal activated and malignant cells of many lineages, they are useful to understand antigenic changes that occur during T-cell ontogeny. With maturation, thymocytes lose T9, retain T10, and coexpress antigens defined by anti-T4 and anti-T8 (see below). Thymocytes coexpressing T4 and T8 account for approximately 70% of the thymic population. At the stage of mature thymocytes prior to exportation into the circulation, T cells segregate into $T4^+$ and $T8^+$ subsets. Immunological competence is acquired at this stage but is not fully developed until thymic lymphocytes emigrate from the thymus (58). Outside the thymus, the T4 antigen is expressed on approximately 55-65% of peripheral T cells (18).

A series of functional studies on isolated subpopulations of peripheral T lymphocytes demonstrates that the specific program of T cells is linked to the expression of particular cell-surface molecules. For example, only the $T4^+$ population responds to soluble antigen and is capable of providing inducer function in T-T, T-B, and T-macrophage interactions (59).

More recently, in vitro studies employing cloned populations of antigen-specific human T lymphocytes indicated that expression of the T4 molecule does not correlate with a particular regulatory or effector function, but rather allows a T cell to interact with other cells expressing class II gene products of the major histocompatibility complex (53). Thus, it was concluded that the 54 Kd T4 glycoprotein represents a receptor molecule employed by T cells for binding to a monomorphic portion of class II determinants (39). Although many functional data support this view, it remains to be proven that T4 in fact binds to class II molecules during cell-cell interactions. However, molecular cloning of the T4 gene and the demonstration that T4 belongs to the MHC/immunoglobulin/T-cell receptor supergene family provides an additional piece of evidence for this notion (60).

By means of monoclonal antibodies a number of discrete epitopes of the T4 glycoprotein have been defined. Importantly, one of these epitopes serves as a receptor which is critically involved in HTLV-III/LAV (human T lymphotropic virus type III/lymphadenopathy-associated virus) infection of T4$^+$ T lymphocytes (61). Moreover, absence of one or the other T4 epitope may render an individual more susceptible to particular types of autoimmune disease (62).

VI. CD8-T8. A SUBSET-RESTRICTED CELL-CELL INTERACTION MOLECULE

The 62 Kd T8 glycoprotein is expressed on approximately 20-30% of peripheral T lymphocytes. As mentioned above (17), T cells during maturation coexpress T8 and T4 at a particular stage. When immunological competence is acquired, T cells segregate into the T8$^+$ and the T4$^+$ subsets. In vitro studies employing purified T-cell subpopulations demonstrated that the T8 subset contains a mature population of cells with cytotoxic and suppressor function. Although cytotoxic T lymphocytes are contained within the T4$^+$ subset as well, the vast majority of cytotoxic effector cells generated in a mixed lymphocyte reaction are T8$^+$ (59). Moreover, the isolated T8 subset cannot respond to soluble antigens. The functional heterogeneity found to exist within the T8$^+$ subpopulation demonstrated that the capacity to express this glycoprotein is unrelated to a particular biological T-cell activity. Employing cloned populations of human T lymphocytes derived from either the T4$^+$ or the T8$^+$ subpopulation indicated that, whereas the former are generally specific for class II MHC determinants, the latter preferentially recognize class I MHC gene products during cellular interactions (53). Therefore, a similar functional role, as proposed for the T4 molecule (see above), has been assigned to the T8 homodimer. Thus, it was suggested that T8 represents an associative recognition structure which interacts with a monomorphic portion of class I determinants on target cells. Since viral gene products preferentially associate with MHC class I molecules, it is not surprising that the majority of cytotoxic cells observed in antivral responses is T8$^+$. That T8 represents a receptor structure is supported by molecular cloning experiments which demonstrated that the T8 gene bears considerable sequence homology with MHC, immunoglobulin, T-cell receptor, and T4 (60,63).

VII. CD1-T6; CD5-T1; CD6-T12. T-CELL STRUCTURES WITH UNKNOWN FUNCTION

Expression of the T6 glycoprotein characterizes an intermediate step of human T-cell ontogeny (64). Within the thymus, T6 reactivity is acquired at a stage where T cells coexpress T4 and T8 and is lost prior to exportation from the thymic environment into the peripheral compartment. T6, which is not homologous to the murine TL antigens, has some interesting molecular characteristics. This 45 Kd structure is associated with β_2 microglobulin on the surface of cortical thymocytes (65). Moreover, there appears to exist a linkage between T6 and T8 on these cells. Both its molecular mass and its association with β_2 microglobulin indicate that T6 may represent a member of the MHC class I family of molecules (66).

Two additional surface structures are expressed by the majority of mature T lymphocytes. These structures, as defined by monoclonal antibodies, have been termed T1 (CD5) and T12 (CD6), respectively (67,68). It should be noted that T1 and T12 are not T-lineage specific but are also expressed on human B lymphocytes at particular stages of B-cell ontogeny. Although the functional significance of the 69 Kd T1 and the 120 Kd T12 glycoprotein is not yet understood, monoclonal antibodies directed at T12 have been successfully employed for removal of mature T cells in the course of bone marrow transplantation. One rationale for employing anti-T12 for T-cell manipulation is that following binding of anti-T12—unlike that found in the case of T1 and T3—modulation of the corresponding surface structure does not occur (27,68).

VIII. CD25-Tac. THE RECEPTOR FOR INTERLEUKIN 2

A number of recently produced monoclonal antibody reagents define a 52-55 Kd surface glycoprotein which is only expressed on human T lymphocytes following their activation by antigens or mitogens. Using biosynthetically labeled IL2, it was demonstrated that monoclonal antibodies directed at this surface receptor, termed Tac, block surface binding of interleukin 2 to the T-cell membrane (69,70). Moreover, such antibodies inhibit T-cell growth, since they interfere with the central mechanism which enables T lymphocytes to proliferate following triggering. Interestingly, both high and low affinity binding sites for interleukin 2 appear to exist on the receptor molecule (71). The physiological role of these two sets of receptors is as yet not known. An intriguing question related to this 55 Kd molecule originated from recent studies in which it was demonstrated that cells lacking the Tac protein can respond to interleukin 2 and that IL2 responsiveness can exist on mature human T lymphocytes prior to the acquisition of surface reactivity with anti-CD 25 antibodies (35). It should be also noted that the capacity to express receptor structures for interleukin 2 is not a unique property of T lymphocytes. For example, human B lymphocytes, upon activation, clearly respond to interleukin 2 by expression of the Tac molecule (72,73). Analogous findings have now been reported for cells of the human monocyte/macrophage lineage (74).

IX. LFA. A FAMILY OF MOLECULES INVOLVED IN CELL-CELL INTERACTIONS

A novel family of leucocyte-differentiation antigens participating in cell-cell interactions has been identified by a set of monoclonal antibodies and extensively studied with regard to both biochemistry and functional significance. Antigens belonging to this family are selectively expressed on some leucocytes, such as macrophages and lymphocytes. These glycoproteins are composed of distinct α subunits with molecular weights of 180 Kd (LFA1), 170 Kd (MAC1), and 150 Kd, which are nonconvalently associated with 95 Kd β subunits. These β subunits are identical for all three molecular species (75).

The human LFA 1 antigen appears to participate in several types of cell-cell interaction. Monoclonal antibodies against LFA 1 block both antigen-specific T-cell-mediated killing and natural killing (76,77). This effect was found to be due to binding of anti-LFA 1 to the effector cell rather than to the target cell. The same antibodies also inhibit T-cell proliferative responses to antigens and mitogens.

Monoclonal antibodies directed against the human MAC 1 antigen were shown to block the human receptor for C3bi, the complement receptor type 3 (CR3) (78). The function of the third member of this family, the p150, 95 molecule, is not known at present.

X. CONCLUSIONS

The possibility of producing monoclonal antibodies directed at surface components of human lymphoid cells has provided a tremendous amount of new information regarding the molecular basis of lymphocyte function. In concert with novel cell culture systems and modern technologies for the separation of pure populations of lymphocytes, monoclonal antibodies have not only been useful in delineating functionally important cell-surface structures; employing such reagents for functional in vitro studies, it has also become possible to recognize the physiological significance of critical determinants involved in the immune response. Besides the fact that the basis of antigen recognition and discrimination as well as the molecular basis of clonal T-cell growth are now known, the approach to study cell function employing monoclonal antibodies has demonstrated its potential for the discovery of previously unknown mechanisms of immunoregulation. Thus, an alternative pathway of T-cell activation which is independent of antigen recognition has been delineated solely on the basis of monoclonal antibody effects, whereas a natural ligand that could engage this mode of T-cell activation remains yet to be identified.

The surface molecules and the corresponding monoclonal antibodies described in this chapter will be crucial tools for further studies of immunoregulatory mechanisms, such as the process of T-cell activation and its abnormalities, which may be underlying disorders of the immune response in autoimmunity and immunodeficiency. With regard to application of these serological reagents to human diseases, many of the above described monoclonal antibodies have become useful typing reagents to detect abnormalities of differentiation as they exist in leuke-

2
In Situ Characterization of Human Lymphoid Cells Using Monoclonal Antibodies

ATUL K. BHAN
Harvard Medical School and Massachusetts General Hospital, Boston, Massachusetts

INA BHAN
Tufts University School of Medicine and New England Medical Center, Boston, Massachusetts

I. INTRODUCTION

The various components of the human lymphoid system (lymphocytes, monocytes/macrophages, and dendritic cells) occupy distinct anatomical compartments, where they mature, differentiate, and function (1-9). Thus, T cells following intrathymic maturation localize in well-defined anatomical sites in peripheral lymphoid tissue, such as paracortical and interfollicular areas in tonsils, lymph nodes, and Peyer's patches of intestine, and in the periarteriolar lymphoid sheath in the spleen. In addition, a unique population of T cells is closely associated with mucosal epithelium (intestine, bronchus) (10). B cells are primarily located in the lymphoid follicles, where they divide and differentiate into mature B cells. Like the progenitors of other hematopoietic cells, the stem cells of B and T cells are located in the human fetal liver in early stages of development and later in the bone marrow.

Most of the information regarding the development and migration of the lymphoid cells has been obtained by studies carried out in animals (1,2,11-13). Examination of immunodeficient states in humans has also contributed considerably to our understanding of human lymphoid tissues. In situ characterization of various components of the lymphoid system was first made possible by the development of rosetting techniques to detect cell-surface receptors (Fc, C3, and sheep erythrocyte receptors), application of histochemical techniques, and the use of specific heteroantisera against cell-surface (or cytoplasmic) antigens (14-17). However, most of the markers detected by these techniques were neither specific nor restricted to one lineage of hematopoietic cells. Furthermore, rosetting techniques, although helpful in defining large groups of cells (such as B cells in follicles), did not allow characterization of individual cells when mixed with other cell types in lymphoid tissues. Similarly, most conventional antisera contained a broad range of reactivities, thus limiting their usefulness in the characterization of cells in tissue sections. The development of monoclonal antibodies against lymphocyte-differentiation antigens has provided molecular markers for precise characterization of the lymphoid subsets in their normal microenvironment (4). Moreover, application of monoclonal antibodies to tissue diagnosis has made possible the immunophenotyping of lymphoproliferative disorders, analysis of inflammatory cell reactions, and the definition of close association of lymphoid cells with other cells in normal and diseased states (4,18).

Since monoclonal antibodies recognize a limited number of antigenic determinants, and only a part of the cell membrane is available for binding with antibodies in tissue sections, it is essential that sensitive immunohistochemical techniques be applied to define the cell populations in tissues (4). Immunofluorescence techniques, although very useful in the analysis of cells in suspension, are generally insensitive when applied to tissue sections to stain lymphocyte subsets. For example, $T4^+$ cells can be convincingly demonstrated in tissue sections by immunoperoxidase techniques but not by immunofluorescence methods (5). The use of enzyme (horseradish peroxidase, alkaline phosphatase)-labeled antibodies has allowed development of sensitive immunohistochemical techniques (19-21). Furthermore, by using different substrates for the enzymes it is possible to develop contrasting reaction products and simultaneously localize two antigens in the tissue sections (20,22). The recent introduction of hapten-labeled antibodies (23,24) and the avidin-biotin system (25-27) has further improved the sensitivity of immunohistochemical techniques.

As most cell-surface antigens are altered by fixatives and the tissue processing used in the preparation of paraffin-embedded sections, immunohistochemical studies for the characterization of lymphoid cells have generally been performed on frozen tissue sections (4). Certain fixatives, including acetone and paraformaldehyde, have been found to preserve the reactivity of most cell-surface antigens with antibodies (4,28,29). This has enabled the performance of immunoelectron microscopy to precisely localize the antigens on the cell surface or in the cytoplasm of cells and to identify ultrastructural characteristics of the stained cells (10,30). Recently, monoclonal antibodies have been developed that are capable of reacting with antigens associated with lymphoid cells that resist procedures used in obtaining paraffin-embedded sections (31).

Immunohistochemical techniques have also provided a means of investigating the specificity of monoclonal antibodies, both during the initial screening and after cloning of hybrid cells.

II. MONOCLONAL ANTIBODIES

In the last several years a large number of immunohistochemical studies have been performed to characterize lymphoid cells in normal lymphoid tissue,

Table 1 Characteristics of Selected Monoclonal Antibodies Against Human Lymphoid Cells

		Antigen[b]		
Antibody[a]	Class	CD code	Molecular weight (Kd)	Major cell reactivity
OKT6 anti-Leu-6 (anti-T6)[c]	IgG1 IgG2b	CD1	49	Cortical thymocytes; Langerhans/indeterminate cells
OKT11 anti-Leu-5b (anti-T11)	IgG2a IgG2a	CD2 (antigen associated with sheep erythrocyte receptor)	45-50	All T cells: some natural killer cells
OKT3 anti-Leu-4 (anti-T3)	IgG2a IgG1	CD3 (three polypeptide chains associated with T cell antigen receptor)	20,20,25	All T cells
OKT1 anti-Leu-1 (anti-T1)	IgG1 IgG2a	CD5	67	All T cells; some B cells in lymphoid tissue
OKT4 anti-Leu-3a (anti-T4)	IgG2b IgG1	CD4	55	T cells which recognize antigen in association with class II MHC antigens (helper/inducer T cells); monocytes/macrophages
OKT 8 anti-Leu-2a (anti-T8)	IgG2a IgG1	CD8	32,43	T cells which recognize antigens associated with class I MHC antigens (cytotoxic/suppressor T cells); sinus lining cells in spleen.

Table 1 *continues*

Table 1 (*continued*)

Antibody[a]	Class	Antigen[b] CD code	Antigen[b] Molecular weight (Kd)	Major cell reactivity
anti-Leu-8	IgG2a		80	A large fraction of T cells (Leu-3+, Leu-8+ cells induce T suppressor cells); B cells; granulocytes; monocytes; natural killer cells
OKM1	IgG2b	CD11	170	Granulocytes; monocytes; natural killer cells
anti-Leu-M3	IgG2b	CDW14		Monocytes/macrophages; Langerhans cells
anti-Leu-7 (HNK-1)	IgM		110	Natural killer cells; certain nonlymphoid normal tissues (endocrine cells)
anti-Leu-11a anti-Leu-11b	IgG1 IgM	CD16 (IgG Fc receptor)		Natural killer cells; granulocytes
OKT9 (anti-T9)	IgG1		90,94 dimer (transferrin receptor)	Reactivity not restricted to any lineage; activated and proliferating cells
OKT10 (anti-T10)	IgG1		46,12	Cortical thymocytes; activated T cells, plasma cells and some B cells; natural killer cells
OKIa1 anti-HLA-DR	IgG2 IgG2a		28,34 (Ia-like antigens)	B cells; monocytes/macrophages; dendritic cells (Langerhans cells, interdigitating reticulum cells); activated T cells; endothelial cells; certain epithelial cells

Table 1 *continues*

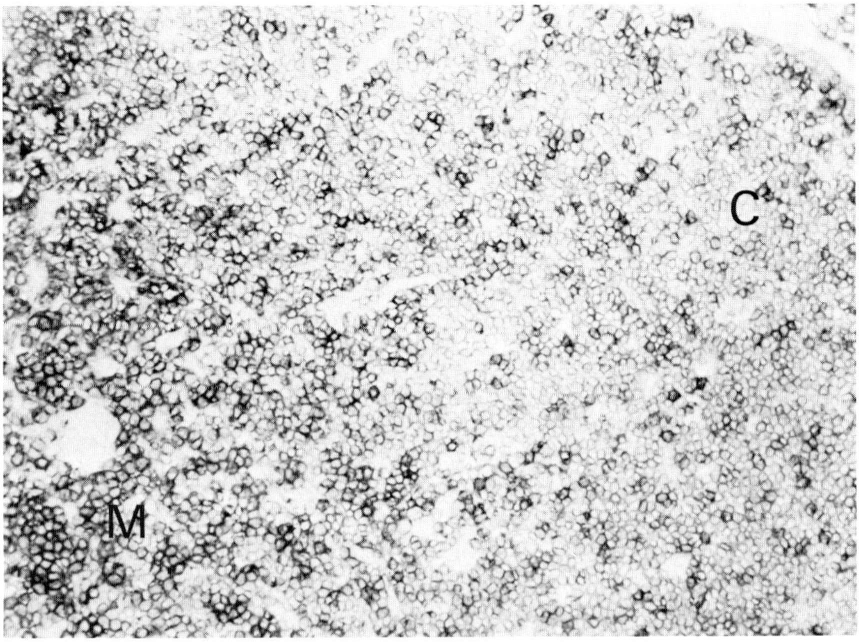

Figure 2 Human thymus stained with anti-Leu-4 antibody. Most of the thymocytes in the medulla (M) are intensely stained. Many intensely stained cells are scattered among lightly stained thymocytes in the cortex (C). (Immunoperoxidase, X 250.)

The expression of T1 and T3 antigens by the majority of cortical thymocytes suggests that the maturation of thymocytes into immunocompetent T cells starts in the cortex. Moreover, as thymocytes staining intensely for T1 or T3 are scattered throughout the cortex and are not concentrated near the corticomedullary junction, mature T cells may be exported into the circulation without passing through the medulla (5). Functional immunocompetence of $T1^+$ cortical thymocytes has been demonstrated following separation of cortical thymocytes from medullary thymocytes by staining thymocyte cell suspensions with fluoresceinated peanut agglutinin (PNA); PNA binds to cortical but not medullary thymocytes (58). PNA^+, $T1^+$ cells (cortical thymocytes staining intensely for T1) showed similar response to PHA or alloantigen in the presence of interleukin-2 as the medullary thymocytes (PNA^-, $T1^+$), whereas PNA^+, $T1^-$ cells (cortical thymocytes staining faintly or not staining for T1) did not respond (58).

The presence of immunocompetent cells that express high levels of a receptor that mediates the homing of bloodborne lymphocytes into peripheral lymph nodes has recently been demonstrated in the cortical region of the murine thymus (59). Thus, these studies further support the possibility that cortical thymocytes may be capable of migrating into peripheral lymphoid tissue without the need for further maturation in the medulla.

Experimental studies in the mouse indicate that small thymocytes are derived from large and rapidly dividing cells in the subcapsular region (60). In the human thymus, subcapsular thymocytes cannot be easily differentiated from other cortical thymocytes but may be more conspicuous in the fetal thymus (56). $T9^+$ cells are mostly confined to the subcapsular region; only a small number of cortical thymocytes (10-30%) and rare medullary thymocytes stain for T9 (56). Differences in the staining between cortical and medullary thymocytes have also been observed for other antigens, including terminal deoxynucleotidyl transferase (TdT) and common acute lymphoblastic leukemia antigen (CALLA); the cortical thymocytes stain for these antigens but only a few cells stain in the medulla (56).

The thymocytes are supported by a reticulum of nonlymphoid cells, most of which are epithelial in nature. Electron microscopic examination of thymic tissue and cell suspensions obtained following enzymatic treatment of thymus has revealed the presence of large lymphoepithelial cell complexes in humans as well as experimental animals (mice, rats) (5,61-63). Thymocytes can be demonstrated either within the cytoplasm or in the deep cytoplasmic invaginations of these cells (also called "nurse cells"). It has been proposed that the "nurse cells," by their close association and secretion of thymic hormones, are involved in the maturation of thymocytes (61-63). Thymic epithelial cells express both class I and class II (HLA-DR) antigens (5,62,63). Staining of human thymus with anti-HLA-DR antibodies produces a patchy pattern of staining in the cortex and more diffuse staining in the medulla, consistent with staining of the epithelial cells (5). At times, groups of thymocytes or individual thymocytes can be seen to be surrounded by a ring of staining, most likely reflecting staining of cytoplasmic processes of the epithelial cells. Certainly, some HLA-DR staining is related to staining of macrophages and dendritic cells. Staining with anti-T6 antibody reveals the presence of intensely stained dendritic cells (Langerhans cells/indeterminate cells) in the medulla (64)

Phenotypic and functional characterization of thymic epithelial cells and other nonlymphoid cells (dendritic cells, macrophages) has not been extensively carried out. Studies so far indicate that there are differences in the antigenic phenotype of subcapsular, cortical, and medullary epithelial cells (52,62,65,66).

IV. DISTRIBUTION OF LYMPHOCYTE SUBSETS IN THE PERIPHERAL LYMPHOID TISSUE

The various cellular components of the peripheral lymphoid tissue (lymph nodes, tonsils, spleen, gut, and bronchial-associated lymphoid tissue) are arranged in distinct anatomical compartments. B cells are primarily located in the lymphoid follicles. The primary lymphoid follicles, which contain mostly small lymphocytes, develop germinal centers following antigenic stimulation and are then called secondary lymphoid follicles. The germinal centers contain B lymphocytes (centroblasts, centrocytes), T lymphocytes, dendritic reticulum cells, and macrophages, and are surrounded by a mantle of small lymphocytes (mantle zone). Histologically, two zones have been recognized in germinal centers: the dark zone, composed primarily of centroblasts; and the light zone, containing mostly centrocytes, dendritic reticulum cells, and a few plasma cells (15). The interfollicular and paracortical areas represent thymus-dependent regions and contain mostly T cells, dendritic reticulum cells, and high endothelial venules. The periarteriolar lymphoid sheath of the malpighian corpuscles represents the thymus-dependent area in the spleen.

Characterization of stages of B-cell differentiation has been greatly facilitated by the use of antibodies against immunoglobulin heavy chain isotypes and by the availability of monoclonal antibodies against B-cell-associated antigens (35, 36,46,48). The earliest defined B cell (pre-B cell) contains cytoplasmic μ heavy chains, and expresses HLA-DR, CALLA, and a B-cell-associated antigen B4 (46, 48,67). Pre-B cells are present in small numbers in the fetal liver and normal adult bone marrow (68). These cells differentiate into immature B cells, which express surface immunoglobulin (IgM and IgD). Further differentiation can be induced by antigenic exposure (or by mitogenic activation) and leads to expression of individual immunoglobulin isotypes (IgM, IgG, IgA), loss of IgD, and development of plasma cells. The differentiation to plasma cells is also associated with loss of surface immunoglobulin and HLA-DR antigens, the presence of cytoplasmic immunoglobulin, and acquisition of new antigens, T10 and PCA-1 (a plasma cell-associated antigen (46,48). The B-cell-associated antigens, B1 and B2, have also been found to be useful in defining stages of B-cell differentiation; B1 antigen is expressed by pre-B cells and by all B cells until the plasma cell stage, while B2 antigen appears at the immature B-cell stage and is lost soon after antigenic (or mitogenic) stimulation of B cells (67).

Immunohistochemical studies of peripheral lymphoid tissue with monoclonal antibodies reveal that most of the lymphocytes in the primary follicle and mantle zone stain for IgM (Fig. 3), IgD, HLA-DR, B1, and faintly for B2, an antigenic phenotype similar to that of circulating B cells in blood (8,69). However, many cells in the mantle zone (not peripheral blood B cells) stain for Blast-2, an early cell-surface marker of human B-cell activation (70). Germinal center B cells (8) stain for IgM, IgG, HLA-DR, B1, and T10 but not for IgD (a few IgD^+ cells are seen in some germinal centers). The acquisition of T10 and IgG and loss of IgD by the germinal center cells is reminiscent of changes occurring after antigenic or mitogenic stimulation of B cells. Anti-T10 stains the cytoplasm of plasma cells intensely. Germinal center cells may also stain for IgA, especially in the gut- and bronchial-associated lymphoid tissue. In one study (71), stains performed on

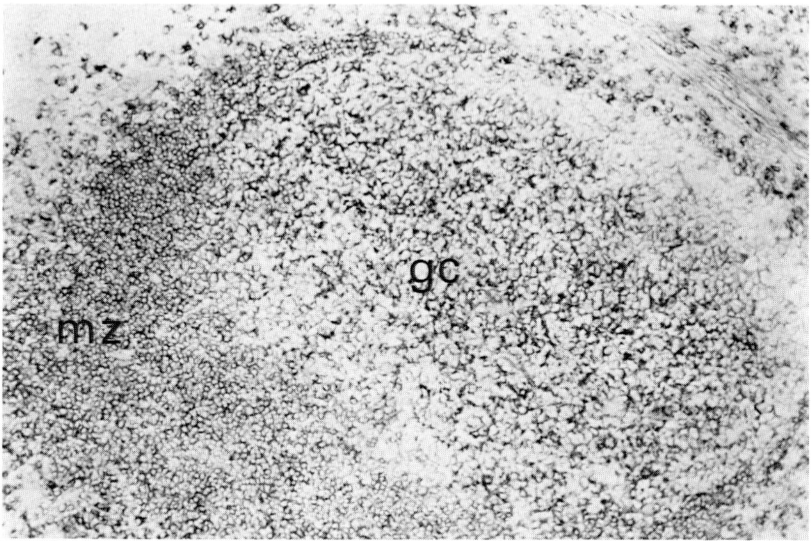

Figure 3 Human tonsil stained with anti-IgM monoclonal antibody. The cells in the mantle zone (mz) show peripheral staining, consistent with cell surface staining. The staining in the germinal center (gc) area is peripheral, cytoplasmic as well as intercellular. (Immunoperoxidase, × 100.)

paraffin-embedded sections indicated that centroblasts stained for surface IgM and IgD, while centrocytes stained for cytoplasmic IgM or IgG. Therefore, it is likely that centroblasts differentiate into centrocytes (71). It is important to note that interpretation of staining of the germinal center area is difficult due to staining of extracellular material, some of which seems to be associated with dendritic reticulum cells. Furthermore, the extent of staining in the germinal center area varies from follicle to follicle, with no recognizable staining of many germinal center cells. Staining with anti-B2 antibody produces marked dendritic staining pattern and intense staining of intercellular material in the germinal center area and, to a lesser extent, in the adjoining mantle zone area (8,9). As this staining pattern is similar to that obtained with an anti-dendritic reticulum cell antibody (72), it is likely that anti-B2 stains dendritic reticulum cells. However, with this staining pattern it is not possible to reliably evaluate the staining of germinal center cells; apparent staining of the cells (dendritic cells, macrophages) may be due not to synthesis of the antigen by the cells but to ingestion or binding of the antigen to the surface of the cells (9).

Immunohistochemical studies performed on human lymph nodes indicate the presence of another B-cell population in the cortical sinuses (73-76). In certain benign lymphoid hyperplasia, which are often associated with a high incidence of seropositivity to toxoplasma gondii, the cells in the cortical sinuses become prominent and, because of their appearance, have been called immature sinus histiocytes. However, these cells stain for B1, immunoglobulins (usually IgG), and do not stain with OKM1 or antibodies to T-cell-associated antigens, indicating the B-cell nature of these cells (73).

The medullary region of the lymph node also contains many B cells (mostly plasma cells) admixed with T cells.

As expected, the majority of cells in the interfollicular and paracortical areas stain for T1, T3, and T11, confirming the T-cell nature of these cells (7,56). In most hyperplastic lymph nodes, $T4^+$ cells are far more numerous than $T8^+$ cells. In addition many cells in the germinal center area stain for T cells (Fig. 4) (7,8, 77). Most of these cells appear to be $T4^+$, and are often arranged in a crescentic pattern at the junction of germinal center with mantle zone (7,8). Generally, only a few $T8^+$ cells are detected in the germinal center area. Both $T4^+$ and $T8^+$

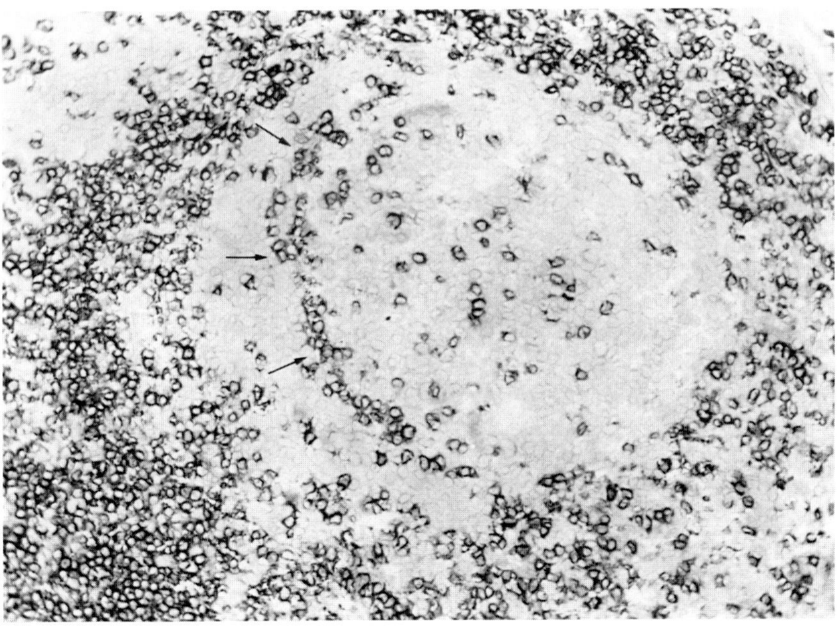

Figure 4 A high magnification of a secondary follicle in a tonsil stained with anti-Leu-4 antibody. Most of the cells surrounding the follicle are stained. In addition, many stained cells are present in the follicle, some of which (arrows) are present at the junction of mantle zone with germinal center. (Immunoperoxidase counterstained with hematoxylin, X 313.)

cells are present in the mantle zone and in primary follicles. The presence of T4$^+$ cells in the germinal center area is consistent with the notion that T cells are involved in the development of germinal center and in the differentiation of B cells (7,8,78). Interestingly, T cells in the germinal center area do not stain for Leu-8, which is expressed by most of the T cells in the paracortical and interfollicular areas, as well as by B cells in the mantle zone (56). As the major helper effect for antibody synthesis resides in the T4$^+$, Leu-8$^-$ population (79,80), the presence of these cells in the germinal center area further supports the role of these cells in the differentiation of B cells in vivo. Double staining techniques indicate that T4$^+$ cells in the germinal center area also express HNK-1, an antigen associated with, but not restricted to, natural killer cells (24,81).

The malpighian follicles (white pulp) of the spleen show a staining pattern similar to that observed in the lymph nodes and tonsils. In the spleen, however, there is a distinct compartment of lymphocytes (marginal zone) located at the junction of lymphoid follicles and red pulp (82,83). The cells in the marginal zone are larger than the mantle zone cells and have been considered to present an intermediate morphologic form between small B lymphocytes and plasma cells. Although the marginal zone B cells, like the mantle zone cells, stain for B4, B1, B2, IgM, and IgD, the staining for B2 and IgM is more intense and staining for IgD considerably less than observed in the mantle zone (82). These findings suggest that marginal zone B cells are more mature (differentiated) than mantle zone B cells (82). In one study (83), unlike mantle zone B cells, the marginal zone cells were shown to express alkaline phosphatase and IL-2 receptor, indicating that marginal zone cells may be activated B cells.

The periarteriolar lymphoid sheath in the spleen contains T cells and shows a distribution pattern of T4$^+$ and T8$^+$ cells similar to that seen in paracortical or interfollicular areas in lymph nodes and spleen. Interestingly, the cells lining sinusoids of red pulp in adult spleen, but not in neonatal spleen, stain for T8 (82).

The well-organized structure of germinal centers can be altered under certain diseased conditions, such as acquired immune deficiency syndrome (AIDS) (84-86). The changes observed in AIDS include: follicular hyperplasia with activated sinus lymphocytes, hypervascular paracortical hyperplasia, and marked lymphocyte depletion (9). In the lymphadenopathy syndrome (pre-AIDS), follicular hyperplasia is characterized by a marked decrease in the T4$^+$ cells in the large reactive germinal centers as well as in the paracortical area, with an apparent increase in the T8$^+$ cells (9,84-86).

A. Interdigitating Reticulum Cells and Macrophages

The thymus-dependent areas contain a distinct type of dendritic reticulum cells, called interdigitating reticulum cells (IDRC) because their cytoplasmic processes tend to interdigitate with each other (15,87). The IDRC stain intensely for HLA-

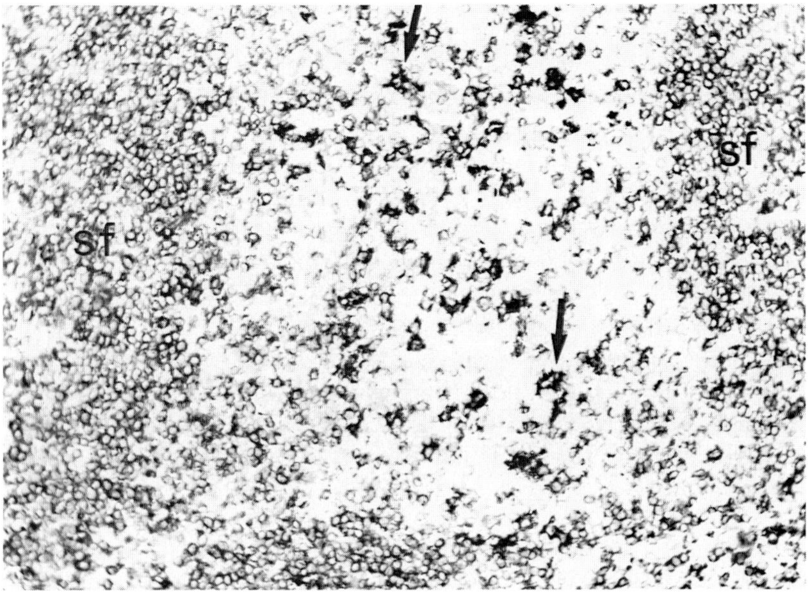

Figure 5 Tonsil stained with anti-HLA-DR antibody. Most of the cells in the secondary follicles (sf) are stained. In addition, many dendritic cells (arrows) in the interfollicular area are intensely stained. (Immunoperoxidase, X 200.)

DR (Fig. 5) and their cytoplasmic processes appear to be in close contact with T cells. The close association of HLA-DR$^+$ IDRC with T cells suggests that the IDRC may be playing a crucial role in the presentation of antigen to T cells, in particular T4$^+$ cells (7). In some lymph nodes, nodular areas can be appreciated in the paracortex due to localized proliferation of T cells (mostly T4$^+$) and IDRC (88). In dermatopathic lymphadenitis, such areas may contain a large number of T6$^+$ dendritic cells, which most likely represent Langerhans cells that have migrated to lymph nodes from the skin (see below) (7,88,89). It is important to note that the paracortex represents an active area of cell migration, therefore, other cells such as B cells may also be present in these areas.

Although dendritic reticulum cells are distinct from mononuclear phagocytes (monocytes/macrophages), these two types of cells share many antigens, indicating a close cytogenic relationship (89,90). The tissue macrophages show a wide variety of variability in their reaction with monoclonal antibodies against monocyte-associated antigens (90,91); the variability is less within an individual anatomical location (macrophages in medullary sinuses of lymph node, Kupffer cells in liver, alveolar macrophages in lung, macrophages in spleen). The commonly used monoclonal antibodies include anti-HLA-DR, -Leu-M1, -Leu-M3, OKM1,

Mo1, Mo2, and antibodies to C3b receptor. The reactivity of many of these antibodies is not restricted to mononuclear phagocytes. Macrophages also stain with anti-T4 (10,92,93). It is of interest that in animals macrophages also express antigens homologous to T4 (W3/25 in rats, L3T4 in mice) (10,94,95).

B. Langerhans Cells

Langerhans cells are antigen-presenting cells in the skin and other stratified squamous epithelia (89,96,97). These cells interact with T cells either locally or after migrating to lymph nodes. Immunohistochemical studies were instrumental in providing evidence that T6 antigen is a highly specific marker for the detection and enumeration of Langerhans cells in tissue sections (Figs. 6, 7) (30,96-98). As cortical thymocytes also express T6, it is important to know whether the antigens recognized by the anti-T6 on cortical thymocytes and Langerhans cells are similar. Biochemical studies confirmed that the antigen recognized by anti-T6 antibody on cortical thymocytes and Langerhans has the same molecular weight (49

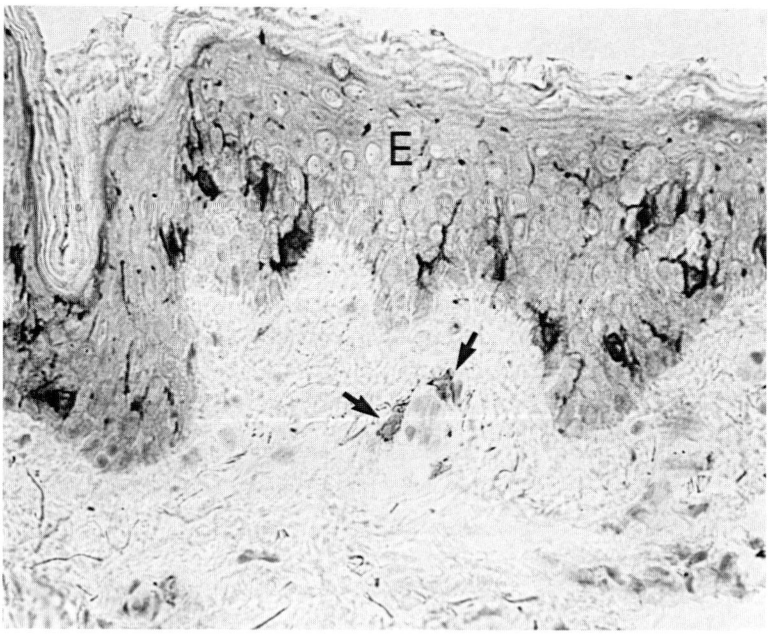

Figure 6 Skin stained with anti-T6 antibody. Many dendritic cells with cytoplasmic processes (Langerhans cells) are stained in the epidermis (E). A few dendritic cells (arrows) in the dermis are also stained. (Immunoperoxidase, counterstained with hematoxylin, X 400.)

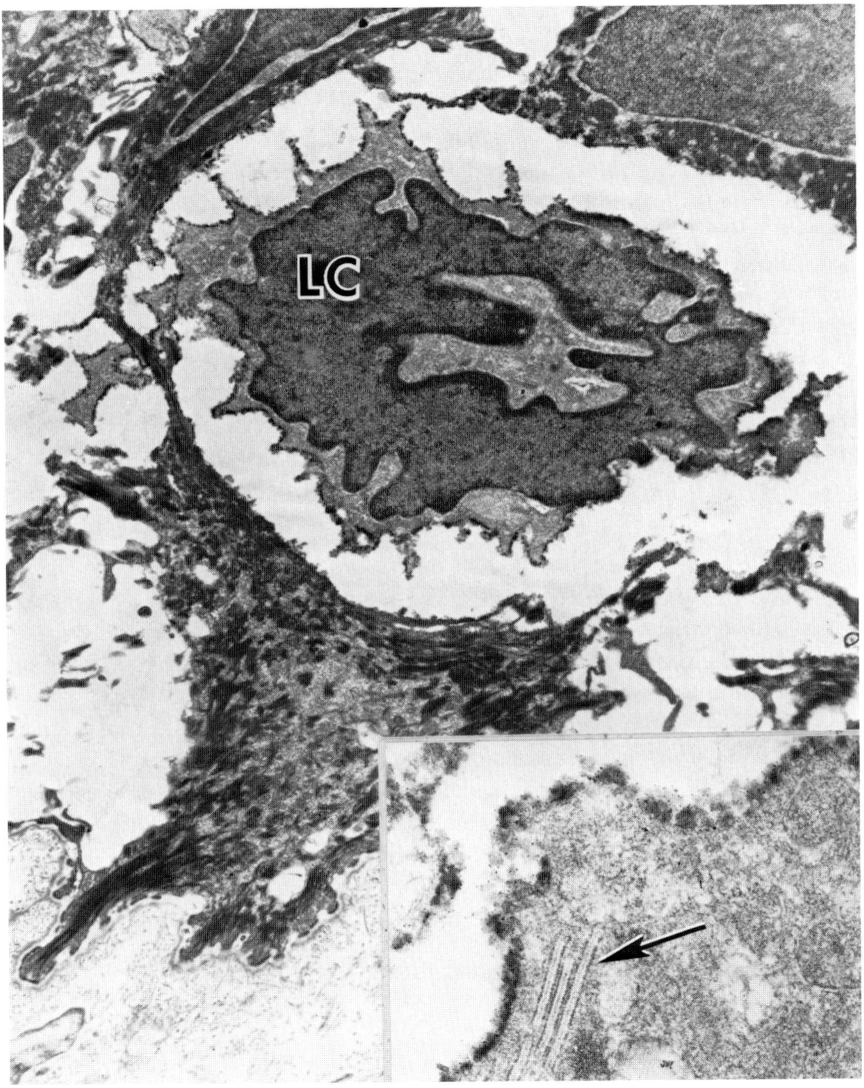

Figure 7 Immunoelectron micrograph of a Langerhans cell (LC), containing characteristic Birbeck granules (arrow, inset), located in the epidermis. The presence of T6 membrane antigen is indicated by the presence of electron-dense deposits along the periphery (inset). (Paraformaldehyde-fixed frozen tissue section of skin stained by immunoperoxidase technique and prepared routinely for electron microscopy; X 10,000; inset X 50,000.) (Courtesy of Dr. George F. Murphy.)

Kd) (64). Similarly, another monoclonal antibody, anti-M241, which also reacts with cortical thymocytes (64) and Langerhans cells (64,99) was also found to recognize an antigen of identical molecular weight (43 Kd) on these two cell types (64). The demonstration of T200, a glycoprotein restricted to hematopoietic cells, on Langerhans cells provided evidence for a bone marrow origin of these cells (100,101). The precursor forms of Langerhans cells, however, have not been recognized in the bone marrow or in the blood. Anti-T6 also reacts with dendritic cells in the dermis, which lack Birbeck granules in the cytoplasm, a characteristic ultrastructure marker of Langerhans cells (102). These cells have been called indeterminate cells and may represent an early form of Langerhans cells (96,102). Like macrophages, Langerhans cells also express Leu-M3 (103) and contain HLA-DR$^+$ and HLA-DR$^-$ subpopulations (104).

Histiocytosis-X cells, which are considered to be abnormal Langerhans cells, also stain for T6, HLA-DR, M241, and Leu-M3 (49,103,105). However, histiocytosis-X cells stain with anti-T4, while most Langerhans cells generally do not (49,93,96,105). In some cases histiocytosis-X cells also react with OKM1 (49).

C. Mucosal Lymphocytes

In addition to localized areas of organized lymphoid tissue (Peyer's patches), the intestine contains a large number of lymphoid cells in the lamina propria, and within the mucosal epithelium (intraepithelial lymphocytes) (10,106). A majority of the T cells in the lamina propria are T4$^+$. In contrast, most of the intraepithelial lymphocytes (IEL) express cytotoxic/suppressor phenotype in humans (T8$^+$) as well as in experimental animals (Lyt2$^+$ in mice, OX8$^+$ in rats) (10,106-108). An increase in IEL has been observed following intraluminal exposure to antigen (109,110) and in enteropathies, including intestinal parasitic diseases and celiac disease (110-112). The function of this cell population remains uncertain. Although the presence of characteristic cytoplasmic granules, similar to the granules present in the large granular lymphocytes in the blood, in 20-50% of IEL suggests that these cells may possess natural killer activity (113, 114), none of the IEL in humans have been shown to express antigens (NHK-1, Leu-11) associated with natural killer cells (10, unpublished observation). It is possible that IEL may regulate epithelial cell functions (108). The presence of unique antigens on mucosal lymphocytes has been suggested by the development of a monoclonal antibody (RGL-1) against IEL, which reacts with a majority of IEL as well as lamina propria lymphocytes of rat intestine, but only with a few cells in blood, lymph nodes, and spleen (115). Monoclonal antibody RGL-1 also reacts with a small number of lymphocytes in other mucosal sites (trachea, bronchi, acini, and ducts in breast). These findings suggest that some of the lymphocytes present in different mucosal sites may share similar antigens (and functions) and, thus, may belong to a common mucosal-associated lymphoid tissue (115,116).

V. IMMUNOHISTOLOGIC ANALYSIS OF CELL-MEDIATED REACTIONS

The availability of monoclonal antibodies against mononuclear inflammatory cells, in particular functionally distinct lymphocyte subsets, permits a more meaningful analysis of cell-mediated reactions than was possible by histological examination. A large number of immunohistological studies have been performed to analyze the cellular infiltrate in a wide variety of inflammatory lesions (mostly skin diseases), allografts, and tumors (4,18,117-128).

Analysis of cellular infiltrate in biopsies obtained from rejecting allografts has attracted the attention of many investigators (119,129-134). As expected, the studies indicate that T cells are the predominant inflammatory mononuclear cells in the cellular infiltrate. There are differences in the distribution of T-cell subsets in the skin as well as renal allografts (119,129,133,134). $T8^+$ cells predominate in the lymphocytes in close contact with epithelial cells (tubular epithelial cells in renal allografts; epidermal and skin appendegeal cells in skin allografts), whereas $T4^+$ cells are more numerous in the large perivascular lymphoid aggregates (119, 129,133). Based on these findings, it has been suggested that $T8^+$ cells may be cytotoxic to epithelial cells, while $T4^+$ cells may be inducing delayed type of hypersensitivity reactions (119). However, as $T4^+$ cells can be cytotoxic to targets with class II antigens (135,136), a direct cytotoxic role of $T4^+$ cells against cells expressing HLA-DR antigens (endothelial cells) cannot be ruled out. Furthermore, tubular epithelial cells also appear to express HLA-DR antigens during graft rejection, possibly due to modulating effect of γ interferon released by the stimulated lymphocytes (137). Predominance of $T4^+$ cells in perivascular infiltrate is also observed in delayed hypersensitivity reactions induced in the skin (138). A similar predominance of $T4^+$ cells is present in the granulomatous lesion of tuberculoid leprosy (121). In contrast, paucity of $T4^+$ cells in the cellular infiltrate has been observed in the lesions of lepromatous leprosy. This observation may be explained by the lack of cell-mediated immunity to *Mycobacterium leprae* in lepromatous leprosy (121).

Most of the studies so far have used anti-T4 (-Leu-3) and anti-T8 (-Leu-2) antibodies to identify functionally distinct populations of cells. However, as indicated above, $T4^+$ cells can function as cytotoxic cells as well as helper cells to B cells in antibody synthesis, and inducers of suppressor cells and delayed hypersensitivity reactions. Therefore, it is not possible to accurately determine the function of $T4^+$ or $T8^+$ cells (which can function as cytotoxic or suppressor cells) in inflammatory reactions. Recently, a number of monoclonal antibodies have become available which can differentiate T cells with limited functional capability within the two major T-cell subsets (139-142). Monoclonal antibody 9.3 can help divide Leu-2^+ cells into subpopulations that include either cytotoxic (9.3^+) or suppressor cells (9.3^-) (139). Similarly, Leu-3^+ population can be separated by anti-Leu-8 into Leu-3^+, Leu-8^+ cells capable of activating Leu-2^+ suppressor cells (140) and a smaller population of Leu-3^+, Leu-8^- cells which provide help antibody synthesis (141). The detection of these subsets in tissue sections requires simultaneous demonstration of two or more antigens on the cells by double staining techniques. With the availability of more discriminating monoclonal antibodies and development of sensitive double staining techniques, the analysis of inflammatory cellular infiltrate will provide more useful information regarding the pathogenesis of immunologically mediated lesions.

VI. CHARACTERIZATION OF LYMPHOPROLIFERATIVE DISORDERS

Immunophenotyping of lymphoproliferative disorders by cell suspension studies as well as by immunohistological methods has permitted characterization of malignant lymphomas and leukemias according to the state of differentiation of their normal counterpart in the immune system (143-153). Thus, with the help of monoclonal antibodies, it has been possible to demonstrate that various T-cell malignancies express antigenic phenotypes corresponding to the stages of thymocyte differentiation (35,145-147); T lymphoblastic leukemia and lymphoblastic lymphoma show a phenotype of immature thymocytes, and antigens associated with mature T cells are expressed by tumor cells from Sézary syndrome, mycosis fungoides, and T chronic lymphocytic leukemia. Similarly, in a recent study (154) tumors of B cells were divided into three major groups: (1) pre-B-cell stage—non-T acute lymphoblastic leukemia and chronic myelocytic leukemia in lymphoid blast crisis; (2) mid-B-cell stage—chronic lymphocytic leukemia and poorly differentiated lymphomas; and (3) secretory B-cell stage—large cell lymphoma and plasma cell tumors.

Immunohistological techniques are now routinely applied in the diagnosis and subclassification of malignant lymphomas. As the majority of adult malignant lymphomas are of B-cell origin, demonstration of immunoglobulins in tumor cells has been helpful in defining the B-cell nature of the tumor. Monoclonality of the B cells in the tumor is manifested by the expression of one type of light chain (κ or λ) by the tumor cells (Fig. 8). Antibodies against B-cell-associated antigens (B1, B4) can be helpful in the recognition of B-cell lymphomas which do not express immunoglobulins (150,154). The B-cell nature of these tumors has been also confirmed by the demonstration of immunoglobulin gene rearrangement in the tumor cells (155). In follicular lymphomas, the neoplastic follicles reproduce the structure of normal lymphoid follicles, including the characteristic dendritic staining pattern of germinal centers obtained with anti-B2 antibody (150). Moreover, the distribution of T cells in follicular lymphomas (small cleaved and mixed cell type) is similar to that seen in secondary follicles of reactive lymphoid tissue (156). It is possible that T cells (in particular $T4^+$ cells) are also involved in the maintenance of follicular structure in these lymphomas.

As lymphoid tumors are considered to represent clonal expansions of specific lymphocyte subsets, immunophenotyping of lymphomas may help identify normal

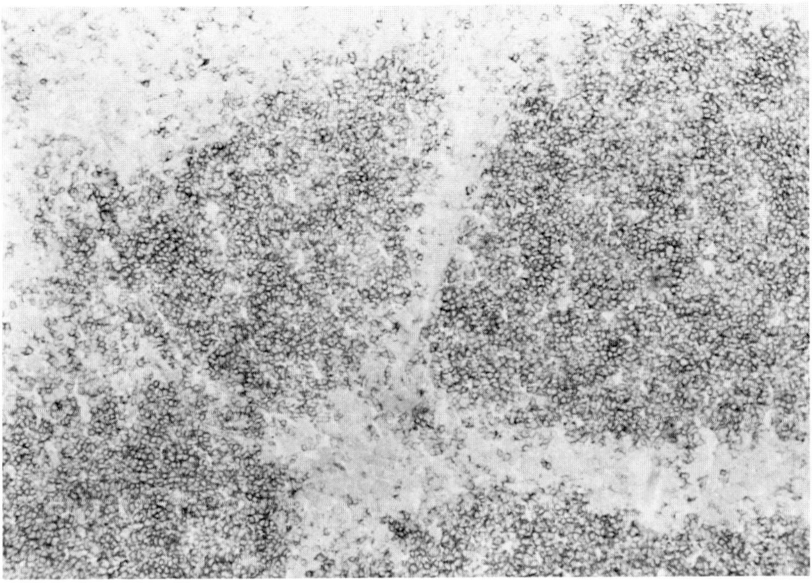

Figure 8 A case of follicular small cleaved cell lymphoma stained for lambda light chain. Most of the cells in the follicles show peripheral staining. (Immunoperoxidase, X 100.)

lymphocyte populations which form a minor component of the lymphoid tissue. For instance, T1, a T-cell-associated antigen, has been found to be expressed by B-cell chronic lymphocytic leukemia cells and by certain other B-cell lymphomas (156-158), raising the possibility that a subpopulation of normal B cells may express the antigen. Studies carried by a number of investigators have confirmed the presence of a small number of B cells reactive with anti-T1 (or anti-Leu-1) in normal lymphoid tissue (154,159).

Immunohistological studies of lymphoma, in particular T-cell neoplasms, indicate that in many instances the tumor cells may not reproduce the antigenic phenotype according to known stages of lymphocyte differentiation (152,160,161). The demonstration of anomalous antigenic phenotype can be useful in differentiating benign from malignant lymphoid cells (162).

Another situation where monoclonal antibodies have been used is in the characterization of cellular constituents in Hodgkin's disease (163-165). However, the exact nature of the Reed-Sternberg cells, which represent the characteristic cells of Hodgkin's disease, has not been clarified so far. Reed-Sternberg cells express HLA-DR and Leu-M1, and bind peanut agglutinin (163,165). A monoclonal antibody (Ki-1), raised against cells cultured from tissue involved with Hodgkin's disease, has been found to react with Reed-Sternberg cells (164). The studies of normal tissue indicate that a small number of Ki-1$^+$ cells can be detected in spleen, thymic medulla, tonsils, and lymph nodes; Ki-1$^+$ cells are usually located at the margin of lymphoid follicles but are sometimes also present in the margin of germinal centers and in the T-cell areas (166). Ki-1 antigen is also expressed by certain peripheral T-cell lymphomas, and by a minority of cells in lymphomatoid papulosis and angio-immunoblastic lymphadenopathy (166).

VII. SUMMARY

The development of monoclonal antibodies against cell surface and cytoplasmic antigens has permitted precise in situ characterization of cells in tissue sections. Thus, immunohistological techniques have allowed identification of cells in areas where the lymphoid cells mature, differentiate and function, and interact with each other in an efficient and orderly fashion. Immunocytochemical methods have been especially useful for the characterization of cells which are either small in number or difficult to obtain in cell suspension. In addition, staining of tissue sections with monoclonal antibodies provides a valuable method of screening of new monoclonal antibodies and defining the tissue distribution of antigens reactive with these antibodies. As new monoclonal antibodies capable of discriminating cells with limited and specific function become available, the immunohistological characterization of lymphoid cells in normal and diseased states will become more meaningful.

REFEFERENCES

1. G. A. Gutman and I. L. Weissman, Lymphoid tissue architecture: experimental analysis of the origin and distribution of T-cells and B-cells, *Immunology, 23*: 465 (1972).
2. R. T. McCluskey and A. K. Bhan, Cell-mediated reaction in vivo, in *Mechanisms of Tumor Immunity* (I. Green, S. Cohen, and R. T. McCluskey, eds.), John Wiley and Sons, New York, 1977, p. 1.
3. H. Stein, A. Bonk, G. Tolksdorf, K. Lennert, H. Rodt, and J. Gerdes, Immunohistologic analysis of the organization of normal lymphoid tissue and non-Hodgkin's lymphoma, *J. Histochem. Cytochem., 28*: 746 (1980).
4. A. K. Bhan, Application of monoclonal antibodies to tissue diagnosis, in *Advances in Immunohistochemistry* (R. A. DeLellis, ed.), Masson Publishing USA, Inc., 1984, p. 1.
5. A. K. Bhan, E. L. Reinherz, S. Poppema, R. T. McCluskey, and S. F. Schlossman, Location of T cell and major histocompatibility complex antigens in the human thymus, *J. Exp. Med., 152*: 771 (1980).
6. G. Janossy, J. Tidman, W. S. Selby, J. A. Thomas, S. Granger, P. C. Kung, and G. Goldstein, Human T lymphocytes of inducer and suppressor type occupy different microenvironments, *Nature, 288*: 81 (1980).
7. S. Poppema, A. K. Bhan, E. L. Reinherz, R. T. McCluskey, and S. F. Schlossman, Distribution of T cell subsets in human lymph nodes, *J. Exp. Med., 153*: 30 (1981).

8. A. K. Bhan, L. M. Nadler, P. Stashenko, R. T. McCluskey, and S. F. Schlossman, Stages of B cell differentiation in human lymphoid tissue, *J. Exp. Med., 154*: 737 (1981).
9. A. K. Bhan and N. L. Harris, The immunohistology of normal and neoplastic lymphoid tissue, in *Lymphoproliferative Disorders of the Skin* (G. F. Murphy and M.C. Mihm Jr., eds.), Butterworth Publishers, Stoneham, MA, 1986, p. 31.
10. N. Cerf-Bensussan, E. E. Schneeberger, and A. K. Bhan, Immunohistologic and immunoelectron microscopic characterization of the mucosal lymphocytes of human small intestine by the use of monoclonal antibodies, *J. Immunol., 130*: 2615 (1983).
11. D. M. V. Parott and M. de Sousa, Thymus-dependent and thymus-independent populations: origin, migratory pattern and life span, *Clin. Exp. Immunol., 8*: 663 (1971).
12. J. C. Howard, S. V. Hunt, and J. L. Gowans, Identification of marrow-derived and thymus-derived small lymphocytes in the lymphoid tissues and thoracic duct lymph of normal rats, *J. Exp. Med., 135*: 200 (1972).
13. J. Sprent, Circulating T and B lymphocytes of the mouse. I. Migratory properties, *Cell Immunol., 7*: 10 (1973).
14. E. S. Jaffe and I. Green, Neoplasms of the immune system, in *Mechanisms of Tumor Immunity* (I. Green, S. Cohen, and R. T. McCluskey, eds.), John Wiley and Sons, New York, 1977, p. 251.
15. K. Lennert, Malignant lymphomas: other than Hodgkin's disease: histology, cytology, ultrastructure, immunology, Springer-Verlag, New York, 1978.
16. R. Schrool, A. Brutel de la Riviere, A. von dem Borne, and T. M. Feltkamp-Vroom, Identification of T and B lymphocytes in human breast cancer with immunohistochemical techniques, *Am. J. Pathol., 84*: 529 (1976).
17. J.-P. Lamelin, N. Thomasset, C. Andre, J. Brochier, and J.-P. Revillard, Study of human T and B lymphocytes with heterologous antisera. III. Immunofluorescence studies on tonsil sections, *Immunology, 35*: 463 (1978).
18. S. E. Kabawat, F. I. Preffer, and A. K. Bhan, Monoclonal antibodies in diagnostic pathology, in *Handbook of Monoclonal Antibodies* (M. P. Dierich and S. Ferrone, eds.), Noyes Publications, Park Ridge, 1985, p. 293.
19. A. G. Farr and P. K. Nakane, Immunohistochemistry with enzyme labeled antibodies: a brief review, *J. Immunol. Methods, 47*:129 (1981).
20. B. Falini and C. R. Taylor, New developments in immunoperoxidase techniques and their application, *Arch. Pathol. Lab. Med., 107*: 105 (1983).
21. J. L. Cordell, B. Falini, W. N. Erber, A. K. Ghosh, Z. Abdulaziz, S. MacDonald, K. A. F. Pulford, H. Stein, and D. Y. Mason, Immunoenzymatic labeling of monoclonal antibodies using immune complexes of alkaline phosphatase and monoclonal anti-alkaline phosphatase (APAAP complexes), *J. Histochem. Cytochem., 32*: 219 (1984).
22. S.-M. Hsu and E. Soban, Color modification of diaminobenzidine (DAB) precipitation by metallic ions and its application for double immunohistochemistry, *J. Histochem. Cytochem., 30*: 1079 (1982).
23. S. Cammisuli, Hapten-modified antibodies specific for cell surface antigens as a tool in cellular immunology, in *Immunological Methods* (I. Lefkovits and B. Pernis, eds.), Vol 2, Academic Press, New York, 1981, p. 139.

24. G. Pizzolo and M. Chilosi, Double immunostaining of lymph node sections by monoclonal antibodies using phycoerythrin labeling and haptenated reagents, *Am. J. Clin. Pathol., 82*: 44 (1984).
25. J. L. Guesdon, T. Ternynck, and S. Avrameas, The use of avidin-biotin interaction in immunoenzymatic techniques. *J. Histochem. Cytochem., 27*: 1131 (1979).
26. R. Warnke and R. Levy, Detection of T and B cell antigens with hybridoma monoclonal antibodies. A biotin-avidin-horseradish peroxidase method, *J. Histochem. Cytochem., 28*: 771 (1980).
27. S.-M. Hsu, L. Raine, and H. Fanger: A comparative study of the peroxidase-antiperoxidase method and an avidin-biotin complex method for studying polypeptide hormones with radioimmunoassay antibodies, *Am. J. Clin. Pathol., 75*: 734 (1981).
28. W. W. Hancock, G. J. Becker, and R. C. Atkins, A comparison of fixatives and immunohistochemical techniques for use with monoclonal antibodies to cell surface antigens, *Am. J. Clin. Pathol., 78*: 825 (1982).
29. I. W. McLean and P. K. Nakane, Periodate-lysine-paraformaldehyde fixative. A new fixative for immunoelectron microscopy, *J. Histochem. Cytochem., 22*: 1077 (1974).
30. G. F. Murphy, A. K. Bhan, S. Sato, T. J. Harrist, and M. C. Mihm Jr., Characterization of Langerhans cells by the use of monoclonal antibodies, *Lab. Invest., 45*: 465 (1981).
31. E. Okon, B. Felder, A. Epstein, R. J. Lukes, and C. R. Taylor, Monoclonal antibodies reactive with B-lymphocytes and histiocytes in paraffin sections, *Cancer, 56*: 95 (1985).
32. E. L. Reinherz and S. F. Schlossman, The differentiation and function of human T lymphocytes, *Cell, 19*: 821 (1980).
33. E. L. Reinherz, P. C. Kung, G. Goldstein, R. H. Levey, and S. F. Schlossman, Discrete stages of human intrathymic differentiation: Analysis of normal thymocytes and leukemic lymphoblasts of T cell lineage, *Proc. Natl. Acad. Sci. USA, 77*: 1588 (1980).
34. K. A. Foon, R. W. Schroff, and R. P. Gale, Surface markers on leukemia and lymphoma cells: Recent advances, *Blood, 60*: 1 (1982).
35. L. M. Nadler, J. Ritz, J. D. Griffin, R. F. Todd III, E. L. Reinherz, and S. F. Schlossman, Diagnosis and treatment of human leukemias and lymphomas utilizing monoclonal antibodies, *Progress in Hematology, 12*: 187 (1981).
36. L. M. Nadler, P. Stashenko, R. Hardy, A. van Agthoven, C. Terhorst, and S. F. Schlossman, Characterization of a human B cell-specific antigen (B2) distinct from B1, *J. Immunol., 126*: 1941 (1981).
37. J. Ritz, L. M. Nadler, A. K. Bhan, J. Notis-McConarty, J. M. Pesando, and S. F. Schlossman, Expression of common acute lymphoblastic leukemia antigen (CALLA) by lymphomas of B cell and T cell lineage, *Blood, 58*: 648 (1981).
38. R. S. Metzgar, M. J. Borowitz, N. H. Jones, and B. L. Dowell, The distribution of common acute lymphoblastic leukemia antigen (CALLA) in nonhematopoietic tissues, *J. Exp. Med., 154*: 1249 (1981).

39. K. Iida, L. Nadler, and V. Nussenzweig, Identification of the membrane receptor for complement fragment C3d by means of a monoclonal antibody, *J. Exp. Med., 158*: 1021 (1983).
40. T. Abo, C. A. Miller, G. L. Gartland, and C. M. Balch, Differentiation stages of human natural killer cells in human lymphoid tissue from fetal to adult life, *J. Exp. Med., 157*: 273 (1983).
41. M. B. Omary, I. S. Trowbridge, and H. A. Battifora, Human homologue of murine T200 glycoprotein, *J. Exp. Med., 152*: 842 (1980).
42. H. Battifora and I. S. Trowbridge, A monoclonal antibody useful for the differential diagnosis between malignant lymphoma and nonhematopoeitic neoplasms, *Cancer, 51*: 816 (1983).
43. A. Dimitri-Bona, G. R. Burmester, S. J. Waters, and R. J. Winchester, Human mononuclear phagocyte differentiation antigens. 1. Patterns of antigenic expression on the surface of human monocytes and macrophages defined by monoclonal antibodies, *J. Immunol., 130*: 145 (1983).
44. R. F. Todd, A. K. Bhan, S. E. Kabawat, and S. F. Schlossman, Human myelomonocytic differentiation antigens defined by monoclonal antibodies, in *Human Leukocytes Markers Detected By Monoclonal Antibodies* (A. Bernard and L. Boumsell, eds.), Springer-Verlag, Berlin, 1984, p. 424.
45. A. L. Bernard, L. Boumsell, and C. Hill, Joint report on the first international workshop on human keukocyte differentiation antigens, in *Leucocyte Typing* (A. Bernard, L. Boumsell, J. Dausett, C. Milstein, and S. F. Schlossman, eds.), Springer-Verlag, Berlin, Heidelberg, 1984.
46. L. M. Nadler, K. C. Anderson, M. Bates, E. Park, B. Slaughenhoupt, and S. F. Schlossman, Human B cell associated antigen: Expression on normal and malignant B cells, in *Leucocyte Typing* (A. Bernard, L. Boumsell, J. Dausett, C. Milstein, and S. F. Schlossman, eds.), Springer-Verlag, Berlin, Heidelberg, 1984, p. 339.
47. S. Pessano, H. Oettgen, A. K. Bhan, and C. Terhorst, The T3/T cell receptor complex: Antigenic distinction between the two 20 kd T3 (T3-δ and T3-ϵ) subunits, *The EMBO J., 4*: 337 (1985).
48. L. M. Nadler, B cell/leukemia panel workshop: Summary and comments, in *Leucocyte Typing II*, Vol. 2 (E. L. Reinherz, B. F. Haynes, L. M. Nadler, and I. D. Berstein, eds.), Springer-Verlag, New York, 1986, p. 3.
49. T. J. Harrist, A. K. Bhan, S. Sato, R. S. Berman, S. E. Gellis, S. Freedman, and M. C. Mihm Jr., Histiocytosis-X: In situ characterization of cutaneous infiltrates with monoclonal antibodies, *Am. J. Clin. Pathol., 79*: 294 (1983).
50. H. Cantor and I. Weissman, Development and function of subpopulations of thymocytes and T lymphocytes, *Prog. Allergy, 20*: 1 (1976).
51. O. Stutman, Intrathymic and extrathymic T cell maturation, *Immunol. Rev., 42*: 138 (1978).
52. G. Tridente, Immunopathology of the human thymus, *Seminar Hematology, 22*: 56 (1985).
53. K. Shortman, The pathway of T-cell development within the thymus, in *Progress in Immunology III* (T. E. Mandel, C. Cheers, C. S. Hosking, I. F. C. McKenzie, and G. J. V. Nossal, eds.), North Holland Publishing Co., Amsterdam, 1977, p. 197.

54. M. P. Bodger, G. Janossy, F. J. Bollum, G. D. Burford, and A. V. Hoffbrand, The ontogeny of terminal deoxynucleotidyl transferase positive cells in the human thymus, *Blood, 61*: 1125 (1983).
55. S. C. Meuer, S. F. Schlossman, and E. L. Reinherz, Monoclonal antibodies as probes to define human T cell surface structures and functions, in *Handbook of Monoclonal Antibodies* (S. Ferrone and M. P. Dierich, eds.), Noyes Publication, Park Ridge, New Jersey, 1985, p. 293.
56. S.-M. Hsu and E. S. Jaffe, Phenotypic expression of T lymphocytes in thymus and peripheral lymphoid tissues, *Am. J. Pathol., 121*: 69 (1985).
57. S. C. Meuer, K. A. Fitzgerald, R. E. Hussey, J. C. Hodgdon, S. F. Schlossman, and E. L. Reinherz, Clonotypic structures involved in antigen-specific human T cell function. Relationship to the T3 molecular complex, *J. Exp. Med., 157*: 705 (1983).
58. T. Umiel, J. F. Daley, A. K. Bhan, R. H. Levey, S. F. Schlossman, and E. L. Reinherz, Acquisition of immune competence by a subset of human cortical thymocytes expressing mature T cell antigens, *J. Immunol., 129*: 1054 (1982).
59. P. J. Fink, W. M. Gallatin, R. A. Reichert, E. C. Butcher, and I. L. Weissman, Homing of receptor-bearing thymocytes, and immunocompetent cortical population, *Nature, 313*: 233 (1985).
60. I. L. Weisman, Thymus cell maturation studies on the origin of cortisone-resistant thymic lymphocytes, *J. Exp. Med., 137*: 504 (1973).
61. H. Wekerle, U.-P. Ketelsen, and M. Ernst, Thymic nurse cells. Lymphoepithelial cell complexes in murine thymuses: Morphological and serological characterization, *J. Exp. Med., 151*: 925 (1980).
62. M. P. Ritter, C. A. Sauvage, and S. F. Cortmore, The human thymus microenvironment: In vivo identification of thymic nurse cells and other antigenically distinct subpopulation of epithelial cells, *Immunology, 44*: 439 (1981).
63. F. P. Van de Wijngaert, L. H. P. M. Rademakers, H.-J. Schuurman, R. A. de Weger, and L. Kater, Identification and in situ localization of the "thymic nurse cells" in man, *J. Immunol., 130*: 2348 (1983).
64. M. van de Rijn, P. G. Lerch, B. R. Bronstein, R. W. Knowles, A. K. Bhan, and C. Terhorst, Human cutaneous dendritic cells express two glycoproteins T6 and M241 which are biochemically identical to those found on cortical thymocytes, *Human Immunol., 9*: 201 (1984).
65. B. F. Haynes and G. S. Eisenbarth, Use of monoclonal antibodies to identify cell surface antigens of human neuroendocrine thymic epithelium, in *Monoclonal Antibodies: Probes for the Study of Autoimmunity and Immunodeficiency*, Academic Press, New York, 1983, p. 47.
66. B. F. Haynes, R. M. Scearce, D. F. Lobach, and L. L. Hensley, Phenotypic characterization and ontogeny of mesodermal derived and endocrine epithelial components of the human thymic microenvironment, *J. Exp. Med., 159*: 1149 (1984).
67. P. Stashenko, L. M. Nadler, R. Hardy, and S. F. Schlossman, Expression of cell surface markers after human B lymphocyte activation, *Proc. Natl. Acad. Sci. USA, 78*: 3848 (1981).

68. M. D. Cooper, Pre B cells: normal and abnormal development, *J. Clin. Immunol., 1*: 81 (1981).
69. S.-M. Hsu and E. S. Jaffe, Phenotypic expression of B lymphocytes: 1. Identification with monoclonal antibodies in normal lymphoid tissue, *Am. J. Pathol., 114*: 387 (1984).
70. D. A. Thorley-Lawson, L. M. Nadler, A. K. Bhan, and R. T. Schooley, BLAST-2 (EBVCS), an early cell surface marker of human B cell activation, is superinduced by Epstein Barr virus, *J. Immunol., 134*: 3007 (1985).
71. S.-M. Hsu and E. S. Jaffe, Phenotypic expression of B-lymphocytes: 2. Immunoglobulin expression of germinal center cells, *Am. J. Pathol., 114*: 396 (1984).
72. M. Naiem, J. Gerdes, Z. Abdulaziz, H. Stein, and D. Y. Mason, Production of a monoclonal antibody reactive with human dendritic reticulum cells and its use in the immunohistological analysis of lymphoid tissue, *J. Clin. Pathol., 36*: 167 (1983).
73. P. Cardoso De Almeida, N. L. Harris, and A. K. Bhan, Characterization of immature sinus histiocytes (monocytoid cells) in reactive lymph nodes by use of monoclonal antibodies, *Hum. Pathol., 15*: 330 (1984).
74. K. Sheibani, R. M. Fritz, C. D. Winberg, J. S. Burke, and H. Rappaport, "Monocytoid" cells in reactive follicular hyperplasia with and without multifocal histiocytic reaction: An immunohistochemical study of 21 cases including suspected cases of toxoplasmic lymphadenitis, *Am. J. Clin. Pathol., 81*: 453 (1984).
75. H. Stein, K. Lennert, D. Y. Mason, S. Liangru, and A. Ziegler, Immature sinus histiocytes: Their identification as a novel B cell population, *Am. J. Pathol., 117*: 44 (1984).
76. J. J. Van den Oord, C. de Wolf-Peeters, R. de Vos, and V. J. Desmet, Immature sinus histiocytis. Light and electron microscopic features, immunologic phenotype, and relationship with marginal zone lymphocytes, *Am. J. Pathol., 118*: 266 (1985).
77. P. Dvoretsky, G. S. Wood, R. Levy, and R. A. Warnke, T lymphocyte subsets in follicular lymphomas compared with those in non-neoplastic lymph nodes and tonsils, *Human Pathol., 13*: 618 (1982).
78. E. B. Jacobson, L. H. Caporale, and G. J. Thorbecke, Effect of thymus cell injections on germinal center formation in lymphoid tissues of nude (thymus less) mice, *Cell Immunol., 13*: 416 (1974).
79. G. S. Kansas, G. S. Wood, and E. G. Engleman, Maturation and functional diversity of human B-lymphocytes delineated with anti-Leu-8, *J. Immunol., 134*: 3003 (1985).
80. G. S. Kansas, G. S. Wood, D. M. Fishwild, and E. G. Engleman, Functional characterization of human T-lymphocyte subsets distinguished by monoclonal anti-Leu-8, *J. Immunol., 134*: 2995 (1985).
81. A. W. S. Ritchie, K. James, and H. S. Micklem, The distribution and possible significance of cells identified in human lymphoid tissue by the monoclonal antibody HNK-1, *Clin. Exp. Immunol., 51*: 439 (1983).

82. W. Timens and S. Poppema, Lymphocytic compartments in human spleen. An immunohistologic study in normal spleen and non-involved spleen in Hodgkin's disease, *Am. J. Pathol., 120*: 443 (1985).
83. S.-M. Hsu, Phenotypic expression of B lymphocytes III. Marginal zone B cells in the spleen are characterized by the expression of Tac and alkaline phosphatase, *J. Immunol., 135*: 123 (1985).
84. L. A. Guarda, J. J. Butler, P. Mansell, E. M. Hersh, J. Reuben, and G. R. Newell, Lymphadenopathy in homosexual men. Morbid anatomy with clinical and immunologic correlations, *Am. J. Clin. Pathol., 79*: 559 (1983).
85. R. L. Modlin, P. R. Meyer, A. J. Amman, T. H. Rea, F. M. Hofman, S. A. Vaccaro, M. A. Conant, and C. R. Taylor, Altered distribution of T and B lymphocytes in lymph nodes from homosexual men with Kaposi's sarcoma, *Lancet, ii*: 768 (1983).
86. R. L. Modlin, P. R. Meyer, F. M. Hofman, M. Mehlmauer, N. B. Levy, R. J. Lukes, J. W. Parker, A. J. Ammann, M. A. Conant, T. H. Rea, and C. R. Taylor, T lymphocyte subsets in lymph nodes from homosexual men, *J. Am. Med. Assoc., 250*: 1302 (1983).
87. E. Kaiserling and K. Lennert, Die interdigitierende reticulum Zelle im menschlichen Lymphoknoten. Eine spezifische Zelle der thymusabhängigen region, *Virchows Arch. B Cell. Pathol., 16*: 51 (1974).
88. J. J. Van Den Oord, C. D. Wolf-Peeters, V. J. Desmet, K. Takahashi, Y. Ohtsuki, and A. Tadaatsu, Nodular alteration of the paracortical area: An in situ immunohistochemical analysis of primary, secondary and tertiary T-nodules, *Am. J. Pathol., 120*: 55 (1985).
89. G. J. Thorbecke, I. Silberberg-Sinakin, and T. J. Flotte, Langerhans cells as macrophages in skin and lymphoid organs, *J. Invest. Dermatol., 75*: 32 (1980).
90. W. A. Franklin, D. Y. Mason, K. Pulford, B. Falini, E. Bliss, K. C. Gatter, H. Stein, L. C. Clarke, and J. O'D McGee, Immunohistological analysis of human mononuclear phagocytes and dendritic cells by using monoclonal antibodies, *Lab. Invest., 54*: 322 (1986).
91. F. M. Hofman, D. Lopez, L. Husman, P. R. Meyer, and C. R. Taylor, Heterogeneity of macrophage populations in human lymphoid and peripheral blood, *Cell Immunol., 88*: 61 (1984).
92. R. A. Moscicki, E. P. Amento, S. M. Krane, J. T. Kurnick, and R. B. Colvin, Modulation of surface antigens of a monocyte cell line, U937, during incubation with lymphocyte-conditioned medium: Detection of T4 antigen and its presence on normal blood monocytes, *J. Immunol., 131*: 743 (1983).
93. G. S. Wood, N. L. Warner, and R. A. Warnke, Anti-Leu-3/T4 antibodies react with cells of monocyte/macrophage and Langerhans lineage, *J. Immunol., 131*: 212 (1983).
94. R. A. H. White, D. W. Mason, A. F. Williams, G. Galfre, and C. Milstein, T lymphocyte heterogeneity in the rat: Separation of functional subpopulations using a monoclonal antibody, *J. Exp. Med., 148*: 664 (1978).
95. D. P. Dialynas, V. S. Quan, K. A. Wall, A. Pierres, J. Quintas, M. R. Loken, M. Pierres, and F. W. Fitch, Characterization of the murine T cell surface

molecule, designated L3T4, identified by monoclonal antibody GK1.5: Similarity of L3T4 to the human Leu-3/T4 molecule, *J. Immunol., 131*: 2445 (1983).
96. G. F. Murphy, Cell membrane glycoproteins and Langerhans cells, *Hum. Pathol., 16*: 103 (1985).
97. A. K. Bhan, L. S. Fujikawa, and C. S. Foster, T-cell subsets and Langerhans cells in normal and diseased conjuctiva, *Am. J. Ophthalmol., 94*: 205 (1982).
98. A. Chu, M. Eisinger, J. S. Lee, S. Takezak, P. C. Kung, and R. E. Edelson, Immunoelectron microscopic identification of Langerhans cells using a new antigenic marker, *J. Invest. Dermatol., 78*: 177 (1982).
99. G. F. Murphy, B. R. Bronstein, R. Knowles, and A. K. Bhan, Ultrastructural documentation of M241 glycoprotein on dendritic cells and endothelial cells in normal human skin, *Lab. Invest., 52*: 264 (1985).
100. T. J. Flotte, G. F. Murphy, and A. K. Bhan, Demonstration of T200 on human Langerhans cell surface membrane, *J. Invest. Dermatol., 82*: 535 (1984).
101. G. S. Wood, V. B. Morhenn, E. C. Butcher, and J. Kosek, Langerhans cells react with panleukocyte monoclonal antibody: Ultrastructural documentation using a live cell suspension immunoperoxidase technique, *J. Invest. Dermatol., 82*: 322 (1984).
102. G. F. Murphy, A. K. Bhan, T. J. Harrist, and M. C. Mihm Jr., In situ identification of T6-positive cells in normal human dermis by immunoelectron microscopy, *Br. J. Dermatol., 108*: 421 (1983).
103. J. H. Beckstead, G. S. Wood, and R. P. Turner: Histiocytosis X cells and Langerhans cells: Enzyme histochemical and immunologic similarities, *Hum. Pathol., 15*: 826 (1984).
104. T. J. Harrist, J. E. Muhlbauer, G. F. Murphy, M. C. Mihm Jr., and A. K. Bhan, T6 is superior to Ia (HLA-DR) as a marker for Langerhans cells and indeterminate cells in normal epidermis. A monoclonal antibody study, *J. Invest. Dermatol., 80*: 100 (1983).
105. G. F. Murphy, T. J. Harrist, A. K. Bhan, and M. C. Mihm Jr., Distribution of cell surface antigens in histiocytosis-X cells. Quantitative immunoelectron microscopy using monoclonal antibodies, *Lab. Invest., 48*: 90 (1983).
106. W. S. Selby, G. Jannossy, G. Goldstein, and D. P. Jewell, T lymphocyte subsets in human intestinal mucosa: The distribution and relationship to MHC-derived antigens, *Clin. Exp. Immunol., 44*: 453 (1981).
107. D. Guy-Grand, C. Griscelli, and P. Vassalli, A mouse gut T lymphocyte, a novel type of T cell: Nature, origin and traffic in mice is normal and graft-vs-host conditions, *J. Exp. Med., 148*: 1661 (1978).
108. N. Cerf-Bensussan, A. Quaroni, J. T. Kurnick, and A. K. Bhan, Intraepithelial lymphocytes modulate Ia expression by intestinal epithelial cells, *J. Immunol., 132*: 2244 (1984).
109. A. Ferguson, Intraepithelial lymphocytes of the small intestine, *Gut, 18*: 921 (1977).

110. J. R. Glaister, Factors affecting the lymphoid cells in the small intestinal epithelium of the mouse, *Int. Arch. Allergy Appl. Immunol., 45*: 719 (1973).
111. A. F. Flores, H. S. Winter, and A. K. Bhan, In situ characterization of T cell subpopulations in gluten sensitive enteropathy (GSE) (Abstract), *Ped. Res., 16*: 161A (1982).
112. W. S. Selby, G. Jannossy, M. Bofill, and D. P. Jewell, Lymphocyte subpopulations in the human small intestine. The findings in normal mucosa and in the mucosa of patients with adult coeliac disease, *Clin. Exp. Immunol., 52*: 219 (1983).
113. A. Tagliabue, A. D. Betus, A. D. Clarke, and J. Bienenstock, Characteristics of natural killer cells in the murine intestinal epithelium and lamina propria, *J. Exp. Med., 155*: 1785 (1982).
114. N. Cerf-Bensussan, D. Guy-Grand, and C. Griscelli, Intraepithelial lymphocytes of human gut: Isolation, characterization and study of NK activity, *Gut, 26*: 81 (1985).
115. N. Cerf-Bensussan, D. Guy-Grand, B. Lsowska-Grospierre, C. Griscelli, and A. K. Bhan, A monoclonal antibody specific for rat intestinal lymphocytes, *J. Immunol., 136*: 76 (1986).
116. M. R. McDermott and J. Bienenstock, Evidence for a common mucosal immunologic system. 1. Migration of B immunoblasts into intestinal, respiratory and genital tissues, *J. Immunol., 122*: 1892 (1979).
117. A. K. Bhan, T. J. Harrist, G. F. Murphy, and M. C. Mihm Jr., T cell subsets and Langerhans cells in lichen planus: In situ characterization using monoclonal antibodies, *Br. J. Dermatol., 105*: 617 (1981).
118. I. A. Lampert, A. J. Suitters, G. Jannossy, J. A. Thomas, S. Palmer, and E. Gordon Smith, Lymphoid filtrates in skin in graft-versus-host disease, *Lancet, 2*: 1352 (1981).
119. A. K. Bhan, M. C. Mihm Jr., and H. F. Dvorak, T cell subsets in allograft rejection: In situ characterization of T-cell subsets in human skin allografts by the use of monoclonal antibodies, *J. Immunol., 129*: 1578 (1982).
120. O. Duke, G. S. Panayi, G. Jannossy, and L. W. Poulter, An immunohistological analysis of lymphocyte subpopulations and their microenvironment in the synovial membranes of patients with rheumatoid arthritis using monoclonal antibodies, *Clin. Exp. Immunol., 49*: 22 (1982).
121. W. C. Van Vorrhis, G. Kaplan, E. N. Sanno, M. A. Horwitz, R. M. Steinman, W. R. Levis, N. Nogueira, L. S. Hair, C. R. Gattas, B. A. Arrick, and Z. A. Cohn, The cutaneous infiltrate of leprosy: Cellular characterization and the predominant T cell phenotype, *N. Eng. J. Med., 307*: 1593 (1982)
122. J. E. Muhlbauer, A. K. Bhan, T. J. Harrist, J. D. Bernhard, and M. C. Mihm Jr., Papular polymorphous light eruption: An immunoperoxidase study employing monoclonal antibodies, *Br. J. Dermatol., 108*: 153 (1983).
123. D. Y. M. Leung, A. K. Bhan, E. E. Schneeberger, and R. S. Geha, Characterization of the mononuclear cell infiltrate in atopic dermatitis using monoclonal antibodies, *J. Allergy Clin. Immunol., 108*: 47 (1983).

124. R. J. Margolis, M. G. Tonnesen, T. J. Harrist, A. K. Bhan, B. U. Wintroub, M. C. Mihm Jr., and N. A. Soter, Lymphocyte subsets and Langerhans/indeterminate cells in erythema multiforme, *J. Invest. Dermatol., 81*: 403 (1983).
125. D. J. Ruiter, A. K. Bhan, T. J. Harrist, A. J. Sober, and M. C. Mihm, Jr., Major histocompatibility antigens and mononuclear inflammatory infiltrate in benign nevomelanocytic proliferations and malignant melanoma, *J. Immunol., 129*: 2808 (1982).
126. A. K. Bhan and C. L. Desmarais, Immunohistologic characterization of major histocompatibility antigens and inflammatory cellular infiltrate in human breast cancer, *JNCI, 71*: 507 (1983).
127. S. E. Kabawat, R. C. Bast Jr., W. R. Welch, R. C. Knapp, and A. K. Bhan, Expression of major histocompatibility antigens and nature of inflammatory cellular infiltrate in ovarian neoplasms, *Int. J. Cancer, 32*: 547 (1983).
128. S. E. Kabawat, M. Mostoufi-Zadeh, S. G. Driscoll, and A. K. Bhan, Implantation site in normal pregnancy, *Am. J. Pathol., 118*: 76 (1985).
129. A. K. Bhan, R. B. Colvin, A. B. Cosimi, and R. T. McCluskey, Nature of cellular infiltrate in renal allograft rejection (abstract), *Kidney Int., 21*: 293 (1982).
130. J. L. Platt, T. W. Lebien, and A. F. Michael, Interstitial mononuclear cell population in renal allograft rejection identification by monoclonal antibodies in tissue section, *J. Exp. Med., 155*: 17 (1981).
131. C. C. Marboe, D. M. Knowles 2nd., L. Chess, K. Reemtsma, and J. J. Fenoglio Jr., The immunologic and ultrastructural characterization of the cellular infiltrate in acute cardiac allograft rejection: Prevalence of cells with the natural killer (NK) phenotype, *Clin. Immunol. Immunopathol., 27*: 141 (1983).
132. W. W. Hancock, N. M. Thomson, and R. C. Atkins, Composition of interstitial cellular infiltrate identified by monoclonal antibodies in renal biopsies of rejecting human renal allografts, *Transplantation, 35*: 458 (1983).
133. P. C. Kolbeck, A. H. Tatum, and F. Sanfilippo, Relationship among the histologic pattern, intensity, and phenotypes of T cells infiltrating renal allografts, *Transplantation, 38*: 709 (1984).
134. R. T. McCluskey and A. K. Bhan, Cell mediated immunity in renal disease, *Human Pathol., 17*: 146 (1986).
135. S. C. Meuer, R. E. Hussey, J. C. Hodgdon, T. Hercend, S. F. Schlossman, and E. L. Reinherz, Surface structures involved in target recognition by human cytotoxic T lymphocytes, *Science, 218*: 471 (1982).
136. A. M. Krensky, C. S. Reiss, J. W. Mier, J. L. Strominger, and S. J. Burakoff, Long term human cytolytic T-cell lines allospecific for HLA-DR6 antigen are OKT4+, *Proc. Natl. Acad. Sci. USA, 79*: 2365 (1982).
137. B. M. Hall, G. A. Bishop, G. G. Duggin, J. S. Horvath, J. Phillips, and D. J. Tiller, Increased expression of HLA–DR antigens on renal tubular cells in renal transplants: Relevance to the rejection response, *Lancet, 2*: 247 (1984).

138. J. L. Platt, B. W. Grant, A. E. Eddy, and A. F. Michael, Immune cell populations in cutaneous delayed type hypersensitivity, *J. Exp. Med., 158*: 1227 (1983).
139. N. K. Damle, N. Mohagheghpour, J. A. Hansen, and E. G. Engleman, Alloantigen-specific cytotoxic and suppressor T lymphocytes are derived from phenotypically distinct precursors, *J. Immunol., 131*: 2296 (1983).
140. N. K. Damle, N. Mohagheghpour, and E. G. Engleman, Dissection of immunoregulatory subpopulations of T lymphocytes within the helper and suppressor sublineages in man, *J. Immunol., 129*: 1997 (1982).
141. R. A. Gatenby, G. S. Kansas, C. Y. Xian, R. L. Evans, and E. G. Engleman, Dissection of immunoregulatory subpopulations of T lymphocytes within the helper and suppressor sublineages in man, *J. Immunol., 129*: 1997 (1982).
142. A. Landay, G. L. Gartland, and L. T. Clement, Characterization of a phenotypically distinct subpopulation of Leu-2+ cells that suppresses T cell proliferative responses, *J. Immuno., 131*: 2757 (1983).
143. R. J. Lukes and R. D. Collins, Immunologic characterization of human malignant lymphomas, *Cancer, 34*: 1488 (1974).
144. S. E. Salmon and M. Seligmann, B-cell neoplasia in man, *Lancet, 2*: 1230 (1974).
145. A. Bernard, L. Boumsell, C. Bayle, Y. Richard, H. Coppin, C. Penit, P. Rouget, C. Micheau, B. Clausse, R. Gerard-Marchant, J. Dausset, and J. Lemerle, Subsets of malignant lymphomas in children related to the cell phenotype, *Blood, 54*: 1058 (1979).
146. A. Bernard, L. Boumsell, E. L. Reinherz, L. M. Nadler, J. Ritz, H. Coppin, Y. Richard, F. Valenesi, J. Dausset, G. Flandrin, J. Lemerle, and S. F. Schlossman, Cell surface characterization of malignant T cells from lymphoblastic lymphoma using monoclonal antibodies: evidence for phenotypic differences between malignant T cells from patients with acute lymphoblastic lymphoma, *Blood, 57*: 1105 (1981).
147. L. M. Nadler, K. C. Anderson, E. K. Park, M. P. Bates, R. Leonard, E. L. Reinherz, and S. F. Schlossman, Immunologic heterogeneity of human T and B cell lymphoid malignancies, in *Tumor Cell Heterogeneity: Origins and Implications* (A. H. Owens, Jr., D. S. Coffey, S. B. Baylin, eds.), Academic Press, New York, Vol. 4, 1982, p. 53.
148. H. Stein, J. Gerdes, and D. Y. Mason, The normal and malignant germinal centre, *Clin. Haematol., 11*: 531 (1982).
149. S. M. Hsu, K. Yank, and E. S. Jaffe, Hairy cell leukemia: A B cell neoplasm with a unique antigenic phenotype, *Am. J. Clin. Pathol., 80*: 421 (1983).
150. N. L. Harris, L. M. Nadler, and A. K. Bhan, Immunohistologic characterization of two malignant lymphomas of germinal center type (centroblastic/centrocytic and centrocytic) with monoclonal antibodies: Follicular and diffuse lymphomas of small cleaved cell type are related but distinct entities, *Am. J. Pathol., 117*: 262 (1984).

151. C. J. L. M. Meijer, F. Albeda, P. Van Der Valk, P. J. Spaander, and J. Jansen, Immunohistochemical studies of the spleen in hairy cell leukemia, *Am. J. Pathol., 115*: 266 (1984).
152. R. S. Doggett, G. S. Wood, S. Horning, R. Levy, R. F. Dorfman, J. Bindl, and R. A. Warnke, The immunologic characterization of 95 nodal and extranodal diffuse large cell lymphomas in 89 patients, *Am. J. Pathol., 115*: 245 (1984).
153. N. L. Harris and A. K. Bhan, B cell neoplasia of lymphocytic, lymphoplasmacytoid, and plasma cell type: Immunohistologic analysis and clinical correlation, *Human. Pathol., 16*: 829 (1985).
154. K. C. Anderson, M. P. Bates, B. L. Slaughenhoupt, G. S. Pinkus, S. F. Schlossman, and L. M. Nadler, Expression of human B cell-associated antigens on leukemias and lymphomas: A model of human B cell differentiation, *Blood, 63*: 1424 (1984).
155. M. L. Cleary, R. A. Warnke, and J. Sklar, Monoclonality of lymphoproliferative lesions in cardiac transplant recipients: Clonal analysis based on immunoglobulin gene rearrangements, *N. Engl. J. Med., 310*: 477 (1984).
156. N. L. Harris and A. K. Bhan, Distribution of T cell subsets in nodular and diffuse lymphomas of B cell type, *Am. J. Pathol., 113*: 172 (1983).
157. C. Y. Wang, R. A. Good, P. Ammirati, G. Dymbort, and R. L. Evans, Identification of a P69,71 complex expressed on human T cells sharing determinants with B-type chronic lymphatic leukemic cells, *J. Exp. Med., 151*: 1539 (1980).
158. B. F. Burns, R. A. Warnke, R. S. Doggett, and R. V. Rouse, Expression of a T-cell antigen (Leu-1) by B-cell lymphomas, *Am. J. Pathol., 113*: 165 (1983).
159. F. Caligaris-Cappio, M. Gobbi, M. Bofill, and G. Janossy, Infrequent normal B lymphocytes express features of B-chronic lymphocytic leukemia, *J. Exp. Med., 155*: 623 (1982).
160. M. P. Link, M. Roper, R. F. Dorfman, W. M. Crist, M. D. Cooper, and R. Levy, Cutaneous lymphoblastic lymphoma with pre-B markers, *Blood, 61(5)*: 838 (1983).
161. L. M. Weiss, G. S. Crabtree, R. Rouse, and R. A. Warnke, Morphologic and immunologic characterization of 50 peripheral T-cell lymphomas, *Am. J. Pathol., 118*: 316 (1985).
162. L. M. Weiss, G. S. Wood, and R. A. Warnke, Immunophenotypic differences between dermatopathic lymphadenopathy and lymph node involvement in mycosis fungoides, *Am. J. Pathol., 120*: 179 (1985).
163. S. Poppema, A. K. Bhan, E. L. Reinherz, M. R. Posner, and S. F. Schlossman, In situ immunologic characterization of cellular constituents in lymph nodes and spleens involved by Hodgkin's disease, *Blood, 59*: 226 (1982).
164. U. Schwab, H. Stein, J. Gerdes, H. Lemke, H. Kirchner, M. Schaadt, and V. Diehl, Production of a monoclonal antibody specific for Hodgkin and Sternberg-Reed cells of Hodgkin's disease and a subset of normal lymphoid cells, *Nature, 299*: 65 (1982).

165. S.-M. Hsu and E. S. Jaffe, Leu M1 and peanut agglutinin stain the neoplastic cells of Hodgkins disease, *Am. J. Clin. Pathol., 82*: 29 (1984).
166. H. Stein, D. Y. Mason, J. Gerdes, N. O'Connor, J. Wainscoat, G. Pellesen, R. Gatter, B. Falini, G. Delsol, H. Lemke, R. Schwarting, and R. Lennert, The expression of the Hodgkin's disease associated antigen Ki-1 in reactive and neoplastic lymphoid tissue: Evidence that Reed-Sternberg cells and histiocytic malignancies are derived from activated lymphoid cells, *Blood, 66*: 848 (1985).

3
Structural and Functional Aspects of HLA Class II Genes

YUKIO KOIDE AND TAKATO O. YOSHIDA
Hamamatsu University School of Medicine, Hamamatsu, Japan

I. INTRODUCTION

Class II molecules encoded by genes in the major histocompatibility complex (MHC) function as restriction elements in cell-to-cell interactions in the immune response (1). Helper T cells can recognize nominal antigens in association with MHC class II antigens on the surface of antigen-presenting cells (APC). This associative recognition also occurs between helper T cells and B cells (2), referred to as the cognate interaction.

HLA class II antigens are highly polymorphic cell-surface glycoproteins encoded in the D region of the HLA complex on the short arm of chromosome 6. The high complexity of the HLA class II system is now generally recognized at both the DNA and protein levels (3,4). At least three distinct HLA class II antigens, designated HLA-DR, -DQ, and -DP, exist although only two class II antigens, called I-A and I-E, have been identified in the mouse.

In the following we describe the structure, gene organization, expression, and function of HLA class II antigens.

II. STRUCTURE OF HLA CLASS II ANTIGENS

All class II antigens consist of two noncovalently linked subunits, the α chain (33-35 Kd) and the β chain (26-29 Kd) (5; Fig. 1). In addition, a third chain of ~ 33 Kd, called the invariant (Ii) chain, is transiently associated with the α and β subunits during their transport to the cell surface (6). Both α and β chains are composed of four domains: (a) an N-terminal (α 1 or β 1) domain of 85-95 amino acids, (b) a membrane proximal (α 2 or β 2) domain of 95 amino acids, (c) a con-

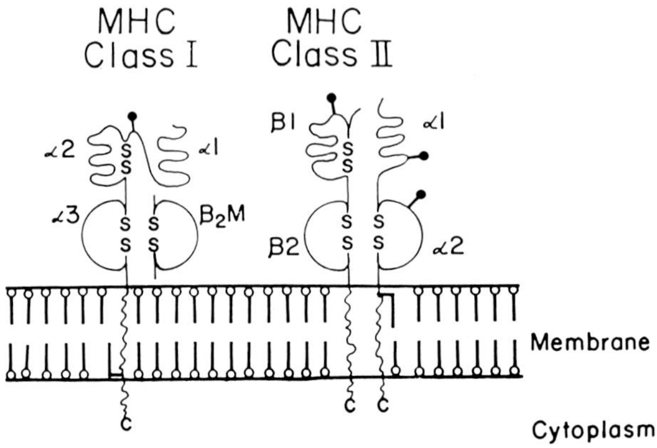

Figure 1 Models MHC class I and class II antigens. S-S indicates disulfide bonds between cysteine residues. C indicates carboxyl terminus, (●) indicates N-linked carbohydrate side chains (from Kaufman et al. (5)).

necting peptide (11-13 amino acids) and a transmembrane region (23 amino acids), and (d) an intracytoplasmic domain (8-15 amino acids). The extracellular portion of the α and β chains appears to be folded into two approximately equally large domains. α 2, β 1, and β 2 domains are each stabilized by a single disulfide bridge. The β 1 domains are more polymorphic than the domains closest to the membrane. In contrast, the α 1 domains, except for DQ antigens, are not polymorphic (7,8). The α 2 and β 2 domains display significant sequence homology. They also display homologies to immunoglobulin light and heavy chains and to T-cell-receptor α and β chains. Thus, the class II antigens are considered to belong to the immunoglobulin superfamily (5).

Class II antigens undergo several posttranscriptional modifications. Each domain of the α chain contains one asparagine-linked carbohydrate moiety, and the β chain contains a single asparagine-linked carbohydrate moiety whose position appears invariable.

Several class II α and β genes have been cloned and their structures elucidated (3,5). The exon-intron organization of class II α and β genes is shown in Figure 2. The α genes are composed of five exons encoding: (a) the 5' untranslated region and signal sequence, (b) the α 1 domain, (c) the α 2 domain, (d) the connecting peptide, transmembrane region, cytoplasmic tail, and part of the 3' untranslated region, and (e) the remainder of the 3' untranslated region.

The β genes are composed of six exons. The organization of the β genes differs from that of the α genes only as regards an extra intracytoplasmic exon between the transmembrane exon and the exon encoding the last four amino acids of the protein and 3' untranslated region.

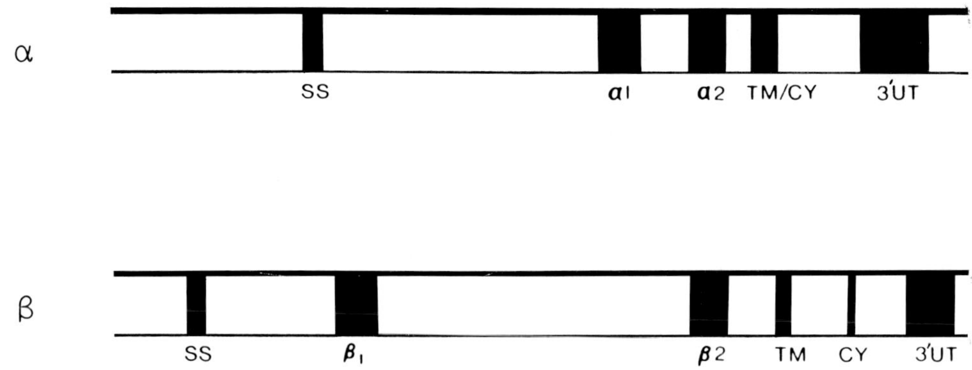

Figure 2 Genomic architecture of the class II genes. SS, signal sequence; TM, transmembrane region; CY, intracytoplasmic region; UT, untranslated sequence (3).

III. HLA CLASS II GENE ORGANIZATION

Figure 3 shows the organization of the class II genes. This work, done by Spies et al. (9) and Okada et al. (10,11), is based on the use of overlapping cosmid and phage clones from the cell line Priess (DR 4, 4, DQw3, w3, DP3, 4).

Regarding the DR region, there appears to be a single DR_{α} chain gene and 3 DR_{β} chain genes. One of the 3 DR_{β} genes, ψ DR_{β}, is revealed to be a pseudogene. This gene contains a *Kpn I* repeat inserted 5' to the promoter, suggesting an implication in the genesis of this pseudogene by means of transcription inactivation (12). Two other DR_{β} genes have been identified by comparison of DNA and protein sequence data. They encode the β chains carrying the DR4 and MT3 serological specificities, respectively (9).

As shown in Table 1, each DR locus appears to contain varying numbers of β chain genes (13). It is suggested that DR8 homozygous cells are comprised of only one β chain gene.

The DQ region consists of two pairs of α and β genes. In contrast to DR_{β} genes, the number of DQ_{β} genes is constant (13). One of the two α-β pairs encodes to the DQ antigen, and the remaining α-β pair, centromeric to DQ, has been termed DX_{α} and DX_{β}.

Although DR_{α} is not polymorphic, both DQ_{α} and DQ_{β} are highly polymorphic in their coding sequence.

The expressed products of DX genes have not yet been identified. Utilizing an oligonucleotide probe specific for DX_{α}, the expression of DX_{α} has not been detected in at least two different B lymphoblastoid cell lines (3). However, sequence analysis of the DX_{α} and DX_{β} genes has not revealed any obvious characteristics that make them pseudogenes. In addition, the DX_{α} gene has been proved

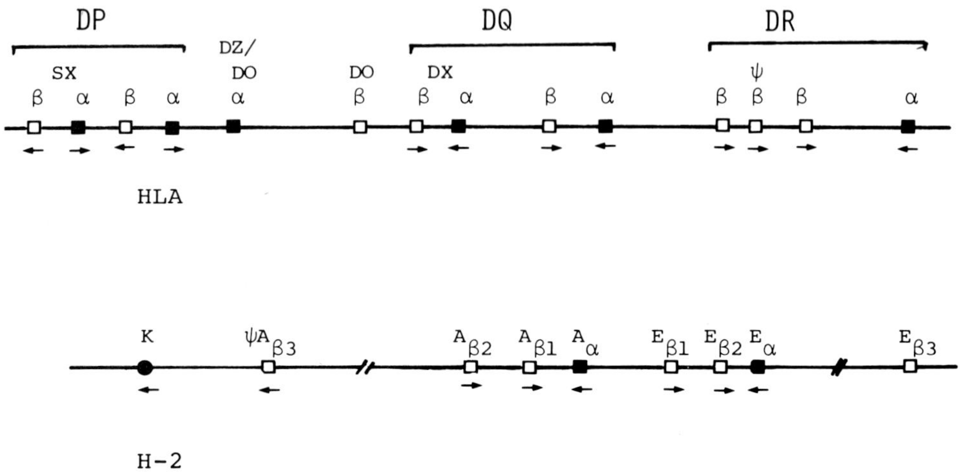

Figure 3 Schematic map of the human and murine class II regions based on the data of various authors, reviewed by Korman et al. (3), Trowsdale et al. (4), Hardy et al. (17), and Steinmetz et al. (18). The arrows indicate the direction of transcription of genes. Slashes indicate that subregion or genes have not been linked.

to be capable of being spliced using the DX_α gene inserted in a retrovirus vector (3). Since the DQ and DX genes are as similar to each other as are alleles of a single segregated series, it is possible that hybrid molecules of the types DQ_α-DX_β and DX_α-DQ_β may exist.

The DP region also consists of two α-β gene pairs, which include the genes for the DP antigens. The second α-β pair has been termed SX_α and SX_β. These genes are in "tail-to-tail" orientation, unlike other MHC α-β gene pairs in the human and the mouse. Structure analysis of SX_α and SX_β has revealed that both SX_α and SX_β are pseudogenes by several features: (a) single base-pair (bp) deletions in the $\alpha 1$ and transmembrane exons which would alter the reading frame, (b) a

Table 1 Estimated Number of DR β Genes in Different DR Specificities

	DR1	DR2	DR3	DR4	DR5	DRw6 = DR3	DR7	DRw8	DRw9 = DR5
Estimated β gene number	2	3	3	3	2 or 3	3	3	1	2 or 3

Source: based on data from Böhme et al. (13).

splice donor mutation at the end of the $\alpha 1$ domain, and (c) a frame-shift mutation in the $\beta 2$ domain which results in a stop codon 18 amino acids away (3).

Sequence analysis of DP_α chains revealed that this polypeptide displays a low degree of genetic polymorphisms (only about 3% of the residues differ) like DR_α chains (4) and that the polymorphism of DP exists in β chains.

DZ_α and DO_α have been independently isolated by Speilman et al. (14) and Inoko et al. (15), respectively. Over the short region compared, the two genes have almost identical exon sequences. Thus, DZ_α and DO_α could be alleles of the same gene.

A cDNA named DO_β has been isolated by Tonnelle et al. (16). DO_β mRNA expression is low in B-cell lines. Unlike other class II genes, DO_β is not induced by interferon (IFN)-γ in fibroblast lines. It is not known whether DZ/DO_α and DO_β are functional. The DZ/DO_α chain seems not to be associated with the DO_β chain since DZ/DO_α RNA is not coordinately expressed with DO_β mRNA.

The precise genomic organization of DZ/DO_α and DO_β genes has been difficult to determine. Recently, Hardy et al. (17) determined the order of these loci using pulse-field gel electrophoresis. The order of the class II subregion was confirmed as DP-DZ/DO_α-DO_β-DX-DQ-DR_β-DR_α (Fig. 3).

Because of lack of linkage disequilibrium between DR and DP in contrast to strong linkage disequilibrium between DR and DQ, a "hot spot" for recombination seems to exist at the right of DP (4). Support for this hypothesis is the high recombination frequency (1-3%) between DP and DQ and the observation that no recombination between DQ and DR genes has yet been reported (4).

IV. COMPARATIVE INTERSPECIES ASPECTS

There is an overall analogous gene organization of the MHC in the human and the mouse (Fig. 3). There are two α genes and four β genes in the murine I region, all clearly assigned to I-A or I-E (18). The A_α, A_β, and E_α, and E_β genes code for the polypeptides of the I-A and I-E molecules, respectively. Although the $A_{\beta 2}$ and $E_{\beta 2}$ genes appear to be transcribed at low levels in spleen cells (19, 20), protein products by the $A_{\beta 2}$ and $E_{\beta 2}$ genes have so far not been identified. $A_{\beta 3}$, linked to the K region, has been analyzed in detail by Widera and Flavell (21). The sequence analysis of $A_{\beta 3}$ reveals that this gene is a pseudogene. Recently, $E_{\beta 3}$ has been mapped into the S region by Wake et al. (20).

Sequence comparisons of human and murine class II β genes reveal that the DP_β, DO_β, and DR_β genes are the counterparts to the murine $A_{\beta 3}$, $A_{\beta 2}$, A_β, and E_β genes, respectively (Table 2). It is of particular interest that the gene order, DP-DO-DQ-DR, is the same as that of the mouse counterparts.

Sequence comparisons of α chain genes indicate that the human DQ_α and DR_α genes are homologous to the A_α and E_α genes, respectively (Table 3).

Table 2 Nucleotide and Amino Acid Sequence Homology (%) Between Mouse and Human Class II β Chain Exons Encoding the Second External Domain

	Nucleotides				Amino Acids			
	DP	DO	DQ	DR	DP	DO	DQ	DR
$A^b_{\beta 3}$	83	–	73	70	75	–	68	60
$A^b_{\beta 2}$	69	83	71	73	62	79	63	65
A^b_{β}	75	67	83	71	70	65	81	67
E^b_{β}	78	70	75	83	69	54	70	83

Source: based on data from Tonelle et al. (16) and Wake et al. (20).

Table 3 Amino Acid Sequence Homologies (%) Between Mouse and Human Class II α Chain Exons Encoding the Second External Domain

	DP_α	DQ_α	DR_α
A_α	60	68	55
E_α	63	60	76

Source: based on data from Auffray et al. (55).

V. TRANSCRIPTIONAL REGULATION OF HLA CLASS II GENES

Class II antigens are expressed on B cells, macrophages, dendritic cells, and certain epithelial cells, indicating that class II gene expression is controlled in a cell-type-specific manner. The expression of class II genes is controlled by *trans*-acting elements as well as *cis*-acting promoter and enhancer sequences. Somatic cell hybrids between class II-negative T-cell lines and class II-positive B-cell lines express class II antigens derived from T-cell lines as well as those derived from B-cell lines (22), suggesting that there is a *trans*-acting element required for regulations of the class II genes. The presence of a *trans*-acting element for expression of class II genes is also suggested by the formation of somatic cell hybrids between class II negative mutants and other B-cell lines; in these hybrids the class II specificities of the mutant are reexpressed (23,24). De Preval et al. (25) also suggested the presence of *trans*-acting elements required for the expression of class II genes by family studies. Some severe combined immunodeficiency (SCID) patients do not express HLA class II antigens on peripheral blood lymphocytes (HLA class II-deficient SCID). In these patients, mRNA for the α and β chains of HLA-DR, -DQ, and -DP are absent. Family studies indicate that the genetic defect does not segregate with MHC, and that the expression of the entire family of class II genes is normally controlled by a *trans*-acting class II regulatory gene which is unlinked to the MHC.

A comparison of the 5' ends of DR_{α} and $I\text{-}E_{\alpha}$ reveals that approximately 100 bp upstream of the transcriptional start are identical except for a single 15 bp gap (26,27). The promoter region of 11 different class II genes shows extensive sequence conservation of the two elements as well as the distance between them (19 bp for α and 20 bp for β) (3). The conservation of these promoter elements suggests that they have a functional role in class II gene expression. In addition, conserved sequences upstream of the genes, expression of which is regulated by IFN, have been identified (28). The consensus IFN response sequence is found upstream of HLA-A3, metallothionein-II, and HLA-DR_{α} genes (Fig. 4). The consensus sequence lies 142 bp, 600 bp, and 567 bp upstream of HLA-A3, metallothionein-II, and HLA-DR_{α} genes, respectively.

Induction of class II antigens by IFN-γ is not confined to hematopoietic cells. It has been demonstrated that fibroblasts (29), endothelial cells (30), astrocytes (31), and melanoma cells (32) can be induced to express class II antigens in response to IFN-γ. Inducible MHC class II antigen expression may confer some of the function of APC to these cells (33,34).

We have investigated the IFN-γ-induced intracellular signaling molecules which are involved in the induction of class II antigen expression, using HL-60 cells (35).

HLA-DR	G**T**GTTGA**ACCTC**-AG**AGTTTCTC**C**TCT**-**C**AT
HLA-A3	A**TTC**CCC**A**A**CTC**C**GCAGTTTCT**TT**TCT**-**CT**C
MT-2	TC**TC**TGG**ACCT**--**GCAGTTTCTC**C**TCT**-**CT**A
Consensus	**TTC**N$\genfrac{}{}{0pt}{}{G}{C}$N**ACCTC**N**GCAGTTTCTC**$\genfrac{}{}{0pt}{}{C}{T}$**TCT-CT**

Figure 4 Homologous 5' sequences flanking the HLA and the metallothionein genes. Boldface letters indicate nucleotides conserved in at least three of the four examples. N any nucleotide (from Friedman and Stark (28)).

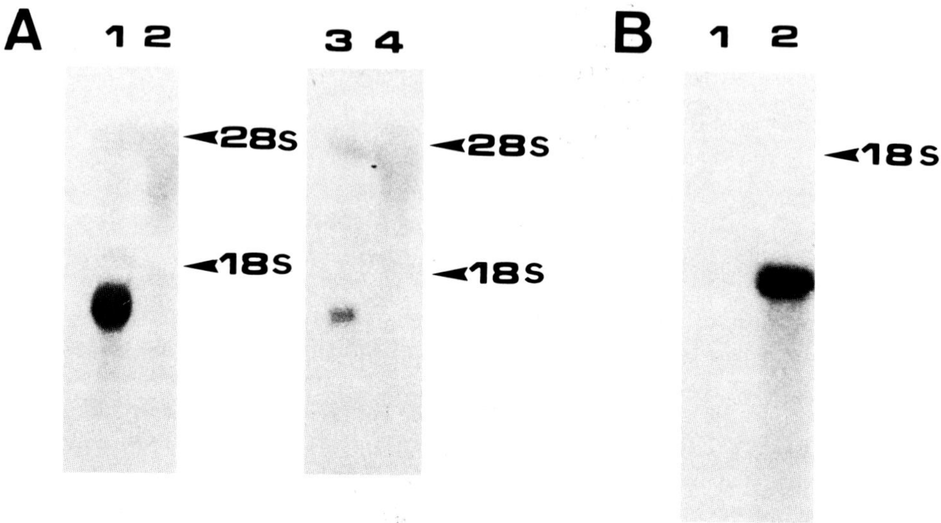

Figure 5 RNA blot analysis of HL-60 exposed to IFN-γ. (A) 20 μg (Daudi; lane 1 & 3) or 40 μg (HL-60; lane 2 & 4) of total RNA was electrophoresed in a 1.0% agarose-formaldehyde gel and transferred to a nylon membrane and hybridized with ^{32}P-labeled cDNA inserts. Lane 1 & 2: DRβ, lane 3 & 4: DQβ. (B) HL-60 cells were cultured without (lane 1) or with 10^3 U/ml recombinant IFN-γ for 48 hr (lane 2); 20 μg of poly $(A)^+$ RNA was applied and hybridized with a DRβ probe.

We observed that IFN-γ-induced expression of class II antigens on HL-60 cells was regulated at the mRNA level (Fig. 5). Toward elucidation of intracellular signaling molecules responsible for this, we employed N-(6-amino-hexyl)-5-chloro-1-naphthalensulfonamide (W-7), a potent calmodulin (CaM) antagonist, and 1-(5-isoquinolinyl sulfonyl)-2-methylpiperazine (H-7), a protein kinase C (PKC) inhibitor (36,37). As shown in Figure 6, the simultaneous addition of W-7 inhibited the IFN-γ-induced DR antigen expression at 20-30 μM. However, H-7 showed no effect on the expression even at 20 μM. The primary effect of W-7 has been shown to be mediated through a competitive inhibition of enzyme activation by interacting with CaM or phospholipid. Since *K*i values of W-7 for CaM-dependent phosphorylation and phospholipid-dependent protein kinase were 12 μM and 110 μM, respectively (38), the effect of W-7 we obtained is attributed to the inhibition of CaM. On the other hand, Hidaka et al. (37) reported that the *K*i value of H-7 for PKC was 6 μM. Therefore, our results obtained with H-7 indicate that PKC is not involved in the IFN-γ-induced expression of class II antigens. This was

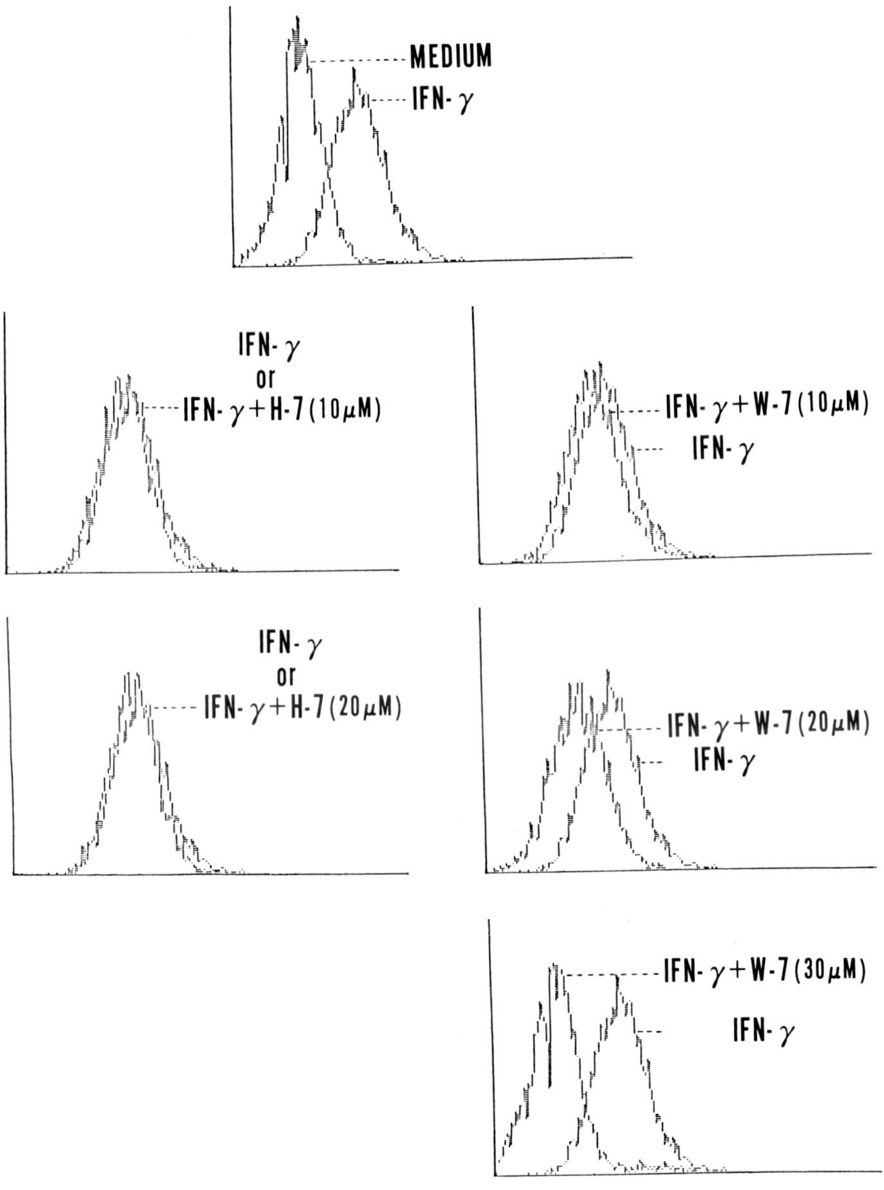

Figure 6 Effect of H-7 or W-7 on the ability of IFN-γ to induce DR antigen expression. HL-60 cells were cultured with IFN-γ (10^3 U/ml) and indicated concentrations of H-7 or W-7 for 48 hr and analyzed for DR expression by EPICS V. The data are presented as histograms, Log_{10} fluorescence intensity (x axis) versus number of cells (y axis).

further confirmed by the use of phorbol myristate acetate (PMA), which is known as a direct activator of PKC (39). The pretreatment of HL-60 with PMA failed to induce class II antigens. It is noteworthy in our experiments that IFN-γ induced class II antigens via a Ca^{2+}-CaM pathway but not via a PKC pathway.

Since a Ca^{2+}-CaM pathway appeared to be involved in IFN-γ-induced class II antigen expression, an increase in the intracellular free calcium ((Ca^{2+})i) level should be involved in induction of the antigen. Using $^{45}CaCl_2$, IFN-γ was demonstrated to evoke calcium influx in HL-60 cells (Fig. 7). In addition, calcium ionophore A23187 was able to induce class II antigen expression (Fig. 8).

The two most likely possibilities for the mechanisms of the elevation of (Ca^{2+})i are extracellular calcium influx and calcium release from intracellular stores, which is presumably provoked by inositol 1,4,5-triphosphate, a product of phosphatidylinositol (PtdIns) hydrolysis (39). Two lines of evidence suggest that calcium influx is primarily responsible for IFN-γ-induced class II antigen expression. First, dantrolene, an inhibitor of intracellular Ca^{2+} release from the endoplasmic reticulum (40), was not able to suppress the induction of class II antigen expression by IFN-γ. Second, depletion of Ca^{2+} from culture medium by EGTA resulted in failure of IFN-γ to induce class II antigen expression. These results suggest that IFN-γ evokes calcium influx by a so-called "receptor-mediated calcium channel" and induces class II antigen expression by activating the CaM

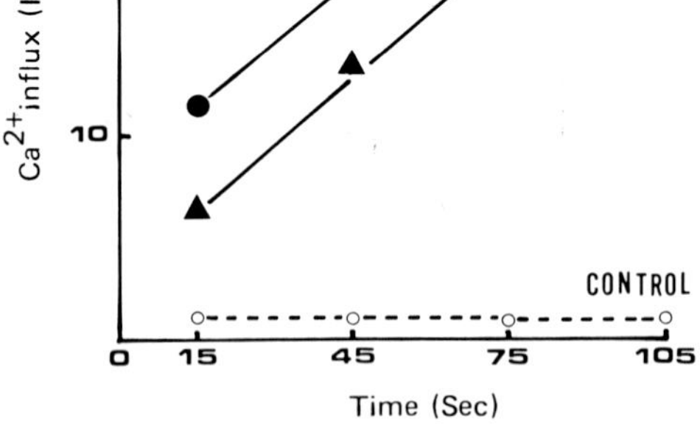

Figure 7 Calcium influx into HL-60 cells. $^{45}Ca^{2+}$ and IFN or PLC were added to HL-60 cell suspensions at time 0, and calcium uptake was examined at 15, 45, 75, and 105 sec. Results were expressed as an influx index. Influx index = cpm stimulated sample at time T/cpm unstimulated sample at time T.

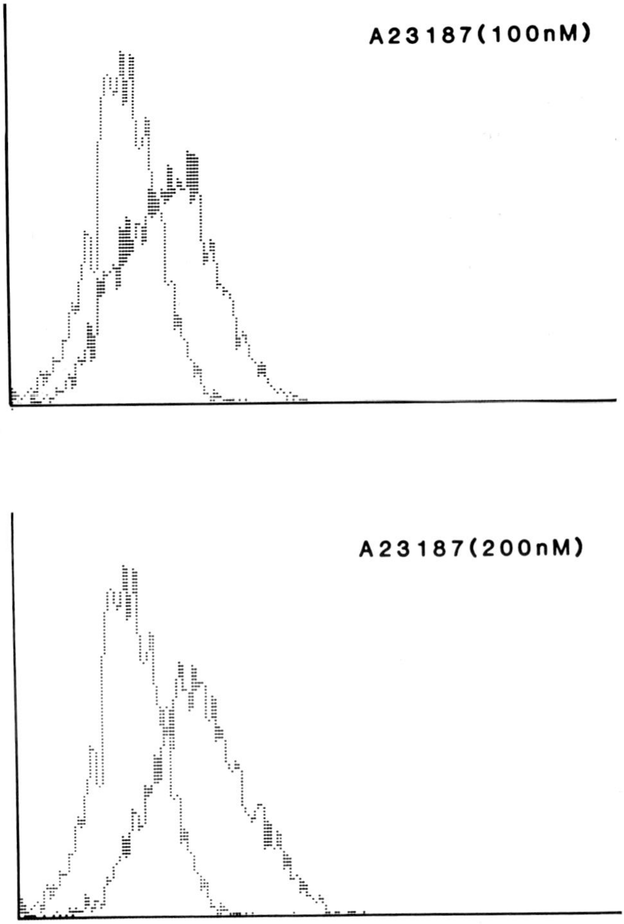

Figure 8 Effect of A23187 on the induction of DR antigen expression. Cells were cultured with indicated concentrations of A23187 for 24 hr and then analyzed for DR expression by EPICS V.

branch of the calcium messenger system. Whether the receptor-mediated calcium influx is operated by direct opening of the calcium channel or PtdIns hydrolysis-mediated induction of calcium influx (41) is still obscure. However, support for the latter possibility comes from our demonstration with bacterial phospholipase C (PLC), which induced both calcium influx (Fig. 7) and class II antigen expression. PLC is known to hydrolyze membrane PtdIns (39). Furthermore, the finding that both IFN-γ-induced calcium influx and class II antigen expression were inhibited in the presence of theophylline and dibutyryl cAMP supports the latter possibility.

Taken together, our results indicate that the binding of IFN-γ to the receptor provokes calcium influx and induces the transcription of class II antigens by activating the CaM branch of the calcium messenger system.

VI. FUNCTION OF HLA CLASS II ANTIGENS

T cells can recognize foreign antigens only when presented together with autologous MHC class I or class II antigens, which is called MHC restriction (1). Class II-positive APC present nominal antigens to regulatory T cells. Most soluble antigens require intracellular "processing" before recognition by T cells, and this processing pathway appears to require the low pH environment of endosomes or lysosomes (42). Recently, invariant (Ii) chains have been suggested to play a role in determining the association of soluble antigens with class II antigens in the intracellular compartment (43).

In T-cell recognition, HLA-DR, -DQ, and -DP antigens on APC are suggested to play distinct roles since a clear functional dichotomy exists for antigens encoded for by I-A and I-E in the mouse (44). In a study of the inhibitory effect of anti-class II antibodies, we showed that the monoclonal antibodies (mAb) against DR antigens were capable of inhibiting T-cell proliferative responses to purified protein derivative (PPD)- and herpes simplex virus antigen-pulsed APC, autologous B-cell lines and alloantigens. However, mAb against DQ antigens showed no inhibitory effect on the proliferative responses of T cells to the antigens (Fig. 9) (45). Furthermore, we isolated and propagated PPD-reactive T-cell clones using interleukin-2. The clones were restricted to DR molecules, and no clone was demonstrated which was restricted to DQ molecules (46).

Qvigstad and Thorsby also reported that most of the *Chlamydia*-specific proliferative T-cell clones were restricted by DR or MT molecules (48). They also established a *Chlamydia*-specific T-cell clone restricted to DP molecules (49). However, neither they nor we have ever found evidence of elements on DQ molecules restricting the response. It was shown that mAb against DQ can effectively block generation of cytotoxic T cells, although neither proliferation of T cells in response to allo- or soluble antigens nor the production of immunoglobulin were affected (50). These data indicate a possible differential function of DQ and the other class II molecules, DR and DP. In fact, it has been shown that the addition of the DQw1 antibody blocked the specific induction of suppressor cells in the mixed lymphocyte culture (51).

Recently we assessed the function of DQ antigens by transfecting two genomic clones, one a phage clone containing a DQα gene and the other a clone containing a DQβ gene, to L cells with pSV2-neo as a selection marker (47). The DQ-positive L-cell transformants showed the ability to induce proliferations in the

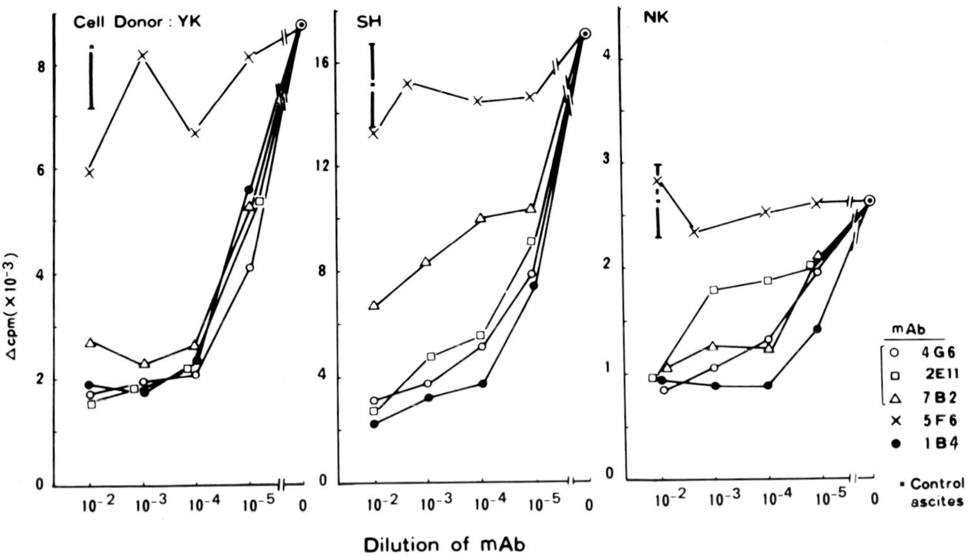

Figure 9 Inhibitory effect of MAb on proliferative response of T cells to PPD-pulsed APC. T cells (1×10^5) from three individuals were cultured with autologous PPD-pulsed APC (1×10^4) for 5 days in the presence of the mAb at different dilutions. Results are expressed as cpm ^{3}H-TdR incorporation. Vertical bars represent ± SD. mAb, 4G6, 2E11, and 7B2 react with DR molecules. 5F6 reacts with DQ molecules and 1B4 reacts with class II molecules distinct from DR or DQ molecules.

mixed lymphocyte culture and this proliferative response was inhibited by a mAb to DQ antigens (Fig. 10).

Lamb and Feldman (52) established DQ-restricted proliferative T-cell clones as well as DR- and DP-restricted clones. The clones were specific to influenza A virus antigens, and the restriction molecules were demonstrated by L cells transfected by cosmid clones containing HLA class II genes.

Although sequence analysis has shown that the DR antigen and the DQ antigen are homologous to the I-E antigen and the I-A antigen of the mouse, respectively, the functional difference of class II antigens between the human and the mouse became apparent. The DR antigen is a dominant restriction molecule in the human. However, it is known that the I-A antigen, which is structurally homologous to DQ, is a dominant restriction molecule in the mouse. These discrepancies observed between the human and the mouse could be explained by the work of Ishii et al. (53), which demonstrated that both I-A and I-E antigens are involved in T-cell responses when restricted by allogeneic class II antigens. They suggested that the germ line repertoire of T-cell receptors contains

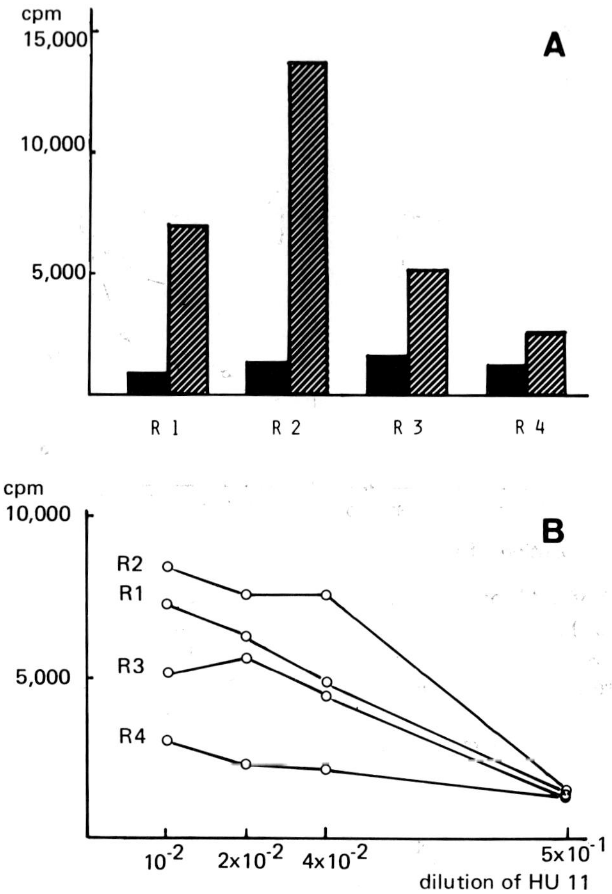

Figure 10 (A) Lymphocyte-stimulating activity of transfected L cells. Hatched columns indicate cpm obtained when the transfected cells were used as stimulators, while the solid columns indicate cpm obtained when the parental cells were used as stimulators. R1-4 indicate peripheral lymphocyte donors. (B) Inhibition of lymphocyte proliferative responses induced by transfected L cells by a mAb against DQ molecules, HU 11 (from Nakatsuji et al. (47)).

both anti-I-A + X (the foreign antigen) and anti-I-E + X, and that probably either anti-I-A + X or anti-I-E + X cells are eliminated during T-cell ontogeny in the mouse. Alternatively, the nature of the antigenic determinant recognized by T cells may be dependent not only on an associative interaction between foreign antigens and class II antigens, but also on the availability of specific receptors in the T-cell repertoire. Therefore, it is quite likely that homologous class II molecules between the human and the mouse have distinct functions.

VII. CONCLUDING REMARKS

Most HLA class II genes seem to have been identified, although some may still be undiscovered. The structure of these genes is also well worked out. However, precise mechanisms underlying the regulation of class II expression, the tissue-specific regulation, and the induction by IFN-γ, is still being unraveled.

Regarding the function of class II antigens, gene transfer experiments will still be useful. The possible existence and the function of hybrid class II antigens will be able to be examined by the transfected cells. Furthermore, exon-shuffling experiments will no doubt be useful in order to identify functionally important regions of class II antigens as has been done in the mouse (54).

REFERENCES

1. B. Benacerraf, *Science, 212*: 1229 (1981).
2. K. Rock, B. Benacerraf, and A. Abbas, *J. Exp. Med., 160*: 1102 (1984).
3. A. J. Korman, J. M. Boss, T. Spies, R. Sorrentino, K. Okada, and J. L. Strominger, *Immunol. Rev., 85*: 45 (1985).
4. J. Trowsdale, J. A. T. Young, A. P. Kelly, P. J. Austin, S. Carson, H. Meunier, A. So, H. A. Erlich, R. S. Spielman, J. Bodmer, and W. F. Bodmer, *Immunol. Rev., 85*: 5 (1985).
5. J. F. Kaufman, C. Auffray, A. J. Korman, D. A. Shackelford, and J. L. Strominger, *Cell, 36*: 1 (1984).
6. E. O. Long, *Surv. Immunol., 4*: 27 (1985).
7. J. F. Kaufman and J. L. Strominger, *Nature, 297*: 694 (1982).
8. J. F. Kaufman and J. L. Strominger, *J. Immunol., 130*: 808 (1983).
9. T. Spies, R. Sorrentino, J. M. Boss, K. Okada, and J. L. Strominger, *Proc. Natl. Acad. Sci. USA, 82*: 5165 (1985).
10. K. Okada, J. M. Boss, H. Prentice, T. Spies, R. Mengler, C. Auffray, J. W. Lillie, D. Grossberger, and J. L. Strominger, *Proc. Natl. Acad. Sci. USA, 82*:3410 (1985).
11. K. Okada, H. Prentice, J. Boss, D. Levy, D. Kappes, T. Spies, R. Raghupathy, R. Mengler, C. Auffray, and J. L. Strominger, *EMBO J., 4*: 739 (1985).
12. D. Larhammar, B. Servenius, L. Rask, and P. A. Peterson, *Proc. Natl. Acad. Sci. USA, 82*: 1475 (1985).
13. J. Böhme, M. Andersson, G. Andersson, E. Möller, P. A. Peterson, and L. Rask, *J. Immunol., 135*: 2149 (1985).
14. R. Spielman, J. S. Lee, W. F. Bodmer, J. Bodmer, and J. Trowsdale, *Proc. Natl. Acad. Sci. USA, 81*: 3461 (1984).
15. H. Inoko, A. Ando, M. Kimura, S. Ogata, and K. Tsuji, in *Histocompatibility Testing 1984* (E. Albert and W. Mayr, eds.), Springer-Verlag, Berlin, Heidelberg, New York, Tokyo, 1984, p. 559.
16. C. Tonnelle, R. DeMaris, and E. O. Long, *EMBO J., 4*: 2839 (1985).
17. D. A. Hardy, J. I. Bell, E. O. Long, T. Lindsten, and H. O. McDevitt, *Nature, 323*: 453 (1986).
18. M. Steinmetz, K. Minard, S. Horrath, J. McNicholas, J. Frelinger, C. T. Wake, E. O. Long, B. Mach, and L. Hood, *Nature, 300*: 35 (1982).

19. N. Braunstein, R. Germain, in *Advances in Gene Technology: Molecular Biology of the Immune System* (J. W. Streilein, F. A. Ahmad, S. Black, B. Blomberg, and R. W. Voellmy, eds.), Cambridge University Press, Cambridge, 1985, p. 119.
20. C. T. Wake, G. Widera, and R. A. Flavell, in *Advances in Gene Technology: Molecular Biology of the Immune System* (J. W. Streilein, F. A. Ahmad, S. Black, B. Blomberg, and R. W. Voellmy, eds.), Cambridge University Press, Cambridge, 1985, p. 33.
21. G. Widera and R. A. Flavell, *Proc. Natl. Acad. Sci. USA, 82*: 5500 (1985).
22. D. N. Howell, A. E. Berger, and P. Cresswell, *Immunogenetics, 15*: 199 (1982).
23. R. S. Acolla, G. Carra, and J. Guardiola, *Proc. Natl. Acad. Sci. USA, 82*: 5145 (1985).
24. P. Gladstone and D. Pious, *Somatic Cell Genet., 6*: 285 (1980).
25. C. de Préval, B. Lisowska-Grospierre, M. Loche, C. Griscelli, and B. Mach, *Nature, 318*: 291 (1985).
26. D. J. Mathis, C. O. Benoist, V. E. Williams II, M. R. Kanter, and H. O. McDevitt, *Cell, 32*: 745 (1983).
27. A. Schamboeck, A. J. Korman, A. Kamb, and J. L. Strominger, *Nuc. Acids Res., 11*: 8663 (1983).
28. R. L. Friedman and G. R. Stark, *Nature, 314*: 637 (1985).
29. T. Collins, A. J. Korman, C. T. Wake, J. M. Boss, D. L. Kappes, W. Fiers, K. A. Ault, M. A. Gimbrone, J. L. Strominger, and J. S. Pober, *Proc. Natl. Acad. Sci. USA, 81*: 4917 (1984).
30. J. S. Pober, M. A. Gimbrone, R. S. Cotran, C. S. Reiss, S. J. Burakoff, W. Fiers, and K. A. Ault, *J. Exp. Med., 157*: 1399 (1983).
31. G. H. W. Wong, I. Clark-Lewis, A. W. Harris, and J. W. Schrader, *Eur. J. Immunol., 14*: 52 (1984).
32. A. N. Houghton, T. M. Thomson, D. Gross, H. F. Ottenger, and L. J. Old, *J. Exp. Med., 160*: 255 (1984).
33. A. Fontana, W. Fiers, and H. Wekerle, *Nature, 307*: 273 (1984).
34. C. R. Wagner, R. M. Vetto, and D. R. Burger, *Immunobiology, 168*: 453 (1984).
35. Y. Ina, Y. Koide, Y. Fujishima, T. Hori, H. Inoko, A. Ando, K. Tsuji, and T. O. Yoshida, in *HLA IN ASIA-OCEANIA 1986* (M. Aizawa, ed.), Hokkaido University Press, Sapporo, 1986, p. 898.
36. H. Hidaka, Y. Sasaki, T. Tanaka, T. Endo, S. Ohno, Y. Fujii, and T. Nagata, *Proc. Natl. Acad. Sci. USA, 78*: 4354 (1981).
37. H. Hidaka, M. Inagaki, S. Kawamoto, and Y. Sasaki, *Biochemistry, 23*: 5036 (1984).
38. T. Tanaka, T. Ohmura, T. Yamamoto, and H. Hidaka, *Mol. Pharmacol., 22*: 408 (1982).
39. Y. Nishizuka, *Nature, 308*: 693 (1984).
40. J. W. Putney and C. P. Branchi, *J. Pharmacol. Exp. Ther., 189*: 202 (1974).
41. D. M. Salmon and T. W. Honeyman, *Nature, 284*: 344 (1980).
42. E. Unanue, *Ann. Rev. Immunol., 2*: 395 (1984).
43. P. Cresswell, *Proc. Natl. Acad. Sci. USA, 82*: 8188 (1985).

44. M. E. Dorf, in *The Role of Major Histocompatibility Complex in Immunobiology* (M. E. Dorf, ed.), Gerland STPM Press, New York, 1982, p. 221.
45. Y. Koide, F. Awashima, T. O. Yoshida, T. Takenouchi, A. Wakisaka, J. Moriuchi, and M. Aizawa, *J. Immunol., 129*: 106 (1982).
46. Y. Koide and T. O. Yoshida, *Human Immunol., 10*: 203 (1984).
47. T. Nakatsuji, H. Inoko, A. Ando, T. Sato, Y. Koide, T. Tadakuma, T. O. Yoshida, and K. Tsuji, *Immunogenetics, 25*: 1 (1987).
48. E. Qvigstad and E. Thorsby, *Scand. J. Immunol., 18*: 299 (1983).
49. E. Qvigstad, T. Moen, and E. Thorsby, *Immunogenetics, 19*: 455 (1984).
50. G. Corte, A. Moretta, M. E. Cosulich, D. Ramarli, and A. Bargellesi, *J. Exp. Med., 156*: 1539 (1982).
51. H. Festenstein, L. Fainboim, D. Jaraquemada, and C. Navarrete, in *HLA Class II Antigens* (B. G. Solheim, E. Møller, and S. Ferrone, eds.), Springer-Verlag, Berlin, New York, Tokyo, 1986, p. 314.
52. J. R. Lamb and M. Feldman, *Nature, 308*: 72 (1984).
53. N. Ishii, Z. A. Nagy, and J. Klein, *J. Exp. Med., 156*: 622 (1982).
54. D. H. Germain, J. D. Ashwell, R. I. Lechler, D. H. Margulies, K. M. Nickerson, G. Suzuki, and J. Y. L. Tou, *Proc. Natl. Acad. Sci. USA, 82*: 2940 (1985).
55. C. Auffray, J. W. Lillie, D. Arnot, D. Grossberger, D. Kappes, and J. L. Strominger, *Nature, 308*: 327 (1984).

4

Cell-Surface Differentiation Antigens Expressed on Thymocytes and T Cells of the Mouse

BONNIE J. MATHIESON
Division of Cancer Treatment, National Cancer Institute–Frederick Cancer Research Center, Frederick, Maryland

SUSAN O. SHARROW
Immunology Branch, National Cancer Institute, National Institutes of Health, Bethesda, Maryland

I. INTRODUCTION

A series of more or less discrete steps are apparent in the differentiation of T cells from uncommitted bone marrow precursors to functionally mature and activated T cells. These stages can be recognized at the cell surface of differentiating thymocytes or T cells by unique patterns or displays of cell-surface markers. We have approached this review by addressing the following questions.

1. What antigenic markers are known to be selectively expressed on thymocytes and/or T cells at some stage in their differentiation? i.e., What antigens can be used to distinguish T cells from other types of lymphoid or hemopoietic cells?
2. What markers are available that identify subsets of thymocytes and T cells? And how are the subsets distinct? Do the markers identify different activation, functional, or developmental stages in the T-cell pathways? i.e., What markers permit us to distinguish some thymocytes or T cells from others?
3. Do the markers have any function themselves? Are they receptors, adhesion molecules, or components of complex receptors? What biochemical characteristics have been defined for the antigens?
4. And finally because genetics has been one of the most useful aspects in the the characterization of cell-surface antigens in the mouse, What is known about the genetics of these antigenic markers? i.e., How are these antigens inherited? Are they associated with a family of antigens or closely linked to other antigens? Where have genes been isolated, and what are the important molecular features?

With these questions, we have limited the scope of the review to deal only with immunogenic markers expressed at the cell surface and identifiable by serological reagents. We have particularly focused on antigens detected by monoclonal antibodies (mAbs) recognizing specific components displayed on the cell surface. At the same time we have excluded B-cell antigens and the conventional major histocompatability complex (MHC) antigens, H-2 and Ia (MHC class I antigens and class II antigens), except where there is an unusual expression relevant to T-cell differentiation. We also have not reviewed viral antigen expression. We have included a number of markers widely expressed on lymphocytes or leukocytes in addition to T cells, which may be useful in extending our knowledge of T-cell differentiation. Finally, we have indicated the homologous cluster determinant (CD) antigen group where some relationship has been established.

II. TL AND Thy-I ANTIGENS: THE ORIGINAL THYMOCYTE AND T-CELL ANTIGENS

Historically the study of T-cell differentiation antigens was established in the early 1960s by the serological characterization of two unrelated markers: TL, the thymus leukemia antigen(s) (1-3) and Thy-1 (4,5). The goals which spurred the discovery of these antigens are very similar to the rationale behind many of the current approaches defining new antigens. Boyse and colleagues were seeking tumor-specific markers that would distinguish leukemias from normal tissue (thymocytes) (3). By immunizing one mouse strain with leukemias from a second mouse strain, they were able to define the TL antigens because of the genetically restricted pattern of expression on thymocytes and thymus-derived leukemias and lymphomas. The proposed homologous CD1 antigens in humans have also been characterized using mAb generated from murine immunizations with human leukemias. See Amiot et al. (6) for a recent discussion of the epitopes of human CD1 antigens where mAb have been generated in a very similar approach.

The second approach is exemplified by the early studies of Reif and Allen (4, 5), wherein they described the strain and tissue distribution of alternative allelic forms of the Thy-1 (Θ, Theta) antigen. Reif and Allen defined Thy-1 in the course of serological analyses to detect genetically disparate histocompatibility markers using normal thymocytes as the immunogen.

Most of the mAb to cell-surface antigens that are currently available have been generated by attempts to obtain either tumor-specific or tissue-specific antibodies. Several advances have permitted more direct immunizations with isolated membrane proteins or glycoproteins instead of cell suspensions. Also, rats have been used for xenogenic immunizations with mouse antigens prior to somatic cell fusion for mAb-producing hybridomas. This has extended the list of detectable systems beyond the somewhat limited alloantigenic variant molecules recognized by inbred strains of mice.

A. TL Antigens (CD1?)

The TL antigens and regulation of their expression have continued to pose intriguing problems for many investigators. The biology, genetics, and biochemistry of the TL antigens have been extensively reviewed elsewhere (7-10), and we will only note the following points:

1. Expression on Thymocytes

TL antigens are preferentially expressed, in TL^+ strains of mice, at high levels on the surface of cortisone-sensitive, small, cortical-type thymocytes of high buoyant density (11-13). Most of these cells appear to be destined for cell death (reviewed in 14).

2. Determinants and Alleles

At least 7 serologically distinct determinants have been recognized by sera or mAb (8,15,16). These distinguish six allelic configurations. At least several of these determinants are expressed on the same molecule as determined by immunoprecipitation and blocking studies (17-20).

3. Molecular Characterization of TL Antigens

TL antigens are biochemically similar to other MHC class I antigens because of their 45-Kd [45-46] apparent molecular weight and association with β_2-microglobulin as detected by immunoprecipitation (17-22).

4. Selective Tissue Expression

The TL antigens are notably dissimilar from the H-2, MHC class I antigens in their selective tissue expression, because TL is restricted to thymocytes and T-cell leukemias or lymphomas (3,7,8,10). In addition, synthesis of the antigen appears to be restricted to proliferating populations within the thymus (23), although the small cortical-type thymocytes express the highest levels of TL antigen on the cell surface.

5. Antigenic Modulation

The TL system has provided a valuable model for antibody-induced modulation of cell-membrane components, i.e., capping and internalization of cell-surface antigen occurs in the presence of antibody or even Fab fragments of immunoglobulin (Ig) binding to the TL antigen. This process converts the cells to phenotypically negative cells (2,3,24-26). This mechanism was proposed as the escape mechanism for tumors growing in the presence of a humoral response generated by the host (1-3).

6. Quantitative Regulation of Antigen

Regulation of the quantitative cell-surface expression of TL antigens appears to be genetically complex. A number of determinants distinguished by strain distribution are expressed on all the molecules in a TL^+ mouse thymus. In addition, many if not all of the epitopes are expressed but at a much decreased level in TL^- strains (at as little as 1/1000 of the TL^+ level) (20). Variable polyadenylation of the mRNA described in this system (27) may account for this differential expression.

7. The Genes of the *T1a* Locus

The number of complete genes coding for TL structural information is not precisely known. However, the mapping and cloning of the *T1a* region genes by Steinmetz et al. (28) indicated that there are several genes closely linked to H-2D (9). At least three distinct genes of the *T1a* cluster are expressed in the TL^+ leukemia ASL1 (27), and the number of genes has been estimated as high as 13 in B10 mice, a TL^-, *T1a*^{b} strain (29), and five genes were assigned to the *T1a* region of BALB/c (*T1a*^{c}) mice (30).

B. Thy-1 Antigens

Antibodies to Thy-1 antigen in the mouse detect two alternative alleles: Thy-1.1 and Thy-1.2 (5). This antigen has proven especially useful for separation of lymphocyte subsets in the mouse because it is expressed on all T cells in the periphery, thymocytes in different stages of differentiation, as well as brain. However, Thy-1 is absent on sIg^+ B cells (31-34). This is in contrast to the rat where the same Thy-1.1 determinant is expressed on all known rat strains, but it is found on early lymphohemopoietic cells, on thymocytes, and on brain but not on T cells (35 and this volume-36). Because a much more extensive review of Thy-1 antigen and its expression will be published later this year, we will review only a few salient points, which should be noted for comparisons in other antigen systems.

1. Differential Cytotoxicity with mAb

In the Thy-1 system, a positive correlation of the ability to kill a cell with mAb plus complement (mAb + C'), relative to the total antigen expressed by the cell and/or antigen density, has been observed (34). In thymocytes this differential expression and cytotoxic susceptibility is inversely correlated with the relative maturity of the cells assessed by functional activities (12,33,34).

2. Thy-1 Expression on Non-T Leukocytes

In the mouse a number of leukocyte subsets other than T cells express Thy-1 antigen. Most notably these include natural killer (NK) cells (37-39) and specifically T-cell-depleted large granular lymphocytes (40), dendritic cells from mouse epidermal tissue (41-43), and some bone marrow cells, which have been shown to express Thy-1 antigen internally (44). Bone marrow-derived donor-type cells (41, 42) have been shown to repopulate epidermis and yield Thy-1^+ dendritic cells. Further, the Thy-1^+ cells of the epidermis may be related to NK cells (41-43).

3. Thy-1 and T-cell Activation

While it is not clear how the Thy-1 molecule is anchored in T-cell membranes in the mouse (see below), Thy-1 has been implicated in membrane signal transduction and T-cell activation (45-48). Thy-1 has been associated with the T-cell activation complex via stimulation of T cells after treatment with a rather unique mAb to a monomorphic determinant of Thy-1 or with xenogeneic Ab (46,47). More recent measuring of changes in calcium influx has shown that Thy-1 can function specifically as a signal transduction molecule in T lymphocytes and B lymphocytes transfected with the Thy-1 gene (48). Thy-1 cannot be a universal signal transduction molecule for T cells in other species, because mice are the only known species with high expression on both thymocytes and T cells.

4. The Immunochemistry and Genetics of Thy-1

The Thy-1 antigen in the mouse, as in the rat, is a 25-Kd glycoprotein whose amino acid sequence (35,49) and complementary DNA sequences (50) suggest that it has a structure similar to an isolated variable region domain of Ig (35), which puts Thy-1 into the Ig superfamily (35,49,51). However, the DNA sequence of mouse Thy-1 (50) initially suggested that there were an additional 31 amino acids at the carboxy-terminus in the mouse. Recently, it has been shown that the rat Thy-1 has a glycophospholipid tail attached at the end of the protein molecule and lacks the 31 amino acids predicted from the mouse DNA sequence (52). It has been proposed that the tail functions to anchor the molecule in the membrane (49,52). It has previously been proposed that the hydrophobic amino acids for the carboxy terminus, encoded in the DNA, could function to insert the mouse protein into the membrane (50). This discrepancy may be explained by a labile mRNA or by protein processing after the total genetic sequence is transcribed or translated. Alternatively, this molecular/biochemical difference may reflect the variable tissue distribution seen between the two species, since rat (and human) Thy-1 is not expressed on peripheral T cells but is restricted to brain and thymus (35,36).

III. LY-1, LY-2/3, LY-4: THE BASIC SUBSET ANTIGENS

A. An Introduction to the Ly Antigens

There are now nearly 50 Ly (lymphocyte) antigens which have been described in allogeneic systems and/or with mAb. There are currently 32 antigens designated Ly-1 to Ly-32, and an additional series of Lyb-2 to Lyb-8, where the antigens are so designated because of their primary, if not exclusive, expression on B cells. In addition, there are a series of antigens with miscellaneous names, such as PC-1, Thy-2, Lna, T_{su}, T_{ind}, and T_{thy}. We will use the recently proposed nomenclature for discussion of the various serologically defined Ly antigens expressed on T cells (53). In particular, we will delete the "t" in the formerly proposed Lyt-2/3 usage, and Ly-1 has already reverted from the earlier Lyt-1 designation (54) (see below). We will also use Ly-4 when referring to the formerly designated L3T4 to avoid confusion with Ly-3 and to bring this antigen into alignment with the homologous CD4 group of human leukocyte antigens.

The early characterization of the Ly antigens has been thoroughly reviewed in several publications. In particular, see Schlesinger (55), McKenzie and Potter (56), Old and Stockert (7), and Hogarth and McKenzie (57). The expression of various markers on thymocyte subsets in particular has been reviewed in Scollay and Shortman (58) and Mathieson and Fowlkes (14). And more recently Stutman (59) and Sprent et al. (60) have reviewed the expression of some of the more commonly used markers on subsets of T cells in relation to their maturity and function.

Ly-1, Ly-2/3, and Ly-4 have been the most useful systems in the mouse for distinguishing subsets within both thymocytes and peripheral T lymphocytes. Ly-1 and Ly-2, initially described as Ly-A and Ly-B, were the first alloantigens which appeared to subset mouse T lymphocytes from spleen and lymph node (61). Ly-3 (Ly-C) was later described as an additional antigen with cell-surface expression characteristics similar to Ly-2 (62). Ly-4 (L3T4) was described only much later in the mouse (63, see below), and this has led to a clarification of some of the controversial data generated earlier with serum Ab + C' lysis.

While MHC restriction is the major functional distinction which appears to divide T cells with a similar phenotype, this aspect of functional differentiation has not yet been absolutely correlated with any surface antigen. It was initially claimed that Ly-1 and Ly-2 distinguished separate populations of cells on the basis of C'-mediated depletion of helper and cytolytic activity (64-66). In addition, these two subsets and activities were initially claimed to be correlated with MHC class restriction (66). Thus Ly-1$^+$ cells were supposed to be Ia-restricted helpers, and Ly-2$^+$ cells were supposed to be H-2 K/D restricted cytolytic T lymphocyte (CTL). With further experimentation it was noted that Ly-2 was also expressed on T-cell suppressors as well as cytotoxic cells (67,68). Other investigators raised questions about the distinction of the subsets on the basis of Ly-1$^+$: helpers and Ly-2/3$^+$: cytotoxic cells because Ly-1 was clearly found on a number of cytolytic cells as well as CTL precursors (69-73). In addition, using the same source of antisera and testing on congenic strains of mice, we demonstrated by quantitative flow cytometry analysis (FCA) of immunofluorescence (IF) that all thymocytes, including "mature" cortisone resistant thymocytes, expressed Ly-1 (74). More importantly, in contrast to the data from C-dependent lysis (64,65), the "mature" cells expressed higher levels of Ly-1 by IF than the majority of thymocytes (74). This was subsequently confirmed by our group and others using mAb on various thymocyte subpopulations (75-76). With two-color IF, this subset distinction was further called into question for peripheral T cells (77). The subsequent work of Swain and colleagues (78,79) clearly demonstrated that Ly phenotype was more highly correlated with MHC restriction than with function, i.e., Ly-1$^+$ (later characterized as Ly-4$^+$, 80) helper cells were Ia/MHC class II-restricted but H-2K, D/ MHC class I-restricted helper cells were Ly-1$^+$, Ly-2$^+$.

Each of these antigen systems will be discussed in more detail with reference to their cellular expression, biochemistry, and genetics. We will also draw attention to areas where mAbs have been particularly useful to study or clarify the function of cell subsets.

B. Ly-1 Antigen (CD5)

Ly-1 has also been called Ly-A (61) and Lyt-1 (54). As indicated above, antibody to Ly-1 has been used extensively because of its somewhat selective ability to facilitate lysis of the subset now recognized as Ly-4$^+$ (L3T4$^+$) cells (62,80). In addition, because of its differential expression on thymocytes, the lymphocyte-specific Ly-1 antigen has continued to be useful for identification and isolation of a subpopulation of precursor thymocytes (14,81-83).

1. Characterization of Ly-1 Antigen

Ly-1 was one of the first cell-surface antigens recognized in two allelic forms by alloantisera (61). The initial report indicated that Ly-1 was expressed in a genetically controlled manner on most thymocytes, i.e., Ly-1 of donor-type was detected on bone marrow-derived thymocytes in irradiated hosts. Further extensive work characterizing this antigen during differentiation has been made possible by congenic mice for the Ly-1, 2, and 3 antigens produced by Boyse and colleagues (see Ref. 84).

Ly-1 has been characterized as a 67-Kd [65-70 Kd] molecule with a variable extent of glycosylation (85,86), which can also be seen on a number of other antigens.

2. Cellular Distribution of Ly-1 on Cells of the T-cell Lineage

As indicated above, lytic studies with serum Ab + C' suggested that Ly-1 was expressed only on "immature" cortical thymocytes and helper T cells and not on cytotoxic T cells (64-66). Although this latter point was rapidly shown to be a questionable conclusion (69-73,87,88), this concept remained firmly established in the literature for some time. Once quantitative techniques that depended only on Ab binding were applied to subset phenotyping studies, it became apparent that Ly-1 was a pan-T-cell antigen (74-77). It is still not apparent why anti-Ly-1 + C' fails to lyse all T cells, because Ly-1 is expressed on *both* Ly-2$^+$ and Ly-4$^+$ subsets at much higher levels than on most cortical-type thymocytes, which are easily lysed with anti-Ly-1 + C'. However, it has been noted that Ly-2$^+$ T cells express slightly less Ly-1 than Ly-2$^-$ (Ly-4$^+$) T cells (77). Finally, there is weak expression of Ly-1 on even precursor thymocytes detected as dull Ly-1 IF by FCA (81-83) (i.e., dLy-1 cells).

Ly-1 has also been described on some natural killer (NK) cells (39), although this antigenic expression has not been more precisely characterized. There is some question whether contaminating T cells with broad cytotoxic activity account for this antigenic expression, or whether only a subset of NK cells expresses Ly-1.

3. Expression of Ly-1 on B Cells

Using mAb, Ly-1 expression was subsequently demonstrated as a glycoprotein on some B-cell lymphomas in culture (89). This antigenic expression was similar in molecular weight to the antigen seen on T cells, but after enzymatic digestion its reexpression could be detected. Other studies demonstrated Ly-1 on a subset of normal B cells and B cells from autoimmune mice (90). These data were repeated and extended further to demonstrate the absence of Ly-1^+ B cells in CBA/N mice with limited B-cell responses (91). Subsequently "normal" lymphoblastoid cell lines (92) and a number of rather unique B-cell tumor lines, derived either from virus-infected mice or from spontaneous lymphomas in a congenic strain of mice carrying a murine leukemia virus genome, were shown to express Ly-1 (93). These data were consistent with parallel studies in man, which demonstrated that the CD5 antigen (T65) was expressed on most B-cell, chronic lymphocytic leukemias (94).

4. The Effects of Antibody in Vivo and in Vitro

Administration of large amounts of anti-Ly-1 IgG in vivo has produced profound immunosuppressive effects which appeared to be relatively striking against helper T-cell populations, partially effective against cytotoxic T cells, and did not affect LPS-responsive B cells (95). However it is not clear that one would expect this subpopulation of B cells to be affected by such in vivo treatment. Thus Ly-1 is truly a pan-T-cell antigen, but it is also expressed on some B-cell subsets representing either different lineages or different stages of differentiation.

Using mAb to Ly-1, it was demonstrated that the antibody in certain conditions could deliver an inductive signal to T cells (96). More recently, binding of anti-Ly-1 to T cells has been demonstrated to result in the stimulation of IL-2 production (97,98). The antibody presumably mimics a ligand interaction, as yet undefined, which leads to the stimulatory response by T cells.

These contrasting results in vivo and in vitro probably reflect the ability of a mouse to clear antibody-coated cells by several mechanisms before the stimulatory effects observed in vitro are produced.

5. Genetics of Ly-1

There are a number of Ly antigens which are associated with other antigens in genetic clusters. Ly-1 is one of these, and its linkage on chromosome 19 and very close association of expression of Ly-10 in congenic B6-*Ly-1*^{a} mice (99 and see below) is the first non-MHC-associated antigen cluster that we encounter in this review.

It has been suggested that a highly conserved peptide found in the N-terminal domain of class I and class II MHC α chains might be the recognition interaction site for Ly-2 and Ly-4 molecules (144). In exploring this possibility, Golding et al. (145) have recently shown that anti-IA^k-specific cytotoxic T cells kill transfected L cells expressing a chimeric class I/class II molecule composed of the N-terminal domain of IA^k β chain linked to the membrane domains of H-2D^d. In addition, this killing is blocked by anti-Ly-4, thus demonstrating that the rest of the IA antigen domains need not be present for IA^k-specific cytolysis (145).

3. In Vivo Effects of Treatment with Anti-Ly-4

In vivo treatment with mAb to Ly-4 leads to a rapid deletion of Ly-41 cells from the blood, spleen, and lymph nodes (146). It also produces a profound suppressive effect on the immune response. Treatment of mice with rat mAb to Ly-4 not only fails to elicit a humoral response to itself (147,148), but it also blocks humoral immunity to other antigens that are administered concomitantly (146,149). And if mAb is administered at the same time as a second antigenic mAb, anti-Ly-4 can even induce tolerance to the second mAb (150). This has raised extensive possibities for new strategies with xenogeneic mAb therapy.

4. Biochemistry and Molecular Biology of Ly-4

The early description of Ly-4 indicated that the antigen detected on thymocytes or T-cell clones was about 52 Kd (63), and thus equivalent to the homologous antigens from both rat and human cells. In this determination it was necessary to chemically modify the amino acids of the protein to facilitate labeling with radiolabeled iodine.

The genetic sequence of Ly-4 has also been described (151). Like Ly-2 the gene product is a member of the Ig supergene family (151,152) with a leader sequence, exons for the extracellular domains which contain cysteines for disulfide bonding, a transmembrane sequence, and an intracytoplasmic sequence (151). However unlike the Ly-2 molecule, there appear to be four similar extracellular protein regions that are homologous with the Ig-variable domain (151). These additional components may account for the more complex functional aspects described above.

IV. LY-5: THE LEUKOCYTE COMMON ANTIGENS (LCA), MAC-1, LYMPHOCYTE FUNCTION-ASSOCIATED ANTIGEN (LFA-1), AND LY-15

For discussion purposes, we have grouped these high molecular weight antigens together because they share antigenic determinants (Ly-5 and LCA) and/or polypeptide chains (Mac-1, LFA-1, and Ly-15). Also, historically these markers were studied together, although it is now clear that the Ly-5/LCA antigens are biochemically and genetically distinct from Mac-1 and LFA-1.

A. The *Ly-5* Allelic System

The Ly-5 allelic antigens have been detected because of the high levels of expression of the LCA molecules on several different leukocyte populations. This allelic system permits the further characterization of the antigen expression on subsets differentiating in vivo after adoptive transfers of bone marrow (or other leukocyte populations) into irradiated hosts.

1. Cellular Distribution of Ly-5 Expression

Ly-5 was originally reported as a T-cell-specific antigen (153). Because of the selective cytotoxicity seen on T cells with antisera, it was once proposed that this antigen be called Lyt-4 (54). This nomenclature was never really adopted because it was rapidly determined that NK cells (154) and many other types of leukocyte populations, including different functional T-cell populations and yolk sac cells, expressed this antigen (155-158). It is now known that all leukocytes and many of their immediate progenitors, but not erythrocytes, express Ly-5 in one of several discrete molecular forms.

2. Use of The Allelic System

Mice congenic with C57BL/6 (B6) for this antigen were developed by Dr. E. A. Boyse and colleagues and their use was first reported in the characterization of the biochemistry and cell-surface expression of Ly-5 (156,159). Because a high level of expression of Ly-5 can be detected by FCA of IF on nearly all hemopoietic cells, the examination of the progeny of precursor cells transferred into congenic recipients has been greatly facilitated (83). Thymocytes, splenic lymphocytes, macrophages, and NK cells can be obtained in appropriate combinations and examined for developmental kinetics with a coordinate transfer (Mathieson, Mason, and Overton, unpublished observations).

3. Molecular Characterization of the Allelic Difference

The allelic difference in Ly-5 has been characterized by immunoprecipitation of the cell-membrane protein antigens. These studies have demonstrated that at least three molecular species are precipitated by the antibodies to the two different alleles (159-163). These studies have reported significant structural differences in the molecules where different isoforms were detected in the tissues examined: 195-200 Kd on thymocytes; 200-210 Kd on T cells; and 220 Kd on B cells (159-163). The nonglycosylated forms are 160 Kd and 190 Kd and closely related by two-dimensional peptide mapping (163). Finally, the Ly-5/LCA molecules represent transmembrane proteins which are phosphorylated at serine residues (164).

4. The Genetics of Ly-5 and a Change of Allelic Designation

The *Ly-5* locus is located on chromosome 1 in the mouse (see 165) with three alleles encoding the polymorphic specificities (153,165). *Ly-5* is linked centromeric to the *Ly-9* locus (166) as discussed below.

The allelic names for the loci which govern the expression of this antigen have recently been reversed to put the Ly-5 antigen nomenclature into the conventional format for all Ly antigens (53). Thus the locus expressed in B6 mice is designated as the *Ly-5^b* locus and its antigen is denoted by Ly-5.2. SJL/J mice and the B6 congenic strain, previously known as B6-Ly-5.2, which obtained its *Ly-5* genes from SJL, will henceforth be known as *Ly-5^a* mice which express Ly-5.1 antigens. Thus in this new nomenclature, nearly all mouse strains express Ly-5.2, from the *Ly-5^b* allele, which is seen on leukocytes of B6 mice.

Recently the cDNA for Ly-5 has been cloned and sequenced (165,167). The Ly-5 polymorphism seen at the serological level extends to the DNA to yield a restriction fragment length polymorphism (RFLP) between B6 (*Ly-5^b*) and the B6-*Ly-5^a* congenic or STS mice (165) (note the allele names have been reversed here.) Further RFLP analysis has detected a third allele in ST/bJ mice now denoted as *Ly-5^c* (165). Finally, sequencing of the gene for *Ly-5* has shown that isoforms of Ly-5 seen on different cell types are the result of differential processing of the transcripts of a single gene rather than multiple *Ly-5* genes (167).

B. T200-B220 and Lineage-Restricted LCA

Because they have been directly compared, it is now apparent that the allelic Ly-5 determinants are expressed on the members of the family of antigens which comprise the LCA group (160-162). The T200 molecule and its related isoforms, which are expressed on various cell types, have been extensively characterized.

The molecular variation in this group of antigens was described first with xenogeneic antisera as a difference between the high molecular weight proteins of B and T cells (168,169). This work and early work with mAb (170-173) was conducted in parallel with studies in the rat by A. F. Williams and colleagues, which are discussed elsewhere in this volume.

Other laboratories have further characterized this family of antigens by immunoprecipitation with anti-B-cell mAb which recognize the B220 molecule in the mouse (174-176). Further characterization has yielded an selected group of anti-B220 mAb which also recognize a high molecular weight antigen on Ly-2$^+$ T cells (176-180). The antigens that this type of antibody recognizes are referred to as lineage-restricted LCA.

1. T200

T200 is so named because it is expressed on T cells, thymocytes, and T-cell leukemias (160-162,168-173). It has been noted in several of these studies that the LCA molecules which are expressed on thymocytes and T cells are heterogenous. In particular, a lineage-restricted mAb has been described which detects a T200 determinant selectively expressed on proliferating T cells (173). This distinction has not been seen with the Ly-5 allelic reagents.

2. B220

This isoform has been detected by several mAb which recognize LCA (indicated above) but also by lineage-restricted mAb which detect only the B220 molecule (174-177). In addition, a group of mAb have been characterized which detect a determinant expressed on Ly-2$^+$ T cells in addition to B cells (176-180). It is apparent from some of these studies that the normal expression of this antigen on T cells is much lower than on B cells (178-180). However lymph node cells from *lpr/lpr* mice with lymphoproliferative disease may have increased levels of this antigen on their abnormal cells (180-182).

C. Mac-1, LFA-1, and Ly-15 Antigens

These antigens have been grouped together because Mac-1 and LFA share a polypeptide chain. Also, there is now evidence that the mAb to Ly-15.2 recognizes a polymorphic site on the molecule known as LFA-1 (183).

1. LFA-1 and Mac-1

These high molecular weight antigens have been identified in several species. The most important feature of these antigens is that they are heterodimers that apparently share a common 95-Kd β chain. This β chain associates with different higher molecular weight α chains detected by several mAb (173,183-188).

The LFA-1 antigen is expressed at high levels on mature, functional T cells and was originally defined by the ability of mAb to this antigen to block CTL function (184,185). In contrast, Mac-1 is an antigen preferentially expressed on macrophages and myelocytic cells (186,188). The LFA-1 antigen has a 180-Kd α chain, whereas the α chain of Mac-1 is only 170 Kd (173,188,189).

From mRNA translation studies, it is apparent that the difference in chain length of the α subunits of LFA-1 and Mac-1 is reflected in differences in the polypeptide backbone. The backbones are 130 Kd for Mac-1 and 140 Kd for LFA-1 before extensive glycosylation to the final high molecular weight cell-surface glycoproteins (190).

The most important feature of these molecules is that they appear to be integral parts of the membrane reflecting the functional nature of the cells. It has recently been shown that anti-LFA-1 mAb binding to the cell surface can mimic the function of a B-cell growth-stimulating factor, BSF-1 (191), whereas it has previously been established that Mac-1 is the receptor for the C3bi complement component in both mouse and man (188,192). Finally, in humans, the genetic deficiency of these high molecular weight proteins can produce a life-threatening disease state (193). In patients with monocytic cells lacking homologous Mac-1 and LFA-1 antigens (as well as a third, p150/95, glycoprotein complex), the cells are incapable of effectively clearing foreign bacterial or viral antigens (see Ref. 193).

2. Ly-15

The *Ly-15* locus had previously been characterized as a locus with two alleles coding for membrane antigens Ly-15.1 and Ly-15.2, with the latter specificity identified by a mAb (194). The initial serological characterization with this mAb had indicated that Ly-15 antigen was detected on thymocytes and all T and B cells. But no genetic map or function had been ascribed to this antigen. More recent studies (183,195) indicate that Ly-15 analyzed in parallel with LFA-1 shows an identical tissue distribution, being present on all thymocytes, lymphocytes, and neutrophils (182). Furthermore, these two cell-surface markers co-precipitate, and the LFA α and β chains are identical to the α and β chains of Ly-15 (183). Thus the Ly-15.2 antigen appears to be a polymorphism of the LFA-1 α chain. However the polymorphic determinant may be formed by the association of the LFA-1 α chain and the shared β chain.

V. THE CLUSTER OF ACTIVATION AND NONLYMPHOID ANTIGENS

The *Ly-6* locus has a surprising number of determinants which have been defined by mAb. This probably reflects the fact that many investigators have attempted to obtain mAb against structures which are expressed on functionally activated cells. This approach might be expected to yield mAb to molecules associated with growth receptors, signal transduction molecules, and antigen receptors—all of which might be expressed at higher levels on activated cells. Closely linked to the *Ly-6* locus are several other markers which are expressed on kidney and other nonlymphoid tissues (see Ref. 196).

A. Ly-6, Ala-1, "Old" Ly-8, and One Ly-11

Ly-6 antigens are a cluster of genetically linked, lymphocyte-associated alloantigens (reviewed in 53,56,197,198). One of the first characterizations of an antigen in this cluster indicated that an activated lymphocyte antigen (Ala-1) was expressed on both B and T lymphoblasts but not on lectin-activated thymocytes (199). Other characterizations with anti-Ly-6 sera and later mAb led to either a broader or to a more confined cellular expression depending on the serological subtype that was examined. The most consistent finding is that Ly-6 antigen expression delineates functional activated lymphocytes by its presence or increased expression on these cells.

Because of similar characteristics of "old" Ly-8 antigen (200) with the antigens detected by mAb for Ly-6, this antigen has been assimilated into the Ly-6 grouping (53,197,198). It also appears that one of the Ly-11 antigens, Ly-11.2 (201), still defined only by antisera should be placed in this cluster. Although this Ly-11 antigen is only poorly defined by the serological characteristics we have reviewed, it has both a similar strain distribution and a comparable pattern of tissue expression to that of Ly-6.

1. Cellular Characterization of the Ly-6 Antigens

There are currently five proposed groupings of mAb to Ly-6, indicated by the designations Ly-6A to Ly-6E (197,198). These groupings are divided by the characteristics of cellular and tissue distribution of the antigen. These range from selective expression on bone marrow and granulocytes (e.g., Ly-6B, Gm-2.2) (202) to expression on nearly all lymphocytes and granulocytes (Ly-6C, H9/95) (53, 197). An additional granulocyte marker, initially reported as MG-1 (203), should also be placed in the Ly-6B group (Shen and Mathieson, unpublished data). Quantitative differences in cellular expression result in bimodal or trimodal histogram peaks on FCA (204). These patterns indicate a further complexity in the expression of this antigen on subsets of normal cells.

2. Variable Characteristics of the Molecules of the *Ly-6* Locus

The molecular characterization has been variable between laboratories and even within laboratories, depending on the antigenic cluster grouping examined (see Refs. 56,198). Molecules ranging from 12-18 Kd, 34-39 Kd, and 78 Kd have been reported (56,198,202,205,206). Palfre et al. (198) have suggested that some of the Ly-6 antigen subgroups may be reduced, if one takes into account the overlapping molecular characterization seen with electrophoretic mobility of Ly-6 antigen in gels containing octylglucoside. Additional comparative FCA studies, such as those reported by Dumont et al. (204), may further resolve some of the arbitrary differences related to typing by Ab + C' cytotoxicity methodology with mAb of different isotype.

It is also not clear whether the differences in molecular weight seen for this antigen reflect differences in the protein backbone molecules or differences in glycosylation. Other variation may be due to variable mRNA transcription or splicing of gene products in this region which has recently been demonstrated for Ly-5 and Ly-2 molecules (see discussions above). Finally, although less interesting, the differences may occasionally reflect the differing affinities of the mAb used and different analytical tests applied in different laboratories.

3. Genetics of *Ly-6*

Although these Ly-6 antigens analyzed in recombinant inbred (RI) mice cluster to the same genetic region, the map assignment is still unclear. The heterogeneity may reflect a secondary level of antigen expression such as glycosylation or other modifications of proteins by products of unlinked loci. [Note that Ly-27.2 and Ly-28.2 of Hogarth et al. (207) have been reassigned to the Ly-6D.2 and Ly-6C.2 clusters, respectively (53).]

In summary, *Ly-6* is still one of the more complex genetic loci. Despite the large number of mAb, the complexity has not been satisfactorily resolved. However, this may be one of the most interesting antigen systems, because, as noted by others (56), the expression of Ly-6 on T cells appears to be higher or more easily detected on activated, functional T cells, and this appears to be one of the hallmarks of the Ly-6 locus.

B. ThB

ThB antigen has been described both by conventional antisera and by mAb (208-210). This antigen has consistently been associated with the Ly-6 locus, although the pattern of reactivity is different (210). Some thymocytes and most B cells express this antigen, but no peripheral T cells do (208-210). There appears to be an inverse relationship with Ly-6 expression, where T cells are more strongly positive. An inverse quantitative difference in the amount of two cell-surface differentiation antigens, which are genetically linked, has been noted above for TL and H-2, as well as for Ly-1 and Ly-10 or TL and Qa (see below).

The variable detection of this antigen as well as Ly-6 antigens has been discussed by Eckert et al. (210), where nearly all of the mAb against the ThB were an IgG_3 isotype which may be preferentially generated against carbohydrate determinants. The implication is that ThB may be a carbohydrate antigen on several different protein backbones.

VI. Ly-9 (T100, Lgp100): THE COMMON LYMPHOCYTE ANTIGEN

Ly-9 is a pan-lymphocyte or common lymphocyte antigen expressed as one of two allelic forms: Ly-9.1 and Ly-9.2 (211-213). Both of the known alleles are expressed in commonly used mouse strains, e.g., *Ly-9^a^* in BALB/c mice and *Ly-9^b^* in B6 mice. Therefore *Ly-9* phenotypic analysis has proved useful in a number of studies involving cell transfers of different genetic backgrounds (see Refs. 211,214,215). In particular, the ability to monitor both T cells and B cells in peripheral lymphoid organs as well as thymocytes presented us with a very useful model to study the development of MHC antigen restriction and thymocyte differentiation (215).

A. The Expression of Ly-9 on Different Lymphocytes

Ly-9 (T100, Lgp 100) was independently characterized in several different laboratories (211-213,216). In two cases, the antigen was detected as a contaminant in anti-Ly sera (211,216). In other studies, Ly-9-specific mAb were obtained from xenogeneic immunization (212) or from immunization with genetically disparate lymphocytes (213).

We first detected anti-Ly-9 antibodies as contaminants in other Ly antisera because the antisera produced weak but homogeneous IF staining by FCA on all thymocytes of a strain negative for the allelic form of the Ly-2,3 antigen being tested. Once the strain distribution was determined, appropriate immunizations yielded highly specific antisera (211).

FCA demonstrated that anti-Ly-9 bound to all of the lymphoid subsets in different lymphoid tissues and blood (211,212). Functional analyses (of T helper and suppressor cells, and antigen-primed B cells) indicated that the anti-Ly-9 + C' was highly effective at cytotoxic elimination of functional lymphocyte populations. Furthermore, only lymphoid cells and not myelomonocytic cells or their precursors (Mathieson, unpublished data) in the bone marrow were Ly-9$^+$ with either xenogeneic mAb or anti-Ly-9 sera (211,212). Thus Ly-9 antigen is a pan-lymphocyte, but not pan-leukocyte, antigen like Ly-5.

Only lymphoid tissues appeared to be Ly-9$^+$, and no nonlymphoid tissues absorbed Ly-9 serum antibodies. There were several minor differences observed with solid tissue (kidney and liver) absorptions between the Ly-9.2 mAb and the serum reagents for the same antigen which have never been resolved (211, 213). However the xenogeneic Lgp 100 mAb appeared to have the same strain and tissue distribution as anti-Ly-9.1 serum (211,212).

B. Biochemical Characterization of Ly-9

The Ly-9 molecule was first reported as a T100 protein because it immunoprecipitated a 100-Kd glycoprotein from thymocytes and T-cell lymphomas (216). With the subsequent use of the Lgp 100 mAb which detected the Ly-9.1 antigen, other studies indicated that Lgp 100 was a glycosylated monomeric protein in the surface membrane of different types of lymphocytes (212).

C. *Ly-9* Linkage with *Ly-17* and Other Chromosome 1 Antigen Genes

Like *Ly-5*, the locus for *Ly-9* is found on chromosome 1. One of the most important features of this antigenic system is its relatively close linkage to a number of other antigens on chromosome 1 of the mouse. This includes both antigens expressed selectively on T cells or on B cells, such as Ly-17 (217) (discussed below Section VIII.C) and viral-associated lymphocyte antigens (218). Ly-9 has also been useful as a tool for genetic studies of closely linked immune response markers (219).

VII. SUBSETS WITHIN SUBSETS

A number of serological reagents have been reported to selectively subset populations of Ly-2$^+$ (Ly-4$^-$) or Ly-4$^+$ (Ly-2$^-$), indicated in earlier literature as Ly-1$^+$ cells. For example, some of these studies with (220,221) xenogeneic reagents have indicated that it is possible to distinguish T cytotoxic precursors in the thymus from the majority of "mature" Ly-2⁺ cells and peripheral CTL. Comparable mAb reagents have not yet been described in the literature. However, both Ly-m22 and Ly-24 (Pgp-1, 9F3) reagents have been shown to distinguish subsets of cells within the Ly-2⁺ subset (222,223). In addition, anti IL-2-R antibodies distinguish subsets within the immature thymocytes and Ly-4⁺ cells (see Section VIII). A third antigen (or group of antigens), called Heat Stable Antigens (HSA), appears to be recognized by a number of mAb which delineate subsets of thymocytes and B cells (discussed below). Finally, several laboratories have used anti-Ia or anti-Qa-1 to identify subsets of cells in immune regulatory pathways. Because positive selections of cells with these reagents have either not been successful and/or not reported, these are mentioned only briefly in the discussions below.

A. Ly-22

Ly-22 (originally called Ly-m22) is defined by a mAb which detects cell-surface expression limited to T cells (224). The Ly-22 antigen was initially described as an antigen primarily expressed on lymph node and spleen cells, but detectable in small quantites on bone marrow and thymus (224). By complement lysis the mAb to this antigen was subsequently characterized as a highly selective reagent against suppressor T cells but not reactive with helper or cytotoxic T cells (222).

The genetic linkage of *Ly-22* to *M1s* and other markers on chromosome 1 (222,224) makes it unlikely that it is identical to putative anti-"IJ" reagents previously reported by several investigators to be effective against suppressor T cells (see Section XI.C).

B. Ly-24 (Pgp-1, 9F3)

It is now apparent that several antibodies have been detected which recognize this antigen. The first of these reagents were described as mAb that detected allelic forms of the antigen on leucocytes, particularly granulocytes and macrophages (225,226). These first reports referred to the antigen as Pgp-1, to denote phagocytic glycoprotein.

In other studies the 9F3 marker was described, and it was shown to be expressed on a subset of T cells and at high levels on the lymph nodes of *1pr/1pr* mice (223). This finding was confirmed and extended in other mice with different lymphoproliferative disease (228). Furthermore, it was shown that this antigen was selectively expressed on Ly2⁺ T cells and this led to the conclusion that the Ly-2⁺ cells are abnormal in the *1pr/1pr* mice (223). In studies analyzing immature thymocytes, it has been shown that this antigen is expressed on the cells of a thymus-homing progenitor (229,230).

Anti-Pgp-1 reagents were shown to identify a 90-95-Kd protein (225-227). Additional biochemical studies have demonstrated that the different xenogeneic antibodies detect either framework or allelic determinants on the same glycoprotein (223,226). Studies that further characterized the 9F3 mAb indicated that it also detected a framework determinant on the Ly-24/Pgp-1 molecules (228).

Using anti-Ly-24 (Pgp-1) and the mAb to β_2-microglobulin ("old" Ly-m11), Ly-24 was shown to be genetically linked to β_2-microglobulin (226). These data were consistent with the data from others that showed that the gene order on chromosome 4 was *Hc* . . . *pgp* . . . $\beta_2 m$ . . . *a* (250).

C. Heat-stable Antigen (HSA)

The first mAb to HSA were reported by Springer et al. (171). That work described several mAb which bound antigens stable to glutaraldehyde fixation and autoclaving at 120°C for 15 min, suggesting a carbohydrate-antigenic determinant. All mAb detecting HSA bound to mouse erythrocytes (RBC). However, M1/69, one of these mAb which was selected for further study, also bound to thymocytes, but subset information was previously not provided (171).

The second antibody placed in this group, J11d, was shown to discriminate between subsets of T and B cells (231). Thymocytes were nearly all positive by mAb + C lysis but J11d was not detectable on mature, peripheral T cells. This antibody was shown to be strongly cototoxic for red blood cells (RBCs) and highly lytic for most bone marrow cells but not for the precursors yielding 7-day spleen colony-forming units (CFU-S) in lethally irradiated mice.

Differential expression of J11d on B cells at different stages of development was also reported (231). Virgin B cells were J11d$^+$, but primed memory B cells were J11d$^-$ by mAb + C' lysis. Furthermore, Ab-forming cells early in the immune response were sensitive to anti-J11d + C', but later in the response not all Ab-forming cells were sensitive. Subsequent studies by others (232) extended these observations of B-cell heterogeneity by analysis of positively selected J11d cells activated by different methods.

For purposes of our discussion, HSA became more important with the description of the differential quantitative IF (233) and differential cytolysis (234, 235) of thymocytes. By deduction from correlated IF of other thymocyte antigens, Scollay and Shortman (235) have claimed that a very similar antigen detected by the mAb B2A2 (236) is present on cells in early stages of both cortical and medullary thymic development. They have further inferred from analysis of thymus repopulation at 15 days after transfer of bone marrow treated with anti-B2A2 + C' (234) and the IF data on thymocytes (235) that two separate lineages of thymocytes exist. However, appropriate transfer experiments with positively selected cells to test this hypothesis have not been reported.

Thus it appears that HSA can be used to distinguish different stages of maturation, activation, and/or lineages, in both thymocyte and B-cell differentiation.

In addition, the failure to eliminate CFU-S at 7 days and the high cytolysis of bone marrow with Ab + C' lysis (231,236) suggests that this antigen is also expressed differentially on the macrophage/granulocyte lineage.

Biochemical characterization of the HSA antigen(s) has been hampered because the mAb are all IgMs and do not easily immunoprecipitate a distinct glycoprotein. See further comments above in this (VI) section regarding the possible carbohydrate nature of the antigen detected by the M1/69 antibody (171). Early attempts to immunoprecipitate the relevant antigen(s) with J11d failed to yield a unique band upon gel electrophoresis of the immunoprecipitate (231). However, subsequent studies have reported that the J11d antibody detects a glycoprotein of 50 Kd (237).

Finally, this group of antibodies, which detect HSA expressed on thymocytes, B cells, RBCs, and possibly granulocytes, do not detect any known allelic differences between strains of mice but recognize a species-specific antigen (171).

VIII. THE RECEPTOR ANTIGENS

In this section, we will discuss the thymocyte and T-cell-surface expression of several receptor antigens which have recently been characterized. It is apparent from the preceding discussion of Ly antigens that the function of most of the Ly antigens is still unknown. However, the receptor antigens that we have included have known functions and are expressed differentially on subsets of thymocytes and T cells.

A. The T-cell Receptor (TcR)

A number of laboratories have raised murine clone-specific, anti-idiotype (anti-Ti) or heterologous antibodies to the TcR (238-241). Studies with these reagents have identified molecules with an apparent MW of 75-85 Kd which can be reduced to demonstrate a disulfide-linked heterodimeric glycoprotein containing an acidic α chain and a neutral to slightly basic β chain, each 40-45 Kd.

Two mAb, reported to have broader reactivity to the β chain, have been useful for more extensive cell-surface studies of the TcR (242,243). The first of these mAb to the TcR, KJ16, is a rat mAb prepared by immunizing rats with a complex of anti-idiotype mAb and the mouse TcR to which is was bound (242). Although it was initially proposed that KJ16 recognized an "allotypic" determinant, it now appears that KJ16 is not a true allotype but recognizes a determinant on a family of variable regions of the TcR β chain ($V_\beta 8$) (244-246). This family is present in most but not all mouse strains (it is absent in C57BR, C57L, SJL, and SWR) (244,245). The $V_\beta 8$ family of TcR genes appears to be preferentially expressed on mouse T cells, and thus KJ16 identifies the TcR on approximately 20% of mature thymocytes and peripheral T cells, including T cells restricted by either class I or class II MHC (247).

The second mAb to the TcR, F23.1, was raised by immunizing a mouse from a strain lacking expression of the KJ16 epitope with TcR from a "positive" strain (243). F23.1, like KJ16, detects the β chain of the TcR on the surface of approximately 20% of mouse T cells, and like KJ16 it is expressed on both Ly-2$^+$ and Ly-4$^+$ cells (244,243). F23.1 apparently detects the same $V_\beta 8$ family of molecules as KJ16, because its strain distribution pattern is identical and it detects an antigen with a similar cell-surface distribution (247,248).

Use of KJ16 has permitted the visualization of the anatomical localization of TcR expression in the perinuclear cytoplasm of cortical thymocytes (249). This lends support to the notion that the β chain of the TcR is productively rearranged and first expressed normally within thymocytes, including immature intrathymic precursors (250-253). This TcR expression occurs during T-cell differentiation in the apparent absence of antigen exposure and coincident with selective differentiation events that determine the MHC restriction pattern of the mature cells (see Ref. 254 for further discussion).

In addition, use of the antibodies to the TcR has demonstrated that only Ly-2$^+$ cells can be stimulated by anti-TcR plus IL-2 (248,255), whereas accessory cells are also required for stimulation of Ly-4$^+$ cells (255). This implies that activation via the TcR may be less complex in Ly-2$^+$ cells than in Ly-4$^+$ cells.

By analogy with the CD3 system in man (see Chapter 1, this volume) and by two-dimensional gel analysis of receptor-associated proteins (256), it is now known that there are a number of other components in the murine TcR complex in addition to the α and β chains. Therefore it is expected that studies of receptor activation will profit greatly by the development of new mAb that recognize these other components of the TcR.

B. Interleukin 2 Receptor (IL-2R)

Several laboratories have reported the production of mAbs to mouse IL-2-R (257-259). All of these mAb have been shown to block T-cell proliferation and growth supported by IL-2. This inhibition of IL-2-dependent proliferation can be caused by mAb binding in the IL-2 binding site (e.g., 3C7) or by steric inhibition of mAb binding to other epitopes on the receptor molecule (e.g., 7D4, PC61) (258,259). From the studies of cell-surface binding of anti-IL-2R mAb, it has been determined that several types of cells express IL-2R depending on their state of differentiation and/or activation (257-263). These and many other studies have recently been reviewed extensively elsewhere (263).

1. Expression of IL-2-R on Thymocytes and T Cells

Using anti-IL-2R mAb it has been reported that IL-2R is expressed on activated T-cell blasts (257,259,261), a subset of immature thymocytes (137,264-269), and activated B cells (258,262). From these studies and others, it appears that the

IL-2R is expressed in higher numbers and has a higher affinity on cells which are activated by antigenic or mitogenic stimuli.

It is not clear how IL-2 and the IL-2-R function in the immature thymocyte population because studies with exogeneous IL-2 have presented conflicting data (266-269). It is possible that the cells use more than one IL-2-binding growth receptor and/or that the currently available mAb only recognize one of these receptors. This is particularly important in light of other studies that have demonstrated an antigen receptor-driven, IL-2 independent pathway for proliferation in T-cell clones (270).

It was earlier shown that when unselected T cells were grown in IL-2 or IL-2 containing supernatants, both Ly-2^+ and Ly-4^+ cells could be grown in vitro. However, it first appeared that resting T cells did not express easily detectable levels of IL-2R (257,258,260,261). Recent studies, however, have demonstrated that a subset of Ly-4^+ cells isolated from normal mice express high levels of the IL-2R detected by mAb (271).

2. Biochemical Characterization of the IL-2R

The receptor recognized by the available mAb has been reported to be a 48-62 Kd membrane protein (137,258,260). More extensive immunoprecipitation studies have demonstrated that three molecular species are co-precipitated with the mAb: 20-25 Kd, 50-60 Kd, and 100-120 Kd (258). However, it has not been determined whether all three species bear this IL-2R epitope, or whether these additional proteins simply represent other components of a receptor complex on activated cells.

3. Genetics of the Regulation of IL-2R

Recent studies have indicated that several genes in the mouse regulate the expression of IL-2R on Ly-4^+ cells (271). These studies have reported that genes on chromosome 7 and possibly also chromosome 4 may be involved in its regulation. The localization of the receptor gene is not yet defined.

C. FcγR/Ly-17 (CD16?)

There has been a xenogeneic (rat) mAb (2.4G2) available for some time to the Fc receptors for IgG (FcγR) in the mouse (272). However, the demonstration that FcγR was expressed on a small subset of T cells in mice had only been characterized by sensitive FCA (273). In separate studies, Ly-17 was described as a B-cell alloantigen (274). Further direct serological characterization of this alloantigen, with reciprocal antisera (217) and a mAb initially reported for "Ly-m20," demonstrated that Ly-17 antigen was expressed on B cells, bone marrow, and by absorption on thymocytes (217,275).

Recent studies of this receptor antigen have reported that the FcγR is expressed on a few thymocytes as well as T cells (166). Furthermore, these and other studies have demonstrated by reciprocal cross-blocking that anti-Ly-17 and 2.4G2 can at least partially cross-block cell-surface binding of each other and both appear to recognize the FcγR as shown by blocking of IgG dimer binding and by immunoprecipitation (166,276).

The assignment of the FcγR/Ly-17 to the CD16 group is somewhat arbitrary because of the tissue distribution. The xenogeneic 2.4G2 mAb was shown to bind to a trypsin-resistant FcRII (272), which is not the predominant FcR on granulocytes (i.e., CD16-like). However, like the homologous human CD16 mAb, 2.4G2 can bind, but at low levels, to purified NK cells (Mathieson, unpublished data). Finally, the molecule detected by the FcγR mAb has been characterized as a 55-60 Kd glycoprotein (166).

As discussed above (in Section VI.), the polymorphic determinant detected by anti-Ly-17 (and also by a mAb formerly called anti-Ly-m20) has been shown to map to mouse chromosome 1 (275). Furthermore, *Ly-17* is closely linked to *Ly-9* and *M1s* (217,275).

IX. THE Qa ANTIGENS

The Qa cell-surface antigens share several general properties which will be summarized here and which have been reviewed in greater detail elsewhere (8,9,277, 279,281). These antigens are primarily expressed on mature lymphocytes or leukocytes at different stages in differentiation. In this regard, the expression of Qa antigen is more similar to H-2 and is inversely related to the high level of expression of TL antigen on thymocytes (see Section II.A). Also, like H-2, Qa antigens are expressed on 40-45-Kd molecules associated with β_2-microglobulin. In addition, Qa antigens have striking DNA and protein sequence homology with other MHC class I genes and proteins and can serve as targets for cytotoxic T cells.

The genes for the Qa antigens are clustered telomeric to the H-2D,L region of the mouse chromosome 17 in the region serologically defined as the *Qa-Tla* region. Of the nearly 30 genes in this region, approximately 10 genes for expression of Qa antigens are closely linked and similar by restriction enzyme mapping and sequence homology (27-30). However the exact number of functional or expressed genes has not been determined, and this may vary between strains (27-30,278,280). In contrast to H-2, and despite the apparently large number of genes, the Qa antigens display a limited polymorphism between strains, in addition to a restricted cellular expression.

The Qa nomenclature has been complicated by genetically controlled, quantitative differences in expression, which has led to Qa-2^{+hi}, Qa-2^{+lo}, and Qa-2^{-} phenotypes (8,281) or Qa-1^{+} and Qa-1^{-} phenotypes (282). The nomenclature has been further complicated by variable tissue distribution, the different analytical tests used in different laboratories, and the variability in the affinity of serological reagents and mAb. The Qa numbers assinged to mAb, Qa-2 to Qa-11, are largely historical and are therefore somewhat arbitrary. At this time there is no definitive relationship between the specificities and the gene numbers Q1-Q10 (30).

It is particularly intriguing that there is almost a complete inverse relationship for the thymocyte/T-cell expression of the Qa antigens and the *Tla* locus antigens. As discussed above, both TL and Qa antigens appear to have MHC class I-like structures but limited polymorphism. Thus, these two types of MHC class I antigens are closely linked and produce extremely similar gene products that are expressed differentially during various stages of T-cell development.

A. Qa-1

The Qa-1 antigen was initially recognized as a lymphocyte cell-surface antigen by sera raised against antigens of the *T1a* region (283). By serological absorption experiments with cells from recombinant mice, Qa-1 expression was observed on lymph node cells, in contrast to the expected expression of TL restricted to thymocytes.

1. Expression of Qa-1 on T Cells

Because no mAb is yet available for this marker, definitive analysis of the cellular distribution is still incomplete. However, anti-Qa-1 sera has been used by several laboratories (a) to detect Qa-1 antigen on mitogen-stimulated and normal T cells (284,285) and (b) to eliminate a subset of Ly-2^- (Ly-1^+) helper T cells which appear to down regulate suppressor T cells (286,287). These data are reviewed more extensively elsewhere (8).

2. Biochemical Characterization

Immunoprecipitation of Qa-1 alloantigens has demonstrated that the antigen is similar to other MHC class I molecules with a 45-47-Kd molecular weight and association with β_2-microglobulin (288-290). In addition, it has been shown that Qa-1 differs from TL glycoprotein because of its shorter polypeptide backbone and extra sites for glycosylation (289). It has also been shown that Qa-1 expression on activated T cells is hyposialyated relative to normal, resting T cells (291).

In addition, biochemical data indicate that three alleles can be defined by immunoprecipitation and preclearing (290). These data demonstrate that anti-Qa-1.1 or anti-Qa-1.2 sera can detect molecules of two different sizes, 40 Kd and 46 Kd (with a possible third band at 69 Kd). Thus these reagents recognize the *Qa-1^a* and *Qa-1^b* genotypes. A third genotype, *Qa-1^d*, which also expresses proteins of both 40 and 46 Kd, has been described by biochemical analysis (290). T cells of the *Qa-1^d* genotype apparently express an additional 46-Kd molecule not precleared with anti-Qa-1.2 immunoprecipitation (290).

3. Qa-1 as a CTL Target

It has been shown by several investigators that anti-Qa-1-specific CTL can be generated, and these CTL are not restricted by other MHC antigens (292-295). Furthermore, the complexity observed in the serology and biochemistry of Qa-1 is reflected in the cytolysis pattern of cloned CTL, which demonstrated that there are at least four *Qa-1* genotypes (296).

Although Qa-1 is like MHC class I antigens in its ability to serve as a target antigen, response to Qa-1 antigens requires in vivo priming. Furthermore, these antigens have not been shown to restrict other nominal antigen responses (8,292-296).

4. Genetics of Qa-1 Expression

Because of the tissue distribution and the detection of Qa-1 in recombinant mice, *Qa-1* was first believed to be controlled by genes closely linked but distinct from the *Tla* genes (283). This was later modified when additional serum samples were examined, and it now appears that all Tla^a, Tla^d, and Tla^e strains are $Qa\text{-}1^a$, and only Tla^b and Tla^c are $Qa\text{-}1^b$ (8). Thus, the strain distribution analyses now indicate no separation between the *Qa-1* and *Tla* loci.

Finally, it appears that Qa-1 antigen expression is regulated such that cells from H-2D^k mice are less susceptible to lysis with anti-Qa-1 sera (282). This regulation of $Qa\text{-}1^b$ expression appears to map to a dominant gene in the region between *H-2S* and *Tla* (282).

B. The Qa-2 Family

The Qa-2 region antigens will be collectively discussed for the following reasons: (a) Although there have been multiple determinants described by sera or mAb, it is not clear how many of these determinants are expressed as shared or different molecules on T cells; (b) some of the antigenic distinctions were based on the detection on different lymphoid subsets in different strains. Because quantitative variation in Qa-2 expression is seen, qualitative differences, types as different specificities, may only reflect quantitative differences; (c) Finally, there is still no formal genetic evidence that more than one of the genes in the *Qa-2* locus controls many of the determinants. Each of these points will be discussed in more detail below

1. Serological Complexities of the Qa-2 Family of Antigens

Some of the complexity of the Qa-2 family of antigens is related to the serological reagents and how they have been tested. Secondly, additional complexity is introduced by the multiple Qa-2 structural genes and other genes which regulate expression of very similar or identical molecules. When these factors are considered, the Qa-2 through Qa-11 and the Qa/H-2 cross-reactive (CR) antigens can be divided into three basic groups of cell-surface antigens: the "Qa-2"-like group of antigens, the "Qa-6"-like group, and the Qa/H-2 CR group. Finally, molecular complexity of Qa-2 is observed in glycosylation but not in protein structure by immunoprecipitation (discussed further below). It is not known if glycosylation contributes to the serological complexities, but a secreted product shares some of the Qa determinants.

Qa-2 was first detected by antisera as an antigenic marker on lymph node cells: showing a positive phenotype on B6.K2 but a negative phenotype on B6.K1 congenic mice (297). Several mAb are now available which have been useful for other studies (281,298,299). The definition of the Qa-3 antigen depended on the failure of thymocytes from some strains of mice to absorb all of the lymph node reactivity of anti-Qa-2 sera (8,300). In addition, Qa-3 was demonstrated only on some Qa-2^+ strains and not detected on any Qa-2^- strains (300). Qa-3 primarily depends on a quantitative difference in expression and has never been genetically separated from Qa-2 expression (8).

Like Qa-3, the Qa-4,5,7, and 8 specificities were only detected on Qa-2^+ mice and were distinguished from Qa-2 either by decreased tissue reactivity or expression on fewer strains of mice. Qa-4 and Qa-5 specificities, which were defined by mAb and originally reported as T-cell antigens (301), may also belong to the Qa-2-like group of antigens. However, because they have mainly been studied on NK cells and not T and B cells, they will be discussed briefly in a separate section.

The Qa-m7 and Qa-m8 antigens were defined by using mAb to demonstrate that fewer strains of mice react with these reagents than with an anti-Qa-2 mAb (302). Since these three mAb were of different isotype, the quantitative differences observed by cytotoxicity may fail to distinguish truly new antigens. Furthermore, we have observed only limited differences with these reagents by flow cytometry (Sharrow, unpublished data). Thus we have placed these antigens into the first group of Qa-2-like specificities.

A second grouping of antigens in the Qa-2 family includes Qa-6, Qa-m9, and Qa-11 antigenic specificities. The Qa-6 and Qa-11 antigenic specificities were identified by antisera (303,304), and Qa-m9 was defined by a mAb (305). These specificities all appear to be related but different from other members of the Qa-2 family because their expression is not detected on thymocytes and is controlled by a gene in the *Tla* or *H-2D* region (303,304,306). In addition, the specificities for Qa-m9 and Qa-11 appear to be expressed only in the presence of the β_2-microglobulin "b" allele (304,305). However, when the molecules detected by Qa-6 or Qa-11 antisera were studied further, they could not be distinguished biochemically from Qa-2 (304,306).

It was initially shown that some anti-H-2 sera might contain antibodies that recognized Qa determinants (300,307). Subsequently, several anti-H-2 mAb have been studied which detect a Qa-2 cross-reactive (CR) specificity. One anti-H-2 k^d and two anti-H-2K^b antibodies were reported to detect a Qa-2 CR specificity with selective expression on T cells and some thymocytes (308,309). Antibody-blocking studies with 20-8-4 (K^b) and 34-1-2 (K^d) demonstrated that the epitope detected by the CR reagents was spatially distinct from the Qa-2 epitope detected by the anti-Qa-2 mAb (D3.262) (308).

A third mAb, 6.3.4 (specific for K^b), was also shown to bind to antigens determined by the Qa-2 region (309). In this second study, the Qa CR antigen Qa-m208 was detected on L cells transfected either with a cosmid containing two Qa-T1a region genes (LB2.11.2) or with a K^b region cosmid (LH8), but not with a D^b transfected line (309). Antigen redistribution studies on K^kD^b T cells demonstrated that the CR determinant was co-capped by the anti-Qa-2 mAb, D2-362 (309). Finally, using the anti-Qa-2 mAb and a sandwich blocking technique, binding of the Qa/CR was inhibited, suggesting that the Qa-2 and Qa CR determinants were on the same molecule (309). In addition, the tissue distribution pattern was strikingly different for theQa-2 mAb versus the Qa/H-2 CR antigen. The CR antigen was predominantly limited to T cells with only low levels on non-T cells from lymphoid and hemopoietic tissues, whereas Qa-2 was expressed on all of these tissues (308).

In summary, there appear to be three general patterns of Qa-2 expression. The first pattern is comparable to the initial serological description of Qa-2, where the antigen is preferentially expressed on all or most T cells, a small subset of mature thymocytes, most B cells, and some bone marrow cells (8,281). There is a quantitative variation on this pattern of expression, which appears to limit expression to T cells which may reflect the assays used. The second pattern of expression ("Qa-6"-like) indicates that there is complex genetic control of closely related or identical antigens. This control is seen as a regulation of presense or absence of Qa-2 antigens by the appropriate β_2-microglobulin gene, compounded with quantitative regulation by genes in the Tla region. In this pattern of expression, Qa antigen appears to be limited only to T cells in peripheral lymphoid tissue.

Finally, there is an intriguing pattern of CR antigen expression detected with some anti-H-2K reagents (308,309). This confirms the close relationship of MHC clss I products and further delineates a pattern of Qa-2 expression limited primarily to T cells and a subset of thymocytes with low amounts of the antigen on non-T cells (308,309). This Qa/H-2K CR antigen expression has been directly linked to gene products of Qa region genes by analysis of transfectants (309).

2. Cellular Expression of Qa-2 Antigen

Initial studies (297) showed that Qa-2 was expressed on lymphocytes from several lymphoid tissues, including lymph node, spleen, thymus, bone marrow, and liver. However it was absent on RBCs, epidermal cells, brain, and kidney. These and additional studies (reviewed in 8,279,281) have shown the presence of Qa-2 on normal and both lectin-activated and MHC-responsive T-cell subsets (291,310,

311). In addition, Qa-2 has been reported on pre-B colony-forming cells (312), LPS-stimulated blasts (300), and some antibody-forming cells (310-312). In addition to its presence on pre-B cells, Qa-2 has been demonstrated on other early stem cells by several laboratories (298,312-314). Furthermore, it appears that Qa-2 is expressed at a higher level on committed stem cells (313).

Finally, several of the Qa-2 specificities, as reviewed above, have been detected on thymocytes, whereas others have not (8,281). Recent evidence has demonstrated that Qa-2 family of antigens are subset markers expressed only on some of the most mature cells in the thymus (279). Thus, elimination of a very small subset of thymocytes depletes functional activity.

3. Biochemical Characterization of Qa-2 Molecules

Like the other MHC class I antigens, the Qa-2 antigen resides on a 40-Kd glycoprotein associated with β_2-microglobulin (315). Even using the complex anti-Qa-2 antisera and isoelectric focusing, no genetic polymorphism has been detected between Qa-2 molecules (316). In addition, attempts to detect different molecular species between Qa-2 and the Qa-6-like group [i.e., Qa-6 (306), Qa-m9 (305), and Qa-11 (304)] or the H-2/Qa CR mAb, 20-8-4 (306), have failed. Extensive, reciprocal, sequential precipitation or blocking experiments have produced no evidence that the molecules detected by these reagents could be distinguished from the Qa-2 molecules detected by antisera (304,306). Thus, although there are multiple serological specificities, there is no evidence that more than one species of Qa-2 protein molecule is expressed on normal lymphocytes.

In contrast, there is evidence that the Qa-2 cell-surface molecule is differentially glycosylated on normal LN cells (316) and activated T cells (291,317). Biosynthesis experiments indicate that although there is no increase in the cell-surface levels of Qa-2 on activated T cells, there is a 2- to 3-fold increase in total Qa-2 molecules (318), with evidence for enhanced secretion of a soluble, glycosylated, hyposialyated form of Qa-2 in activated T cells (291,317,318).

4. Functional Analysis of Qa-2

It has been established that, like other MHC class I molecules, Qa-2 can function as a target antigen. However, like Qa-1 and unlike H-2K or H-2D, anti-Qa-2 responses require antigen-specific priming. In addition, the Qa-2 antigen(s) do not serve as restricting elements for other nominal antigen responses (8,319).

5. Genetics of the Qa-2 Region and Regulation of Qa-2 Antigen Expression

We have alluded to the genetics of the regulation of Qa-2 in the sections above. Serological analysis of congenic and recombinant inbred mice maps the Qa-2 family of genes to two regions in the MHC: the *Qa* region and the *Tla-H-2D* region with a regulatory control associated with β_2-microglobulin. However, biochemical analysis of the three types of Qa-2 antigens (Qa-2, Qa-6, and Qa/H-2 CR) indicates that the molecules on which these antigenic specificities reside are very similar or identical.

The organization and the number of Qa region genes (and pseudogenes) differs between the two strains [C57BL/10 (B10) and BALB/c] that have been analyzed extensively (29,30). The gene names, Q1-Q10, that have been assigned do not coincide with the Qa serological specificities nor do they necessarily coincide between strains; see Weiss et al. (30) for the alignment between B10 and BALB/c. Both conserved and polymorphic segments have been identified in the Qa region. The latter have been suggested to result from deletions, insertions, and translocations within the MHC (9,29,30).

Although most of the Qa region genes have a truncated 3' end relative to other MHC class I genes, at least one of the Q genes (Q10) has a transmembrane region. Its gene product is a glycoprotein presumably secreted into the serum from the liver in normal mice (320). Furthermore, this product may be related to the secreted Qa-2 seen with activated T cells. The Q10 protein has been successfully obtained as a secreted product from transfected cell lines in vitro (321). Furthermore, Mellor et al. (277,322) have proposed that the lack of polymorphism for the Q10 gene between strains may indicate selective pressure which prevents accumulation of mutations at this locus. They have concluded that the Qa region acts as a stable genetic reservoir for the MHC.

The Q6 gene of BALB/c was first analyzed by exon shuffling to construct hybrid Q6 genes with a 5' Q6 and a 3' K^d, D^d, or L^d sequence (323). This maneuver permitted expression of the Q6 gene product on the surface of transfected L cells (323). Subsequent analysis with Q5, Q7, and Q8 genes of BALB/c demonstrated that the 5' half of Q5 and Q8 could be expressed, whereas the 5' half of Q7 could not (324). Immunoprecipitation analyses of the transfected cells with the 20-8-4 CR mAb has detected a 40-Kd molecule with the characteristic truncated cytoplasmic tail of a Qa-2 molecule (323). Furthermore the 3' portion of the Q6 gene appears to be responsible for the "tissue-specific" lack of expression of the unmodified Q6 gene sequence in L cells (323).

Finally, analysis of the Qa genes of BALB/cBy variant mice has demonstrated that the loss of Qa-2 expression is a direct consequence of a gene loss or conversion to pseudogenes by gene fusion. Initial gene fusion of the B10 Q8 and Q9 genes, followed by fusion of B10 Q6 and Q7 genes, gave rise to the one nonfunctional gene in BALB/c and subsequently two nonfunctional genes in BALB/cBy mice. The alignment between the B10 genes and BALB/c is such that the BALB/c Q7 gene was proposed as a gene fusion product of $H\text{-}2^b$ Q8 and $H\text{-}2^b$ Q9 genes (30). In turn, it was shown that neither the 5' nor the 3' half of the Q7 gene could be expressed in L cells by the exon shuffling that produced Qa products of Qa-5 and Qa-8 detected by a Qa/H-2 CR mAb (324). Although this has not been analyzed extensively on other $H\text{-}2^d$ strains, the sequential loss in gene number by gene fusion resulting in loss or pseudogenes may account for some of the quantitative phenotype variation seen in different strains of mice. This is seen as: *H-2*^{b}, Qa-2$^+$ high; *H-2*^{d,q,s}, Qa-2$^+$ low, and Qa-2$^-$, particularly on a number of *H-2*^{k} strains (8,279,281,300).

C. Qa-4,5

These two Qa antigens detected by mAb (301) were described as Qa region specificities different from Qa2/3 based on the differential strain reactivity and, in particular, a decreased reactivity when the *H-2D*^{d} allele was present. Qa-4,5 were originally thought to be T-cell-specific, because direct cytotoxicity with these IgM mAb gave selective killing of sIg$^-$ spleen and lymph node cells. FCA first reported for these specificities indicated low levels of binding with the mAb on sIg$^-$ cells (301).

Over the next few years it became apparent that Qa-4,5 specificities were detected on a variety of other cell types (8), but in particular on naturally occurring or interferon-activated NK cells (39,325-327). Furthermore, the Qa-5 marker became useful for distinguishing between NK cells (Qa-5$^+$) and natural cytotoxic (NC) cells Qa-5$^-$ (328,329). This latter type of cytotoxic activity has now been shown to be mediated by TNF (330), potentially released from several types of cells.

More recently, comparative phenotypic characterization of Qa-5 on NK cells and T cells, separated by Percoll density gradients from liver-derived nonparenchymal cells, has been reported (40). These studies have shown that the large granular lymphocyte population, containing cells enriched for NK activity, expresses a much higher level of Qa-5 than do low density T cells. Further, these studies demonstrate that the selective cytotoxicity against NK cells observed with anti-Qa-5 + C' is based on an increased level of expression.

Studies with the transplantation of bone marrow precursors for NK activity in the spleen have demonstrated that NK precursors are not eliminated by anti-Qa-5 pretreatment but can be eliminated by anti-Qa-2 (331). We have confirmed these data in a transfer system where the NK cells can be recovered from the recipient animal and analyzed for donor phenotype as well as activity (Mathieson and Mason, manuscript in preparation). While this difference between Qa-5 and Qa-2 may be only quantitative, it is a useful marker in these types of studies.

X. Ia EXPRESSION ON THYMOCYTES

Ia expression was observed on thymic lymphocytes only when sufficiently sensitive FCA was available for detection (332). This level of antigen is not detected by cytolytic methods even with mAb. We will not discuss the antigen in extensive detail because it is beyond the scope of this review. We will restrict our discussion to several important details about thymic Ia expression.

A. IA/IE and Nongenetic Acquisition

1. Ia Expression on Thymic Cells

Using mAb to both IA and IE subregions, it was possible to demonstrate these antigens at low levels on thymic lymphoid populations (332). However, this antigenic expression did not appear to be limited to subsets differing in size or maturity (332). At the same time, analysis of histological sections of thymus demonstrated that epithelial cells and other stromal cells appeared to be the primary cells in the thymus which expressed Ia (333-337). In addition, thymic lymphocytes adjacent to Ia^+ epithelial cells appeared to express the highest levels of Ia antigen(s) (334,337).

2. Nongenetic Acquisition of Ia

In studies with irradiation, bone marrow-transfer chimeras, it was demonstrated that after thymic repopulation by donor-derived lymphoid cells, thymocytes expressed largely, but not exclusively, Ia of the host type (338). This Ia was sufficiently integrated into the membrane of the thymocytes to require pronase to remove it, and overnight cultures of the antigen-stripped cells did not regenerate the Ia, whereas Ly-2 surface antigen was regenerated in this same time period (338). Thus it appeared that most of the Ia antigen on the thymic lymphocytes was acquired from surrounding stromal cells at the same time that the thymic cells acquired their MHC restriction.

B. Blocking of Differentiation

1. Anti-Ia Treatment in Vivo

Studies with anti-Ia treatment in vivo have demonstrated a loss of Ia from the cell surface of thymocytes of the treated animals (339). In addition, deletion of the $Ly\text{-}4^+$ ($Ly\text{-}2^-$) subset in the thymus as well as the periphery has been observed with anti-Ia treatment (340). Since other data has indicated that at least three distinct cellular types of stromal cells express Ia (337), it remains to be determined whether all or only some of these nonlymphoid components are determining the limitation in the differentiation of $Ly\text{-}4^+$ lineage. Further, it is not known precisely when this block in differentiation occurs since $Ly\text{-}2^+$, $Ly\text{-}4^+$ cells are generated in these thymuses (340). It is also possible that the $Ly\text{-}4^+$ cells are generated in low numbers but the population is unable to expand because a critical type of stromal cell capable of producing required factor(s) has been depleted.

2. Blocking of Thymocyte Differentiation in Vitro

Additional data from in vitro experiments indicates that anti-Ia treatment of fetal thymus lobes in organ cultures causes a severe depletion of lymphocytes and Ia^+ stromal cells and a concomitant loss of cells capable of an allogeneic response in vitro (341). More recent data indicates that administration of interleukin 1 (IL-1) to the organ cultures bypasses this block created by the anti-Ia administration (342).

XI. OTHER ANTIGENS DEFINED BY MONOCLONAL ANTIBODIES

A number of antigens expressed on T cells have been defined in the literature by mAb. We will discuss these in several groups, organized primarily by the genetic linkage that has been reported for them. We have grouped several antigens whose genetic association fits them into one of these patterns or which are defined by nonpolymorphic determinants where this appears appropriate. The strain distribution pattern of the polymorphic Ly antigens has been reviewed and tabulated elsewhere (53).

A. *Igh*-Linked Chromosome 12 Antigens Expressed on Thymocytes and/or T Cells: Ly-7, Ly-16, Tsu, Tind, Tthy, and Tpre

In this section, we will review several antigens that have been reported to be linked to the Ig heavy chain locus (*Igh*) on chromosome 12 in the mouse. These antigens are not themselves Ig heavy chain markers and are weakly or variably expressed on thymocytes and T cells during differentiation or activation. Ly-16 has not been defined by mAb but fits into this group because of its *Igh* linkage.

1. Ly-7: An *Igh-1*-linked Antigen on Mature T and B Cells

Ly-7 has been characterized with alloantisera raised between recombinant inbred (RI) strains of mice (343,344) and two mAb raised against a B-cell lymphoma (345,346). These studies on lymphoid populations and other tissues have indicated that Ly-7 has features that make it (a) a lymphocyte but not leukocyte antigen, (b) a T-cell subset and differentiation antigen, and (c) a "blood group" type of antigen.

Cytotoxicity and IF studies of Ly-7 antigen expression on lymphoid populations (76,343-346) have indicated that both T and B lymphocytes express Ly-7, but Ly-7 is expressed at a somewhat higher level on B cells than on T cells. Quantitative FCA of Ly-7 antigen expression in F_1 animals indicates that, unlike the genetically linked Ig markers, expression of Ly-7 is not allelically excluded (345). Other leukocytes and hemopoietic cells, including erythrocytes, granulocytes, and most bone marrow cells, are negative (76,343-346).

Thymocytes express Ly-7 only at low levels (76,344-346), and apparently only on the more mature, cortisone-resistant cells express Ly-7 (76). By C'-dependent cytotoxicity, T helper cells are Ly-7^+ but CTL and suppressor T cells are Ly-7^-, and all T-cell blasts have an increased sensitivity to anti-Ly-7 + C' compared to resting T cells (56). Thus Ly-7 shows characteristics which suggest that it is a differentiation antigen with increased expression on mature and activated T cells. It was also noted that only some T-cell lines and no pre-B lymphomas or plasmacytomas express Ly-7 (345), supporting the contention that Ly-7 is preferentially expressed on cells at different states of maturity, further distinguishing the expression of Ly-7 from the pan-lymphocyte antigen, Ly-9 (described above).

The function of Ly-7 has not been reported, and the biochemistry has not been well defined. However, it was reported that Ly-7.2 and Ly-7.3 antigens were trypsin-sensitive (346). The genetics and unique strain distribution for expression of this antigen reveal another interesting feature of Ly-7. All strains tested are either *Ly-7^a^* or *Ly-7^c^* (346,347), except for B6, B10, and C58, which are *Ly-7^b^*. [Note that the revised designation for Ly-7.2 is Ly-7.1/*Ly-7^a^* (53).] The gene(s) for expression of Ly-7 antigen is linked 19 cM telomeric to the *Igh-1* locus on chromosome 12 (347). No antisera has ever been successfully raised to the Ly-7.2 specificity of the *Ly-7^b^* allotype (56), and an H-2-linked immune response gene controls the response to the Ly-7.1 specificity by *Ly-7^b^* mice (344). This raises interesting parallels to the Qa-2 system described above and to the human ABO blood group antigens. In the blood group antigens, the backbone antigen (O type) is not normally recognized as a foreign antigen within the species but the A or B types which have complex carbohydrates added to the backbone are detected as foreign "allotypes." Furthermore, the Ly-7.3 antigenic specificity is only expressed when Ly-7.1 antigen is present (346); i.e., mouse strains are commonly found which express either Ly-7.1 with Ly-7.3 or Ly-7.1 without Ly-7.3. However, no Ly-7.1$^-$, Ly-7.3$^+$ mice are found (346). This is also similar to the expression observed for some members of the Qa-2 family, where a second restricted antigenic specificity has been observed when a more common, genetically related antigenic specificity is expressed (discussion above).

2. Thymocyte and T Subset Antigens: Epitopes on a Second Type of T-Cell Receptor?

A series of alloantigens linked to *Igh-1* have been reported on thymocytes or functionally active T cells (348-351). The first of these markers, Tsu^d, was detected only in *Igh-1^d* allotype mice (352,353), and it was initially proposed that the Tsu antigen was a T-cell receptor constant region gene because of the ability of alloantisera to Tsu^d to polyclonally trigger suppressor T cells for T-dependent antigens (354). A second antigen, Tind, was detected on T suppressor inducer cells and was also shown to be linked to *Igh-1* (355). The third antigen, originally reported as Ly-18 (356) and now referred to as Ly-16 (53), has only been detected by alloantisera. Ly-16 antigen was detected on CTL, but antisera to Ly-16 did not block cytotoxicity. Furthermore, Ly-16 was not detected on proliferating cells in response to alloantigens, Ig plaque-forming cells, or resting lymphocytes. Ly-16 was linked to the V_H gene complex by its selective expression in *Igh-1^d*

allotype mouse strains (356). It is now clear that this family of antigens bears no similarity to the α or β chains of the MHC-restricted T-cell antigen receptor discussed above. In addition, the β chain of the TcR is linked to Ig κ light chain and Ly-2 on chromosome 6 (357,358).

Additional mAb were subsequently produced that recognized two *Igh-1*-linked antigens expressed on subsets of normal adult or fetal thymocytes (348,350). Tpre and Tthy antigens are expressed at different times during ontogeny and may reflect transitional states of thymocyte differentiation. Tpre is expressed in fetal liver and early fetal thymocytes whereas Tthy is expressed only on a subset (20-30%) of thymocytes in postnatal animals (350). The sequence for expression is Tpre/fetal –> Tthy, 1-2 days postnatal –> Tind, 2-3 days postnatal, and finally –> Tsu, 5-6 days postnatal (349). The appearance of the latter three antigens requires the presence of a thymus because nude mice lack these three types of cells.

Immunoprecipitation of Tthy from a T-cell line has indicated that two proteins of about 30 and 48 Kd are detected with the anti-Tthy mAb (350). Anti-Tsu immunoprecipitations from culture supernatant revealed a 33-Kd protein, whereas anti-Tind yielded protein bands of 45 and 17 Kd. From these studies, a model was proposed that suggested that transitional cells expressing both of the mature markers, Tind and Tsu, as well as the earlier thymocyte marker, Tthy, could be found (350). The function of all of these markers is still undefined.

B. Chromosome 19 Antigens: Ly-10, An Ly-1-Associated Antigen, the Alloantigens Ly-12 and Ly-13, and Murine "4F2" Equivalents

These antigens are grouped together because genetic, biochemical, or serological criteria used to define these antigens indicate that the reagents are detecting at least related, if not identical, molecules.

1. The Alloantigens Ly-10, Ly-12, and Ly-13

Ly-10 has been defined by a mAb to the Ly-10.1 specificity (359). This mAb detects an antigen expressed on thymocytes, splenic T and B cells, bone marrow lymphocytes, and a cell line, 416B, with stem cell characteristics (359). In addition, Ly-10 expression has been detected on several nonlymphoid tissues–brain, kidney, and liver–but not on red blood cells (359). The characterization of lymphoid expression was extended to demonstrate that Ly-10 was expressed on T helpers, T suppressors, and alloreactive CTL (222). Furthermore, the functionally activated cells were more sensitive to lysis than the precursors or resting cells (360).

From the expression of Ly-10.1 on the B6-*Ly-1*^{a} congenic strain, Ly-10 was shown to be closely linked to Ly-1, with its expression separated from Ly-1 by only two strains, C57BR and C57L (359). These two strains were also used in other studies defining Ly-12 and Ly-13 (361); the other Ly-10.1$^+$ strains used to define Ly-12 and Ly-13 were strains that would have co-absorbed Ly-10 with some of the other specificities in the complex alloantisera used. We raise the possibility of overlap with one or both of these antigens, because Morse et al. (53) have indicated that Ly-12 expression is also genetically associated with chromosome 19, and the FCA profiles shown for Ly-12 and Ly-13 on thymocytes (361) are essentially identical to those of Ly-10.1 and Ly-1 (B.J. Mathieson, S.O. Sharrow, and U. Hammerling, unpublished data). In addition, the reported nonlymphoid expression for Ly-13 (361) is similar to that reported for Ly-10 (359); however, Ly-12 expression is restricted to lymphocytes (361).

Immunoprecipitation of Ly-10 reveals a disulfide-linked heterodimer with a glycosylated 80-Kd heavy chain (with a 60-Kd protein backbone) and a nonglycosylated 34-Kd light chain (360). These data and the cellular expression characteristics led to the suggestion that Ly-10.1 was an alloantigenic determinant on the murine equivalent of human 4F2 antigen (360). Human 4F2 was previously reported to be an antigen expressed at high levels on monocytes and activated lymphocytes with similar biochemical characteristics (362). Attempts to immunoprecipitate Ly-12 and Ly-13 using the alloantisera were unsuccessful (361).

Further genetic characterization of the expression of Ly-10.1 indicated no negative genetic control of antigen expression in F_1 animals and very close linkage to *Ly-1* in RI strains and backcross mice (recombination frequency 0.023-0.029) (363).

2. Murine "4F2" Equivalents and Activation Antigens

Three rat mAb to a variant subline of the mouse EL4 thymic lymphoma have been produced that could substitute for IL-1 in the stimulation of the production of IL-2 by the subline (364). Two of the mAb, RL119 and RL73, could competitively inhibit binding of labeled RL119 mAb to EL4-6.1. Binding of a third mAb, RL388, was not cross-inhibited. However, IF profiles by FCA indicated very similar staining between RL119 and RL388; i.e., low intensity IF on most thymocytes, negligible IF on most cortisone-resistant thymocytes (CRT), and high intensity staining on Con A-activated CRT. Once again, the IF profiles on thymocytes of RL388 very closely resemble the IF profiles of Ly-10. RL73 demonstrated an inverse pattern of IF, with a higher intensity on normal thymocytes and lower intensity of IF on Con A-activated CRT, but undetectable IF on unstimulated CRT (364). In addition, various T-cell, B-cell, macrophage, and fibroblast cell lines were positive for the "4F2"-like expression detected by RL388 (364).

Like the anti-human 4F2 and anti-mouse Ly-10, RL388 immunoprecipitates a disulfide-linked heterodimer composed of a glycosylated, 86-Kd heavy chain and a nonglycosylated 39-Kd light chain (365). However, RL119 and RL73 detect a different, heavily glycosylated protein of 55 Kd (365). The relationship of this latter activation antigen to Ly-10 or 4F2 is undetermined. Further studies with the mAb to the murine human 4F2 antigens have compared the peptide maps of the proteins detected by RL388 and 4F2, respectively, demonstrating the existence of a highly conserved protein between man and mouse (366).

The function of the Ly-10/4F2 antigens has not been defined. However, from studies on human cardiac and skeletal muscle, it appears that a related 4F2-like mAb, 44D7, inhibits Na^{+}/Ca^{++} fluxes (367). This is particularly relevant since the RL388 Ab can stimulate IL-2 production by the poised EL4-6.1 subline but not on normal T cells (364). Bron et al. (366) cite further unpublished data that calcium ionophore can also induce IL-2 production in the EL4 subline and that the RL388 mAb can mimic this by inducing a significant calcium ion flux.

Thus RL388 appears to detect a nonpolymorphic determinant on the Ly-10/4F2 antigen complex in the mouse. The functional data suggest that the Ly-10/4F2 equivalents in the mouse may provide highly selective tools to dissect ligand interactions involved in lymphocyte transmembrane signaling by lymphokines.

C. A Cluster of Genetic Loci on Chromosome 4 Controls Diverse Ly Antigens: Ly-19, Ly-20, Ly-29, Ly-31, J_t, and Several B-cell Antigens

This diverse grouping of antigens is clustered for the purposes of our discussion because of their reported linkage to loci for a coat color marker, *b*, a urinary protein, *Mup-1*, and/or *Lyb-2* on chromosome 4. Several of these antigens have also been reported to be linked to retroviral genes. A listing of the genetically linked loci for Ly alloantigens and additional comments on the B-cell alloantigens, Lyb-2, Lyb-4, and Lyb-6, which are closely clustered on chromosome 4, are presented elsewhere (53,56,57).

1. Ly-19

This antigen is defined by a single mAb, Ly-19.2, which detects a relatively undefined antigen on most T cells, B cells, lymphoid bone marrow, and <15% of thymocytes (368). By Ab + C' cytotoxicity, Ly-19 has been shown to be variably expressed on functionally activated T-cell subpopulations (222,368). Ly-19 was easily detected on Con A blasts, and weakly expressed on alloantigen-reactive blasts (368). However, Ly-19 was not detected on antigen-specific T helper cells, Con A-induced suppressor cells, or alloreactive CTL (222). These data are remarkable because most T cells in lymph node or normal spleen express Ly-19 (368). In addition, Ly-19 was demonstrated to have variable expression on several T-cell leukemia lines, a B-cell lymphoma, and the pre-B-cell line which was used for the hybridoma/mAb immunization (368). However, several unrelated hybridomas, myelomas, and a sarcoma cell line were Ly-19^{-}. Furthermore, brain, liver, kidney, and erythrocytes did not absorb anti-Ly-19 antibody (368). Thus the antigen expression appears to be restricted to lymphocytes.

Ly-19 was linked to the *Lyb-2* locus on chromosome 4 by typing with the mAb on spleen cells of AKXL RI mouse strains (368). It was noted that the

Lyb-2.3 phenotype was highly correlated with the Ly-19.2⁻ strains, whereas Ly-19.2⁺ strains included Lyb-2.1, Lyb-2.2, and Lyb-2.4 strains of mice.

2. Ly-20 (old Ly-22.2)

Ly-20 has been only poorly defined by antisera (369), but is has been reported as an antigen whose expression is largely confined to lymphoid tissues. Some cells from lymph nodes, spleen, bone marrow, and thymus all express Ly-20. However, the characteristics of cells expressing Ly-20 in each of these tissues was not defined (369).

A unique strain distribution pattern distinguishes Ly-20 from many other Ly alloantigens; i.e., Ly-20 is present on lymphocytes of B6 and on most strains of mice, whereas it is absent from cells in the closely related B10 strain of mice (369). It was claimed that Ly-20 antigen expression was controlled by two genes, one of which was on chromosome 4 (369). However, examination of the reported genetic marker data on the RI strains of mice suggests only a linkage to an endogenous retroviral cell-surface antigen, XenCSA, whose expression is itself complex, and to another retroviral susceptibility marker, *Fv-1* (370). No convincing genetic linkage to other chromosome 4 markers, such as *b, Mup-1,* or *Lyb-4,* was demonstrated (369).

3. Ly-29

Ly-29 antigen is defined by a single mAb to an alloantigenic determinant, Ly-29.2, found on most B cells (87%), some T cells (66%), and only 30% of Ig^-, $Ly\text{-}2^-$ spleen cells, 30% of thymocytes, and 40% of bone marrow (371). Nonlymphoid tissues fail to absorb antibody activity.

Ly-29 antigen displays a unique strain distribution pattern from other antigens in this linkage group. It also has a intriguing, close linkage to both *Lyb-2* and another retroviral marker, *Mtv-20* (371). Further characterization of the biochemistry and function of Ly-29 antigen has not been reported.

4. Ly-31

Ly-31 is also defined by a single mAb to an alloantigenic determinant, Ly-31.1 (372). This antigen is expressed widely on both T and B lymphocyte lineages, however only some cells in all lymphoid tissues appear to be positive for Ly-31 antigen by Ab + C' lysis; i.e., 55% of thymocytes, 20% of spleen, lymph node or bone marrow cells and 10-15% of peripheral blood leukocytes are lysed by Ab + C'.

Ly-31 is linked to *Fv-1* (372), like *Ly-20* as mentioned above; however, the strain distribution pattern is not correlated with that reported for *Ly-20*. Furthermore, there is complete concordance of *Ly-31* with the *Akp-20* locus, an enzymatic (alkaline phosphatase) marker found in nonlymphoid tissues, although the interrelationship of these two genetic markers is unknown.

5. J_t and I-J

I-J was first defined as determinant on suppressor T cells controlled by the I region of the MHC (373). An extensive discussion of I-J antigen expression on functional cells and factors is beyond the scope of this review, and a number of reviews are available on this subject (see Ref. 374). Therefore, we will confine our discussion to several recent developments in this area of investigation and in particular to the characterization of a related cell-surface antigen, J_t, determined at least in part by genes on chromosome 4.

Extensive controversy has evolved over whether MHC-associated I-J molecules exist. The antisera originally used to define I-J were heavily contaminated with antibodies binding to lymphocytes of many strains of mice, and the reagents for I-J have been difficult to obtain or unavailable to many investigators. A more serious problem arose for 'I-J' when Steinmetz and co-workers (375) demonstrated that the DNA from B10.A(3R) and B10.A(5R) mice was identical by restriction site polymorphism mapping. Since these congenic mice had been used to map the location of *I-J*, these data strongly suggested that *I-J* had been incorrectly mapped.

Subsequently, expression of a T-cell marker, J_t, was reported to be highly correlated with expression of an antigen detected by an anti-I-J mAb (376). However, it was shown that B6-H-2^k mice, which have MHC region genes derived from AKR mice, had some T cells that were J_t^+, whereas no J_t^+ cells were found in either B6 or AKR mice. In addition, (B10xAKR)F_1 mice did have J_t^+ cells, suggesting genetic complementation. It was further demonstrated that the expression of the J_t marker was controlled by a gene on chromosome 4, and it was proposed that J_t together with the *H-2* locus controlled 'I-J^k' expression (376).

Because only 10-15% of T cells are lysed with anti-J_t + C', techniques to make T cells more susceptible to Ab + C' were devised (377). From these studies, up to 20% of T cells in a J_t +/− heterozygote were lysed, whereas up to 50% of the T cells from (B6xB6-H-2^k)F_1 mice could be lysed in Ab + C' assays after the cells had been treated with neuraminidase. In these same studies, it was shown that J_t was not reexpressed after proteolytic removal of the antigen if glycosylation or protein synthesis was blocked. In addition, *a* mannosidase treatment of neuraminidase-treated T cells apparently destroyed the epitope recognized by anti-J_t, implying that a carbohydrate moiety constitutes the J_t antigenic determinant.

The previously reported studies of J_t do not resolve the issues surrounding the detection of I-J on functional cell populations involved in T-cell suppressor circuits. In addition, subsequent studies demonstrate that the production of T suppressor factors binding to an anti-'I-J' mAb can be found in I-E^k mice expected to be negative for the chromosome 4 region antigen (378).

D. Additional Chromosome 7 Antigens: Ly-14 and Ly-21

We have previously discussed LFA-1, the cellular adhesion family of molecules and Ly-15 which apparently detects a specificity on the heavy chain of LFA-1. Expression of Ly-15/LFA-1 is linked to the *Hbb* locus on chromosome 7 (379). A B-cell alloantigen locus *Lyb-8,* which controls the expression of a 95-105-Kd glycoprotein is also found on chromosome 7 (380). It is not known whether this protein is related to the 95-Kd light chain of the Ly-15/LFA-1 family of antigens, but the tissue and strain distribution patterns of Lyb-8 and Ly-15 are distinct. Two other Ly antigens, Ly-14 and Ly-21, which are also controlled by genes on chromosome 7, have been reported.

1. Ly-14

The specificity Ly-14.1 was detected by antibodies in complex alloantisera as a weakly expressed antigen on thymocytes using an antibody rosetting technique (361). Antibody to the reciprocal specificity was not generated. By absorption, Ly-14 antigen was shown to be expressed on all tissues tested (including lymphoid cells, brain, liver, and kidney), but not on red blood cells. Immunoprecipitation with the anti-Ly-14 antisera detected a 73-Kd protein that was not further characterized. Genetic linkage studies indicated that Ly-14 was linked to albinism, *C* (361).

2. Ly-21

Ly-21 is defined by a single mAb detecting the Ly-21.2 antigenic specificity expressed on all strains of mice except A/J and A strain congenics (381). The antigen was shown to be on thymocytes, at least T cells of spleen and lymph node and 70% of bone marrow by visual IF with a reagent that also detected B cells.

Ly-21 was linked to the albino/color locus, *c*, on chromosome 7. A unique strain distribution distinguished it from other antigens controlled by genes on chromosome 7. It was further suggested in the initial report that there was a correlated susceptibility to Friend virus-induced erythroleukemia (381).

E. Additional Chromosome 2 Antigens: Ly-23 and Ly-25

Several markers whose expression is seen on diverse populations of leukocytes have been reported to be linked to markers on chromosome 2. The Ly-24/Pgp-1 antigen was previously discussed in Section VII. This marker and several other antigens have been linked to the β_2-microglobulin gene, *B2m*. The genetics of *B2m* has been reviewed elsewhere (382) and its importance in cell-surface expression of MHC-associated antigens has been widely recognized. One of the Ly-11 antigens, previously described as Ly-m11 (382), has now been shown to be β_2-microglobulin (53,383). A second Ly-11 antigen was initially claimed to be linked to both *Ly-6* (on chromosome 15) and *B2m*/coat color markers on chromosome 2 (201). The weak linkage to chromosome 2 markers and the cellular expression of Ly-11 antigen has led us to propose that this is not a chromosome 2 antigen, but rather an antigen in the Ly-6 family. For completeness, we mention here the report of a granulocyte/macrophage alloantigen, Gm-3.2, whose expression is also linked to *B2m* and *H-3* on chromosome 2 (384).

1. Ly-23

Ly-23 has been defined by two mAb apparently recognizing the same alloantigenic specificity, Ly-23.2 (385). Expression of Ly-23 has been reported on lymph node cells, lymphoid tumor lines, and both T-cell-enriched and B-cell-enriched lymphoid populations (385). Furthermore, mAb activity could be partially removed by absorption with liver, brain, and kidney, but not by lung or melanoma cells.

Ly-23 antigen expression was shown to be independent of β_2-microglobulin on cell lines deficient in the latter protein and in one RI strain with a genetic crossover for *B2m* (385). However, Ly-23 is closely linked to *B2m* and *H-3*, and the B10.C-$H\text{-}3^c$ congenic mouse strain lacks Ly-23.2 and thus serves as a congenic for both markers.

2. Ly-25

The Ly-25.1 specificity is detected only on hemopoietic cells by the single mAb that defines this alloantigenic system (386). The initial report indicated that 60% of Ig-depleted spleen cells were Ly-25$^+$ whereas >90% of the Ig$^+$ cells were Ly-25$^+$ The antigen is also expressed on thymocytes which were used as the target in screening the Ly-25 mAb. Bone marrow analysis indicated expression on both lymphoid and nonlymphoid cells of hemopoietic origin. However, kidney, liver, and red cells failed to absorb subsequent Ly-25 mAb binding to thymocytes (386).

The strain distribution is unique with only C57BR/cd, SWR, SJL, STS, and CE mice expressing this antigen out of 40 strains tested. Finally, typing on the CXS RI strains derived from BALB/c and STS/A indicated very close linkage to *Ly-24/Pgp-1*, with only one of 14 strains showing a discordance between the typing for *Ly-24* and *Ly-25* (386).

F. Other Lymphocyte Antigens Expressed on T Cells or Other Lymphocytes: Ly-18, Ly-26, Ly-27, Ly-30, Leugp90, MEL-14, FT-1, and FT-2

This group of Ly antigens is a very heterogeneous group of antigens representing a wide range of specificities. Many of these alloantigens are largely uncharacterized by many of the criteria that we have reviewed above.

1. Ly-18

A mAb to the Ly-18.2 specificity defines an antigen expressed on all thymocytes, about 50% of T and B cells, in both lymph node and spleen and is more weakly expressed on mitogen- or alloantigen-stimulated blast populations (387). Furthermore, Ly-18 appears to be absent, by Ab + C', from functionally active T-cell helper and suppressors and CTL (222). Ly-18 is also expressed on about 50% of bone marrow and was detected on pre-B and lymphocyte stem cell lines; However it was indicated that depletion of Ly-18$^+$ cells from bone marrow did not affect subsequent lymphocyte repopulation in irradiated hosts or CFU-S formation (387). Several nonlymphoid tissues (brain, liver, and kidney) absorbed mAb to Ly-18, whereas red blood cells did not.

The strain distribution patterns, segregating about evenly in commonly used strains of mice, and linkage to *Ltw-2* (387) separate this antigen from others that we have discussed. Thus, Ly-18 is a lymphoid antigen distinguished by a higher level of expression on immature precursors or resting "differentiated" cells.

2. Ly-26

Three mAb from the same hybridoma fusion were produced that bound only to B lymphocytes from NZB, NZB-*Igh* congenic, CE, and LP.RIII mice, thus detecting a new alloantigen, Ly-26 (388). Ly-26 expression is largely confined to B cells and lymphocyte precursors in bone marrow and possibly sIg$^-$, Thy-1$^-$ (null) cells, whereas thymocytes and T cells appear to be negative.

The binding to the LP.RIII congenic is notable because the antigen did not appear to be MHC-linked but was not expressed on either LP/J or RIII, the parental mouse strains from which LP.RIII was derived (388). Similarly genetic complementation of genes on chromosomes 4 and 11, for the expression of J_t has been discussed above and more fully elsewhere (376,377). Another example of potential genetic complementation has also been seen with Ly-10.1 expression, where B6 and C3H, the parental stocks, are negative but B6-*Ly*-^{a} congenic mice are Ly-10.1$^+$ (359,363). In contrast, it has been noted that B10.S mice, an MHC congenic strain, are negative for expression of Ly-18.2, but the parental strains are Ly-18.2$^+$ (387). These several examples suggest that gene complementation to produce new antigens (or lose expression) may not be that uncommon.

3. Ly-27

The antigen designation "Ly-27" has been reassigned to a new antigen which is expressed on >60% of thymocytes, about 50% of lymphocytes in spleen and lymph node, 65% of T cells including Con A or alloantigen responsive cells, and 40% of B cells including LPS or pokeweed mitogen-responsive cells (389). Ly-27 has not been detected on bone marrow and was only weakly positive or not detected by Ab + C' lysis on blasts stimulated by mitogens or on activated allo-CTL (389). [Ly-27 was previously assigned to an antigen (207), now recognized as Ly-6D (53).] The reported characterization of Ly-27.2 contrasted its detection with a different Ly-6A mAb (389). This comparison demonstrated only a weak reactivity on various blast populations with anti-Ly-27, but a strong reactivity with anti-Ly-6.

The strain distribution of Ly-27 indicated that over 20 of the strains tested were Ly-27.2$^+$ with only A/J, BALB/c, C3H, CBA/CaJ, CE/J, and SM/J being negative. Typing on the CXB RI strains indicated that Ly-27 was linked to two markers not assigned to chromosomal maps (389). Together these data indicated the detection of a new Ly antigen, which may be selectively expressed on the maturing Ly-4$^+$ (CD4$^+$) T cell subset.

4. Ly-30

Ly-30 is a newly characterized polymorphic antigen, which is defined by a mAb to the Ly-30.2 determinant (390). The cellular pattern of reactivity is reminiscent of that seen with some of the T200/B220 antibodies which react with B cells and a subset of Ly-2$^+$ T cells. Ly-30 is detected on most B cells and bone marrow, 35% of T cells in lymph node and spleen, but not on thymocytes or PBL. It has not been determined which subset of T cells is expressing Ly-30. Ly-30 does not appear to be directly associated with Ly-5/T200 expression because both B6 and B6-Ly-5.1 (congenic) mice are expressing Ly-30.2, and the strain distribution, with only three negative strains (CE, C58, and SJL) (390), is discrepant from that of Ly-5.

5. Leugp90

Leugp90, defined by a xenogeneic mAb, has several characteristics which make it similar to Ly-7 (see discussion above). However, Leugp90 is expressed on bone marrow whereas Ly-7 is not (391). Leugp90 also shares many characteristics with Ly-10, except that most thymocytes are Ly-10$^+$ but only 9% are Leugp90$^+$ (391). Furthermore, immunoprecipitations with anti-Ly-10 characteristically co-precipitate a 34-39-Kd molecule as well as an 80-85-Kd molecule (360,365,366). The function of this antigen has not been reported and the original strain distribution analysis was relatively limited (391).

6. MEL-14

MEL-14 antigen was originally characterized by a mAb selected to block binding of lymphoma cells to high endothelial venules (HEV) of peripheral lymph nodes but not Peyer's patch HEV (392). The mAb recognized an antigen that was expressed on mesenteric lymph node cells and T- and B-cell lymphomas that selectively bound HEV but was absent on T-cell clones. MEL-14 antigen was originally reported to be weakly expressed on thymus and absent on pre-B cells of bone marrow (392). Subsequent reports have either claimed that MEL-14 was on a population of immunocompetent cortical cells which were cortisone-resistant (393-396), fetal thymocytes at a specific point in ontogeny (397), or subsets within all of the major subsets defined by Ly-2 and Ly-4/CD4 (395). Subsequent analyses have raised questions about the correlation of flow cytometry analysis with cell membrane staining in situ (398) and have suggested that MEL-14 is only expressed on thymocytes with a medullary phenotype (398). Furthermore, the reported functional characterization of CTL precursors as cortical phenotype with MEL-14 expression has been questioned because the intensity is highly variable for the Ly-2$^+$ cells containing the CTL precursors (399). The relationship of MEL-14 antigen to either a state of differentiation or to one or more functional lineages has been postulated in these several reports but has not been directly assessed. No data has been provided to exclude expression on nonlymphoid populations, and no strain distribution analysis was reported.

The molecule immunoprecipitated by the MEL-14 mAb was originally indicated as an 80- or 92-Kd molecule which appeared to become larger when the analytical gel was run under reducing conditions (392). This was later modified to claim that the mAb identified a 90-Kd ubiquitinated branched-chain glycoprotein (400). Questions about whether this antigen can transmit transmembrane signals when functioning as a ligand binding to its "homing" receptor on HEV have not been addressed.

7. Fetal Thymocyte Antigens: FT-1 and FT-2

Two antigens, FT-1 and FT-2, have been defined which are restricted to a limited expression on some fetal thymocytes and some leukemia cells (401-403). The ontogeny of the expression of these two antigens is similar but fewer cells express FT-2, and there is a higher proportion of FT-1$^+$ cells in the day 15 than in the day 17 fetal thymus (403). An extensive strain distribution of this antigen has not been reported, but T-cell lymphomas from several strains were positive for FT-1, whereas, only one GR and one A/J lymphoma were positive for FT-2 (402). FT-1 has been identified as a 130-Kd glycoprotein with extensive charge heterogeneity (401). It has been suggested that these antigens may prove very useful in identifying early stem cells from fetal liver or possibly bone marrow in the adult (403).

G. Murine CD3 and Additional T-Cell Receptor or Activation Antigens

During the final stages of revision of this review, two mAb detecting cell-surface determinants of the TcR were reported. The first of these is an anti-CD3 mAb from a hamster-mouse fusion which recognizes the CD3ϵ component of the TcR (404). The second mAb defines a subset of thymocytes and T cells that express a newly defined Vβ17 family for the TcR (405). This new Vβ gene product appears to recognize IE and reflect a bias in the germline TcR repertoire for recognition of MHC proteins (405). Finally a further mAb may recognize components of a second class of T-cell γ receptor (406) whose function is not defined.

Several other mAb have also recently been described that may recognize additional components of T-cell activation pathways. One of these recognizes an 85-Kd protein composed of a disulfide-linked, 43-Kd homodimer (407). It has been suggested that this mAb, which recognizes cell-surface antigens on two T-cell lymphomas, may recognize a clonotypic determinant on the murine homologue of the human 9.3/Tp44 activation antigen (408). A rat mAb reported earlier, YE1/48.10, may recognize this same antigen (409).

XII. ANTIGENS STILL DEFINED ONLY BY ANTISERA

In this final section, we will briefly review several antigens that have been characterized only by alloantisera. These include Ly-8, Ly-11, Ly-12, Ly-13, Ly-14, Ly-16, Ly-20, Ea-7, Thy-2, and Lna-1. Some of these have been discussed in the chromosome cluster groups.

A. Ly-8 (One of the "Old" Ly-11 Antigens)

As mentioned in the discussion of Ly-6, the antigen originally designated as Ly-8 has been assimilated into the Ly-6 antigen family (53). Ly-8 has now been assigned to one of the antigens originally called Ly-11 (361). These Ly-8 ("old" Ly-11) serological specificities were detected in complex antisera by Ab + C' lysis or anti-Ig rosetting on thymocytes and by absorption on kidney cells. The thymocyte reactivity of the antisera were not absorbed by brain, liver, or erythrocytes. Ly-8.1 (Ly11.1) antiserum, raised between two RI strains [B10,RIII(71IN) anti-LP.RIII], was shown to be positive only on thymocytes from two relatively uncommon strains of mice (129 and 101) and the RI strain (LP.RIII) against which the animals were immunized. An additional complex antiserum, from the immunization of 129 mice with C57L lymphoid cells, generated antibodies to the reciprocal Ly-8.2 (Ly11.2) antigen detected on thymocytes of many commonly used strains of mice.

Immunoprecipitation analyses of ^{125}I-labeled cell-surface membrane proteins revealed an 18-20-Kd band (361) which was ascribed to this antigen. Genetic linkage studies performed with the reciprocal antisera indicated no linkage of *Ly-8* to *Ly-1, Ly-2/3, Ly-5,* or *Thy-1* loci (361).

B. Antigens Included in Other Cluster Groups

The antigenic name Ly-11 is retained by one of the three antigens that were originally called Ly-11 (201). However, this antigen, as indicated above, has been tentatively included in the Ly-6 family.

Ly-12 and Ly-13 have been described in the section on chromosome 19 antigens and their similarities to Ly-10, 4F2, and possibly other related activation antigens has been noted.

Ly-14 has been described in the section on chromosome 7 antigens, while Ly-16 (formerly Ly-18) has been described in the section on *Igh*-linked antigens. And finally, Ly-20 (formerly Ly-22.2) has been discussed in the section on chromosome 4 antigens.

C. Ea-7

The erythrocyte antigen, Ea-7.1, was also detected in the complex RI alloantisera (361). Ea-7 is included here because of its detection on thymocytes. The characterization of this antigen as a marker shared by red blood cells and thymocytes rests on two pieces of information: first, the cross-absorption of the red cell antigen by thymocytes, and second, on the detection of the thymic antigen in the B10.*Ea2^a Ea7^a* congenic mice and all Ea-7.1-bearing strains tested. Further characterization of this antigen was not reported.

D. Thy-2

Thy-2 was identified by a "contaminant" antibody in an anti-H-2.4 serum (410). The "Thy" designation was applied because, like Thy-1, the antigen was selectively expressed on thymocytes, brain tissue, and bone marrow with lower levels on spleen; Thy-2 antigen was not detected on lymph node, liver, or red blood cells. This tissue distribution is also similar to a number of xenogeneic rabbit anti-mouse brain sera that have been raised in a number of laboratories. Immunoprecipitation analyses of thymocyte extracts indicated that the antigen was unrelated to Thy-1 and was 150 Kd with semidominant expression on heterozygotes (410). Analysis of the genetics by congenics and RI mouse strains indicated that Thy-2 expression was linked to *H-2D, T1a,* and *Pgk-2* on chromosome 17 (410). It is noteworthy that, unlike the Qa-2/CR antigen detected as a cross-reactivity seen with mAbs to H-2, Thy-2 alloantisera did not detect an MHC class I molecule but detected an antigen with quite different biochemical characteristics.

E. Lna-1

Although this antigen has only been detected by alloantisera, it is nonetheless one of the more unusual and intriguing antigens which has been reported (411). The "Lna" designation was applied because antigen-positive cells were only detected in lymph nodes but not in spleen, thymus, or bone marrow. Furthermore, lymph nodes from various anatomical sites appeared to have similar numbers of Lna-1$^+$ cells. Lna-1, however, was not detected in lymph nodes of *Dh*/+ mutant "spleenless" mice, suggesting the requirement of splenic maturation events in the differentiation of Lna-1$^+$ cells (411). Finally, about 30% of both T and B lymphocytes from the lymph node express Lna-1. Because cultured tumor (I.29) cells apparently lose the expression but in vivo transferred cells maintain Lna-1 expression, one can draw a parallel with MEL-14 antigen expression discussed above. However, no further biochemical or functional analysis of the cells expressing the antigen has been reported.

XIII. CONCLUDING REMARKS

We have discussed a number of the rapidly growing series of Ly antigens and other cell-surface markers which have proven useful in the analysis of T-cell differentiation. Much of the complexity for some of the antigens, such as Ly-6, remains to be resolved, and several of the newer antigens and markers need to be compared to determine their interrelationships. It is our hope that this review serves to clarify some of the complexities produced by application of various serological techniques in different laboratories and provides a framework for continuing investigations. Toward this end we have compiled a summary table (Table 1) of the characteristics of T-cell antigens detected by mAb that have been reported in the literature. While this listing does not ensure availability of all of these reagents, it may serve to alert interested colleagues to potential sources and provide an outline for description of new antigens or specificities useful for the study of T-cell differentiation.

ACKNOWLEDGMENTS

We especially wish to thank Theresa Gregorio, Susan Charbonneau, Julie Masiello, and the members of the Leukocyte Differentiation Section and Laboratory of Experimental Immunology, who have tolerated the aberrant behavior of B. J. M. during the generation of this chapter. We also are indebted to Drs. John Ortaldo, Margaret Beckwith, and Kristin Komschlies, who have patiently corrected errors at various stages of preparation of this manuscript. We are particularly indebted to the Editors for their patience and kindness.

ABBREVIATIONS

B6	C57BL/6.
B10	C57BL/10.
C	complement.
CD	cluster determinant.
CFU-S	colony-forming unit in the spleen.
CR	cross-reactive (determinant).
CRT	cortisone-resistant thymocytes.
CTL	cytotoxic T lymphocyte.
FCA	flow cytometry analysis.
$Fc\gamma$-R	receptor for the Fc portion of immunoglobulin.
HEV	high endothelial venules.
HSA	heat-stable antigen.
IF	immunofluorescence.

Table 1 Monoclonal Antibodies (mAbs) to Cell-Surface Markers

				mAbs[a]			
Antigen	CD	MW x 10^{-3}	Major cell reactivity	Clones	Specificity	Ig Isotype	Ref.
TL	(CD1?)	45(12)[b]	Thymocytes, Lymphomas, Leukemias	TL.1;12/190	TL.1	IgG2aκ	16
				TL.2;18/407	TL.2	IgG2aκ	16
				TL.3;18/20	TL.3	IgG2aκ	16
				TL.4;G	TL.4	IgG2aκ	15
				TL.5	TL.5	IgG2κ	15
				TL.6;79	TL.6	IgG2κ	15
				TL.7;F	TL.7	IgMk	15
				TL.8;129	TL.8	IgMk	15
				TL.9;I	TL.9	IgG2aλ	15
Thy-1 (Θ) (Theta)		25	Thymocytes T cells, NK cells, brain	G7	Framework Thy-1	rIg2c[c]	46
				30-H12	Thy-1.2	rIgG2b	86
				J1j.10	Thy-1.2	rIgM	231
				AT83A	Thy-1.2	rIgM	412
				4D11	Thy-1.2	rIgM	97
				F7D5	Thy-1.2	IgM	413
				HO-13-4[d]	Thy-1.2	IgM	414
				23-64.10	Thy-1.2	IgG1κ	415
				6/68	Thy-1.2	IgM	416
				37-3-1	Thy-1.2	IgM	417
				HO-22-1	Thy-1.1	IgM	414
				T11D7e2[d]	Thy-1.1	IgM	413
				T32B11	Thy-1.1	IgG2	413

Ly-1	CD5	67	Thymocytes	53-7.313	Framework Ly-1	rIgG2a	86
				2F10	Framework Ly-1	rIgM	97
(Ly-A)			T cells	39/3	Ly-1.1	IgG_3[e]	417
(Lyt-1)			Subset of T cells	39/107	Ly-1.1	IgM	39
				W3	Ly-1.1		359
				18.2.3	Ly-1.1	IgG2κ	417
				41-16.5	Ly-1.1	IgMκ	417
				7-20.6/3	Ly-1.1	IgG2aκ	73
				3-3.1	Ly-1.2	IgG2aκ	417
				C3PO	Ly-1.2	IgM	418
Ly-2	CD8a	34,38	Subsets of	53-6.72	Framework Ly-2	rIgG2b	86
			thymocytes	H35-17.2	Framework Ly-2	rIgG2b	419
(Ly-B)			and T cells	3.155[d]	Framework Ly-2	rIgM	109
(Ly-2)				2.43[d]	Ly-2.2	rIgG2b	109
				19/178	Ly-2.2	IgG2aκ	301
				HO-2.2 [AD4(15)][d]	Ly-2.2	IgM	420
				41-3.48	Ly-2.2	IgM	76
				116-13.1	Ly-2.1	IgG2a	417
				49-11.1[d]	Ly-2.1	IgG2aκ	415
				49-14.2[d]	Ly-2.1	IgG1κ	415
				49-31.1	Ly-2.1	IgG3κ	415
				49-19.1	Ly-2.1	IgMκ[f]	415
Ly-3	CD8b	30	Subsets of	HO-3.1 [F9(1)]	Ly-3.1	IgM	420
(Ly-C)			thymocytes	53-5	Ly-3/Ly-3.2	rIg	118
(Lyt-3)			and T cells				
Ly-4	CD4	55	Subsets of	GK1.5	Ly-4a (Framework)	rIgG2b	63,80

(Continued)

Table 1 *(Continued)*

Antigen	CD	MW x 10^{-3}	Major cell reactivity	mAbs[a] Clones	Specificity	Ig Isotype	Ref.
(L3T4)			thymocytes and	H129.19	Ly-4a (Framework)	rIgG	104
			T cells	RL172-4	Ly-4 (Framework)	rIgM	137
				2B6	Ly-4b (Framework)	rIgm	97
Ly-5	CD45	195,200,	All leukocytes	A-20	Ly-5.1[h]	IgG2aκ	417
(LCA)		220[g]		104-2	Ly-5.2[h]	IgG2aκ	417
(T200)		220[g]	T cells/B cells	13/2	T200-B220	rIgG2b	170
				M1/9.3	T200/B220	rIgG2a	171
				M1/89	T200/B220	rIgG2b	171
	CD45R	T195-205	Subset of T cells only	B5-528E	T195-205	rIgM	173
(B220)		220	B cells only	RA3-3A1	B220	rIgM	174
		220	$Ly-2^+$ T cells	14.8.8	B220	rIgG2b	176
			and B cells	14D10	B220	rIgG2b	175
				100C5	B220	rIgG2b	180
				6B2	B220	r?	174
Ly-15	CD11a	180(95)[i]	Lymphocytes	H35-89.9	LFA-1	rIgG	185
				M14/7	LFA-1	rIgG2a	184
				8-6.2	Ly-15.2	IgG2a	194
Mac-1	CD11b	170(95)[i]	Macrophages	M1/70	Mac-1	rIgG	186
Ly-6		34	Blasts, LN[j],	S8.106	Ly-6A.2	IgG2aκ	421
(old Ly-8)			Spl, T > B, non-	S7.81	Ly-6A.2	IgG2bκ	421
(DAG)			lymphoid cells	34-11-3S	Ly-6A.2	IgG2aκ	422
			(Thc, BM low)	162	Ly-6A.2	?	389

(Gm-2.2)		Granulocytes	SK38.86	Ly-6B.2	IgG2aκ	197
		and BM	5119-4/7	Ly-6B.2	IgG3	202
(MG-1/Gma-1.2)			B38	Ly-6B.2	IgG2aλ	203[k]
	12-15	LN, Spl, BM	H0/25	Ly-6C.2	IgM	423
		blasts, PMNs	SK140.112	Ly-6C.2	IgMk	197
		(Thc low)	SK.142.446	Ly-6C.2	IgM	197
(old Ly-28.2)			5075-3.6	Ly-6C.2	IgG2b	207
			5075-12.1[d]	Ly-6C.2	IgG2a	207
			5095-16.6	Ly-6C.2	IgM	207
			34-2-11S	Ly-6C.2	IgG2a	422
			34-10-7S	Ly-6C.2	IgG2b	422
			6-C-3	Ly-6C Framework	rIgG2a	204
	12-15	Blasts, Thc,	SK142.476	Ly-6D.2	IgMk	197
(old Ly-27.2)		LN, Spl, BM	5075-19.1	Ly-6D.2	IgG1	207
	34,56		5041-24.2	Ly-6D.2	IgG2a	424
(Ala-1)	12-18 kd	Blasts, low on	SK70.94	Ly-6E.1	IgG2a	197
		normal lymphoid	SK70.36	Ly-6E.1	IgM	197
		tissues, non-	HD-42	Ly-6E.1	IgG2a	425
		lymphoid cells	D7	Ly-6E.1,2/A.2	rIgG	198[l]
(MALA-1)			YE3/19.1	Ly-6E.1,2/A.2	rIgG	426
ThB		Thymocytes,	41-h4[d]	ThB	rIgG2c	210
		B cells, BM	53-9.2	ThB	rIgG2c	86
			17C9	ThB	rIgG2a	175
			4B9	(?ThB)	rIgG2c	175
Ly-9	100	All lymphocytes	30C7	Lgp100/Ly-9.1	rIgG2a	212
(Lgp100)			M7/83	Lgp100	rIgG2b	184
(T100)			20-1.5[d]	Ly-9.2	IgG2a	213
Ly-22		Suppressor	T28.45	Ly-22.2	IgG2bκ	224
		T cells				

(continues)

Table 1 *(Continued)*

Antigen LC-24	CD	MW x 10^{-3}	Major cell Reactivity	mAbs[a] Clones	Specificity	Ig Isotype	Ref.
Ly-24		100	PMNs, macs	142/5	Ly-24 Framework	rIgGa	227
(Pgp-1)			Thc and T cell	IM7	Ly-24 Framework	rIgG2b	227
(9F3)			subsets	9F3	Ly-24 Framework	IgG2b	427
				RAMBM44	Ly-24.1	rIgM	226
				AMF-8	Ly-24.2	rIgG2a	225
				C71/26	Ly-24.2	rIgM	226
HSA		35-40	Thc BM RBC,	M1/69	HSA	rIgG	171
		48, 52[g]	B-cell subset	J11d	(HSA)	rIgGm	231
				B2A2	(HSA)	rIgM	236
TcR		40-45	T cells	KJ16-133.18	Vβ8	rIgG	242
(Ti)				F23.1	Vβ8	IgG2aκ	243
				KJ23a	Vβ8	IgG	405
IL-2-R	CD25	55(20,110)	Activated T	7D4	IL-2-R	rIgM	258
(TAC)			and B cells,	2E4	IL-2-R	rIgG	258
			Ly-4$^+$ T subset,	PC61.5.18	IL-2-R	rIgG1	259
			The precursors	3C7	IL-2-R[m]	rIgG	258
				AMT-13	IL-2-R[m]	rIgG2a	257
Ly-17	(CD16)	52	B cells, macs,	2.4G2	FcγR	rIgG[n]	267
(FcγR)			NK cells	K7.234[d]	Ly-17.2[o]	IgMκ	270
(Ly-m20)			T cells	K9.361[d]	Ly-17.2[o]	IgG2aκ	270
Qa-2	—	40(12)[b]	T and B cells,	D3.262	Qa-2	IgM	298
			NK cells,	141-15.8	Qa-2	IgG2bκ	299

		Thc and BM subsets	141-16.6	Qa-2	IgG2bκ	299
			Y-7	Qa-2	IgM	281
			B16-146	Qa-4	IgM	301
			B16-167	Qa-5	IgM	301
			5035-50.1	Qa-m7	IgM	302
			5035-24.1	Qa-m8	IgG3	302
			5034-54.8	Qa-m9	IgG1	305
			20-8-4	Qa/CR H-2K^{b},D^{b} K^{d},H-2^{sr}	IgG2aκ	308
			34-1-2	Qa/CR H-2K^{d},D^{d}, K^{b},H-2$^{s\ r\ p\ q}$	IgG2aκ	308
(Qa-m208)			6.3.4	Qa/CR H-2K^{b},K^{d} H-2$^{p\ r\ s}$	IgM	309
Ly-7		T < B cells, blasts,	BD5-334.5	Ly-7.1^{h}	IgG1κ	345
		(Thc low)	BD5-96.6	Ly-7.3	IgG1κ	346
Tpre	28,33,38	Fetal Thc	F.6.9.1	Tpre	IgMκ	350
Tthy	18,28,38,47	Thc subset	17IIC6^{d}	Tthy^{d}	IgMκ	348
Tsu	18,28,33	T suppressors	13IIIB4	Tsu^{d} factor	IgG1κ	349
Tind	18-28,45,62	T inducers	9IIIA2	Tind^{d}	IgG1κ	349
Ly-10	80,34	Thc, macs, BM	3/214	Ly-10.1/4F2	IgM	359
(murine 4F2)	86,39	Blasts, T and B lymphocytes, (brain, liver, kidney)	RL388	4F2/Ly-10?	rIg	364

(continues)

Table 1 *(Continued)*

Antigen	CD	MW x 10^{-3}	Major cell Reactivity	mAbs[a] Clones	Specificity	Ig Isotype	Ref.
Activation antigen CELL-SURFA		55	Thc, T and B cells, macs, fibroblasts	RL119	??	rIg	364
				RL73	??	rIgG2a	364
Ly-18			Thc, subsets of T and B cells, BM (brain, liver, kidney)	S8.261	Ly-18.2	IgM	387
Ly-19			T and B cells Thc and BM subsets	K10.6	Ly-19.2	IgG2bκ	368
Ly-21			Thc, T cells, and BM	—	Ly-21.2	IgG2a	381
Ly-23			Lymphocyte subsets and non-lymphoid tissue	BP/12	Ly-23.2	IgM	385
				BP/32	Ly-23.2	IgM	385
Ly-25			Lymphocytes, BM	5069-1.1	Ly-25.1	IgG2a	386
Ly-26			B cells, BM and null cells	5075-17.10	Ly-26.1	IgG2a	388
				5075-7.10[d]	Ly-26.1	IgM	388
Ly-27			Thc, T and B cells	1.13	Ly-27.2	IgG2a	389
β_2-microglobulin		12	B cells, etc.		β_2-M	IgG2b	382
Ly-29			B cells, Thc BM and T cell subsets	S-459-77.2	Ly-29.2	IgG2bκ	371

Ly-30			Subsets of T cells, B cells, and BM, liver and kidney	S-459-24.1	Ly-30.2	IgG/κ	390
Ly-31			Subsets of Thc	N1.10	Ly-31.1	IgG2bκ	372
			T and B cells, BM and PBL				
J_t			T-cell subset	Jk.18[d]	J_t/I-J	IgM	375
Leugp90		90	B > T	3MB1		rIgG	391
MEL-14 (Homing-receptor)			T and B cells, Thc subsets	MEL-14	Homing receptor	rIgG2a	392
FT-1		130	Fetal Thc	M6	FT-1	IgM	401
FT-2		–	Fetal Thc	C21	FT-2	IgM	402
	CD3	20	T cells, Thc	145-2C11	Framework CD3e	hIgG[p]	404

[a]Commercial sources for mAb are not indicated because equivalent reagents are often available from the American Type Tissue Culture Collection (ATCC) or individual investigators. This table lists most reagents reported in the literature. Several mAb not available outside of the reporting laboratory have not been listed, and listing here does not assure current availability.

[b]The 12-Kd protein co-precipitated with MHC class I antigens is β_2-microglobulin (see text). This molecule can be detected by a mAb originally called Ly-m11 (382).

[c]An "r" before the isotype of the mAb indicates that it is the Ig product of a rat-mouse or rat-rat hybridoma.

[d]Other hybridoma clones with similar specificity and isotype were reported by these same investigators. (Note *d* in Table indicates the allelic specificity detected.)

[e]The isotype previously indicated in the older ATCC listing is erroneous.

[f]This IgM mAb was reported to be noncytotoxic.

[g]The molecular weight of the antigen is dependent on the type of cells used in the precipitation.

[h]Note that the allelic nomenclature has been revised.

[i]The 95-Kd protein co-precipitated is the β chain shared by this family of molecules.

(continues)

(Table 1 footnotes--continued)

[j]Abbreviations for tissue sources or cells used in this table: LN, lymph node; Spl, spleen; Thc, thymocytes; BM, bone marrow; macs, macrophages; PMNs, polymorphonuclear leucocytes; "blasts" refers to lymphocyte blast cells activated by mitogens or alloantigens. T > B is used to indicate a higher expression of the antigen on T cells than on B cells.
[k]Dr. F. -W. Shen and G. Viamontes, unpublished data.
[l]This antibody, described by R.G.E. Palfree et al., was obtained from Drs. T.R. Malek and E.M. Shevach, NIAID, Bethesda, Maryland.
[m]mAb 3C7 and AMT-13 can inhibit binding of the IL-2 ligand to its receptor, implying that the Ab recognizes the receptor-binding site.
[n]Extensive contamination of mouse fusion-partner light chain is produced by this hybridoma.
[o]Previously reported as Ly-m20.2.
[p]The designation 'h' is for the hamster-derived mAb.

Ig	immunoglobulin.
Igh	Ig heavy chain allotype gene locus.
IL-1, IL-2	interleukin 1, interleukin 2.
IL-2-R	interleukin 2 receptor.
Kd	kilodalton.
LCA	leukocyte common antigen.
LFA-1	lymphocyte function-associated antigen-1.
mAb	monoclonal antibody.
mAb + C'	mAb (Ab) plus complement for antibody-dependent complement-mediated lysis.
MHC	major histocompatibility complex.
NK cells	natural killer cells.
RFLP	restriction fragment length polymorphism.
RI	recombinant inbred (strains of mice).
TcR	T-cell receptor (also Ti).
TL	thymus leukemia antigen.

REFERENCES

1. L. J. Old, E. A. Boyse, and E. Stockert, Antigenic properties of experimental leukemias. I. Serological studies *in vitro* with spontaneous and radiation-induced leukemias, *J. Natl. Cancer Inst., 31*: 977 (1963).
2. E. A. Boyse, L. J. Old, and S. Luell, Antigenic properties of experimental leukemias. II. Immunological studies *in vivo* with C57BL/6 radiation-induced leukemias, *J. Natl. Cancer Inst., 31*: 987 (1963).
3. E. A. Boyse, L. J. Old, and E. Stockert, TL (thymus leukemia) antigen: A review, in *Immunopathology IVth International Symposium* (P. Grabar and P. A. Miescher, eds.), Schwabe & Co, Basel, Switzerland, 1965, pp. 23-40.
4. A. E. Reif, and J. M. V. Allen, Specificity of isoantisera against leukemic and thymic lymphocytes, *Nature, 200*: 1332 (1963).
5. A. E. Reif, and J. M. V. Allen, The AKR thymic antigen and its distribution in leukemias and nervous tissues, *J. Exp. Med., 120*: 413 (1964).
6. M. Amiot, A. Bernard, B. Baynal, W. Knapp, C. Deschildre, and L. Boumsell, Heterogeneity of the first cluster of differentiation: Characterization and epitopic mapping of three CD1 molecules on normal human thymus cells, *J. Immunol., 136*: 1752 (1986).
7. L. J. Old, and E. Stockert, Immunogenetics of cell surface antigens of mouse leukemias, *Annu. Rev. Genet., 17*: 127 (1977).
8. L. Flaherty, T1a-region antigens, in *The Role of the Major Histocompatibility Complex in Immunobiology* (M. E. Dorf, ed.), STPM Press, Garland, New York, 1981, pp. 33-57.
9. L. Hood, M. Steinmetz, and B. Malissen, Genes of the major histocompatibility complex of the mouse, *Annu. Rev. Immunol., 1*: 529 (1983)
10. E. A. Boyse, The biology of T1a, *Cell, 38*: 1 (1984).

11. E. Leckband, and E. A. Boyse, Immunocompetent cells among mouse thymocytes: A minor population, *Science, 172*: 1258 (1971).
12. S. Konda, Y. Nakao, and R. T. Smith, Immunologic properties of mouse thymus cells: Identification of T cell functions within a minor, low-density subpopulation, *J. Exp. Med., 136*: 1461 (1972).
13. S. Konda, E. Stockert, and R. T. Smith, Immunologic properties of mouse thymus cells: Membrane antigen patterns associated with various cell subpopulations, *Cell. Immunol., 7*: 275 (1973).
14. B. J. Mathieson, and B. J. Fowlkes, Cell surface antigen expression on thymocytes: Development and phenotypic differentiation of intrathymic subsets, *Immunol. Rev., 82*: 141 (1984).
15. H. Lemke, G. J. Hammerling, and U. Hammerling, Fine specificity analysis with monoclonal antibodies of antigens controlled by the major histocompatibility complex and by the Qa/TL region in mice, *Immunol. Rev., 47*: 175 (1979).
16. F.-W. Shen, M. J. Chorney, and E. A. Boyse, Further polymorphism of the *Tla* locus defined by monoclonal TL antibodies, *Immunogenetics, 15*: 573 (1982).
17. K. R. McIntyre, E. S. Vitetta, U. Hammerling, J. Michaelson, L. Flaherty, and J. W. Uhr, Analysis of thymus-leukemia (TL) antigens with monoclonal antibodies, *J. Immunol., 125*: 601 (1980).
18. K. R. McIntyre, U. Hammerling, J. W. Uhr, and E. S. Vitetta, Structural analysis of thymus-leukemia (TL) antigens in the mouse, *J. Immunol., 128*: 1712 (1982).
19. J. Michaelson, J.-S. Tung, L. Flaherty, U. Hammerling, and Y. Bushkin, The biochemical genetics of TL antigens on mouse thymocytes, *Eur. J. Immunol., 12*: 257 (1982).
20. J. Michaelson, E. A. Boyse, L. Ciccia, L. Flaherty, E. Fleissner, E. Garnick, U. Hammerling, M. Lawrence, P. Mauch, and F.-W. Shen, Biochemical genetics of TL antigens, *Immunogenetics,* in press.
21. E. S. Vitetta, J. W. Uhr, and E. A. Boyse, Association of a β_2-microglobulin-like subunit with H-2 and TL alloantigens on murine thymocytes, *J. Immunol., 114*: 252 (1975).
22. H. Anundi, L. Rask, L. Ostberg, and P. A. Peterson, The subunit structure of thymus leukemia antigens, *Biochemistry, 14*: 5046 (1975).
23. E. Rothenberg, Specific biosynthetic marker for immature thymic lymphoblasts: Active synthesis of thymus-leukemia antigen restricted to proliferating cells, *J. Exp. Med., 155*: 140 (1982).
24. E. A. Boyse, E. Stockert, and L. J. Old, Modification of the antigenic structure of the cell membrane by thymus-leukemia (TL) antibody, *Proc. Natl. Acad. Sci. USA, 58*: 954 (1967).
25. M. E. Lamm, E. A. Boyse, L. J. Old, B. Lisowska-Bernstein, and E. Stockert, Modulation of TL (thymus-leukemia) antigens by Fab-fragments of TL antibody, *J. Immunol., 101*: 99 (1968).
26. C. W. Stackpole, J. B. Jacobson, and M. P. Lardis, Antigenic modulation *in vitro*. I. Fate of thymus-leukemia (TL) antigen-antibody complexes follow-

ing modulation of TL antigenicity from the surfaces of mouse leukemia cells and thymocytes, *J. Exp. Med., 140*: 939 (1974).
27. Y. T. Chen, Y. Obata, E. Stockert, and L. J. Old, Thymus-leukemia (TL) antigens of the mouse. Analysis of TL mRNA and TL cDNA TL^+ and TL^- strains, *J. Exp. Med., 162*: 1134 (1985).
28. M. Steinmetz, A. Winoto, K. Minard, and L. Hood, Clusters of genes encoding mouse transplantation antigens, *Cell, 28*: 489 (1982).
29. A. Winoto, M. Steinmetz, and L. Hood, Genetic mapping in the major histocompatibility complex by restriction enzyme site polymorphisms: Most mouse class I genes map to the *Tla* complex, *Proc. Natl. Acad. Sci. USA, 80*: 3425 (1983).
30. E. H. Weiss, L. Golden, K. Fahrner, A. L. Mellor, J. J. Devlin, H. Bullman, H. Tiddens, H. Bud, and R. A. Flavell, Organization and evolution of the class I gene family in the major histocompatibility complex of the C57BL/10 mouse, *Nature, 310*: 650 (1984).
31. M. C. Raff, Theta isoantigen as a marker of thymus-derived lymphocytes in mice, *Nature (Lond.), 224*: 378 (1969).
32. M. C. Raff, Evidence for subpopulation of mature lymphocytes within mouse thymus, *Nature (New Biology, London), 229*: 182 (1971).
33. C. G. Fathman, M. Small, L. A. Herzenberg, and I. L. Weissman, Thymus cell maturation. II. Differentiation of three "mature" subclasses *in vivo, Cell. Immunol., 15*: 109 (1975).
34. K. Shortman, D. S. Linthicum, F. L. Battye, I. Goldschneider, A. Liabeuf, P. Golstein, E. A. Clark, and P. Lake, Cytotoxic and fluorescent assays for thymocyte subpopulations differing in surface Thy-1 level, *Cell Biophys., 1*: 255 (1979).
35. D. G. Campbell, J. Gagnon, K. B. M. Reid, and A. F. Williams, Rat brain Thy-1 glycoprotein, *Biochem. J., 195*: 15 (1981).
36. W. Jefferies, et al., in *Comparative Aspects of Differentiation Antigens in Lymphohemopoietic Tissues* (Z. Trnka and M. Miyasaka, eds.), Marcel Dekker, Inc., New York, 1988.
37. R. B. Herberman, M. E. Nunn, and H. T. Holden, Low density of Thy 1 antigen on mouse effector cells mediating natural cytotoxicity against tumor cells, *J. Immunol. 121*: 304 (1978).
38. M. J. Mattes, S. O. Sharrow, R. B. Herberman, and H. T. Holden, Identification and separation of Thy-1 positive mouse spleen cells active in natural cytotoxicity and antibody-dependent cell-mediated cytotoxicity, *J. Immunol., 126*: 2851 (1979).
39. G. C. Koo, J. B. Jacobson, G. J. Hammerling, and U. Hammerling, Antigenic profile of murine natural killer cells, *J. Immunol., 125*: 1003 (1980).
40. R. H. Wiltrout, B. J. Mathieson, J. E. Talmadge, C. W. Reynolds, S.-R. Zhang, R. B. Herberman, and J. R. Ortaldo, Augmentation of organ-associated natural killer activity by biological response modifiers: Isolation and characterization of large granular lymphocytes from the liver, *J. Exp. Med., 160*: 1431 (1984).

41. P. R. Bergstresser, R. E. Tigelaar, J. H. Dees, and J. W. Streilein, Thy-1 antigen-bearing dendritic cells populate murine epidermis, *J. Invest. Dermatol., 81*: 286 (1983).
42. P. R. Bergstresser, R. E. Tigelaar, and J. W. Streilein, Thy-1 antigen-bearing dendritic cells in murine epidermis are derived from bone marrow precursors, *J. Invest. Dermatol., 83*: 83 (1984).
43. N. Romani, G. Stingl, E. Tschachler, M. D. Witmer, R. M. Steinman, E. M. Shevach, and G. Schuler, The Thy-1-bearing cell of murine epidermis: A distinctive leukocyte perhaps related to natural killer cells, *J. Exp. Med., 161*: 1368 (1985).
44. M. A. Ritter, R. J. Morris, and I. Goldschneider, Hidden Thy-1 antigen in a subpopulation of mouse bone marrow cells, *Immunology, 39*: 375 (1980).
45. V. C. Maino, M. A. Norcross, M. S. Perkins, and R. T. Smith, Mechanism of Thy-1-mediated T cell activation: Roles of Fc receptors, T200, Ia, and H-2 glycoproteins in accessory cell function, *J. Immunol., 126*: 1829 (1981).
46. K. C. Gunter, T. R. Malek, and E. M. Shevach, T cell-activating properties of an anti-Thy-1 monoclonal antibody, *J. Exp. Med., 159*: 716 (1984).
47. H. R. MacDonald, C. Bron, M. Rousseaux, C. Horvath, and J.-C. Cerottini, Production and characterization of monoclonal anti-Thy-1 antibodies that stimulate lymphokine production by cytolytic T cell clones, *Eur. J. Immunol., 15*: 495 (1985).
48. R. A. Kroczek, K. C. Gunter, R. N. Germain, and E. M. Shevach, Thy-1 functions as a signal transduction molecule in T lymphocytes and transfected B lymphocytes, *Nature, 322*: 181 (1986).
49. A. F. Williams, and J. Gagnon, Neuronal cell Thy-1 glycoproteins: Homology with immunoglobulin, *Science, 216*: 696 (1982).
50. T. Seki, H.-C. Chang, H. Ploegh, and J. Silver, A hydrophobic transmembrane segment at the carboxyl terminus of Thy-1, *Science, 227*: 649 (1985).
51. A. F. Williams, Immunoglobulin-related domains for cell surface recognition, *Nature, 314*: 579 (1985).
52. A. G. D. Tse, A. N. Barclay, A. Watts, and A. F. Williams, A glycophospholipid tail at the carboxyl terminus of the Thy-1 glycoprotein of neurons and thymocytes, *Science, 230*: 1003 (1985).
53. H. C. Morse, III, F.-W. Shen, and U. Hammerling, Genetic nomenclature for loci controlling murine lymphocyte antigens, *Immunogenetics,* in press.
54. E. A. Boyse, H. Cantor, F.-W. Shen, and I. F. C. McKenzie, Nomenclature for antigens demonstrable on lymphocytes, *Immunogenetics, 5*: 189 (1977).
55. M. Schlesinger, Antigens of the thymus, *Prog. Allergy, 16*: 214 (1972).
56. I. F. C. McKenzie, and T. Potter, Murine lymphocyte surface antigens, *Adv. Immunol., 27*: 179 (1979).
57. P. M. Hogarth, and I. F. C. McKenzie, Lymphocyte antigens, in *Fundamental Immunology* (W. E. Paul, ed.), Raven Press, New York, 1985, pp. 457-477.
58. R. Scollay, and K. Shortman, Thymocyte subpopulations: An experimental review, including flow cytometric cross-correlations between the major murine thymocyte markers, *Thymus, 5*: 245 (1983).
59. O. Stutman, Postthymic T-cell development, *Immunol. Rev., 91*: 159 (1986).

60. J. Sprent, M. Schaefer, D. Lo, and R. Korngold, Functions of purified L3T4$^+$ and Lyt-2$^+$ cells *in vitro* and *in vivo, Immunol. Rev., 91*: 195 (1986).
61. E. A. Boyse, M. Miyazawa, T. Aoki, and L. J. Old, Ly-A and Ly-B: Two systems of lymphocyte isoantigens in the mouse, *Proc. R. Soc. Lond.* (*Biol.*), *170*: 175 (1968).
62. E. A. Boyse, K. Itakura, E. Stockert, C. A. Iritani, and M. Miura, Ly-C: A third locus specifying alloantigens expressed only on thymocytes and lymphocytes, *Transplantation, 11*: 351 (1971).
63. D. P. Dialynas, Z. S. Quan, K. A. Wall, A. Pierres, J. Quintans, M. R. Loken, M. Pierres, and F. W. Fitch, Characterization of the murine T cell surface molecule, designated L3T4, identified by monoclonal antibody GK1.5: Similarity of L3T4 to the human Leu-3 T4 molecule, *J. Immunol., 131*: 2445 (1983).
64. P. Kosielow, J. A. Hirst, H. Shiku, P. C. L. Beverley, M. K. Hoffman, E. A. Boyse, and H. F. Oettgen, Ly antigens as markers for functionally distinct subpopulations of thymus-derived lymphocytes of the mouse, *Nature* (*Lond*), *253*: 219 (1975).
65. H. Cantor, and E. A. Boyse, Functional subclasses of T lymphocytes bearing different Ly antigens. I. The generation of functionally distinct T-cell subclasses is a differentiative process independent of antigen, *J. Exp. Med., 141*: 1376 (1975).
66. H. Cantor, and E. A. Boyse, Functional subclasses of T lymphocytes bearing different Ly antigens. II. Cooperation between subclasses of Ly$^+$ cells in the generation of killer activity, *J. Exp. Med., 141*: 1390 (1975).
67. M. Feldmann, P. C. L. Beverley, M. Dunkley, and S. Kontiainen, Different Ly antigen phenotypes of *in vitro* induced helper and suppressor cells, *Nature, 258*: 614 (1975).
68. J. Jandinski, H. Cantor, T. Tadakuma, D. L. Peavy, and C. W. Pierce, Separation of helper T cells from suppressor T cells expressing different Ly components. I. Polyclonal activation: Suppressor and helper activities are inherent properties of distinct T-cell subclasses, *J. Exp. Med., 143*: 1382 (1976).
69. H. Shiku, P. Kiseilow, M. A. Bean, E. A. Takahashi, E. A. Boyse, H. F. Ottegen, and L. J. Old, Expression of T-cell differentiation antigens on effector cells in cell-mediated cytotoxicity *in vitro*: Evidence for functional heterogeneity related to the surface phenotype of T cells, *J. Exp. Med., 141*: 227 (1975).
70. O. Stutman, F.-W. Shen, and E. A. Boyse, Ly phenotype of T-cells cytotoxic for syngeneic mouse mammary tumors: Evidence for T-cell interactions, *Proc. Natl. Acad. Sci. USA, 74*: 5667 (1977).
71. P. J. Wettstein, D. W. Bailey, L. E. Mobraaten, J. Klein, and J. A. Frelinger, T lymphocyte response to H-2 mutants. I. Proliferation is dependent on Ly-1+, 2+ cells, *J. Exp. Med., 147*: 1395 (1978).
72. J.-C. Cerottini, and H. R. MacDonald, Limiting dilution analysis of alloantigen-reactive T lymphocytes. V. Lyt phenotype of cytolytic T lymphocyte presursors reactive against normal and mutant H-2 antigens, *J. Immunol., 126*: 490 (1981).

73. P. M. Hogarth, T. A. Potter, F. N. Cornell, R. McLachlan, and I. F. C. McKenzie, Monoclonal antibodies to murine cell surface antigens. I. Lyt-1.1, *J. Immunol., 125*: 1618 (1980).
74. B. J. Mathieson, S. O. Sharrow, P. S. Campbell, and R. Asofsky, An Lyt differentiated thymocyte subpopulation detected by flow microfluorometry, *Nature, 277*: 478 (1979).
75. I. Betel, B. J. Mathieson, S. O. Sharrow, and R. Asofsky, Distribution of Lyt phenotypes in thymocyte subpopulations as measured by flow microfluorometry: Selective enrichment of Lyt $1^{+}23^{-}$ thymocytes. *J. Immunol., 124*: 2209 (1980).
76. T. A. Potter, P. M. Hogarth, and I. F. C. McKenzie, Flow microfluorometric analysis of alloantigen expression during T cell development, *Eur. J. Immunol., 10*: 899 (1980).
77. J. A. Ledbetter, R. V. Rouse, H. S. Micklem, and L. A. Herzenberg, T cell subsets defined by expression of Lyt- 1, 2, 3 and Thy-1 antigens. Two-parameter immunofluorescence and cytotoxicity analysis with monoclonal antibodies modified current views, *J. Exp. Med., 152*: 280 (1980).
78. S. L. Swain, A. Bakke, M. English, and R. W. Dutton, Ly phenotypes and MHC recognition: The allohelper that recognizes K or D is a mature Ly123 cell, *J. Immunol., 123*: 2716 (1979).
79. S. L. Swain, Significance of Lyt phenotypes: Lyt-2 antibodies block activities of T cells that recognize class 1 major histocompatibility complex antigens regardless of their function, *Proc. Natl. Acad. Sci. USA 78*: 7101 (1981).
80. D. P. Dialynas, D. B. Wilde, P. Marrack, A. Pierres, K. A. Wall, W. Havran, G. Otten, M. R. Loken, M. Pierres, J. Kappler, and F. W. Fitch, Characterization of the murine antigenic determinant, designated L3T4a, recognized by monoclonal antibody GK1.5: Expression of L3T4a by functional T cell clones appears to correlate primarily with class II MHC antigen-reactivity, *Immunol. Rev., 74*: 29 (1983).
81. W. M. Leiserson, B. J. Fowlkes, T. M. Chused, and B. J. Mathieson, Analysis of a new thymus subpopulation delineated by Ly-1 and Ly-2 surface markers, in *Intracellular Communication in Leukocyte Function* (J. W. Parker and R. L. O'Brien, eds.), J. Wiley and Sons Ltd, Chichester, England, 1983, pp. 181-184.
82. B. J. Fowlkes, L. Edison, B. Mathieson, and T. M. Chused, Differentiation *in vitro* of an adult precursor thymocyte, in *Regulation of the Immune System* (H. Cantor, L. Chess and E. Sercarz, eds.), Alan R. Liss, Inc., New York, 1984, pp. 275-293.
83. B. J. Fowlkes, L. Edison, B. J. Mathieson, and T. M. Chused, Early T lymphocytes. Differentiation *in vivo* of adult intrathymic precursor cells, *J. Exp. Med., 162*: 802 (1985).
84. J. Klein, List of congenic lines of mice. I. Lines with differences at alloantigen loci, *Transplantation, 15*: 137 (1973).
85. P. J. Durda, C. Shapiro, and P. D. Gottlieb, Partial molecular characterization of the Ly-1 alloantigen on mouse thymocytes, *J. Immunol., 120*:53 (1978).
86. J. A. Ledbetter, and L. A. Herzenberg, Xenogeneic monoclonal antibodies to mouse lymphoid differentiation antigens, *Immunol. Rev., 47*: 63 (1979).

87. N. Watanabe, S. Kojima, F.-W. Shen, and Z. Ovary, Suppression of IgE antibody production in SJL mice. II. Expression of Ly-1 antigen on helper and nonspecific suppressor T cells, *J. Immunol., 118*: 485 (1977).
88. K. Pickel, and M. K. Hoffmann, The Ly phenotype of suppressor T cells arising in mice subjected to a graft-versus-host reaction, *J. Exp. Med., 145*: 1169 (1977).
89. L. L. Lanier, N. L. Warner, J. A. Ledbetter, and L. A. Herzenberg, Expression of Lyt-1 antigen on certain murine B cell lymphomas, *J. Exp. Med., 153*: 998 (1981).
90. V. Manohar, E. Brown, W. M. Leiserson, and T. M. Chused, Expression of Lyt-1 by a subset of B lymphocytes, *J. Immunol., 129*:532 (1982).
91. K. Hayakawa, R. R. Hardy, D. R. Parks, and L. A. Herzenberg, The "Ly-1" B cell subpopulation in normal, immunodefective, and autoimmune mice, *J. Exp. Med., 157*: 202 (1983).
92. J. Braun, Spontaneous *in vitro* occurrence and long-term culture of murine B lymphoblast cell lines, *J. Immunol., 130*: 2113 (1983).
93. W. F. Davidson, T. N. Frederickson, E. K. Rudikoff, R. L. Coffman, J. W. Hartley, and H. C. Morse III, A unique series of lymphomas related to the Ly-1$^+$ lineage of B lymphocyte differentiation, *J. Immunol., 133*: 744 (1984).
94. I. Royston, J. Majda, S. Baird, B. Meserve, and S. Griffiths, Human T cell antigens defined by monoclonal antibodies: The 65,000 dalton antigen of T cells (T65) is also found on chronic lymphocytic leukemia cells bearing surface immunoglobulin, *J. Immunol., 125*: 725 (1980).
95. M. Michaelides, P. M. Hogarth, and I. F. C. McKenzie, The immunosuppressive effect of monoclonal anti-Lyt-1.1 antibodies *in vivo, Eur. J. Immunol. 11*: 1005 (1981).
96. N. Hollander, E. Pillemer, and I. L. Weissman, Effects of Lyt antibodies on T-cell functions: Augmentation by anti-Lyt-1 as opposed to inhibition by anti-Lyt-2, *Proc. Natl. Acad. Sci. USA, 78*: 1148 (1981).
97. L. Logdberg, and E. M. Shevach, Role of the Ly 1 antigen in interleukin 1-induced thymocyte activation, *Eur. J. Immunol., 15*: 1007 (1985).
98. T. Stanton, T. L. Stevens, J. A. Ledbetter, and F. Wofsy, Anti-Ly-1 antibody induces interleukin 2 release from T cells, *J. Immunol., 136*: 1734 (1986).
99. S. Kimura, N. Tada, and U. Hammerling, A new lymphocyte alloantigen (Ly-10) controlled by a gene linked to the Lyt-1 locus, *Immunogenetics, 10*: 363 (1980).
100. K. Itakura, J. J. Hutton, E. A. Boyse, and L. J. Old, Genetic linkage relationships of loci specifying differentiation alloantigens in the mouse, *Transplantation, 13*: 239 (1972).
101. M. Mage, B. Mathieson, S. Sharrow, L. McHugh, U. Hammerling, C. Kanellopoulos-Langevin, D. Brideau Jr., and C. A. Thomas, III, Preparative non-lytic separation of Lyt2$^+$ and Lyt2$^-$ T lymphocytes, functional analysis of the separated cells and demonstration of synergy in graft-vs.-host reaction of Lyt2$^+$ and Lyt2$^-$ cells, *Eur. J. Immunol. 11*: 228 (1981).
102. D. H. Raulet, P. D. Gottlieb, and M. J. Bevan, Fractionation of lymphocyte populations with monoclonal antibodies specific for Lyt-2.2 and Lyt-3.1, *J. Immunol., 125*: 1136 (1980).

103. D. B. Wilde, P. Marrack, J. Kappler, D. P. Dialynas, and F. W. Fitch, Evidence implicating L3T4 in class II MHC antigen reactivity; monoclonal antibody GK1.5 (anti-L3T4a) blocks class II MHC antigen-specific proliferation, release of lymphokines, and binding by cloned murine helper T lymphocyte lines, *J. Immunol., 131*: 2178 (1983).
104. A. Pierres, P. Naquet, A. Van Agthoven, F. Bekkhoucha, F. Denizot, Z. Mishal, A.-M., Schmitt-Verhulst, and M. Pierres, A rat anti-mouse T4 monoclonal antibody (H129.19) inhibits the proliferation of Ia-reactive T cell clones and delineates two phenotypically distinct ($T4^+$, Lyt-$2,3^-$, and $T4^-$, Lyt-$2,3^+$) subsets among anti-Ia cytolytic T cell clones, *J. Immunol., 132*: 2775 (1984).
105. S. L. Swain, D. P. Dialynas, F. W. Fitch, and M. English, Monoclonal antibody to L3T4 blocks the function of T cells specific for class II major histocompatibility complex antigens, *J. Immunol., 132*: 1118 (1984).
106. E. Nakayama, H. Shiku, E. Stockert, H. F. Oettgen, and L. J. Old, Cytotoxic T-cells: Lyt phenotype and blocking of killing activity by Lyt antisera, *Proc. Natl. Acad. Sci. USA, 76*: 1977 (1979).
107. N. Shinohara, and D. H. Sachs, Mouse alloantibodies capable of blocking cytotoxic T-cell function. I. Relationships between the antigen reactive with blocking antibodies and the *Lyt*-2 locus, *J. Exp. Med., 150*: 432 (1979).
108. N. Hollander, N. Pillemer, and I. L. Weissman, Blocking effect of Lyt-2 antibodies on T cell function, *J. Exp. Med. 152*: 674 (1980).
109. M. Sarmiento, A. L. Glasebrook, and F. W. Fitch, IgG or IgM monoclonal antibodies reactive with different determinants on the molecular complex bearing Lyt-2 antigen block T cell-mediated cytolysis in the absence of complement, *J. Immunol., 125*: 2665 (1980).
110. H. R. MacDonald, A. L. Glasebrook, and J. C. Cerottini, Clonal heterogeneity in the functional requirement for Lyt-2/3 molecules on cytolytic T lymphocytes: Analysis by antibody blocking and selective trypsinization, *J. Exp. Med., 156*: 1711 (1982).
111. N. Shinohara, and M. Kojima, Mouse alloantibodies capable of blocking cytotoxic T cell function. V. The majority of I region-specific CTL are Lyt-2^+ but are relatively resistant to anti-Lyt2 blocking, *J. Immunol. 132*: 578 (1984).
112. G. Moller, T cell subsets and MHC restriction, *Immunol. Rev., 74*:1 (1984).
113. N. Hollander, Lyt-2^+ suppressor T cells are resistant to anti-Lyt-2 antibody blocking, *J. Immunol., 134*: 2205 (1985).
114. P. J. Durda, and P. D. Gottlieb, The Ly-3 antigens on mouse thymocytes: Immune precipitation and molecular weight characterization, *J. Exp. Med., 144*: 476 (1976).
115. P. J. Durda, and P. D. Gottlieb, Sequential precipitation of mouse thymocyte extracts with anti-Lyt-2 and anti-Lyt-3 sera. I. Lyt-2.1 and Lyt-3.1 antigenic determinants reside on separable molecular species, *J. Immunol., 121*: 983 (1978).
116. E. B. Reilly, K. Auditore-Hargreaves, U. Hammerling, and P. D. Gottlieb, Lyt-2 and Lyt-3 alloantigens: precipitation with monoclonal and conven-

tional antibodies and analysis on one and two dimensional polyacrylamide gels, *J. Immunol., 125*: 2245 (1980).

117. T. A. Ledbetter, W. E. Seaman, T. T. Tsu, and L. A. Herzenberg, Lyt-2 and Lyt-3 antigens are on two different polypeptide subunits linked by disulfide bonds. Relationship of subunits to T cell cytolytic activity, *J. Exp. Med., 153*: 1503 (1981).
118. J. W. Goding, and A. W. Harris, Subunit structure of cell surface proteins: Disulfide bonding in antigen receptors, Ly2/3 antigens, and transferrin receptors of murine T and B lymphocytes, *Proc. Natl. Acad. Sci. USA, 78*: 4530 (1981).
119. I. D. Walker, P. M. Hogarth, B. J. Murray, K. E. Lovering, B. J. Classon, G. W. Chambers, and I. F. C. McKenzie, Ly antigens associated with T cell recognition and effector function, *Immunol. Rev. 82*: 47 (1984).
120. I. D. Walker, B. J. Murray, P. M. Hogarth, A. Kelso, and I. F. C. McKenzie, Comparison of thymic and peripheral T cell Lyt2/3 antigens, *Eur. J. Immunol., 14*: 906 (1984).
121. P. D. Gottlieb, Genetic correlation of a mouse light chain variable region marker with a thymocyte surface antigen, *J. Exp. Med. 140*: 1432 (1974).
122. D. M. Gibson, S. J. MacLean, D. Anctil, and B. J. Mathieson, Recombination between kappa chain genetic markers in the mouse, *Immunogenetics., 20*: 493 (1984).
123. J. L. Claflin, B. A. Taylor, M. Cherry, and M. Cubberley, Linkage in mice of genes controlling an immunoglobulin kappa chain marker and the surface alloantigen Ly-3 on T-lymphocytes, *Immunogenetics, 6*: 379 (1978).
124. J. A. Laskin, A. Gray, A. Nisonoff, N. R. Klinman, and P. D. Gottlieb, Segregation at a locus determining an immunoglobulin genetic marker for the light chain variable region affects inheritance of expression of an idiotype, *Proc. Natl. Acad. Sci. USA, 74*: 4600 (1977).
125. D. M. Gibson, B. A. Taylor, and M. Cherry, Evidence for close linkage of a mouse light chain marker with the *Ly-2,3* locus, *J. Immunol. 121*: 1585 (1978).
126. D. M. Gibson, and S. J. MacLean, Ef2: A new Ly-3-linked light chain marker expressed in normal mouse serum immunoglobulin, *J. Exp. Med., 149*: 1477 (1979).
127. R. Riblet, L. Claflin, D. M. Gibson, B. J. Mathieson, and M. Weigert, Antibody gene linkage studies in (NZB x C58) recombinant inbred lines, *J. Immunol. 124*: 787 (1980).
128. C. Lazure, W.-T. Hum and D. M. Gibson, A major subgroup of mouse kappa chains controlled by the chromosome 6 locus *IgK-Ef2, J. Exp. Med., 152*: 555 (1980).
129. P. D. Gottlieb, H. C.-W. Tsang, D. M. Gibson, and L. E. Cannon, Unique V_k subgroup associated with two mouse light chain genetic markers, *Proc. Natl. Acad. Sci. USA, 78*: 559 (1981).
130. D. M. Gibson, S. J. MacLean, and M. Cherry, Recombination between kappa chain genetic markers and the *Lyt-3* locus, *Immunogenetics, 18*: 111 (1983).

131. R. Zamoyska, A. C. Vollmer, K. C. Sizer, C. W. Liaw, and J. R. Parnes, Two Lyt-2 polypeptides arise from a single gene by alternative splicing patterns of mRNA, *Cell, 43*: 153 (1985).
132. C. W. Liaw, R. Zamoyska, and J. R. Parnes, Structure, sequence, and polymorphism of the *Lyt-2* T cell differentiation antigen gene, *J. Immunol., 137*: 1037 (1986).
133. G. D. Snell, M. Cherry, I. F. C. McKenzie, and D. W. Bailey, Ly-4 a new locus determining a lymphocyte cell-surface alloantigen in mice, *Proc. Acad. Sci. USA, 70*: 1108 (1973).
134. I. F. C. McKenzie, and G. D. Snell, Ly 4.2: A cell membrane alloantigen of murine B lymphocytes. I. Population studies, *J. Immunol., 114*: 848 (1975).
135. N. Tada, S. Kimura, A. Hatzfeld, and U. Hammerling, Ly-M11: The H-3 region of mouse chromosome 2 controls a new surface alloantigen, *Immunogenetics, 11*: 441 (1980).
136. L. Logdberg, P. Wassmer, and E. M. Shevach, Role of the L3T4 antigen in T cell activation. I. Description of a monoclonal IgM antibody to a distinct epitope (L3T4b) of the L3T4 antigen and its effect on interleukin-1-induced thymocyte proliferation, *Cell. Immunol., 94*: 299 (1985).
137. R. Ceredig, J. W. Lowenthal, M. Nabholz, and H. R. MacDonald, Expression of interleukin-2 receptors as a differentiation marker on intrathymic stem cells, *Nature, 314*: 98 (1985).
138. R. Ceredig, D. P. Dialynas, F. W. Fitch, and H. R. MacDonald, Precursors of T cell growth factor producing cells in the thymus: ontogeny, frequency, and quantitative recovery in a subpopulation of phenotypically mature thymocytes defined by monoclonal antibody GK-1.5, *J. Exp. Med., 158*: 1654 (1983).
139. B. J. Mathieson, S. O. Sharrow, Y. Rosenberg, and U. Hammerling, Lyt $1^{+}23^{-}$ cells appear in the thymus before Lyt 123^{+} cells, *Nature* (*London*), *289*: 179 (1981).
140. A. Truneh, F. Albert, P. Golstein, and A-M. Schmitt-Verhulst, Calcium ionophore plus phorbol ester can substitute for antigen in the induction of cytolytic T lymphocytes from specifically primed precursors, *J. Immunol., 135*: 2262 (1985).
141. R. DeKruyff, C. Clayberger, H. Cantor, and M. E. Dorf, Activation requirements of cloned inducer T cells. I. Differential inhibition by anti-L3T4 or anti-I-A is determined by the accessory cell population, *J. Immunol., 135*: 2243 (1985).
142. M. E. Katz, J. P. Tite, and C. A. Janeway, Jr., The immunobiology of T cell responses to *M1s*-locus-disparate stimulator cells. III. Helper and cytolytic functions of cloned, *M1s*-reactive T cell lines, *J. Immunol., 136*: 1 (1986).
143. P. Wasserman, C. Chan, L. Logdberg, and E. M. Shevach, Role of the L3T4 antigen in T cell activation. II. Inhibition of T cell activation by monoclonal anti-L3T4 antibodies in the absence of accessory cells, *J. Immunol., 135*: 2237 (1985).
144. J. Goverman, T. Hunkapillar, and L. Hood, A speculative view of the multicomponent nature of T cell antigen recognition, *Cell, 45*: 475 (1986).

145. J. Golding, H. McCluskey, T. I. Munitz, R. N. Germain, D. H. Margulies, and A. Singer, T cell recognition of a chimaeric class II/class I MHC molecule and the role of L3T4, *Nature, 317*: 425 (1985).
146. D. Wofsy, D. C. Mayes, J. Woodcock, and W. E. Seaman, Inhibition of humoral immunity *in vivo* by monoclonal antibody to L3T4: Studies with soluble antigens in intact mice, *J. Immunol., 135*: 1698 (1985).
147. D. Wofsy, and W. E. Seaman, Successful treatment of autoimmunity in NZB/NZW F_1 mice with monoclonal antibody to L3T4, *J. Exp. Med., 161*: 378 (1985).
148. S. P. Cobbold, A. Jayasuriya, A. Nash, T. D. Prospero, and H. Waldmann, Therapy with monoclonal antibodies by elimination of T cell subsets *in vivo, Nature, 312*: 548 (1984).
149. P. G. Coulie, J.-P. Coutelier, C. Uyttenhove, P. Lambote, and J. V. Snick, *In vivo* suppression of T-dependent antibody responses by treatment with a monoclonal anti-L3T4 antibody, *Eur. J. Immunol., 15*: 638 (1985).
150. N. L. Gutstein, W. E. Seaman, J. H. Scott, and D. Wofsy, Induction of immune tolerance by administration of monoclonal antibody to L3T4, *J. Immunol., 137*: 1127 (1986).
151. D. R. Littman, and S. N. Gettner, Unusual intron in the Ig domain of the newly isolated CD4 (L3T4) gene, submitted for publication.
152. A. Williams, A. N. Barclay, J. Gagnon, and M. L. Thomas, Cloning of the leucocyte-common antigen (T200): Unusual antigenic heterogeneity and a cytoplasmic domain of 80,000 M_r. *Advances in Gene Technology*: *Molecular Biology of the Immune System, Vol. 2* (J. W. Streilein, F. Ahmad, S. Black, B. Blomberg, and R. W. Voellmy, eds.), Cambridge University Press, New York, 1985, pp, 89-91.
153. K. Komuro, K. Itakura, E. A. Boyse, and M. John, A new T-lymphocyte antigen system, *Immunogenetics, 1*: 452 (1975).
154. M. Kasai, J. C. Leclerc, F.-W. Shen, and H. Cantor, Identification of Ly5 on the surface of 'natural killer' cells in normal and athymic inbred mouse strains, *Immunogenetics, 8*: 153 (1979).
155. J. N. Woody, M. Feldmann, P. C. L. Beverly, I. F. C. McKenzie, Expression of alloantigens Ly-5 and Ly-6 on cytotoxic effector cells, *J. Immunol., 118*: 1739 (1977).
156. M. P. Scheid, and D. Triglia, Further description of the *Ly-5* system, *Immunogenetics, 9*: 423 (1979).
157. D. Triglia, Expression of Ly-5 on yolk sac and fetal liver cells of the mouse, *Immunogenetics, 11*: 303 (1980).
158. A. R. Al Adra, L. M. Pilarski, C. A. Ross, and I. F. C. McKenzie, Expression of Ly-5.1 antigens on the effector and regulatory cells involved in cytotoxic T cell response to transplantation antigens, *Transplantation, 32*: 67 (1981).
159. J. M. Michaelson, M. Scheid, and E. A. Boyse, Biochemical features of Ly-5 alloantigen, *Immunogenetics, 9*: 193 (1979).
160. B. M. Omary, I. S. Trowbridge, and M. Scheid, T200 cell surface glycoprotein of the mouse polymorphism defined by the Ly-5 system of alloantigens, *J. Exp. Med., 151*: 1311 (1980).

161. A. W. Siadak, and R. C. Nowinski, Identification of Ly-5 and T200 antigens on identifical cell surface proteins, *J. Immunol., 125*: 1400 (1980).
162. J.-S. Tung, M. P. Scheid, M. A. Palladino, Different forms of Ly-5 within the T-cell lineage, *Immunogenetics, 17*: 649 (1983).
163. J.-S. Tung, M. C. Deere, E. A. Boyse, Evidence that Ly-5 product of T and B cells differ in protein surface, *Immunogenetics, 19*: 149 (1984).
164. A. J. Watson, Ly-5 (T200) structural polymorphism: The identification of intramolecular sites of phosphorylation, *Immunogenetics, 16*: 485 (1982).
165. F.-W. Shen, Y. Saga, G. Litman, G. Freeman, J.-S. Tung, H. Cantor, and E. A. Boyse, Cloning of Ly-5 cDNA. *Proc. Natl. Acad. Sci. USA, 82*: 7360 (1985).
166. K. L. Holmes, R. Palfree, U. Hammerling, and H. C. Morse, III, Alleles of the Ly-17 alloantigen define polymorphisms of the murine IgG Fc gamma receptor, *Proc. Natl. Acad. Sci. USA, 82*: 7706 (1985).
167. Y. Saga, J.-S. Tung, F.-W. Shen, and E. A. Boyse, Sequences of Ly-5 cDNA: Isoform-related diversity of Ly-5 mRNA, *Proc. Natl. Acad. Sci., USA, 83*: 6940 (1986).
168. I. S. Trowbridge, P. Ralph, M. J. Bevan, Differences in the surface proteins of mouse B and T cells, *Proc. Natl. Acad. Sci. USA, 72*: 157 (1975).
169. I. S. Trowbridge, Immunological properties of murine thymus-dependent lymphocyte surface glycoproteins, *Eur. J. Immunol., 6*: 557 (1978).
170. I. S. Trowbridge, Interspecies spleen-myeloma hybrid producing monoclonal antibodies against mouse lymphocyte surface glycoprotein, T200, *J. Exp. Med., 148*: 313 (1978).
171. T. Springer, G. Galfre, D. S. Secher, and C. Milstein, Monoclonal xenogeneic antibodies to murine cell surface antigens: Identification of novel leukocyte differentiation antigens, *Eur. J. Immunol., 8*: 539 (1978).
172. B. Dunlap, P. F. Mixter, B. Koller, A. Watson, M. B. Widmer, and F. H. Bach, Molecular relationships between large membrane proteins (LMP) expressed on T and B lymphocytes, *J. Immunol., 125*: 1829 (1980).
173. M. Sarmiento, M. R. Loken, I. S. Trowbridge, R. L. Coffman, and F. W. Fitch, High molecular weight lymphocyte surface proteins are structurally related and are expressed on different cell populations at different times during lymphocyte maturation and differentiation, *J. Immunol., 128*: 1676 (1982).
174. R. L. Coffman, and I. L. Weissman, B220: A B cell specific marker of the T200 glycoprotein family, *Nature, 289*: 681 (1981).
175. J. T. Kung, S. O. Sharrow, C. A. Thomas, and W. E. Paul, Analysis of B lymphocyte differentiation antigens by flow microfluorometry, *Immunol. Rev., 69*: 51 (1982).
176. P. W. Kincade, G. Lee, T. Watanabe, L. Sun, and M. P. Scheid, Antigens displayed on murine B lymphocyte precursors, *J. Immunol., 127*: 2262 (1981).
177. M. P. Scheid, K. S. Landreth, J.-S. Tung, and P. W. Kincade, Preferential but nonexclusive expression of macromolecular antigens on B-lineage cells, *Immunol. Rev., 69*: 141 (1982).

178. J. T. Kung, S. O. Sharrow, M. G. Mage, and W. E. Paul, Detection of a common antigen on murine B cells and Lyt2$^+$ T cells by a rat monoclonal antibody, 14D10, *J. Immunol., 129*: 81 (1982).
179. H. C. Morse, III, W. F. Davidson, R. A. Yetter, and R. L. Coffman, A cell-surface antigen shared by B cells and Ly2$^+$ peripheral T cells, *Cell. Immunol., 70*: 311 (1982).
180. F. J. Dumont, R. C. Habbersett, E. A. Nichols, J. A. Treffinger, and A. S. Tung, A monoclonal antibody (100C5) to the Lyt-2$^-$ T cell population expanding in MRL/Mp-*1pr*/*1pr* mice detects a surface antigen normally expressed on Lyt-2$^+$ cells and B cells, *Eur. J. Immunol., 13*: 455 (1983).
181. H. C. Morse, III, W. F. Davidson, R. A. Yetter, E. D. Murphy, J. B. Roths, and R. L. Coffman, Abnormalities induced by the mutant gene 1pr: Expression of a unique lymphocyte subset, *J. Immunol., 129*: 2612 (1982).
182. R. C. Budd, MacDonald, H. R., Lowenthal, J. W., Davignon, J-L. Izui, S., and Cerottini, J-C, Growth and differentiation in vitro of the accumulating Lyt-2$^-$/L3T4$^-$ subset in 1pr mice, *J. Immunol., 135*: 3704 (1900).
183. P. M. Hogarth, I. D. Walker, I. F. C. McKenzie, and T. Springer, The Ly-15 alloantigenic system: A genetically determined polymorphism of the murine lymphocyte function-associated antigen-1 molecule, *Proc. Natl. Acad. USA, 82*: 529 (1985).
184. D. Davignon, E. Martz, T. Reynolds, K. Kurzinger, and T. A. Springer, Lymphocyte function-associated antigen 1 (LFA-1): A surface antigen distinct from Lyt-2,3 that participates in T lymphocyte-mediated killing, *Proc. Natl. Acad. Sci. USA, 78*: 4535 (1981).
185. M. Pierres, C. Goudis, and P. Golstein, Inhibition of murine T cell-mediated cytolysis and T cell proliferation by a rat monoclonal antibody immunoprecipitating two lymphoid cell surface polypeptides of 94,000 and 180,000 molecular weight, *Eur. J. Immunol., 12*: 60 (1982).
186. T. Springer, G. Galfre, D. S. Secher, and C. Milstein, Mac-1: A macrophage differentiation antigen identified by monoclonal antibody, *Eur. J. Immunol., 9*: 301 (1979).
187. I. S. Trowbridge, and M. B. Omary, Molecular complexity of leukocyte surface glycoproteins related to the macrophage differentiation antigen Mac-1, *J. Exp. Med., 154*: 1517 (1981).
188. K. Kurzinger, and T. A. Springer, Purification and structural characterization of LFA-1, a lymphocyte function-associated antigen, and Mac-1, a related macrophage differentiation antigen associated with the type three complement receptor, *J. Biol. Chem., 257*: 12412 (1982).
189. F. Sanchez-Madrid, P. Simon, S. Thompson, and T. A. Springer, Mapping of antigenic and functional epitopes on the α- and β-subunits of two related mouse glycoproteins involved in cell interactions, LFA-1 and MAC-1, *J. Exp. Med., 158*: 586 (1983).
190. L. Sastre, T. K. Kishimoto, C. Gee, T. Roberts, and T. A. Springer, The mouse leukocyte adhesion proteins Mac-1 and LFA-1: Studies on mRNA translation and protein glycosylation with emphasis on Mac-1. *J. Immunol., 137*: 1060 (1986).

191. G. C. Mishra, M. T. Berton, K. G. Oliver, P. H. Krammer, J. W. Uhr, and E. S. Vitetta, A monoclonal anti-mouse LFA-1α antibody mimics the biological effects of B cell stimulatory factor-1 (BSF-1), *J. Immunol., 137*: 1590 (1986).
192. D. I. Beller, T. A. Springer, and R. D. Schreiber, Anti-Mac-1 selectively inhibits the mouse and human type three complement receptor, *J. Exp. Med., 156*: 1000 (1982).
193. S. Kohl, L. S. Loo, F. S. Schmalstieg, and D. C. Anderson, The genetic deficiency of leukocyte surface glycoprotein Mac-1, LFA-1, p150,95 in humans is associated with defective antibody-dependent cellular cytotoxicity *in vitro* and defective protection against *Herpes simplex* virus infection *in vivo, J. Immunol., 137*: 1688 (1986).
194. T. A. Potter, P. M. Hogarth, and F. C. McKenzie, Ly-15: A new murine lymphocyte alloantigenic locus, *Transplantation, 34*: 339 (1981).
195. I. D. Walker, P. M. Hogarth, B. J. Murray, K. E. Lovering, B. J. Classon, G. W. Chambers, and I. F. C. McKenzie, Ly antigens associated with T cell recognition and effector function, *Immunol. Rev., 82*: 47 (1984).
196. P. F. Halloran, D. Dutton, H. Chance, and Z. Cohen, An Ly-like specificity with extensive nonlymphoid expression, *Immunogenetics, 7*: 185 (1978).
197. S. Kimura, N. Tada, Y. Liu-Lam, and U. Hammerling, Studies of the mouse Ly-6 alloantigen system. II. Complexities of the Ly-6 region, *Immunogenetics, 20*: 47 (1984).
198. R. G. E. Palfree, F. J. Dumont, and U. Hammerling, Ly-6A.2 and Ly-6E.1 molecules are antithetical and identical to MALA-1, *Immunogenetics, 23*: 197 (1986).
199. A. J. Feeney, and U. Hammerling, Ala-1: A murine alloantigen of activated lymphocytes. I. Serological analysis of mitogen-stimulated T and B cells, *Immunogenetics, 3*: 369 (1976).
200. J. A. Frelinger, and D. B. Murphy, A new alloantigen, Ly-8, recognized by C3H anti-AKR serum, *Immunogenetics, 3*: 481 (1976).
201. D. Meruelo, A. Paolino, N. Flieger, and M. Offer, Definition of a new T lymphocyte surface antigen, Ly-11.2, *J. Immunol., 125*: 2713 (1980).
202. M. L. Hibbs, P. M. Hogarth, B. M. Scott, R. A. Harris, and I. F. C. McKenzie, Monoclonal antibody to murine neutrophils: Identification of the Gm-2.2 specificity, *J. Immunol., 133*: 2619 (1984).
203. B. J. Mathieson, F.-W. Shen, A. Brooks, and W. M. Leiserson, MG-1, identification of an early differentiation marker for bone marrow cells in a monocytic/granulocytic lineage, in *Macrophage and NK Cell Regulation and Function. Advances in Experimental Biology and Medicine,* Vol. 155 (E. Sorkin and S. Norman, eds.), Plenum Press, New York, 1982, pp. 201-207.
204. F. J. Dumont, L. Z. Coker, R. C. Habbersett, and J. A. Treffinger, Xenogeneic monoclonal antibody to an Ly-6-linked murine cell surface antigen: Differential reactivity with T cell subpopulations and bone marrow cells, *J. Immunol., 134*: 2357 (1985).
205. L. C. Anderson, M. Hurme, M. A. Horton, E. Simpson, and C. G. Gahmberg, Molecular characterisation of the Ly-6.2 antigen, *Cell. Immunol., 64*: 187 (1981).

206. A. Matossian-Rogers, P. Rogers, J. A. Ledbetter, and L. A. Herzenberg, Molecular weight determination of two genetically linked cell surface murine antigen ThB and Ly-6, *Immunogenetics, 15*: 591 (1982).
207. P. M. Hogarth, B. A. Houlden, S. E. Latham, V. R. Sutton, and I. F. C. McKenzie, Definition of new alloantigens encoded by genes in the *Ly-6* complex, *Immunogenetics, 20*: 57 (1984).
208. M. Yutoku, A. L. Grossberg, and D. Pressman, A cell surface antigenic determinant present on mouse plasmacytes and only about half of mouse thymocytes, *J. Immunol., 112*: 1774 (1974).
209. R. D. Stout, M. Yutoku, A. Grossberg, D. Pressman, and L. A. Herzenberg, A surface membrane determinant shared by subpopulations of thymocytes and B lymphocytes, *J. Immunol., 115*: 508 (1975).
210. L. A. Eckhardt, and L. A. Herzenberg, Monoclonal antibodies to ThB detect close linkage of *Ly-6* and a gene regulating ThB expression, *Immunogenetics, 11*: 275 (1980).
211. B. J. Mathieson, S. O. Sharrow, K. Bottomly, and B. J. Fowlkes, Ly-9, an alloantigenic marker for lymphocyte differentiation, *J. Immunol., 125*: 2127 (1980).
212. J. A. Ledbetter, J. W. Goding, T. T. Tsu, and L. A. Herzenberg, A new mouse lymphoid alloantigen (Lgp100) recognized by a monoclonal rat antibody, *Immunogenetics, 8*: 347 (1979).
213. P. M. Hogarth, J. Craig, and I. F. C. McKenzie, A monoclonal antibody detecting the Ly-9.2 (Lgp, 100) cell-membrane alloantigen, *Immunogenetics, 11*: 65 (1980).
214. S. O. Sharrow, A. Singer, U. Hammerling, and B. J. Mathieson, Phenotypic characterization of early events of thymus repopulation in radiation bone marrow chimeras, *Transplantation, 35*: 355 (1983).
215. S. O. Sharrow, B. J. Mathieson, and A. Singer, Cell surface appearance of unexpected host MHC determinants on thymocytes from radiation bone marrow chimeras, *J. Immunol., 126*: 1327 (1981).
216. P. J. Durda, S. C. Boas, and P. D. Gottlieb, T 100: A new murine cell surface glycoprotein detected by Lyt-2.1 serum, *J. Immunol., 122*: 1407 (1979).
217. W. F. Davidson, H. C. Morse III, B. J. Mathieson, C. A. Kozak, and F.-W. Shen, The B cell alloantigen Ly-17.1 is controlled by a gene closely linked to Ly-20 and Ly-9 on chromosome 1, *Immunogenetics, 17*: 325 (1983).
218. C. A. Kozak, W. F. Davidson, and H. C. Morse III, Genetic and functional relationships of the retroviral and lymphocyte alloantigen loci on mouse chromosome 1, *Immunogenetics, 19*: 163 (1984).
219. W. F. Davidson, T. M. Chused, and H. C. Morse III, Genetic and functional analyses of the primary *in vitro* CTL response of NZB lymphocytes to H-2-compatible cells, *Immunogenetics, 12*: 445 (1981).
220. P. Kisielow, H. Shiku, and J. A. Hirst, A new differentiation antigen defining a subpopulation of mouse T cells, *Nature, 261*: 137 (1976).
221. B. J. Mathieson, M. Mage, I. Betel, and S. O. Sharrow, Cytotoxic lymphocyte precursors: Phenotypic analysis and functional activity of peanut lec-

tin fractionated thymocytes, in *Protides of the Biological Fluids,* Vol. 27 (H. Peeters, ed.), Pergammon Press, Oxford, 1980, pp. 535-538.
222. M. M. Chan, N. Tada, S. Kimura, M. K. Hoffmann, R. A. Miller, O. Stutman, and U. Hammerling, Characterization of T lymphocyte subsets with monoclonal antibodies: Discovery of a distinct marker, Ly-m22, of T suppressor cells, *J. Immunol., 130*: 2075 (1983).
223. F. J. Dumont, R. C. Habbersett, and L. Z. Coker, Subsets of Lyt-2+ cells defined by differential expression of the 9F3 antigen: Alterations in mice of the *lpr/lpr* genotype, *J. Immunol., 134*: 196 (1985).
224. N. Tada, S. Kimura, Y. Liu-Lam, and U. Hammerling, Mouse alloantigen system Ly-m22 predominantly expressed on T lymphocytes and controlled by a gene linked to *Mls* region on chromosome 1, *Hybridoma, 2*: 29 (1983).
225. A. Colombatti, E. N. Hughes, B. A. Taylor, and J. T. August, Gene for a major cell surface glycoprotein of mouse macrophages and other phagocytic cells is on chromosome 2, *Proc. Natl. Acad. Sci. USA, 79*: 1926 (1982).
226. J. Lesley, and I. Trowbridge, Genetic characterization of a polymorphic murine cell-surface glycoprotein, *Immunogenetics, 15*: 313 (1982).
227. I. S. Trowbridge, J. Lesley, R. Schulte, R. Hyman, and J. Trotter, Biochemical characterization and cellular distribution of a polymorphic, murine cell-surface glycoprotein expressed on lymphoid tissues, *Immunogenetics, 15*: 299 (1982).
228. W. F. Davidson, F. J. Dumont, H. G. Bedigian, B. J. Fowlkes, and H. C. Morse III, Phenotypic, functional, and molecular genetic comparisons of the abnormal lymphoid cells of C3H-*lpr/lpr* and C3H-*gld/gld* mice, *J. Immunol., 136*: 4075 (1986).
229. I. S. Trowbridge, J. Trotter, and R. Hyman, Thymocyte subpopulation enriched for progenitors with an unrearranged T-cell receptor β-chain gene, *Nature, 315*: 666 (1985).
230. J. Lesley, R. Hyman, and R. Schulte, Evidence that the Pgp-1 glycoprotein is expressed on thymus-homing progenitor cells of the thymus, *Cell. Immunol., 91*: 397 (1985).
231. J. Bruce, F. W. Symington, T. J. McKearn, and J. Sprent, A monoclonal antibody discriminating between subsets of T and B cells, *J. Immunol., 127*: 2496 (1981).
232. P. S. Pillai, S. D. Reynolds, J. H. Chace, and D. W. Scott, Differential expression of a surface antigen recognized by a monoclonal antibody, J11d, on unprimed and primed B cells, *J. Immunol., 137*: 791 (1986).
233. B. J. Fowlkes, Characterization and differentiation of thymic lymphocytes in the mouse, Ph.D. thesis, George Washington University Graduate School of Arts and Sciences, Washington, D.C., 1984.
234. R. Scollay, P. Bartlett, and K. Shortman, T cell development in the adult murine thymus: Changes in the expression of the surface antigens Ly2, L3T4 and B2A2 during development from early precursor cells to emigrants, *Immunol. Rev., 82*: 79 (1984).

235. R. Scollay, and K. Shortman, Identification of early stages of T lymphocyte development in the thymus cortex and medulla, *J. Immunol., 134*: 3632 (1985).
236. P. Bartlett, and A. W. Boyd, The identification and purification of hemopoietic stem cells, *J. Immunol.*, in press.
237. F. W. Symington, and S.-I. Hakamori, Hematopoietic subpopulations express cross-reactive, lineage-specific molecules detected by monoclonal antibody, *Molec. Immunol., 21*: 507 (1984).
238. J. P. Allison, B. W. McIntrye, and D. Bloch, Tumor-specific antigen of murine T-lymphoma defined with monoclonal antibody, *J. Immunol., 129*: 2293 (1982).
239. K. Hashins, R. Kubo, J. White, M. Pigeon, J. Kappler, and P. Marrack, The major histocompatibility complex-restricted antigen receptor on T cells. I. Isolation with a monoclonal antibody, *J. Exp. Med., 157*: 1149 (1983).
240. L. E. Samelson, R. N. Germain, and R. H. Schwartz, Monoclonal antibodies against the antigen receptor on a cloned T-cell hybrid, *Proc. Natl. Acad. Sci. USA, 80*: 6972 (1983).
241. B. W. McIntyre, and J. P. Allison, The mouse T cell receptor: Structural heterogeneity of molecules of normal T cells defined by xenoantiserum, *Cell, 34*: 739 (1983).
242. K. Haskins, C. Hannum, J. White, N. Roehm, R. Kubo, J. Kappler, and P. Marrack, The major histocompatibility complex-restricted antigen receptor on T cells. VI. An antibody to a receptor allotype, *J. Exp. Med., 160*: 452 (1984).
243. U. D. Staerz, H.-G. Rammensee, J. D. Benedetto, and M. J. Bevan, Characterization of a murine monoclonal antibody specific for an allotypic determinant on T cell antigen receptor, *J. Immunol., 134*: 3994 (1985).
244. B. A. Behlke, D. G. Spinella, H. S. Chou, W. Sha, D. L. Hartl, and D. Y. Loh, T-cell receptor β-chain expression: Dependence on relatively few variable region genes, *Science, 229*: 566 (1985).
245. G. K. Sim, and A. A. Augustin, Vβ gene polymorphism and a major polyclonal T cell receptor idiotype, *Cell, 42*: 89 (1985).
246. B. A. Behlke, H. S. Chou, K. Huppi, and D. Y. Loh, Murine T cell receptor mutants with deletions of β-chain variable region genes, *Proc. Natl. Acad. Sci. USA, 83*: 767 (1986).
247. N. Roehm, L. Herron, J. Cambier, D. DiGusito, K. Haskins, J. Kappler, and P. Marrack, The major histocompatibility complex-restricted antigen receptor on T cells. Distribution on thymus and peripheral T cells, *Cell, 38*: 577 (1984).
248. I. N. Crispe, M. J. Bevan, and U. D. Staerz, Selective activation of Lyt-2^+ precursor T cells by ligation of the antigens receptor, *Nature, 317*: 627 (1985).
249. A. Farr, S. Anderson, P. Marrack, and J. Kappler, Expression of antigen-specific, major histocompatibility complex-restricted receptors by cortical and medullary thymocytes *in situ, Cell, 43*: 543 (1985).

250. L. E. Samelson, T. Lindsten, B. J. Fowlkes, P. van den Elsen, C. Terhorst, M. M. Davis, R. M. Germain, and R. H. Schwartz, Expression of genes of the T-cell antigen receptor complex in precursor thymocytes, *Nature, 315*: 765 (1985).
251. W. Born, J. Yagüe, E. Palmer, J. Kappler, and P. Marrack, Rearrangement of T-cell receptor β-chain genes during T cell development, *Proc. Natl. Acad. Sci. USA, 82*: 2925 (1985).
252. D. H. Raulet, R. D. Gasman, H. Saito, and S. Tonegawa, Developmental regulation of T cell receptor gene expression, *Nature, 314*: 103 (1985).
253. H. R. Snodgrass, P. Kisielow, M. Kiefer, M. Steinmetz, H. von Boehmer, Ontogeny of the T cell antigen receptor within the thymus, *Nature, 313*: 592 (1985).
254. B. J. Fowlkes, and B. J. Mathieson, Intrathymic differentiation: Thymocyte heterogeneity and the characterization of early T-cell precursors, *Surv. Immunol. Res., 4*: 96 (1985).
255. M. Bekoff, R. Kubo, and H. M. Grey, Activation requirements for normal T cells: Accessory cell-dependent and -independent stimulation by anti-receptor antibodies, *J. Immunol., 137*: 1411 (1986).
256. L. E. Samelson, J. R. Harford, and R. D. Klausner, The components of the murine T cell antigen receptor complex, in *Leukocytes and Host Defense* (J. J. Oppenheim and D. M. Jacobs, ed.), Alan R. Liss, Inc., 1986, p. 37.
257. H. Osawa, and T. Diamantstein, A monoclonal antibody that binds specifically to mouse T lymphoblasts and inhibits IL-2 receptor functions: A putative anti-IL-2 receptor antibody, *J. Immunol., 132*: 2445 (1984).
258. R. G. Ortega, J. Robb, E. M. Shevach, and T. R. Malek, The Murine IL-2 receptor. I. Monoclonal antibodies that define distinct functional epitopes on activated T cells and react with activated B cells, *J. Immunol., 133*: 1970 (1984).
259. J. W. Lowenthal, P. Corthesy, C. Tougne, R. Lees, H. R. MacDonald, and M. Nabholz, High and low affinity IL-2 receptors: Analysis by IL-2 dissociation rate and reactivity with monoclonal anti-receptor antibody PC61, *J. Immunol., 135*: 3988 (1985).
260. T. Malek, R. Robb, and E. Shevach, Identification and initial characterization of a rat monoclonal antibody reactive with the murine interleukin 2 receptor-ligand complex, *Proc. Natl. Acad. Sci. USA, 80*: 5694 (1983).
261. T. R. Malek, G. Ortega R., J. P. Jakway, C. Chan, and E. M. Shevach, The murine Il-2 receptor. II. Monoclonal anti-IL-2 receptor antibodies as specific inhibitors of T cell function *in vitro*, *J. Immunol., 133*: 1976 (1984).
262. J. Lowenthal, R. Zubler, M. Nabholz, and H. MacDonald, Similarities between interleukin-2 receptor number and affinity on activated B and T lymphocytes, *Nature* (*London*), *315*: 669 (1985).
263. G. Moller, IL-2: Receptors and genes, *Immunol. Rev., 92*: 1 (1986).
264. L. Takacs, H. Osawa, and T. Diamantstein, Detection and localization by the monoclonal anti-interleukin 2 receptor antibody AMT-13 of IL 2 receptor-bearing cells in the developing thymus of the mouse embryo and in the thymus of cortisone-treated mice, *Eur. J. Immunol., 14*: 1152 (1984).

265. D. H. Faulet, Expression and function of interleukin-2 receptor on immature thymocytes, *Nature, 314*: 101 (1985).
266. J. P. Lugo, S. N. Krishnan, R. D. Sailor, P. Koen, T. Malek, and E. Rothenberg, Proliferation of thymic stem cells with and without receptors for interleukin-2: Implications for intrathymic antigen recognition, *J. Exp. Med., 161*: 1048 (1985).
267. C. Hardt, T. Diamantstein, and H. Wagner, Developmentally controlled expression of IL-2 receptors and of sensitivity to IL-2 in a subset of embryonic thymocytes, *J. Immunol., 134*: 3891 (1985).
268. R. Palacios, and H. von Boehmer, Requirements for growth of immature thymocytes from fetal and adult mice *in vitro, Eur. J. Immunol., 16*: 12 (1986).
269. R. L. Moldwin, D. W. Lancki, K. C. Herold, and F. W. Fitch, An antigen receptor-driven interleukin 2-independent pathway for proliferation of murine cytolytic T lymphocyte clones, *J. Exp. Med., 163*: 1566 (1986).
270. R. Ceredig, Proliferation *in vitro* and interleukin production by 14-day fetal and adult Lyt-2^-/L3T4^- mouse thymocytes, *J. Immunol., 137*: 2260 (1986).
271. H. Kawamura, S. O Sharrow, D. W. Alling, D. Stephany, J. York-Jolley, and J. A. Berzofsky, Interleukin 2-receptor expression in unstimulated murine splenic cells: Localization to L3T4^+ cells and regulation by non-H-2-linked genes, *J. Exp. Med., 86*: 1376 (1986).
272. J. C. Unkeless, Characterization of a monoclonal antibody directed against mouse macrophage and lymphocyte Fc receptors, *J. Exp. Med., 150*: 580 (1979).
273. J. A. Titus, F. D. Finkelman, D. A. Stephany, J. F. Jones, and D. M. Segal, Quantitative analysis of Fcγ receptors on murine spleen cell populations by using dual parameter flow cytometry, *J. Immunol., 133*: 556 (1984).
274. F. W. Shen, and E. A. Boyse, An alloantigen selective for B cells: Ly17.1, *Immunogenetics, 11*: 315 (1980).
275. S. Kimura, N. Tada, E. Nakayama, Y. Liu, B. A. Taylor, and U. Hammerling, A new mouse cell-surface antigen (Ly-m20) controlled by a gene linked to *Mls* locus and defined by monoclonal antibodies, *Immunogenetics, 14*: 3 (1981).
276. M. L. Hibbs, P. M. Hogarth, and I. F. C. McKenzie, The murine Ly-17 locus identifies a polymorphism of the Fc receptor, *Immunogenetics, 22*: 335 (1985).
277. A. Mellor, The class I MHC gene family in mice, *Immunol. Today, 7*: 19 (1986).
278. A. L. Mellor, J. Antoniou, and P. J. Robinson, Structure and expression of genes encoding murine Qa-2 class I antigens, *Proc. Natl. Acad. Sci. USA, 82*: 5920 (1985).
279. R. Rabinowitz, S. O. Sharrow, S. Chatterjee-Das, M. J. Rogers, and D. H. Sachs, Qa-2 alloantigen expression on functional T lymphocytes from spleen and thymus, *Immunogenetics, 24*: 391 (1986).

280. P. A. Pontarotti, H. Mashimo, R. A. Zeff, D. A. Fisher, L. Hood, A. Mellor, R. A. Flavell, and S. G. Nathenson, Conservation and diversity in the class I genes of the major histocompatibility complex: Sequence analysis of a Tla gene and comparison with a Tla gene, *Proc. Natl. Acad. Sci. USA, 83*: 1782 (1986).
281. J. Rucker, M. Horowitz, E. A. Lerner, and D. B. Murphy, Monoclonal antibody reveals H-2-linked quantitative and qualitative variation in the expression of a Qa-2 region determinant, *Immunogenetics, 17*: 303 (1983).
282. T. H. Stanton, and S. Carbon, Gene(s) affecting the expression of Qa-1, *Immunogenetics, 16*: 435 (1982).
283. T. Stanton, and E. A. Boyse, A new serologically defined locus in the Tla region of the mouse, Qa-1, *Immunogenetics, 3*: 525 (1976).
284. T. H. Stanton, C. E. Calkins, J. Jandinski, D. J. Shendel, O. Stutman, H. Cantor, and E. A. Boyse, The Qa-1 antigenic system. Relation of Qa-1 phenotypes to lymphocyte sets, mitogen responses, and immune functions, *J. Exp. Med., 148*: 963 (1978).
285. T. H. Stanton, Expression of Qa-1 on mitogen-stimulated cells, *Immunogenetics, 9*: 597 (1979).
286. D. D. Eardley, F.-W. Shen, H. Cantor, and R. K. Gershon, Genetic control of immunoregulatory circuits: Genes linked to the Ig locus govern communication between regulatory T-cell sets, *J. Exp. Med., 150*: 44 (1979).
287. C. E. Calkins, T. A. Stanton, and O. Stutman, Cellular requirements for the *in vitro* induction of specific suppression of antibody responses by immune spleen cells, *Eur. J. Immunol., 10*: 449 (1980).
288. T. H. Stanton, and L. Hood, Biochemical identification of the Qa-1 allo antigen, *Immunogenetics, 11*: 309 (1980).
289. E. Rothenberg, and D. Triglia, Structure and expression of glycoproteins controlled by the Qa-1 allele, *Immunogenetics, 14*: 455 (1981).
290. R. G. Cook, R. N. Jenkins, L. Flaherty, and R. R. Rich, The Qa-1 alloantigens. II. Evidence for the expression of two Qa-1 molecules by the Qa-1 genotype and for cross-reactivity between Qa-1 and H-2K, *J. Immunol., 130*: 1293 (1983).
291. N. F. Landolfi, and R. G. Cook, Activated T-lymphocytes express class I molecules which are hyposialyated compared to other lymphocyte populations, *Molec. Immunol., 23*: 297 (1986).
292. K. Fischer-Lindahl, Unrestricted killer cells recognize an antigen controlled by a gene linked to Tla, *Immunogenetics, 8*: 71 (1979).
293. D. Wernet, and J. Klein, Unrestricted cell-mediated lympholysis to antigens linked to the Tla locus in the mouse, *Immunogenetics, 8*: 361 (1979).
294. D. L. Kastner, R. R. Rich, and F.-W. Shen, *Qa-1*-associated antigens. I. Generation of *H-2*-nonrestricted cytotoxic T lymphocytes specific for determinants of the *Qa-1* region, *123*: 1232 (1979).
295. J. Forman, H-2 unrestricted cytotoxic T cell activity against antigens controlled by genes in the Qa/Tla region, *J. Immunol., 123*: 2451 (1979).
296. R. N. Jenkins, and R. R. Rich, Characterization of determinants encoded by four Qa-1 genotypes and their recognition by cloned cytotoxic T lymphocytes, *J. Immunol., 131*: 2147 (1983).

297. L. Flaherty, The *Tla* region of the mouse: Identification of a new serologically defined locus, *Qa-2*, *Immunogenetics, 3*: 533 (1976).
298. M. A. Lynes, S. Tonkonogy, and L. Flaherty, *Qa-1* and *Qa-2* expression on CFU-s, *J. Immunol., 129*: 928 (1982).
299. P. M. Hogarth, P. E. Crewther, and I. F. C. McKenzie, Description of a Qa-2 like alloantigen (Qa-m2), *Eur. J. Immunol., 12*: 374 (1982).
300. L. Flaherty, D. Zimmerman, and T. H. Hansen, Further serological analysis of the Qa antigens: Analysis of an anti-H-2.28 serum, *Immunogenetics, 2*: 245 (1978).
301. G. J. Hammerling, U. Hammerling, and L. Flaherty, Qat-4 and Qat-5, new murine T cell antigens governed by the *Tla* region and identified by monoclonal antibodies, *J. Exp. Med., 150*: 108 (1979).
302. M. S. Sandrin, P. M. Hogarth, and I. F. C. McKenzie, Two "Qa" specificities: Qa-m7 and Qa-m8 defined by monoclonal antibodies, *J. Immunol., 131*: 546 (1983).
303. L. Flaherty, M. Karl, and C. L. Reinisch, Syngeneic tumor immunizations produce Qa antibodies. Discovery of a new Qa antigen, Qa-6, *Immunogenetics, 16*: 329 (1982).
304. W. van de Meugheuvel, G. van Seventer, and P. Demant, A new T1a region antigen Qa-11, similar to Qa-2 and associated with B-type β_2-microglobulin, *J. Immunol., 134*: 2507 (1985).
305. V. R. Sutton, P. M. Harth, and I. F. C. McKenzie, Description of a new Qa antigen specificity, "Qa-m9," whose expression is under complex genetic control, *J. Immunol., 131*: 1363 (1983).
306. S. M. Widacki, L. Flaherty, and R. G. Cook, Biochemical characterization of the molecules reactive with Qa-6 antiserum and the monoclonal antibody 20-8-4: Evidence for structural similarity with the Qa-2 molecule, *J. Immunol., 135*: 3333 (1985).
307. D. Ivanyi, M. Cherry, and P. Demant, Molecular heterogeneity of D-end products detected by anti-H-2.28 sera, *Immunogenetics, 15*: 477 (1982).
308. S. O. Sharrow, L. Flaherty, and D. H. Sachs, Serologic cross-reactivity between class I MHC molecules and an H-2-linked differentiation antigen as detected by monoclonal antibodies, *J. Exp. Med., 159*: 21 (1984).
309. M. Oudshoorn-Snoek, A. L. Mellor, R. A. Flavell, and P. Demant, A new determinant Qa-m208 detected on T-lymphocytes and transfected L-cells by an anti-K^b monoclonal antibody, *Immunogenetics, 19*: 461 (1984).
310. L. Flaherty, D. Zimmerman, and K. A. Sullivan, *Qa-2* and *Qa-3* antigens on lymphocyte subpopulations. I. Mitogen responsiveness, *J. Immunol., 121*: 1640 (1978).
311. P. M. Hogarth, A. Basten, H. Prichard-Briscoe, M. H. Henning, V. R. Sutton, and I. F. C. McKenzie, The distribution of the Qa-2 alloantigen on functional T lymphocytes, *J. Immunol., 135*: 1632 (1985).
312. P. W. Kincade, L. Flaherty, G. Lee, T. Watanabe, and J. Michaelson, Qa antigen expression of functional lymphoid, myeloid, and stem cells in adult mice, *J. Immunol., 124*: 2879 (1980).

313. R. A. Harris, P. M. Hogarth, L. J. Wadeson, P. Collins, I. F. C. McKenzie, and D. G. Penington, An antigenic difference between cells forming early and late haematopoietic spleen colonies (CFU-S), *Nature, 307*: 638 (1984).
314. I. Bertoncello, S. H. Bartelmez, T. R. Bradley, E. R. Stanley, R. A. Harris, M. S. Sandrin, A. B. Kriegler, I. K. McNiece, S. D. Hunter, and G. S. Hodgson, Isolation and analysis of primitive hemopoietic progenitor cells on the basis of differential expression of Qa-m7 antigen, *J. Immunol., 136*: 3219 (1986).
315. J. Michaelson, L. Flaherty, E. Vitetta, and M. D. Poulik, Molecular similarities between the Qa-2 alloantigen and other gene products of the 17th chromosome of the mouse, *J. Exp. Med., 145*: 1066 (1977).
316. J. Michaelson, L. Flaherty, B. Hutchinson, and H. Yudkowitz, Qa-2 does not display structural genetic polymorphism detectable on isoelectric-focusing gels, *Immunogenetics, 16*: 363 (1982).
317. D. H. Sherman, D. M. Kranz, and H. N. Eisen, Expression of structurally diverse Qa-2-encoded molecules on the surface of cloned cytotoxic T lymphocytes, *J. Exp. Med., 160*: 1421 (1984).
318. M. J. Soloski, J. Vernachio, G. Einhorn, and A. Lattimore, Qa gene expression: Biosynthesis and secretion of Qa-2 molecules in activated T cells, *Immunology, 83*: 2949 (1986).
319. J. Forman, J. Trial, S. Tonkonogy, and L. Flaherty, The Qa-2 subregion controls the expression of two antigens recognized by H-2 unrestricted cytotoxic T cells, *J. Exp. Med., 155*: 749 (1982).
320. D. Cosman, M. Kress, G. Khoury, and G. Jay, Tissue-specific expression of an unusual *H-2* (class I)-related gene, *Proc. Natl. Acad. Sci. USA, 79*: 4947 (1982).
321. J. J. Devlin, A. M. Lew, R. A. Flavell, and J. E. Coligan, Secretion of a soluble class I molecule encoded by the Q10 gene of the C57BL/10 mouse, *EMBO J., 4*: 369 (1985).
322. A. L. Mellor, E. H. Weiss, M. Kress, G. Jay, and R. A. Flavell, A nonpolymorphic class I gene in the murine major histocompatibility complex, *Cell, 36*: 139 (1984).
323. I. Stroynowski, J. Forman, R. S. Goodenow, S. G. Schiffer, M. McMillan, S. O. Sharrow, D. H. Sachs, and L. Hood, Expression and T cells recognition of hybrid antigens with amino-terminal domains encoded by Qa-2 region of major histocompatibility complex and carboxyl termini of transplantation antigens, *J. Exp. Med., 161*: 935 (1985).
324. D. S. Straus, I. Stroynowski, S. G. Schiffer, and L. Hood, Expression of hybrid class I genes of the major histocompatibility complex in mouse L cells, *Proc. Natl. Acad. Sci. USA, 82*: 6245 (1985).
325. M. Chun, V. Pasanen, U. Hammerling, G. F. Hammerling, and M. K. Hoffmann, Tumor necrosis serum induces a serologically distinct population of NK cells, *J. Exp. Med., 150*: 426 (1979).
326. M. Chun, G. Fernandes, and M. K. Hoffmann, Mechanism of NK cell activation: Relationship between $Qa5^+$ NK cells and lymphocytes, *J. Immunol., 126*: 331 (1981).

327. N. Minato, L. Reid, and B. R. Bloom, On the heterogeneity of murine natural killer cells, *J. Exp. Med., 154*: 750 (1981).
328. E. C. Lattime, G. A. Pecoraro, and O. Stutman, Natural cytotoxic cells against solid tumors in mice. III. Comparison of effector cell antigenic phenotype and target cell recognition structures with NK cells, *J. Immunol., 126*: 2011 (1981).
329. E. C. Lattime, G. A. Pecoraro, and O. Stutman, The activity of natural cytotoxic cells is augmented by interleukin 2 and interleukin 3, *J. Exp. Med., 157*: 1070 (1983).
330. J. R. Ortaldo, L. H. Mason, B. J. Mathieson, S.-M. Liang, D. A. Flick, and R. B. Herberman, Mediation of mouse natural cytotoxic activity by tumour necrosis factor, *Nature, 321*: 700 (1986).
331. J. Hackett, Jr., M. Bennett, and V. Kumar, Origin and differentiation of natural killer cells. I. Characteristics of a transplantable NK cell precursor, *J. Immunol., 134*: 3731 (1985).
332. S. O. Sharrow, K. Ozato, and D. H. Sachs, Phenotypic expression of I-A and I-E/C subregion determinants on murine thymocytes, *J. Immunol., 125*: 2263 (1980).
333. R. V. Rouse, W. van Ewijk, P. P. Jones, and I. L. Weissman, Expression of MHC antigens by mouse thymic dendritic cells, *J. Immunol., 122*: 2508 (1979).
334. W. van Ewijk, R. V. Rouse, and I. L. Weissman, Distribution of H-2 microenvironments in the mouse thymus, *J. Histochem. Cytochem. 28*: 1089 (1980).
335. E. J. Jenkinson, W. van Ewijk, and J. J. T. Owen, Major histocompatibility antigen expression on the epithelium of the developing thymus in normal and nude mice, *J. Exp. Med., 153*: 280 (1981).
336. P. G. Natali, C. De Martino, M. A. Pellegrino, and S. Ferrone, Analysis of the expression of IA-like antigens in murine fetal and adult tissues with the monoclonal antibody 10-2.16, *Scand. J. Immunol., 13*: 541 (1981).
337. A. G. Farr, and P. K. Nakane, Cells bearing Ia antigens in the murine thymus: An ultrastructural study, *Am. J. Pathology, 111*: 88 (1983).
338. S. O. Sharrow, B. J. Mathieson, and A. Singer, Cell surface appearance of unexpected host MHC determinants on thymocytes from radiation bone marrow chimeras, *J. Immunol., 126*: 1327 (1981).
339. A. M. Kruisbeek, M. J. Fultz, A. Singer, and J. J. Mond, Early development of the T cell repertoire. Neonatal treatment with anti-Ia antibodies interferes with differentiation of I-restricted T cells but not K/D-restricted T cells, *J. Exp. Med., 157*: 1932 (1983).
340. A. M. Kruisbeek, J. J. Mond, B. J. Fowlkes, J. A. Carmen, S. Bridges, and D. L. Longo, Absence of the $Lyt2^-$, $L3T4^+$ lineage of T cells in mice treated neonatally with anti-I-A correlates with absence of intrathymic I-A-bearing antigen-presenting cell function, *J. Exp. Med., 161*: 1029 (1985).
341. D. DeLuca, Ia-positive nonlymphoid cells and T cell development in murine fetal thymus organ cultures: Monoclonal anti-Ia antibodies inhibit the development of T cells, *J. Immunol., 136*: 430 (1986).

342. D. DeLuca, and S. B. Mizel, I-A-positive nonlymphoid cells and T cell development in murine fetal thymus organ cultures: Interleukin 1 circumvents the block in T cell differentiation induced by monoclonal anti-I-A antibodies, *J. Immunol., 137*: 1435 (1986).
343. I. F. C. McKenzie, J. Gardiner, M. Cherry, and G. D. Snell, Lymphocyte antigens: Ly-4, Ly-6, and Ly-7, *Trans. Proc., 9*: 667 (1977).
344. T. A. Potter, G. M. Morgan, and I. F. C. McKenzie, Murine lymphocyte alloantigens. II. The *Ly-7* locus, *J. Immunol., 125*: 546 (1980).
345. L. L. Lanier, and N. L. Warner, Lym 7.2: Monoclonal antibody defining an alloantigen similar or identical to Ly-7.2, *Hybridoma, 1*: 227 (1982).
346. L. L. Lanier, and N. L. Warner, Lym 7.3: New murine specificity defining third allele of the *Ly-7* locus, *Hybridoma, 2*: 177 (1983).
347. P. M. Hogarth, I. F. C. McKenzie, L. Lanier, D. W. Bailey, and B. A. Taylor, Location of *Ly-7* on mouse chromosome 12, *Immunogenetics, 19*: 539 (1984).
348. F. L. Owen, G. M. Spurll, and E. Pangageas, Tthy^d, a new thymocyte alloantigen linked to Igh-1. Implications for a switch mechanism for T cell antigen receptors, *J. Exp. Med., 155*: 52 (1982).
349. F. L. Owen, Products of the IgT-C region of chromosome 12 are maturational markers for T cells. Sequence of appearance in immunocompetent T cells parallels ontogenetic appearance of Tthy^d, Tind^d, and Tsu^d, *J. Exp. Med., 156*: 703 (1982).
350. F. L. Owen, and G. M. Peterman, Neoplastic model for the differentiation of a subpopulation of lymphocytes bearing IgH-1-linked gene products, *Immunol. Rev., 82*: 29 (1984).
351. F. Owen, and R. Riblet, Genes for the mouse T cell alloantigens Tpre, Tthy, Tind and Tsu are closely linked near Igh on chromosome 12, *J. Exp. Med., 159*: 313 (1984).
352. F. L. Owen, A. Finnegan, E. R. Gates, and P. D. Gottlieb, A mature T lymphocyte subpopulation marker closely linked to the Ig-1 allotype C_H locus, *Eur. J. Immunol., 9*: 948 (1979).
353. F. L. Owen, R. Riblet, and B. A. Taylor, The T suppressor cell alloantigen Tsu^d maps near immunoglobulin allotype genes and may be a heavy chain constant-region marker on a T cell receptor, *J. Exp. Med., 153*: 801 (1981).
354. F. L. Owen, A mature lymphocyte marker closely linked to Igh-1 which is expressed on the precursor for the suppressor T cell regulating a primary response to SRBC, *J. Immunol., 124*: 1411 (1980).
355. G. M. Spurll, and F. L. Owen, A family of T-cell alloantigens linked to Igh-1, *Nature (Lond.), 293*: 742 (1981).
356. A. Finnegan, and F. L. Owen, Ly-18, a new alloantigen present on cytotoxic T cells and controlled by a gene(s) linked to the Igh-V locus, *J. Immunol., 127*: 1947 (1981).
357. N. E. Lee, P. D'Eustachio, D. Pravtcheva, F. H. Ruddle, S. M. Hedrick, and M. M. Davis, Murine T cell receptor, beta chain is encoded on chromosome 6, *J. Exp. Med., 160*: 905 (1984).

358. L. A. D'Hoostelaere, E. Jouvin-Marche, and K. Huppi, Localization of $C_{T\beta}$ and C_{κ} on mouse chromosome 6, *Immunogenetics, 22*: 277 (1985).
359. S. Kimura, N. Tada, and U. Hämmerling, A new lymphocyte alloantigen (Ly-10) controlled by a gene linked to the *Lyt-1* locus, *Immunogenetics, 10*: 363 (1980).
360. M. M. Chan, U. Hammerling, and O. Stutman, Ly-m10 is a marker of activated murine T lymphocytes, the counterpart of human 4F2 antigen, *J. Leuk. Biol., 38*: 106 (1985).
361. T. A. Potter, and I. F. C. McKenzie, Identification of new murine lymphocyte alloantigens: Antisera prepared between C57L, 129, and related strains define new loci, *Immunogenetics, 12*: 357 (1981).
362. B. F. Haynes, M. E. Hamler, D. L. Mann, G. S. Eisenbarth, J. Hamer, H. S. Mostowski, C. A. Thomas, J. L. Strominger, and A. S. Fauci, Characterization of a monoclonal antibody (4F2) that binds to human monocytes and to a subset of activated lymphocytes, *J. Immunol., 129*: 1409 (1981).
363. S. Kimura, N. Tada, Y. Liu-Lam, and U. Hämmerling, Further genetic characterization of mouse Ly-m10 alloantigens, *Immunogenetics, 17*: 211 (1983).
364. H. R. MacDonald, R. K. Lees, and C. Bron, Cell surface glycoproteins involved in the stimulation of interleukin 1-dependent interleukin 2 production by a subline of EL4 thymoma cells. I. Functional characterization by monoclonal antibodies, *J. Immunol., 135*: 3944 (1985).
365. B. Lüscher, M. Rousseaux, R. Lees, H. R. MacDonald, and C. Bron, Cell surface glycoproteins involved in the stimulation of interleukin 1-dependent interleukin 2 production by a subline of EL4 thymoma cells. II. Structure, biosynthesis, and maturation, *J. Immunol., 135*: 3951 (1985).
366. C. Bron, M. Rousseaux, A. Spiazzi, and H. R. MacDonald, Structural homology between the human 4F2 antigen and a murine cell surface glycoprotein associated with lymphocyte activation, *J. Immunol., 137*: 397 (1986).
367. M. Michalak, E. J. Quackenbush, and M. Letarte, Inhibition of Na^{+}/Ca^{2+} exchanger activity in cardiac and skeletal muscle sarcolemmal vesicles by monoclonal antibody 44D7, *J. Biol. Chem., 261*: 92 (1986).
368. N. Tada, S. Kimura, B. Taylor, and U. Hämmerling, Ly-m19: The Lyb-2 region of mouse chromosome 4 controls a new cell surface antigen, *Immunogenetics, 13*: 539 (1981).
369. D. Meruelo, M. Offer, and N. Fleiger, A new lymphocyte cell surface antigen, Ly-22.2, controlled by a locus on chromosome 4 and a second unlinked locus, *J. Immunol., 130*: 946 (1983).
370. H. C. Morse III, T. M. Chused, J. W. Hartley, B. J. Mathieson, S. O. Sharrow, and B. A. Taylor, Expression of xenotropic murine viruses as cell-surface gp70 in genetic crosses between strains DBA/2 and C57BL/6, *J. Exp. Med., 149*: 1183 (1979).
371. L. J. Gonez, M. S. Sandrin, M. M. Henning, J. Hilgers, and I. F. C. McKenzie, Ly-29: A locus closely linked to *Mtv-20* on chromosome 4 codes for a new mouse lymphocyte surface alloantigen, *Immunogenetics, 22*: 305 (1985).

372. N. Tada, S. Kimura, Y. Liu-Lam, U. Hämmerling, A new lymphocyte surface antigen (Ly-m31) controlled by a gene closely linked to the *Akp-2* locus on chromosome 4, *Immunogenetics, 20*: 589 (1984).
373. D. B. Murphy, L. A. Herzenberg, K. Okumura, L. A. Herzenberg, and H. O. McDevitt, A new *I* subregion (I-J) marked by a locus (*Ia-4*) controlling surface determinants on suppressor T lymphocytes, *J. Exp. Med., 144*: 699 (1976).
374. D. B. Murphy, M. C. Horowitz, R. J. Homer, and P. M. Flood, Genetic, serological and functional analysis of I-J molecules, *Immunol. Rev., 83*: 79 (1985).
375. M. Steinmetz, K. Minard, S. Horvath, J. McNicholas, J. Frelinger, C. Wake, E. Long, B. Mach, and L. Hood, A molecular map of the immune response region from the major histocompatibility complex of the mouse, *Nature (Lond.), 300*: 35 (1982).
376. C. E. Hayes, K. K. Klyczek, D. P. Krum, R. M. Whitcomb, D. A. Hullett, and H. Cantor, Chromosome 4 J_t gene controls murine T cell surface I-J expression, *Science, 223*: 559 (1984).
377. K. K. Klyczek, H. Cantor, and C. E. Hayes, T cell surface I-J glycoprotein. Concerted action of chromosome-4 and -17 genes forms an epitope dependent on α-D-mannosyl residues, *J. Exp. Med., 159*: 1604 (1984).
378. C. Waltenbaugh, L. Sun, and H.-Y. Lei, I-J expression is not associated with murine chromosome 4, *Eur. J. Immunol., 15*: 922 (1985).
379. P. M. Hogarth, E. M. Eicher, and I. F. C. McKenzie, Mapping of the murine *Ly-15*(*LFA-1*) locus to chromosome 7, *Immunogenetics, 23*: 348 (1986).
380. F. W. Symington, B. Subbarao, D. E. Mosier, and J. Sprent, Lyb-8.2: A new B cell antigen defined and characterized with a monoclonal antibody, *Immunogenetics, 16*: 381 (1982).
381. J. Kennard, and D. Meruelo, A new murine lymphocyte alloantigen, Ly-21.2, mapping to the seventh chromosome, *Immunogenetics, 15*: 239 (1982).
382. N. Tada, S. Kimura, A. Hatzfield, and U. Hämmerling, Ly-m11: The *H-3* region of mouse chromosome 2 controls a new surface alloantigen. *Immunogenetics, 11*: 441 (1980).
383. J. Michaelson, Genetics of beta-2 microglobulin in the mouse, *Immunogenetics, 17*: 219 (1983).
384. M. L. Hibbs, P. M. Hogarth, R. A. Harris, and I. F. C. McKenzie, Gm-3.2, a new granulocyte/macrophage alloantigen, *Immunogenetics, 21*: 61 (1985).
385. D. L. Gasser, J. Ziebur, and K. Matsumoto, A new lymphocyte antigen encoded by a locus closely linked to *H-3* on the second chromosome of the mouse, *Proc. Natl. Acad. Sci. USA, 80*: 6620 (1983).
386. P. M. Hogarth, A. Rigby, V. R. Sutton, I. F. C. McKenzie, and J. Hilgers, The Ly-25.1 specificity: Definition with a monoclonal antibody, *Immunogenetics, 19*: 83 (1984).
387. S. Kimura, N. Tada, Y. Liu, and U. Hämmerling, A new mouse cell-surface antigen (Ly-m18) defined by a monoclonal antibody, *Immunogenetics, 13*: 547 (1981).

388. P. M. Hogarth, S. E. Latham, and I. F. C. McKenzie, A new murine alloantigen: Ly-26.1, *Immunogenetics, 19*: 355 (1984).
389. G. K. Matsushima, R. C. Harmon, and J. A. Frelinger, A new murine lymphocyte alloantigen, Ly-27.2, *Immunogenetics, 23*: 406 (1986).
390. L. J. Gonez, M. S. Sandrin, M. M. Henning, and I. F. C. McKenzie, Ly-30: A new mouse lymphocyte surface alloantigen defined by a monoclonal antibody, *Immunogenetics, 22*: 301 (1985).
391. G. Moldenhauer, D. Haustein, T. Hüppe, A. Wagner, and K.-U. Hartmann, A new murine cell surface differentiation antigen (Leugp 90) defined by a rat monoclonal antibody: Cellular distribution and biochemical characterization, *J. Immunol., 128*: 2664 (1982).
392. W. M. Gallatin, I. L. Weissman, and E. C. Butcher, A cell surface molecule involved in organ-specific homing of lymphocytes, *Nature, 304*: 30 (1983).
393. P. J. Fink, W. M. Gallatin, R. A. Reichert, E. C. Butcher, and I. L. Weissman, Homing receptor-bearing thymocytes, an immunocompetent cortical subpopulation, *Nature, 313*: 233 (1985).
394. R. A. Reichert, W. M. Gallatin, E. C. Butcher, and I. L. Weissman, A homing receptor-bearing cortical thymocyte subset: Implications for thymus cell migration and the nature of cortisone-resistant thymocytes, *Cell, 38*: 89 (1984).
395. R. A. Reichert, I. L. Weissman, and E. C. Butcher, Phenotypic analysis of thymocytes that express homing receptors for peripheral lymph nodes, *J. Immunol., 136*: 3521 (1986).
396. R. A. Reichert, I. L. Weissman, and E. C. Butcher, Dual immunofluorescence studies of cortisone-resistant thymocytes, *J. Immunol., 136*: 3529 (1986).
397. R. A. Reichert, L. Jerabek, W. M. Gallatin, E. C. Butcher, and I. L. Weissman, Ontogeny of lymphocyte homing receptor expression in the mouse thymus, *J. Immunol., 136*: 3535 (1986).
398. K. Shortman, A. Wilson, W. Van Ewijk, and R. Scollay, Phenotype and localization of thymocytes expressing the homing receptor-associated antigen MEL-14: Arguments for the view that most mature thymocytes are located in the medulla, *J. Immunol., 138*: 342 (1987).
399. A. Wilson, R. Scollay, R. A. Reichert, E. C. Butcher, I. L. Weissman, and K. Shortman, The correlation of lectin-stimulated proliferation and cytotoxicity in murine thymocytes with expression of the MEL-14-defined homing receptor, *J. Immunol., 138*: 352 (1987).
400. M. Siegelman, M. W. Bond, W. M. Gallatin, T. St. John, H. T. Smith, V. A. Fried, and I. L. Weissman, Cell surface molecule associated with lymphocyte homing is a ubiquitinated branched-chain glycoprotein, *Science, 231*: 823 (1986).
401. M. Kasai, T. Takashi, T. Takahashi, and T. Tokunaga, A new differentiation antigen (FT-1) shared with fetal thymocytes and leukemia cells in the mouse, *J. Exp. Med., 159*: 971 (1984).
402. T. Takashi, M. Kasai, N. Tanaka, T. Takahashi, and T. Tokunaga, FT-2 antigen for distinguishing lymphocyte subpopulations in the developing thymus, *Immunol. Lett., 9*: 259 (1985).

403. M. Kasai, T. Takashi, T. Takahashi, and T. Tokunaga, Two new fetal antigens, FT-1 and FT-2, *Immunol. Rev., 82*: 105 (1984).
404. O. Leo, M. Foo, D. H. Sachs, L. E. Samelson, J. A. Bluestone, Identification of a monoclonal antibody specific for a murine T3 polypeptide, *Proc. Natl. Acad. Sci. USA, 84*: 1374 (1987).
405. J. W. Kappler, T. Wade, J. White, E. Kushnir, M. Blackman, J. Bill, N. Roehm, and P. Marrack, A T cell receptor Vβ segment that imparts reactivity to a class II major histocompatibility complex product, *Cell, 49*: 263 (1987).
406. P. Y. Chan, and F. Takei, Expression of a T cell receptor-like molecule on normal and malignant murine T cells detected by rat monoclonal antibodies to nonclonotypic determinants, *J. Immunol., 136*: 1346 (1986).
407. R. Nagasawa, J. Gross, O. Kanagawa, K. Townsend, L. L. Lanier, J. Chiller, and J. P. Allison, Identification of a novel T cell surface disulfide-bonded dimer distinct from the α/β antigen receptor, *J. Immunol., 138*: 815 (1987).
408. P. J. Martin, J. A. Ledbetter, Y. Morishita, C. H. June, P. G. Beatty, and J. A. Hansen, A 44 kilodalton cell surface homodimer involved in interleukin 2 production by activated human T lymphocytes, *J. Immunol., 136*: 3282 (1986).
409. F. Takei, Two surface antigens expressed on proliferating mouse T lymphocytes defined by rat monoclonal antibodies, *J. Immunol., 130*: 2794 (1983).
410. A. W. Siadek, and R. C. Nowinski, Thy-2: A murine thymocyte-brain alloantigen controlled by a gene linked to the major histocompatibility complex, *Immunogenetics, 12*: 45 (1981).
411. F.-W. Shen, G. Viamontes, and E. A. Boyse, A system of alloantigens that selectively identifies lymph-node lymphocytes, *Immunogenetics, 15*: 17 (1982).
412. M. Sarmiento, M. Loken, and F. Fitch, Structural differences in cell surface T25 polypeptides from thymocytes and cloned T cells, *Hybridoma, 1*: 13 (1981).
413. P. Lake, E. A. Clark, M. Khorshidi, and G. H. Sunshine, Production and characterization of cytotoxic Thy-1 antibody-secreting hybrid cell lines. Detection of T cell subsets, *Eur. J. Immunol., 9*: 875 (1979).
414. A. Marshak-Rothstein, P. Fink, T. Gridley, D. H. Raulet, M. J. Bevan, and M. L. Gefter, Properties and applications of monoclonal antibodies directed against determinants of the *Thy-1* locus, *J. Immunol., 122*: 2491 (1979).
415. P. M. Hogarth, J. Edwards, I. F. C. McKenzie, J. W. Goding, and F. Y. Liew, Monoclonal antibodies to murine Ly-2.1 cell surface antigen, *Immunology, 46*: 135 (1982).
416. G. J. Hammerling, H. Lemke, U. Hammerling, C. Hohmann, R. Wallich, and K. Rajewsky, Monoclonal antibodies against murine cell surface antigens: Anti-H-2, anti-Ia and anti-T cell antibodies, in *Current Topics in Microbiology and Immunology*, Vol. 81 Lymphocyte Hybridomas (F. Melchers, M. Potter, and N. Warner, eds.), Springer-Verlag, Berlin, Heidelberg, 1978, p. 100.

417. F. W. Shen, Monoclonal antibodies to mouse lymphocyte differentiation antigens, in *Monoclonal Antibodies and T Cell Hybridomas: Perspectives and Technical Advances* (G. J. Hammerling, U. Hammerling, and J. F. Kearney, eds.), Elsevier/North Holland and Biomedical Press, Amsterdam/New York/Oxford, 1981, pp. 25-31.
418. C. Mark, F. Figueroa, Z. A. Nagy, and J. Klein, Cytotoxic monoclonal antibody specific for the Lyt-1.2 antigen, *Immunogenetics, 16*: 95 (1982).
419. P. Golstein, C. Goridis, A.-M. Schmitt-Verhulst, B. Hayot, A. Pierres, A. van Agthoven, Y. Kaufmann, Z, Eshar, and M. Pierres, Lymphoid cell-surface interaction structures detected using cytolysis-inhibiting monoclonal antibodies, *Immunol. Rev., 68*: 5 (1982).
420. P. D. Gottlieb, A. Marshak-Rothstein, K. Auditore-Hargreaves, D. B. Berkoben, D. A. August, and R. M. Rosche, Construction and properties of new Lyt-congenic strains and anti-Lyt-2.2 and anti-Lyt-3.1 monoclonal antibodies, *Immunogenetics, 10*: 545 (1980).
421. S. Kimura, N. Tada, E. Nakayama, and U. Hammerling, Studies of the mouse Ly-6 alloantigen system. I. Serological characterization of mouse Ly-6 alloantigen by monoclonal antibodies, *Immunogenetics, 11*: 373 (1980).
422. H. Auchincloss, Jr., K. Ozato, and D. H. Sachs, Two distinct murine differentiation antigens determined by genes linked to the Ly-6 locus, *J. Immunol., 127*: 1839 (1981).
423. F. Takei, G. Galfre, T. Alderson, E. S. Lennox, and C. Milstein, H 9/25 monoclonal antibody recognizes a new allospecificity of mouse lymphocyte subpopulations: Strain and tissue distribution, *Eur. J. Immunol., 10*: 241 (1980).
424. V. R. Sutton, C. A. Mickelson, G. H. Tobias, P. M. Hogarth, and I. F. C. McKenzie, Identification of two forms of the Ly-6.2 antigen showing differential expression, *Immunogenetics, 21*: 539 (1985).
425. P. M. Flood, D. B. Murphy, M. Horowitz, K. P. LeClair, F. R. Smith, E. Stockert, M. A. Palladino, Jr., and A. B. DeLeo, A monoclonal antibody that recognizes an Ly-6-linked antigen inhibits the generation of functionally active T cell subsets, *J. Immunol., 135*: 63 (1985).
426. F. Takei, MALA-1: A surface antigen expressed on activated murine T and B lymphocytes, *J. Immunol., 133*: 345 (1984).
427. F. J. Dumont, R. C. Habbersett, and E. A. Nichols, A new lymphocyte surface antigen defined by a monoclonal antibody (9F3) to the T cell population expanding in MRL/Mp-*1pr/1pr* mice, *J. Immunol., 133*: 809 (1984).

5
Mouse B-Cell Differentiation Antigens: Working Toward a Structure-Function Relationship

JOHN P. McKEARN*
E. I. duPont de Nemours and Co., Glenolden, Pennsylvania

I. INTRODUCTION

A. Definition of the B-Cell Lineage

While our understanding of the precise mechanisms of antigen recognition by the cellular components of the immune system still requires investigation, the manner by which B lymphocytes recognize antigen has been established for some time. Two principle findings provided much of the impetus needed to physically describe the component which conferred the exacting range of molecular specificities ($>10^7$ antigenic possibilities) that comprise the humoral arm of the immune system. Porter (1) and Edelman (2) described immunoglobulin (Ig) molecules as dimeric polypeptides in terms which accounted for antibody specificity. Their findings provided a critical framework needed to understand the clonal selection theory of humoral immunity (3). While this work provided the identifying trait which still serves to define the B lymphocyte (i.e., the Ig molecule), the manner by which B lymphocytes generate this tremendously diverse pool of antibodies was still a much-debated issue. It was subsequently demonstrated by Tonegawa and others (4-8) that Ig molecules are encoded by multiple gene segments which recombine during somatic development. Further expansion of the repertoire can be obtained by somatic mutations (9-11) and variation at the joining sites of gene segments (7,12).

These findings not only explained the genetic basis for clonal diversity, but also led to the finding that during somatic development, Ig gene segments encoding the heavy chain and light chain recombine in asynchronous and ordered fashion (13). Since expression of functional or complete Ig protein serves as a well-char-

**Present affiliation*: Searle Research and Development, Monsanto Co., St. Louis, Missouri.

acterized and unequivocal marker of the B-cell lineage, it is important to review Ig gene organization and expression within mouse B lymphocytes.

The first recognizable step toward commitment of multipotential stem cells to the B-lymphocyte lineage involves the rearrangement of Ig heavy chain genes. Specifically, studies examining gene structure in virally transformed pre-B-cell clones suggest that stem cells give rise to progeny which initially rearrange their diversity (D) and joining (J) segment genes in close juxtaposition (13). Four J_H segment genes are located roughly 7 kb upstream of the first μ constant (C) region gene, while 12 D_H genes lie 1-80 kb upstream of the J_H genes (14). In almost every clone examined to date, this rearrangement event occurs on both alleles of chromosome 12. In a significant percentage of virus-transformed clones, a truncated RNA transcript encoding the D-J_H-C_H portion of an Ig molecule could be detected (15). The function of this truncated transcript (16) and its significance to the B-cell lineage is unknown since similar results can be obtained in examination of mature T-lymphocyte clones (17,18).

As shown in Figure 1, the next step in commitment occurs when the precursor cell recombines 1 of 200-1000 variable (V_H) region genes located an unknown distance upstream of the D region genes. Once again, this translocation of H chain gene segments can occur on both chromosomes (13) if the initial recombination is nonproductive. While clones characterized as transcriptionally silent (both alleles defectively joined) were found in a significant percentage of cases, others actively translate IgM heavy chain protein with monoclonality predicted by models of allelic exclusion (19,20). It would appear, on the basis of experiments performed with A-MuLV transformed pre-B-cell clones, that allelic exclusion operates during the transition from progenitor (D-J_H) to pre-B (V_H-D-J_H); i.e., during V_H gene recombination.

V_H-D-J_H rearranged clones can accumulate large amounts of complete heavy chain protein in their cytoplasm without detectable transport of such proteins to the cell surface. This stage of B-cell development generates cells typically referred to as pre-B cells. It is generally believed that mechanisms of Ig gene recombination generate many nonfunctional DNA sequences during these early stages of B-lymphocyte development. Out-of-frame or mismatched gene segments are not expressed in the functional repertoire, and it is believed that the immune system is purged of such clones. This process is generally referred to as abortive rearrangement (21). While frequency estimates of this event have been made (22) and measurements of B-lymphocyte generation in the marrow suggest overproduction (23), the fate of such cells is not known. Answers to these questions will be more easily addressed once the precise mechanisms and enzymes which generate recombination are defined.

The third step of the differentiation scheme shown in Figure 1 depicts the transition from pre-B-cell to B-cell stage. This step involves the successful rearrangement of V and J region light chain genes to encode a functional V_L-J-C_L

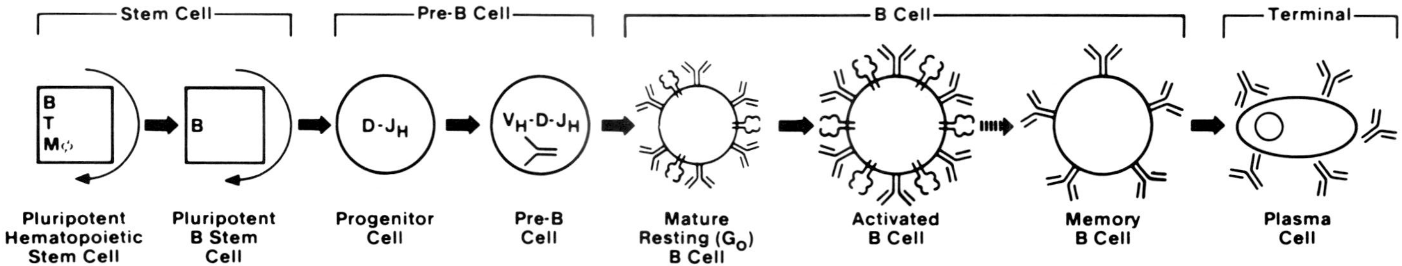

Figure 1 Scheme for differentiation sequence from stem cell to plasma cell.

transcript. In the mouse, the κ locus found on chromosome 6 is the initial light chain locus that attempts successful recombination (24). If reorganization events at both κ alleles fail to generate a successful transcript, the clones can delete the κ locus and attempt to rearrange its λ light chain genes found on chromosome 16 (25,26). Following successful rearrangement of the light chain genes a complete Ig molecule, containing two heavy chains and two light chains, is transported to the plasma membrane where it is displayed on the cell surface at high density ($>10^5$ copies per cell). The display of IgM at the cell surface (sIgM) marks the transition from the pre-B stage to the immature B-cell stage. Immature sIg-positive (sIg$^+$) B cells can be distinguished from mature B cells by the following criteria: high ratio of sIgM:sIgD (27-29), little or no Ia expression (28,30), and the relative ease with which one can render these cells refractory (tolerant) to antigenic stimulation (31-35). In the relative life span of the B lymphocyte, this immature stage does not persist for extended periods. Within a few days following the emergence of such cells, their diminution leads to the accumulation of sIg$^+$ B cells with higher levels of IgD (hence a lower sIgM:sIgD ratio), nearly all sIg$^+$ cells coexpress adult levels of class II MHC (Ia) antigens, and they mature to a stage where they are no longer hypersusceptible to tolerance induction (27-35). These cells probably represent the bulk of the small, resting (G_0) B cells observed in peripheral lymphoid organs. It is likely, despite considerable experimental controversy on this point, that peripheral B cells can persist in the resting state (G_0) for extended periods of time. Some experimental systems have demonstrated that such cells may persist for several months (36-38).

Once B lymphocytes acquire sIg and Ia, they are fully capable of participating in immune functions which serve to protect the host from bacterial, viral, and parasitic (antigenic) invasion. Preventing physiological damage by such antigens is recognized as the major importance of the antibody or humoral response and is therefore a process which demonstrates considerable functional heterogeneity.

The response of mature sIg$^+$ B lymphocytes to antigenic stimulation is a complex series of growth and differentiation events. A brief outline of what is known of these events will be presented since these properties describe the physiology of B lymphocytes at a pivotal stage in the developmental program. Namely, the sIgM$^+$ B cell most likely represents the focal point of the effector arm of the humoral immune system.

Evidence supports the view that sIgM$^+$ B cells initiate the primary phases of the humoral response, i.e., these cells bind ligand (antigen) and are activated to replicate and differentiate. Anti-IgM antibodies suppress B-cell function since primary (IgM) as well as formation of secondary (IgG) responses are obliterated when development of sIgM$^+$ cells is blocked (39-42). Conversely, blockade of IgG$^+$ B cells does not prevent response by IgM$^+$ cells (43). In addition, depletion of mature sIg$^+$ cells does not result in increased frequencies of pre-B cells (23,44).

These results suggest that sIgM+ B lymphocytes serve as the immediate precursors to primary and more diverse secondary responses to antigen. Therefore, a great deal of effort has been placed on understanding the physiology of this cell before and after activation.

Once a G_0 resting B cell is activated as part of a humoral immune response, i.e., through Ig receptor occupancy, the earliest alterations in normal cellular physiology include activation of phosphatydic acid metabolism, mobilization of intracellular or extracellular calcium, and changes in protein phosphorylation. These changes can be charted within 1-10 minutes following B-cell activation. Membrane depolarization occurs with slower kinetics, generally reaching peak levels at 30 minutes or better. Additional changes include increases in total cellular volume, increases in membrane Ia expression, and large increases in total cellular RNA production at 4-8 hours. After a considerable lag period, activated B cells begin DNA synthesis, marked by entry into the S phase of the cell cycle (reviewed in 45).

Once the sIgM+ B cell has been activated, clonal expansion and differentiation-inducing signals force the emergence of B cells, which actively secrete immunoglobulin, and, under appropriate antigenic stimulation, "memory" B cells can also be generated (46,47). These highly T-cell-dependent B-cell responses generate cell populations which greatly augment the ability to mount secondary responses when the host subsequently encounters the same antigen. Improved antibody affinity, faster onset of responses, and increased life span of such cells functionally define secondary or "memory" B cells (48-51). Despite considerable effort on the part of cellular immunologists, physical descriptions of such cells remain widely varied and, in some situations, contradictory. Once "virgin" or "memory" B lymphocytes have been induced to high rate immunoglobulin secretion, they have reached the penultimate stage of their lineage. These terminally differentiated cells probably do not enjoy long life spans (52). Their only obvious function is to secrete enormous amounts of their Ig products. Typically such cells can secrete sufficient Ig to account for 10-12% of their total protein synthesis (53). These cells differ sharply from their precursors with regard to cell-surface phenotype, since most do not express detectable Ia antigens, little or no sIg, and no B220 (54), the B-lineage component of the Ly-5 locus.

B. Monoclonal Antibodies Recognizing B-Cell Differentiation Antigens

While our capacity to quantitate and catalog changes in cellular metabolism and gene activation are continually improving, many aspects of B-cell growth and differentiation are still unclear. Our knowledge of which soluble mediators (interleukins or cytokines) participate in these events is enhanced by refined biochemical and recombinant DNA techniques. Once the relevant molecules are identified, their mechanism of action must be charted. These regulatory influences can be

Table 1 Summary of Monoclonal Antibodies Described in this Review

mAb clone	Pseudonym for antibody specificity	Apparent molecular weight of plasma membrane molecule
AA4	–	2 chains 125 Kd and 55-80 Kd
GF1	–	75-90 Kd
14.8	B220	220 Kd
10.1.D2	Lyb2	45 Kd
MEL-14	–	90 Kd
IR 518	PC-1	Homodimer 115 Kd

quantitated by measuring changes in the growth and differentiation status of the responding cells. For this purpose, monoclonal antibodies (mAb) which recognize differentiation antigens or receptors for growth/differentiation factors would allow us to probe these aspects of B-cell physiology by monitoring changes in the developmental program of B cells, including blocking or enhancing the function of B-cell growth and differentiation factors. These capabilities would not only allow improved understanding of the participating molecules, but information concerning temporal hierarchies could also be derived. Table 1 summarizes those mAb discussed in some detail in this review.

II. STUDIES USING mAb TO DEFINE THE DIFFERENTIATION SEQUENCE

A. The Study of B-Lymphocyte Precursors

This section will deal with four differentiation antigens expressed by various types of B-cell precursors: the cell surface antigens recognized by mAb AA4 (54), GF1 (54), 14.8 (55), and 10.1.D2 (56). These mAb have been extremely useful in identifying cells at a stage previously difficult to manipulate experimentally. Functional studies performed with such mAb have expanded our understanding of early B-lymphocyte differentiation.

Descriptions of these mAb should begin with experiments enumerating precursor cell frequencies in tissues which serve as primary sites of lymphopoiesis, typically fetal liver and adult bone marrow. When frequencies of mAb^+ (differentiation antigen-positive) cells are compared with precursor cell frequency estimates from functional or immunocytological assays, several interesting (and discrepant) observations can be made.

Table 2 Frequencies of mAb-Positive Cells Among Fetal, Newborn, and Adult Lymphoid Organs

Organ analyzed	mAb-positive population analyzed: AA4	GF1 (percent positive nucleated cells)	14.8	κ L-chain	Ia
fetal liver (day 12)	1.3	<1.0	<1.0	<1.0	<1.0
fetal liver (day 14)	2.7	<1.0	<1.0	<1.0	<1.0
fetal liver (day 16)	9.3	5.8	7.1	1.7	2.5
fetal liver (day 19)	10.7	9.3	5.9	<1.0	<1.0
newborn spleen (day 7)	4.4	5.7	7.9	4.5	7.1
adult bone marrow	25.8	7.9	24.2	5.0	N.T.
adult spleen	2.5	3.2	47.3	42.1	43.0

N.T. = not tested.
Frequencies determined by immunofluorescence assays using a FACS as described previously (54).

Initial observations demonstrated that mAb AA4, GF1, 14.8, and 10.1.D2 (or similar anti-Lyb2 mAb) recognize cIgM$^+$ pre-B cells present in adult bone marrow (54,55,57,58). In addition, subsequent experiments (shown in Table 2) demonstrate that mAb AA4 recognizes an infrequent cell population (~0.5-1.0% of nucleated cells) which appears in fetal liver at about the twelfth day of gestation. GF1 and 14.8 do not demonstrate detectable levels of binding at this time. At or near the sixteenth day of gestation, both GF1 and 14.8 bind significant numbers of cells. It is also at this point that a low number of sIg$^+$ B cells can be detected. AA4$^+$ and 14.8$^+$ cells reach plateau levels of roughly 7-11% by the fifteenth day of gestation. GF1-positive cells do not reach peak levels (~6-9%) until late gestation (days 16-19). AA4 recognizes approximately 4% of cells in spleens of 1-week-old mice and 26% of adult bone marrow cells, while GF1 recognizes 6% and 8%, respectively. These values far exceed the frequency of cIgM$^+$ (pre-B) cells measured during these stages of development (57). Likewise, these frequency estimates also exceed clonal frequencies determined in functional B-cell precursor assays by as much as 100-fold (59). However, immunofluorescence experiments and functional assays indicate that these mAb recognize B-lymphocyte precursors and that temporal hierarchies of differentiation antigen expression exist (54). Difficulties in making these absolute assignments include the rare frequency of precursor cells and uncertainties in defining cells only recently committed to the B lineage (the Ig$^-$ D-J_H or V_H-D-J_H rearranged precursor). For this reason we performed a more detailed analysis of Abelson murine leukemia virus (A-MuLV) transformed pre-B-cell clones. These experiments indicated that all pre-B cells express the differentiation antigens recognized by mAb AA4 and 14.8. Approximately 50% of all precursors express the GF1 recognized determinant (60). These results extended our earlier analysis, since some of these cell lines represent the earliest definable stages of commitment to the B-cell lineage. Namely, even Ig^- cells which had only rearranged their D-J_H genes expressed high levels of AA4 and 14.8 antigens.

While these observations were based on immunofluorescence staining assays, independent correlations were also made in functional assays. All four mAb were able to significantly deplete pre-B cells found in adult bone marrow (57,58, and unpublished results). However, other experiments demonstrated an interesting relationship between these differentiation antigens. Specifically, depletion experiments using mAb-coated polystyrene dishes to selectively remove antigen-positive cells demonstrated that AA4 expression precedes the expression of 14.8, which in turn precedes the expression of the 10.1.D2 (Lyb2) determinant among precursors defined in agar colony-forming assays (59). However, a proposed $AA4^-$ B-cell precursor found in day 12 fetal liver (59) seems rather uncertain since no mAb was found to deplete this cell (e.g., anti-class I MHC or mAb recognizing any ubiquitous cell-surface determinant). It is very likely that this observation is related to the efficiency of the depletion technique, i.e., it is likely that the frequency of this precursor (1 in 300,000) is too low for effective removal under the conditions described by Paige et al. (59). These experiments also raise an interesting point concerning the GF1 antigen. This mAb failed to remove precursors at any time in the agar colony-forming assay, but clearly removed immature cells in liquid cultures (54 and unpublished results). Therefore, results from liquid culture and immunofluorescence experiments provide an interesting contrast to the results from agar colony-forming assays. We propose that GF1 marks a subpopulation, which our results demonstrate to be 50% of all precursors (54,60), which does not mature in agar cultures (59).

A different strategy has been used to successfully identify B-lymphocyte precursors in tissues containing low frequencies of such cells. Purification of mAb-positive cells was accomplished using mAb-coated polystyrene dishes (54). Our rationale in these experiments rested mainly on two observations: First, AA4 and GF1 both recognize a significant percentage of bone marrow cells which could not be unambiguously defined as committed B-lymphocyte precursors, since they did not express detectable levels of Ig in their cytoplasm or on the plasma membrane (54); secondly, growth factors capable of supporting multipotential and committed precursors belonging to each of the major hematopoietic lineages were being resolved by improved biochemical separation and gene-cloning techniques. Specifically, it had been shown that a single glycoprotein, identified as IL-3 by Ihle and co-workers (61), was capable of supporting the growth and differentiation of precursors which generate the erythroid, myeloid, and possibly T-lymphocyte lineages (reviewed in 62). Since multiple growth activities previously ascribed to many separate molecules could be accounted for by IL-3 and this molecule was generously made available to us in its purified form, it was then possible to perform in vitro experiments which would support precursor cell development. We then tested whether any mAb would selectively enrich for IL-3-responsive precursors and, if so, we identified the lineage to which the precursor belonged.

MAb AA4, GF1, and 14.8 were tested for their ability to enrich precursors which would respond to IL-3- or WEHI-3-conditioned medium (WEHI-3CM). GF1 and 14.8 showed no enrichment properties when cells were isolated from adult bone marrow or fetal liver at days 13 or 19. However, selection of $AA4^+$ cells resulted in significant enrichment of IL-3- and WEHI-3CM-responsive cells. Enrichment was observed in ^{3}H-thymidine uptake by dividing cells in low density cultures, in methylcellulose colony-forming cell assays for erythroid and myeloid precursors, and in clonal liquid cultures (63). Our results demonstrated that AA4 selection enriched multipotential and restricted colony-forming unit precursors 50-100 fold. This analysis included multipotential precursors which generate all of the erythroid and myeloid lineages (colony-forming unit-mix, CFU-mix) as well as multipotential and restricted precursors which can generate the myeloid or erythroid lineages (colony-forming unit-granulocyte/macrophage, CFU-G/M and burst-forming unit-erythroid, BFU-E). AA4 did not recognize more mature erythropoietin-dependent erythroid precursors (colony-forming unit-erythroid, CFU-E). Similar levels of enrichment were observed when frequencies of IL-3 responsive precursors were quantitated in liquid cultures. Specifically, when colonies were scored after 14 days growth in limiting dilution cultures, AA4-selected cells contained approximately 100 times the number of precursors found in unselected fetal liver. Frequencies of WEHI-3 CM-responsive precursors among AA4-selected cells was 1 in 23, while unselected cells demonstrated frequencies of 1 in 2036 cells (63). IL-3-dependent clones derived from these liquid cultures were subsequently characterized as multipotential B-lymphocyte stem cells. Since these cells could be grown in the absence of filler cells we could establish the following points for each clone. First, their Ig heavy and light chain genes were in germline configuration. Second, these clones expressed high levels of the AA4, GF1, and LGP200 antigens on their surface. These cells also expressed low levels of class I major histocompatibility complex (MHC) antigens, while no B220 (14.8), sIg, Ia, or T lineage markers could be detected. Third, these cells possessed an absolute requirement for IL-3 to support their growth. Fourth, such cells could be induced to generate mature IgM-secreting cells after appropriate stimulation and extended maturation times. Fifth, these Ig responses were polyclonal, i.e., each clone generated antibody-producing cells committed to multiple V region specificities. Sixth, these IL-3-dependent stem cells did not form erythroid or myeloid colonies in methylcellulose cultures. Our ability to distinguish conditions which support growth (clonal expansion) and differentiation provide some insight into several apparent discrepancies raised by the work of other investigators (64,65). It has been suggested by Palacios and Steinmetz (64) that IL-3 supports the long-term growth of cells which reconstitute the B-cell compartment of irradiated hosts. Such IL-3-dependent cells do not contain rearranged Ig genes and apparently give rise to mature B lymphocytes upon adoptive transfer. Reconstitution was monitored by infecting donor cells with a retrovirus vector containing a bacterial gene which confers resistance to the neomycin antibiotic analog G418 (66). These studies, while consistent with the notion that IL-3 supports stem cell growth, fail to address several key points which would firmly establish such conclusions in this experimental system. First, integration and function of the neo resistance gene (neo^r) is only inferred since Southern blot analysis was not used to demonstrate integration into the host cell genome. Secondly, no evidence was presented to demonstrate that a single cell clone could repopulate the recipient's immune system by generating B lymphocytes committed to multiple variable region specificities. This point is crucial in making assignments related to B-lymphocyte stem cells. Thirdly, these precursor cell lines were judged to be $B220^+$ (14.8). This observation is inconsistent with those of several other laboratories (59,63,65). Fourth, genetic markers of Ig specificity were not used to assess the relative contribution of donor vs. host stem cells. This point should be addressed since surprisingly high levels of reconstitution were documented following sublethal doses of radiation. The fact that stem cell reconstitution was readily achieved with sublethal doses of radiation stands at odds with previous studies concerning stem cell reconstitution (67).

The recent report by Paige et al. (65) supports our observation that mAb AA4 selects a WEHI-3 CM-responsive precursor cell which can generate Ig-secreting B-cell clones. While these authors suggest that the ability of IL-3 to support B-cell precursors is indirect, their conclusion would seem premature since our experiments clearly demonstrate that pure IL-3 only supports B-stem cell growth (63). Differentiation (either Ig gene rearrangement or induction of Ig secretion) along the B-lymphocyte pathway could not be detected in the presence of IL-3 (63). This antagonistic relationship of growth- vs. differentiation-inducing signals complicates conclusions drawn from systems which require both events while failing to distinguish such properties (65).

Our experimental protocol (63) offers an avenue to study the rare precursor cells which give rise to committed B lymphocytes. Having established their cell surface phenotype and at least one interleukin (IL-3) whose role is to support growth, it should be possible to devise improved strategies to study their growth and differentiation requirements in vivo and in vitro. In addition, these results demonstrate that differentiation antigens expressed by B-cell precursors can also be found on erythroid and myeloid precursors. Therefore, by starting at a defined point in the B lineage, namely at the level of the cIg^+ pre-B cell (stage 3), it has been possible to trace precursor cell development back to earlier points in the lineage. This effort has provided several basic points of information which should make precursor cell development more amenable to direct analysis. The structure/function relationship of the mAb-defined differentiation antigens is likely to produce insight into the mechanisms of growth factor recognition and novel cell-cell interactions which regulate growth and differentiation.

B. Analysis of sIg^+ B Lymphocytes and Lymphocyte Migration

While it has long been possible to analyze and select mature sIg^+ B lymphocytes, tremendous gaps exist in our understanding of the conditions, soluble factors, and cell-cell interactions which promote their growth and differentiation. B lymphocytes have long stood as enigmas when one considers the relative ease with which growth conditions for T lymphocytes have been described. While this may reflect the functional plasticity of the B lymphocyte, it almost certainly is a reflection of the inadequacies of our description of B-cell growth and differentiation factors. It has been very difficult to establish the purity of factors originally derived from heterogeneous mixtures contained in culture supernatants and even more difficult to establish representative clonal assays which measure B-lymphocyte development. Difficulties in establishing clonal B-cell assays which are limiting only for responding B cells include the fact that such cells require various types of "accessory" cell help to promote the effector cell function they are committed to perform. Therefore, even when soluble factors have been purified to homogeneity or produced in quantity through recombinant DNA techniques, it is difficult to unequivocally demonstrate direct action on B lymphocytes. Despite these difficulties, several laboratories have recently made considerable progress toward defining soluble peptides which modulate B-lymphocyte growth and differentiation (68-78).

Our understanding of the physical properties and biological activities possessed by the B-lymphocyte stimulatory factor designated BSF-p1 (71), BCGF-I (72), BCDF (73), and IL-4 (75) has been greatly enhanced as a result of recent breakthroughs utilizing recombinant DNA techniques. Two different groups have isolated and molecularly cloned a gene encoding a 20 Kd glycoprotein which mediates multiple biological activities when tested among mature B-cell populations (68,69). It has recently been shown that this factor possesses properties previously ascribed to $BCGF_1$ (72), BCDF (73), and BSF-1 (71). Specifically, this B-cell stimulatory factor induces cell division, increased Ia expression, and enhanced Ig secretion among activated B cells. This molecule can also stimulate dramatic increases in surface Ia among small resting (G_0) B cells (68,69,75). These findings are important for several reasons. First, it would appear that isolation and characterization of the gene encoding B-cell stimulatory factor-1 (IL-4) has eliminated much of the confusion surrounding the function and existence of several B-cell factors since these results consolidate a large body of work. Namely, a single lymphokine can mediate a multiplicity of effects by interacting with

B cells poised at different stages of development. This does not rule out that a variety of factors interact with B lymphocytes to differentially influence their growth and maturation. However, these experiments do suggest that this list of candidate molecules may not be as long as we once believed.

Another molecule currently named IL-5 or eosinophil-differentiating factor (EDF) has also been shown to influence B-cell growth and differentiation (76). This molecule is believed to mediate effects previously ascribed to BCGF-II (77), i.e., support of BCL_1 B-lymphoma growth. The genes encoding this protein have not been reported to be molecularly cloned at this time, however careful biochemical and function analysis of this factor would strongly indicate that it is distinct from IL-4. IL-4 has an apparent M_r of 20,000 while IL-5 possesses an M_r of 44,000 (76).

These observations demonstrate a stark contrast between lymphokine regulation of B-cell versus T-cell growth and differentiation. Compelling evidence is accumulating that B-cell growth and differentiation is influenced by at least three soluble mediators or interleukins: IL-3 supports B-lymphocyte stem cell growth (63), IL-4 influences small resting (G_0) B cells and activated B cells (68, 69,71-75), and IL-5 modulates mitogen-activated B cells in the manner of BCGF-II (70,76,77).

It is clear from these studies that a single lymphokine has pleiotropic effects on its target cell. The many changes induced by these molecules and our ability to deduce the mechanism of action of these lymphokines are enhanced by the use of mAb which specifically monitor differentiation antigens, interleukins, and interleukin receptors. A mAb which recognizes IL-4 is a good example of the utility of such reagents (78). In addition, the unresolved complexities of B-lymphocyte activation can be studied with mAb which stimulate or inhibit B-cell growth and differentiation. Studies on the physiology of the immune response demonstrate that B-lymphocyte growth and differentiation is not a static process which can be duplicated in its entirety under typical experimental conditions. Studies on the lymphocyte "architecture" and lymphocyte trafficking support the existence of another level of complexity which most experimental systems have not addressed.

With regard to the issue of B-cell growth and differentiation, several mAb have been shown to influence murine B-cell growth and differentiation. We will focus on one mAb specificity whose functional utility has been characterized extensively. In addition, a mAb that has helped define specific interactions which govern lymphocyte trafficking (extravasation) will be discussed later, since this work has elucidated some of the mechanisms which generate specialized lymphoid "architecture."

Two mAb which define the Lyb-2 glycoprotein, a 45,000 dalton cell-surface molecule, demonstrate that this molecule may be involved in T-cell-dependent B-cell activation (56,79). Analysis of in vitro antibody responses show that anti-

Lyb-2 mAb can specifically block the generation of antibody responses to T-cell-dependent antigens, but not responses to T-cell-independent antigen (56,80). While it is not entirely clear how this molecule functions during B-cell activation, a direct influence on B cells has been suggested by experiments from two laboratories (56,80). Subbarao and Mosier (56) demonstrated that T-cell-depleted B-cell populations can be induced following exposure to anti-Lyb-2 mAb to undergo rapid increase in total cellular volume, incorporate ^{3}H-thymidine (enter S phase), and become receptive to T-cell-derived maturation factors which can ultimately drive the B cells to mature to Ig-secreting cells. While full characterization of the mechanism by which the Lyb-2 molecule participates in activation pathways (reviewed in 56) remains unresolved, it would seem that this molecule represents a prime candidate as one of the few non-Ig plasma membrane molecules which plays an important role in B-lymphocyte growth/differentiation. There are conflicting reports that the 45,000 dalton cell-surface molecule represents the IL-4 receptor (81,82). Perhaps the determinant recognized by anti-Lyb-2 mAb is a receptor for another (as yet undefined) interleukin whose biology is closely linked to IL-4.

It remains an ongoing challenge to understand how many immunoregulatory molecules (interleukins and cytokines) are involved in the humoral immune response. From a physiological standpoint we would like to know how these regulators interact when small resting (G_0) B lymphocytes are induced to grow and differentiate following interaction with antigen, T cells, and antigen-processing cells. Following the early studies describing T- and B-cell interaction (83-85), it became evident that a comprehensive understanding of cognate interaction and activation of B lymphocytes would be an arduous task. Activation and clonal expansion is manifested as a complex cascade of events (45) which also leads to systemic reorganization of the participating cell types (86). Antigen activated B lymphocytes generate high-rate Ig secreting cells and, under appropriate circumstances, long-lived high affinity "memory" B cells (87). The onset of "memory" B-cell production has been associated with the formation of specialized follicular domains called germinal centers (46). While the physiology of germinal center B cells remains an open question, their appearance in specialized microenvironments among spleen, lymph node, and Peyer's patches marks an important transition in the differentiation status of B lymphocytes. While the organizational events which lead to germinal center formation are quite striking, they are preceded by a series of extravasations.

During B-cell differentiation at least two major concerns must be addressed. Microenvironmental associations which promote B-cell maturation during precursor stages (before acquisition of sIg) must support production of tremendous numbers (2-5 $\times$ 10^7/day) of B lymphocytes without coordinate exposure to each specificity within the antigenic repertoire. These "antigen-independent" mechanisms supply the body with a diverse pool ($>10^7$ specificities) of antigen-reactive

sIg^+ B lymphocytes, which in turn interact with another supporting cast of accessory cells to generate the effector arm of the humoral immune system. Somehow this extremely mobile collection of lymphocytes must form proper associations with sessile populations of accessory cells which generate committed progeny from multipotential stem cells found in primary lymphopoietic sites (bone marrow, fetal spleen, and fetal liver), break these associations at the proper moment, and migrate to sites where appropriate interactions with antigen-processing cells and other accessory cells can lead to clonal expansion of antigen-specific B-cell clones. The specificity, timing, and overall mechanisms which control lymphocyte movement are not understood in precise detail. However, classical studies have shown us that lymphocytes are extremely mobile and that nearly all lymphocytes traffic about the body. Recent studies using a well-characterized mAb have contributed a great deal of information toward our understanding of the molecular mechanisms which govern lymphocyte migration and the generation of specialized domains within lymphoid tissues.

Gowans and Knight (88) demonstrated conclusively that lymphocytes recirculate by moving from the bloodstream into lymphoid organs where they eventually are collected in the efferent lymphatics and move back to the bloodstream. While much of the work which documents lymphocyte migration has been performed in animals larger than mice, enough corroborating evidence would suggest that similar mechanisms are used in the immune systems of all mammals. Sprent (89) demonstrated that nearly all small lymphocytes recirculate to some measurable extent. Therefore, the lymphoid compartment must be viewed to be in a constant state of flux which enables the full repertoire of antigen-reactive cells to survey the body for signs of antigenic exposure (infection). This process also would provide the appropriate dynamics for cell-cell interactions which would bring together different cell types required to generate an immune response. Lymphocyte migration appears to be controlled in part by associations between lymphocytes and structures which line specialized areas of postcapillary restrictions termed the high endothelial venules (HEV). An in vitro assay (90) established specific mechanisms which selectively recruit certain cells to privileged sites in the lymphoid architecture and bring such cells into close proximity with the site of antigenic entry or its site of sequestration. This study suggested that specific association between subsets of recirculating lymphocytes and HEV is mediated via "receptorlike" interactions. Lymphocytes homing to lymph nodes express a cell-surface determinant which binds to peripheral node HEV. This determinant was defined with a mAb designated MEL-14 (91) which specifically blocks HEV-binding activity. This mAb only blocks binding to peripheral node HEV and not gut-associated lymphoid tissue HEV. Therefore, distributional preferences of lymphocyte subsets, dictated by HEV-lymphocyte interactions (92), appear to be linked to the expression of molecules like the 90 Kd glycoprotein recognized by MEL-14 (91). This molecule is unusual since it contains at least two N-termini. One protein encodes ubiquitin and the second a unique glycoprotein (minimum mass of core protein equal to roughly 47 Kd) which contains at least three N-glycosylation sites (93). The presence of ubiquitin on the cell surface and its possible role in conferring some degree of specificity to the homing receptor is an unexpected finding. It will be interesting to learn whether similar mechanisms account for lymphocyte homing interactions at other sites.

While MEL-14 specifically inhibits binding of B and T cells to peripheral lymph node HEV, it does not inhibit binding to other HEV sites. However, it would appear that similar mechanisms account for specific binding at these sites (92,94). Interestingly, "homing receptors" (e.g., the MEL-14 antigenic determinant) are not expressed on antigen-activated B lymphocytes (95). Therefore, germinal center B cells, memory B cells, and Ig-secreting plasma cells do not express such receptors (95). The expression of functional receptors for HEV appears to be tightly linked with emigration of newly matured lymphocytes from primary lymphopoietic sites (93). Selective binding to HEV has been invoked as a major determining event which controls influx and composition of B- and T-cell subsets among lymphoid sites (92,94). Stark distributional preferences exist whereby roughly 70% of Peyer's patch lymphocytes are B cells and 10-20% are T cells. A reciprocal distribution is found among lymph nodes. Also, once lymphocytes have emigrated to peripheral sites, it is possible that loss of HEV receptors leads to an arrest of their specific exit (96). This cessation of traffic might help to account for clonal expansion of sessile lymphocyte clones (97). Interestingly, expression of specific homing receptors may also play a major role in the establishment of specialized lymphoid follicles near inflammatory and autoimmune lesions (96,97).

C. Transition to Terminal Differentiation Stages

As stated earlier, B-cell activation is a dynamic process which includes systemic reorganization of the participating cells. Specific binding reactions control movement of lymphocytes from primary lymphopoietic sites to peripheral lymphoid organs (86-97). In order to protect the host from infection, antigen-activated B lymphocytes must generate high-rate Ig-secreting cells, and for further protection, high-affinity, long-lived "memory" B cells. When these aspects of B-cell differentiation function properly, the sites of antigenic exposure are limited significantly.

The generation of antigen-primed "memory" B-cell populations correlates strongly with the appearance of specialized microenvironments, called germinal centers, found in spleen, lymph nodes, and Peyer's patches (46,47). Despite extensive studies devoted to cells which make up these structures and cells which have been functionally identified as "memory" cells (48-51), the developmental relationships of such populations is unresolved. Their relationship remains, in large part, circumstantial despite extensive homology in their physical characteristics. Both germinal center B cells and "memory" B cells are highly T-cell dependent and both express high levels of Ia, higher frequencies of sIgG, lower levels of total sIg, and considerably lower levels of IgD (47-51,98). It should be stressed that not all B-cell activators induce "memory" cell production. T-cell-dependent activators are very good inducers of germinal centers and "memory" B cells (99). Of several major questions which remain unresolved regarding these cell types, one remains prominent. How and when are high affinity "memory" cells selected? To understand how an activated B lymphocyte gives rise to both high-affinity, long-lived "memory" cells and high-rate, short-lived Ig-secreting plasma cells is puzzling.

The penultimate stage of B-lymphocyte maturation is defined as the generation of high-rate Ig-secreting plasma cells. These cells dedicate roughly 10-12% of their total transcriptional activity to the production of a monoclonal (clonally selected) antibody molecule (53). Again, while the life span of such cells is an area of debate, it is likely that most of these cells do not enjoy long life spans (52). The production of enormous titers of Ig is not a necessary requisite of the normal physiology. Thus extended life spans among high-rate Ig producers is unnecessary since Ig molecules can enjoy considerable half-life survival times in the blood, and effective concentrations of Ig can be remarkably low.

Identification of these end-stage cells has been extremely easy at the functional level since unequivocal assays for individual Ig-secreting cells have been available for a number of years (100,101). In addition, a large number of transformed plasmacytoma clones have been available for detailed biochemical analysis.

Terminally differentiated plasma cells lack many of the cell-surface molecules which help to identify less mature members of the B lineage. Namely, these cells express little or no sIg, Ia, or B220 (54). They do acquire a marker encoded by the PC-1 locus which is recognized under three allelic forms which encode a 115 Kd molecule which forms a homodimer on the cell surface (102-104). This gene is being analyzed in considerable detail since cDNA clones have been isolated, and attempts are being made to understand the mechanism(s) which controls its expression (104). This gene has been mapped to chromosome 2 of the mouse (102), but its functional relevance is still undiscovered. The recent results of Goding and van Driel suggest that PC-1 contains a short N-terminal cytoplasmic domain and an extensive C-terminal extracellular domain (104). Overall structure may resemble the transferrin receptor and possible asialoglycoprotein receptors and the Ia invariant chain. As suggested earlier (105), since PC-1 shares some structural properties with these molecules, it is possible that all share similar functional properties, namely transport functions.

III. SUMMARY

B lymphocytes originate from multipotential precursors which, through assymmetric division schedules, replenish themselves and generate committed progeny which proceed through a series of differentiation steps to become surface Ig-positive antigen-responsive B lymphocytes. These cells proliferate and differentiate to become effector cells which produce enormous quantities of Ig whose function is to neutralize and eliminate foreign antigen. Charting their course of differentiation through the use of monoclonal antibodies which recognize novel cell-surface markers of the maturation process combined with our current interest in soluble mediators (interleukins and cytokines) which modulate growth and maturation has greatly expanded our view of the mechanisms which lead to the functional plasticity of B lymphocytes. These studies have served as elegant models of eukaryotic gene regulation.

REFERENCES

1. R. R. Porter, *Biochem. J., 73*: 119 (1959).
2. G. M. Edelman, B. A. Cunningham, W. E. Gall, P. D. Gottlieb, U. Rutishauser, and M. J. Waxdal, *Proc. Natl. Acad. Sci. USA, 63*: 78 (1969).
3. F. M. Burnet, *The Clonal Selection Theory of Acquired Immunity,* The University Press, Cambridge, 1959.
4. C. Brack and S. Tonegawa, *Proc. Natl. Acad. Sci. USA, 74*: 5652 (1977).
5. C. Brack, M. Hirama, R. Lenhard-Schuller, and S. Tonegawa, *Cell, 15*: 1 (1978).
6. H. Sakano, K. Huppi, G. Heinrich, and S. Tonegawa, *Nature, 280*: 228 (1979).
7. E. E. Max, J. G. Seidman, and P. Leder, *Proc. Natl. Acad. Sci. USA, 76*: 3450 (1979).
8. P. Early, H. Huang, M. Davis, K. Calame, and L. Hood, *Cell, 19*: 981 (1980).
9. S. Crews, J. Griffin, H. Huang, K. Calame, and L. Hood, *Cell, 25*: 59 (1981).
10. E. Selsing and U. Storb, *Cell, 25*: 47 (1981).
11. M. Pech, J. Hochtl, H. Schnell, and H. G. Zachau, *Nature, 291*: 668 (1981).
12. M. Weigert, R. Perry, D. Kelley, T. Hunkapiller, J. Schilling, and L. Hood, *Nature, 283*: 497 (1980).
13. F. W. Alt, G. D. Yancopoulos, T. K. Blackwell, C. Wood, E. Thomas, M. Boss, R. Coffman, N. Rosenberg, S. Tonegawa, and D. Baltimore, *EMBO J., 3*: 1209 (1984).
14. Y. Kurosawa and S. Tonegawa, *J. Exp. Med., 155*: 201 (1982).
15. F. W. Alt, N. Rosenberg, V. Enea, E. Siden, and D. Baltimore, *Mol. Cell. Biol., 2*: 386 (1982).
16. M. G. Reth, P. Amirati, S. Jackson, and F. W. Alt, *Nature, 317*: 353 (1985).
17. D. J. Kemp, A. W. Harris, S. Cory, and J. M. Adams, *Proc. Natl. Acad. Sci. USA, 77*: 2876 (1980).
18. Y. Kurosawa, H. von Boehmer, W. Haas, H. Sakano, A. Traunecker, and S. Tonegawa, *Nature, 290*: 565 (1981).
19. B. G. Pernis, G. Chiappino, A. S. Kelus, and P. G. H. Gell, *J. Exp. Med., 122*: 853 (1965).
20. J. Cebra, J. E. Colberg, and S. Dray, *J. Exp. Med., 123*: 547 (1966).

21. R. P. Perry, D. E. Kelley, C. Coleclough, J. G. Seidman, P. Leder, S. Tonegawa, G. Matthyssens, and M. Weigert, *Proc. Natl. Acad. Sci. USA, 77*: 1937 (1980).
22. F. W. Alt, T. K. Blackwell, R. A. DePinho, M. G. Reth, and G. D. Yancopoulos, *Immunol. Rev., 89*: 5 (1986).
23. D. Opelsten and D. G. Osmond, *J. Immunol., 131*: 2635 (1983).
24. S. Lewis, M. Rosenbert, F. Alt, and D. Baltimore, *Cell, 30*: 807 (1982).
25. J. Durdick, M. W. Moore, and E. Selsing, *Nature, 307*: 749 (1984).
26. K. A. Siminovitch, A. Bakhshi, P. Goldman, and S. J. Korsmeyer, *Nature, 316*: 260 (1985).
27. E. S. Vitetta, U. Melcher, M. McWilliams, M. E. Lamm, J. M. Phillips-Quagliata, and J. W. Uhr, *J. Exp. Med., 141*: 206 (1975).
28. J. F. Kearney, M. D. Cooper, J. Klein, E. R. Abney, R. M. E. Parkhouse, and A. R. Lawton, *J. Exp. Med., 146*: 297 (1977).
29. I. Scher, S. O. Sharrow, R. Wistar, R. Asofsky, and W. E. Paul, *J. Exp. Med., 144*: 494 (1976).
30. J. J. Mond, S. Kessler, F. D. Finkelman, W. E. Paul, and I. Scher, *J. Immunol., 124*: 1678 (1979).
31. G. J. V. Nossal and B. L. Pike, *J. Exp. Med., 141*: 904 (1975).
32. J. W. Stocker, *Immunology, 32*: 283 (1977).
33. E. S. Metcalf and N. R. Klinman, *J. Exp. Med., 143*: 1327 (1976).
34. J. P. McKearn and J. Quintans, *J. Immunol., 124*: 77 (1980).
35. J. P. McKearn and J. Quintans, *J. Immunol., 124*: 1983 (1980).
36. J. Sprent and A. Basten, *Cell. Immunol., 7*: 40 (1973).
37. J. Sprent and J. F. A. P. Miller, *Eur. J. Immunol., 2*: 384 (1972).
38. S. Strober, *Transplant. Rev., 24*: 84 (1975).
39. C. W. Pierce, S. M. Solliday, and R. Asofsky, *J. Exp. Med., 135*: 698 (1972).
40. D. D. Manning and J. W. Jutilla, *J. Immunol., 108*: 282 (1972).
41. A. R. Lawton, R. Asofsky, M. B. Hylton, and M. D. Cooper, *J. Exp. Med., 135*: 277 (1972).
42. J. F. Kearney, M. D. Cooper, and A. R. Lawton, *J. Immunol., 116*: 1664 (1976).
43. C. F. Webb, W. E. Gathings, and M. D. Cooper, *Eur. J. Immunol., 13*: 556 (1983).
44. G. Fulop, J. Gordon, and D. G. Osmond, *J. Immunol., 130*: 644 (1983).
45. K. M. Coggeshall, J. G. Monroe, J. T. Ransom, and J. C. Cambier, in *B Lymphocyte Differentiation* (J. C. Cambier, ed.), CRC Press, Boca Raton, Florida, 1986.
46. G. J. Thorbecke, T. J. Romano, and S. P. Lerman, in *Progress in Immunology II*, Vol. 3 (L. Brent and J. Holborow, eds.), Elsevier North-Holland, Amsterdam, 1974.
47. G. Kraal, I. L. Weissman, and E. C. Butcher, *Nature, 298*: 377 (1982).
48. E. Yefenof, V. M. Sanders, E. C. Snow, R. J. Noelle, K. G. Oliver, J. W. Uhr, and E. S. Vitetta, *J. Immunol., 135*: 3777 (1985).
49. R. F. Coico, B. S. Bhogal, and G. J. Thorbecke, *J. Immunol., 131*: 2254 (1983).

50. D. M. Rennick, P. R. Morrow, C. Y. Leung, R. J. Scibienski, and E. Benjamini, *J. Immunol., 125*: 1262 (1980).
51. G. G. B. Klaus and A. Kunkl, Ciba Foundation Symposium *84*: 265 (1981).
52. A. A. Freitas, B. Rocha, and A. A. Coutinho, *Immunol. Rev., 91*: 5 (1986).
53. W. M. Kuehl, *Curr. Topics Microbiol. Immunol., 76*: 1 (1977).
54. J. P. McKearn, C. Baum, and J. M. Davie, *J. Immunol., 132*: 332 (1984).
55. P. W. Kincade, G. Lee, T. Watanabe, L. Sun, and M. P. Scheid, *J. Immunol., 127*: 2262 (1981).
56. B. Subbarao and D. E. Mosier, *Immunol. Rev., 69*: 81 (1983).
57. K. S. Landreth, P. W. Kincade, G. Lee, and E. S. Medlock, *J. Immunol., 131*: 572 (1983).
58. P. W. Kincade, G. Lee, M. P. Scheid, and M. D. Blum, *J. Immunol., 124*: 947 (1980).
59. C. J. Paige, R. H. Gisler, J. P. McKearn, and N. N. Iscove, *Eur. J. Immunol., 14*: 979 (1984).
60. J. P. McKearn and N. Rosenberg, *Eur. J. Immunol., 15*: 295 (1985).
61. J. N. Ihle, J. Keller, L. Henderson, F. Klein, and E. Palaszynski, *J. Immunol., 129*: 2431 (1982).
62. N. N. Iscove, in *Leukemia*, Vol. 30 (I. L. Weissman, ed.), Springer, Berlin, 1985.
63. J. P. McKearn, J. A. McCubrey, and B. Fagg, *Proc. Natl. Acad. Sci. USA, 82*: 7414 (1985).
64. R. Palacios and M. Steinmetz, *Cell, 41*: 727 (1985).
65. C. J. Paige, H. Skarvall, and H. Sauter, *J. Immunol., 134*: 3699 (1985).
66. P. J. Southern and P. J. Berg, *J. Molec. Appl. Genet., 1*: 327 (1982).
67. C. J. Paige, P. W. Kincade, M. A. S. Moore, and G. Lee, *J. Exp. Med., 150*: 548 (1979).
68. Y. Noma, P. Sideras, T. Naito, S. Bergstedt-Lindquist, C. Azumi, E. Severinson, T. Tanabe, T. Kinashi, F. Matsuda, Y. Yaoita, and T. Honjo, *Nature, 319*: 640 (1986).
69. F. Lee, T. Yokota, T. Otsuka, P. Meyerson, D. Villaret, R. Coffman, T. Mosmann, D. Rennick, N. Roehm, C. Smith, A. Zlotnik, and K. Arai, *Proc. Natl. Acad. Sci. USA, 83*: 2061 (1986).
70. C. J. Sanderson, A. O'Garra, D. J. Warren, and G. G. B. Klaus, *Proc. Natl. Acad. Sci. USA, 83*: 437 (1986).
71. M. Howard, J. Farrar, M. Hilfiker, B. Johnson, T. Kiyoshi, K. Takatsu, T. Hamaoka, and W. E. Paul, *J. Exp. Med., 155*: 914 (1982).
72. R. Noelle, P. H. Krammer, J. Ohara, J. W. Uhr, and E. S. Vitetta, *Proc. Natl. Acad. Sci. USA, 81*: 6149 (1984).
73. K. Yoshizaki, T. Nakagawa, K. Fukunaga, T. Kaieda, S. Maruyama, S. Kishimoto, Y. Yamamura, and T. Kishimoto, *J. Immunol., 130*: 1241 (1983).
74. J. Ohara, S. Lahet, J. Inman, and W. E. Paul, *J. Immunol., 135*: 2518 (1985).
75. N. W. Roehm, P. J. Leibson, A. Zlotnik, J. Kappler, P. Marrack, and J. C. Cambier, *J. Exp. Med., 160*: 679 (1984).

76. A. J. O'Garra, D. J. Warren, M. Holman, A. M. Popham, C. J. Sanderson, and G. G. B. Klaus, *Proc. Natl. Acad. Sci. USA, 83*: 5228 (1986).
77. S. L. Swain and R. W. Dutton, *J. Exp. Med., 156*: 1821 (1982).
78. J. Ohara and W. E. Paul, *Nature, 315*: 333 (1985).
79. H. Yakura, F. W. Shen, E. Bourcet, and E. A. Boyse, *J. Exp. Med., 155*: 1309 (1982).
80. H. Yakura, F. W. Shen, H. Kaemmer, and E. A. Boyse, *J. Exp. Med., 153*: 129 (1981).
81. I. Laurindo, F. D. Finkelman, J. Ohara, and J. J. Mond, Abstract, Sixth International Congress of Immunology, p. 266, 1986.
82. H. Yakura, I. Kawabata, T. Ashida, F. W. Shen, and M. Katagiri, *J. Immunol., 137*: 1475 (1986).
83. K. Rajewsky, V. Schirrmacher, S. Nase, and N. K. Jerne, *J. Exp. Med., 129*: 1131 (1969).
84. M. C. Raff, *Nature, 226*: 1257 (1970).
85. N. A. Mitchison, *Eur. J. Immunol., 1*: 18 (1971).
86. Z. Trnka and R. N. P. Cahill, *Mongr. Allergy, 16*: 245 (1980).
87. L. A. Herzenberg, S. J. Black, T. Tokuhisa, and L. A. Herzenberg, *J. Exp. Med., 151*: 1071 (1980).
88. J. L. Gowans and E. J. Knight, *Proc. R. Soc. London, 159*: 257 (1964).
89. J. Sprent, *Cell. Immunol., 7*: 10 (1973).
90. H. B. Stamper and J. J. Woodruff, *J. Exp. Med., 144*: 828 (1976).
91. W. M. Gallatin, I. L. Weissman, and E. C. Butcher, *Nature, 303*: 30 (1983).
92. S. K. Stevens, I. L. Weissman, and E. C. Butcher, *J. Immunol., 128*: 844 (1982).
93. M. Siegelman, M. W. Bond, W. M. Gallatin, T. St. John, H. T. Smith, V. A. Fried, and I. L. Weissman, *Science, 231*: 823 (1986).
94. E. C. Butcher and I. L. Weissman, *Ciba Fdn. Symp., 71*: 265 (1979).
95. R. A. Reichert, W. M. Gallatin, I. L. Weissman, and E. C. Butcher, *J. Exp. Med., 157*: 813 (1983).
96. S. T. Pals, G. Kraal, E. Horst, A. deGroot, R. J. Scheper, and C. J. L. M. Meijer, *J. Immunol., 137*: 760 (1986).
97. S. Jalkanen, A. C. Steere, R. I. Fox, and E. C. Butcher, *Science, 233*: 556 (1986).
98. E. C. Butcher, R. V. Rouse, R. L. Coffman, C. Nottenburg, R. R. Hardy, and I. L. Weissman, *J. Immunol., 129*: 2698 (1982).
99. J. F. A. P. Miller and J. Sprent, *J. Exp. Med., 134*: 66 (1971).
100. N. K. Jerne and A. A. Nordin, *Science, 140*: 405 (1963).
101. E. Gronowicz, A. Coutinho, and F. Melchers, *Eur. J. Immunol., 6*: 588 (1976).
102. J. S. Tung, F. W. Shen, E. A. Boyse, and E. Fleissner, *Immunogenetics, 6*: 101 (1978).
103. P. A. Stearne, I. R. van Driel, B. Grego, R. J. Simpson, and J. W. Goding, *J. Immunol., 134*: 443 (1985).
104. I. R. van Driel, A. F. Wilks, P. A. Pietersz, and J. W. Goding, *Proc. Natl. Acad. Sci. USA, 82*: 8619 (1985).
105. J. W. Goding and F. W. Shen, *J. Immunol., 129*: 2636 (1982).

6

Hemopoietic and T-Lymphocyte Marker Antigens of the Rat Characterized with Monoclonal Antibodies

WILFRED A. JEFFERIES*
Swiss Institute for Experimental Cancer Research, Lausanne, Switzerland

I. GENERAL INTRODUCTION

This review summarizes the current view of comparative hemopoietic differentiation with a particular emphasis on rat T-lymphocyte development. The use of monoclonal antibodies in dissecting the lymphocyte cell surface will be discussed, as will the general characteristics of lymphoid cells including results pertaining to pluripotent and committed T stem cells. Finally, the structure and possible function of particular cell-surface molecules and the functions of lymphocytes that bear them will be described in detail.

II. MARKER ANTIGENS AS TOOLS IN HEMOPOIETIC DIFFERENTIATION

A. Strategy for Using Monoclonal Antibodies to Study Cell-Surface Glycoproteins

A detailed analysis of the lymphocyte cell surface requires a reductionist approach. The main components of the membrane must be identified, isolated, and fully characterized in terms of structure and function, and then an overall picture may emerge regarding lymphocyte differentiation and the interactions of these cells. The cell-surface glycoproteins of lymphocytes cannot readily be identified on the basis of specific biological activities but can be identified antigenically.

**Present affiliation*: Ludwig Institute for Cancer Research, Stockholm, Sweden.

Theoretically, antibodies can be raised against all cell-surface proteins providing the molecules have diverged in sequence during evolution between mammalian species.

Before the discovery of hybridoma technology, both xenogeneic and allogeneic antisera were prepared (1) but were difficult to use in practice. Most molecules diverge in sequence between species, and xenogeneic immunizations result in very complex mixtures of antibodies which must be heavily preabsorbed before use. Even then monospecificity is not necessarily achieved. Conversely, allogeneic immunizations (2) generate low titre and, in some cases, low affinity antibodies. In addition, a surface protein will only be antigenic if it happens to be polymorphic between the strain of recipient and donor used as the inoculum (3). For most molecules, polymorphisms are found at relatively low frequency (2).

Monoclonal antibodies solved the problem of resolving the complexity of the xenogeneic response (4; reviewed in 5) and allowed a systematic approach to the identification of new cell-surface molecules (Fig. 1) (6). In addition, monoclonal antibodies that react with polymorphic determinants are produced in xenogeneic immunizations and can be detected by screening in antibody assays with cells from different inbred strains (7). Furthermore, hybrid cells produced in these fusions can be stored indefinitely and large amounts of antibody can be produced.

The strategy for screening monoclonal antibodies must be established before the fusion is undertaken, and hybridomas worth cloning must be chosen on the basis of appropriate criteria (1). Categories of hybridomas for further characterization usually fall into four groups (see Fig. 1). Antibodies that bind to cell-surface alloantigens can be selected by differential screening using inbred strains of animals. Secondly, antibodies may be selected which perturb in vitro lymphocyte functions. This includes screening for antibodies that inhibit cytotoxic T lymphocyte-mediated lysis (CTL), concanavalin A (Con A) response, the mixed lymphocyte culture (MLC), lymphocyte binding to high-walled endothelium or testing whether antibodies are mitogenic for resting lymphocytes. An example of an antibody that perturbs function is the W3/25 antibody, which binds to the rat CD4 "T helper" molecule and inhibits the MLC (8).

A third category of important monoclonal antibodies includes those that label functionally interesting subsets of lymphocytes. An example of this is the MRC OX22 antibody, which binds to the rat leucocyte-common antigen (L-CA) molecule now called CD45 and labels virtually all B cells, all rat cytotoxic/suppressor T lymphocytes, and the subset of T helper cells that produces interleukin-2 and provides help for cytotoxic T cells but does not provide help for B-cell responses (9).

A fourth category of interesting antibodies includes those that bind antigens with unusual anatomical distributions. The most prevalent in this category appear to be the antigens found on both lymphoid and brain cells. These include the OX2 antigen, which is expressed on rat thymocytes, neurons, B cells, and follicular

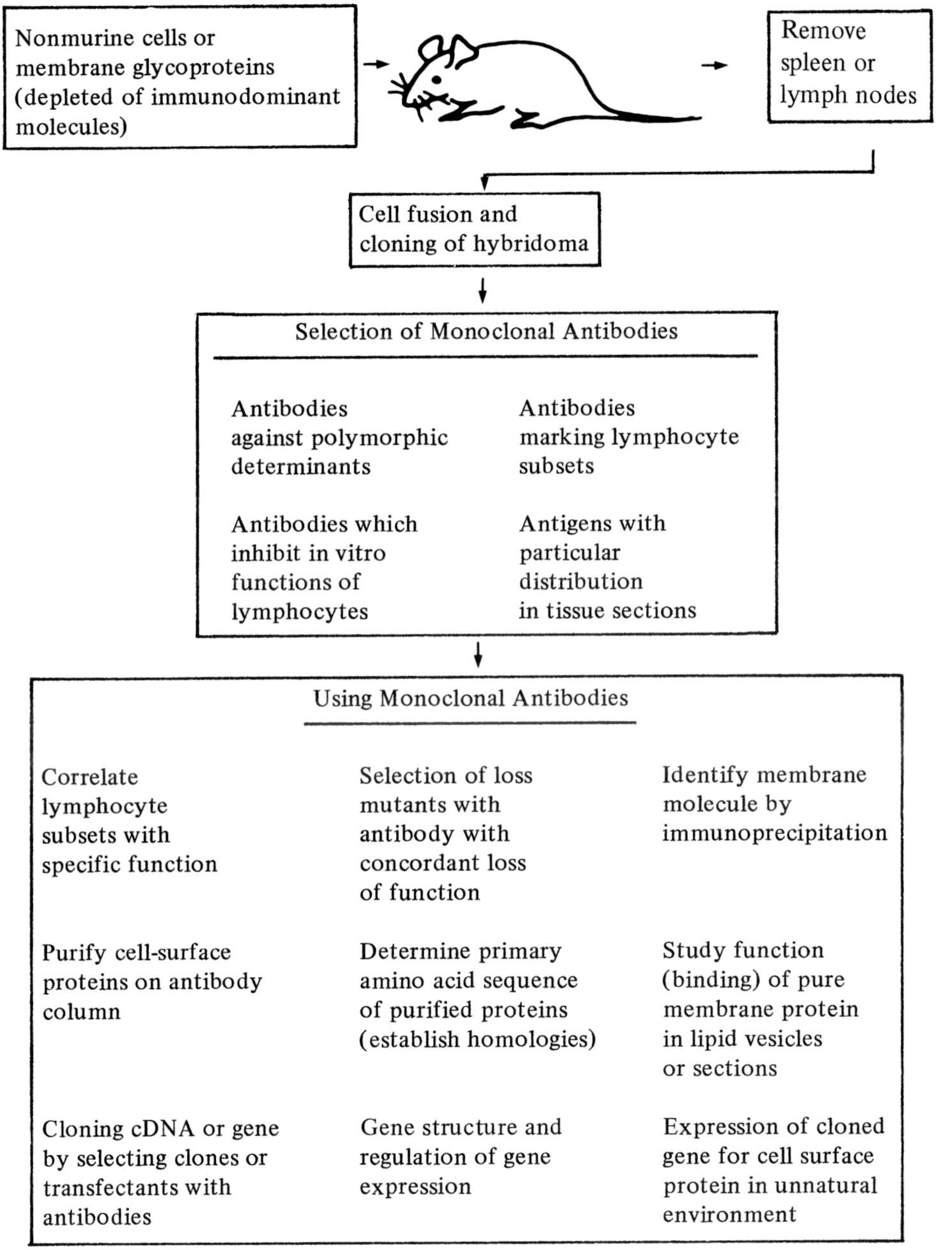

Figure 1 Selection of monoclonal antibodies for use in probing the structure and function of lymphocytes and lymphocyte cell-surface glycoproteins.

dendritic cells, and the Thy-1 antigen, which is found on brain, thymocytes, and hemopoietic stem cells in the rat. At present, it is not clear why there are so many shared lymphoid/brain antigens. The advantage of this final category of interesting antibodies in selecting hybridomas for further analysis and cloning is that large numbers of monoclonal antibodies can be screened on tissue sections or on the fluorescence-activated cell sorter (FACS), and this selection procedure operates independently of assayable functions of lymphocytes.

B. Problems with Derivation of Monoclonal Antibodies

Hybridoma technology has resulted in the identification of a large number of monoclonal antibodies that react with rat lymphocyte antigens, the most well studied of which are summarized in Table 1. Some polemics in the use of antibodies are worth mentioning, for example, cross-reactive monoclonal antibodies have been produced in interspecies immunization that react with unrelated proteins. Examples of this are cross-reactions between a SV-40 protein and a cellular protein (10) and also between Thy-1 and a component of intermediate filaments (11). Another strange cross-reaction has been reported using the UCHT-1 antibody, which reacts with the human CD3 pan-T cell antigen. This antibody also binds to a component of Purkinje cells in the brain and does so in various species (12). Suffice it to say, it is not a trivial point to ensure that the same protein is recognized on two different cell types and is not a spurious cross-reaction (13).

One other anomaly has occurred in the preparation of monoclonal antibodies across species barriers. It appears that certain antibody-reactivities either predominate or are completely absent from interspecies fusions. Examples of the first situation are anti-Thy-1 and anti-lymphocyte function associated antigen-1 (LFA 1) antibodies, which can dominantly appear in rats immunized with mouse T cells (14). Conversely, at least four mouse monoclonal antibodies exist (OKT3, UCHT-1, 83bI, and 38.1) that react with the human CD3 antigen (15), but at present no anti-CD3 antibody has been reported in any other species; the CD3 protein and the mRNA encoding the δ chain of the CD3 complex has been detected in mouse T cells (16,17).

Many important lymphocyte-surface molecules have been defined in the rat, mouse, and human (Table 2), but it seems possible that key molecules remain undiscovered. Problems in generating monoclonal antibodies against previously undefined antigens may be overcome by preparing cell-surface glycoproteins and depleting the immunodominant antigens (1). Alternatively, a different cell type that expresses lower relative amounts of the immunodominant antigen can be used as the immunogen, for example, activated T-cell blasts or perhaps a leukemia cell line (9,13). Another method is to immunize with T cells from another closely related species (i.e., lower primates) and screen for new antibodies on the desired target, human T cells (19). Finally, hamsters instead of mice or rats can be immunized and the spleen cells from these animals used in fusions (20).

Table 1 Monoclonal Antibodies that React with Rat Lymphohemopoietic Cells

			Site numbers[a]					
Antibody	Subclass	Name:nature of antigen	Thym	T	B	Cell types labeled	Functional effects	Ref.
MRC OX1	IgG_1	L-CA, all forms: gp 180-220	52	59	63	All rat leukocytes, not RBC	None	297
MRC OX2	IgG_1	OX2: gp43	30	0	5	Rat thymocyte, brain B cells, dendritic cells, T lympho-cyte blasts, endothelium	None	7
MRC OX3	IgG_1	Ia: gp33; gp29	45[b]	0	100	RT1B polymorphic, ($RTIB^u$) B cells, dendritic cells	ND	7
MRC OX4	IgG_1	Ia: gp33; gp29	45[b]	0	100	RT1B common non-polymorphic (MHC class II products)	ND	7
MRC OX6	IgG_1	Ia: gp33; gp29	45[b]	0	100	As for MRC OX4	Inhibits MLR	7
MRC OX7	IgG_1	Thy-1: gp18	1000	0	0	CFU-S, rat thymocytes, brain, some polymorphs, fibroblasts, pluripotent stem cells, pre-B cells	None	298
MRC OX8	IgG_1	CD8: gp36; gp33	27	100	0	T cytotoxic/suppressor cells and NK cells, thymocytes	Inhibits the generation of cytotoxic T cells	299
MRC OX9	IgG_1	CD8: gp36; gp33	25	ND	0	Competes with MRC OX8	ND	299
MRC OX10	IgG_1	CD8: gp36; gp33	14	ND	0	Same population as MRC OX8, does not compete with MRC OX8 or MRC OX9	ND	299

(Table 1 *continues*)

Table 1 (*continued*)

Antibody	Subclass	Name:nature of antigen	Site numbers[a]			Cell types labeled	Functional effects	Ref.
			Thym	T	B			
MRC OX11	IgG_1[c]	IgK^a chain (kappa[a] allotype) 2x (p25; gp55)	0	0	ND	Rat anti-rat Kappa chain B cells (a allotype)	ND	300
MRC OX12	IgG_{2a}	Ig K chain: 2x (p25; gp55)	0	0	70	Mouse anti-rat Kappa chain (preference for a allotype) B cells	ND	44
MRC OX14	IgG_1	IgG_2: 2x (p25; gp55)	0	0	ND	B cells	ND	317
MRC OX16	IgG_1	IgG_2: 2x (p25; gp55)	0	0	ND	B cells	ND	317
MRC OX17	IgG_1	Ia: gp33; gp29	45[b]	0	100	RT1D not polymorphic (MHC class II products)	Inhibits MLR	136
MRC OX18	IgG_1	MHC class I: gp43; p12	ND	200	200	RT1A non-polymorphic (MHC class I)	ND	136
MRC OX19	IgG_1	CD5: gp67	20	50	ND	Thymocytes, T cells, 2% B cells	Augments T-cell responses in vitro	240
MRC OX22	IgG_1	L-CA subset: gp190, 200, 220	0	12	42	L-CA on B cells, cytotoxic/suppressor T cells, 75% T helper cells, B lymphocytes, NK cells	None	9
MRC OX26	IgG_{2a}	Transferrin receptor: 2x gp95	0	0[d]	0	Leukemias, 30% B.M., 95% fetal liver, brain capillary endothelium, some other tissues	ND	54
MRC OX27	IgG_{2a}	MHC class I: gp43; p12	ND	ND	ND	$RT1A^c$ haplotype specific (not RT1A a, u, or 1 haplotypes)	ND	13

MRC OX28	IgG_1	LCA: all forms: gp 180-220	55	64	57	All rat leukocytes, not RBCs, competes with MRC OX1	None	206
MRC OX29	IgG_{2a}	LCA: all forms: gp 180-220	30	37	33	All rat leukocytes, not RBCs, competes with MRC OX1 and MRC OX28	ND	206
MRC OX30	IgG_{2a}	LCA: all forms: gp 180-220	55	70	52	All rat leukocytes noncompetitive with MRC OX1, 28	ND	206
MRC OX31	IgG_1	LCA: subset gp 190, 200, 220	0	8	44	As MRC OX22, competes with MRC OX22	ND	206
MRC OX32	IgG_{2b}	LCA: subset gp 190, 200, 220	0	32	58	As MRC OX22, noncompetitive with MRC OX22 and MRC OX31	ND	206
MRC OX34	IgG_{2a}	OX34: gp50 (CD2)	18	ND	0	Rat thymocytes, NK cells, T cells, scattered cells in red pulp of spleen	Variably inhibits MLC and Con A response	13
MRC OX35	IgG_{2a}	CD4: gp52	16	40[e]	0	Thymocytes T helper cells, macrophages, dendritic cells, not competitive with W3/25	Inhibits MLC	13
MRC OX36	IgG_{2a}	CD4: gp52	12	35[e]	0	Not competitive with W3/25 competes with MRC OX35	Inhibits MLC	13
MRC OX37	IgG_1	CD4: gp52	9	30[e]	0	Competes with W3/25 and MRC OX38 but not MRC OX35-36	Inhibits MLC	13
MRC OX38	IgG_{2a}	CD4: gp52	12	35[e]	0	Competes with W3/25 and MRC OX37 but not with MRC OX35-36	Inhibits MLC	13

(Table 1 *continues*)

Table 1 (*continued*)

Antibody	Subclass	Name: nature of antigen	Site numbers[a] Thym	T	B	Cell types labeled	Functional effects	Ref.
MRC OX39	IgG_1	IL-2 receptor: gp50	0	0	0	Activated T and B cells, dendritic cells cross-react slightly with mouse IL-2 receptor	Inhibits IL-2 from bind to IL-2 receptor	233
MRC OX40	IgG_{2b}	OX40: gp45	0	0	0	Activated T cells only, GvH lymph node cells	Variably augments MLC	233
MRC OX41	IgG_{2a}	OX41: gp120	0	0	0	All brain cells, polymorphs, granulocytes, dendritic cells, macrophage subset	None	302
MRC OX42	IgG_{2a}	OX42: gp95; 103; 160 (C3bi receptor)	0	0	0	Granulocytes, dendritic cells, macrophages subset, microglia	Inhibits complement mediated rosettes between red blood cells and macrophages	303
MRC OX43	IgG_1	OX43: gp90	0	0	0	Rat peritoneal macrophages and alveolar macrophages, endothelium, not brain endothelium	None	251
MRC OX44	IgG_1	OX44: gp45	ND	ND	ND	40% B.M., 12% thymocytes, peripheral lymphocytes	None	74
MRC OX45	IgG_1	gp44	ND	ND	ND	All hemopoietic cells and endothelium	Inhibits MLC by effect on macrophages	303
MRC OX46	IgG_{2a}	gp44	ND	ND	ND	Competes with MRC OX45	Same as MRC OX45	303
MRC OX47	IgG_1	ND	20	ND	ND	B.M. subset, thymocytes, some TDL, macrophages, dendritic cells	ND	233

MRC OX48	IgG_1	OX48: gp95	7.5	0	0	Activated T and B cells macrophages, hepatocytes, brain endothelium	None	233
MRC OX49	IgG_{2a}	OX49: p85	10	ND	ND	40% B.M., thymocytes T cells, subset of B cells	None	233
MRC OX50	IgG_1	OX50: p85	10	ND	ND	Same as MRC OX49	None	233
MRC OX51	IgG_1	L-CA: gp240	ND	ND	ND	B cells, T cells weak possibly B220	None	184
MRC OX52	IgG_1	OX52: gp120; gp95	ND	ND		T cells thymocytes	None	304
W3/13	IgG_1	Leukocyte Sialoglyco-protein (LSGP): gp95	100	150	0	CFU-S, thymocytes, T cells, plasma cells, polymorphs, brain, Dim on committed T progenitors/stem cells	None	6
W3/15	IgG_1	W3/15: gp135; p95	ND	0	0	B.M. erythroid, thymocytes	ND	6
W3/25	IgG_1	CD4: gp52	10	30[d]	0	Thymocytes, T helper cells, macrophages, dendritic cells, competes with MRC OX37-38	Inhibits MLR	6
ART 18	IgG_1	IL-2 receptor: gp50	0	0[f]	0	Activated T cells, B cells, prothymocytes	Inhibits IL-2 from binding to T blast cells	267
A11	IgG_1	gp135; gp63; gp40	ND	ND	ND	Peripheral lymphocyte	Inhibits lymphocyte adhesion to peripheral lymph node HEVs	92
1B.2.	IgG_1	gp80	ND	ND	ND	Peripheral lymphocyte 8% B.M., 10% thymocytes	Inhibits lymphocyte adhesion to Peyer's patch HEVs	93
R-1-3133	IgG_{2a}	CD5: gp67	ND	ND	ND	Thymocytes, T cells, B cell subset	ND	242

(Table 1 *continues*)

Table 1 (*continued*)

Antibody	Subclass	Name: nature of antigen	Site numbers[a] Thym	T	B	Cell types labeled	Functional effects	Ref.
R-1-12C5	IgG_1	gp95	ND	ND	ND	20% B.M., thymocytes, T cells	ND	242
R-2-1B3	IgG_{2b}	gp32-47	ND	ND	ND	10-20% thymocytes, all leukocytes, probably same as MRC OX44	ND	306
ED-1	IgG_1	ND	0	0	0	Cytoplasmic staining of all macrophage and dendritic cells	ND	307
ED-2	IgG_{2a}	ND	0	0	0	All macrophages, not monocytes	ND	307
ED-3	IgG_{2a}	ND	0	0	0	Spleen, mesenteric and some thymic and peritoneal macrophages	ND	307

5C6-F4	IgG_3	2x p100	0	0	0	Activated T and B lymphocytes	Inhibits Con A and LPS mitogenesis and IL-2 dependent proliferation	308
GY1/12[7]	IgG	RT6.2: p24; p21	0	ND	0	85% of peripheral T cells of DA rat	ND	46
P4/16[7]	IgG	RT6.1	0	ND	0	85% of peripheral T cells of PVG rat	ND	46

The monoclonal antibodies which react with rat cell-surface proteins of lymphohemopoietic cells are summarized. Key references have been included together with the name of the cluster differentiation (CD) groups assigned to the human homologues (15). The molecular weights of the molecules are approximate as determined by polyacrylamide gel electrophoresis in sodium dodecylsulphate. p = protein, gp = glycoprotein, neither g nor gp denotes that the glycosylation is not known. A zero in the site number section indicates there is no binding over background in FACS analysis (>2000 molecules per cell). ND indicates that at least a subset of the cell type is labeled but that the site number has not been determined. NK = not known. Thym = thymocytes, T = T cells, B = B cells.

[a]The number of molecules $\times 10^{-3}$ of the particular protein on the cell surface as determined by the method described in reference 28.

[b]The number of molecules of Ia found on dendritic cells in the thymus.

[c]Rat anti-rat monoclonal antibodies.

[d]The number of transferrin receptors on activated T cells is 60,000 (184).

[e]The peritoneal macrophages express 30,000 molecules of CD4 per cell (184).

[f]The number of interleukin-2 receptors on activated T cells is 75,000 sites per cell (267).

Table 2 Lymphocyte Cell-Surface Marker Molecules

Molecules	Molecular nature	Commonly used names: Human	Mouse	Rat	1	2
Immunoglobulin related						
T cell receptor	gp43; gp40	WT-31	No mAb recognise all receptors		–	±
MHC Class I	gp43; p12	HLA A,B,C	H-2 K,D.L	RT1A	±	–
MHC Class II	gp33; gp29	HLA DR, DQ DP (SB)	H-2 I-A, I-E	RT1B, RT1D	±	–
TL	gp43; p12	ND	TL	ND	–	+
Qa	gp43; p12	ND	Qa	ND	+	ND
Thy-1	gp18	Thy-1	Thy-1	Thy-1	±	+
OX2	gp47	OX2[a]	OX2[a]	OX2	±	+
CD1	gp45; p12	HTA1/T6	ND	ND	–	+
CD4	gp55	T4, Leu3	L3T4	W3/25	–	+
CD8	gp38; gp34 or 2xgp34	T8, Leu2	Ly2,3	OX8	–	+
Heavily glycosylated proteins						
L-CA	gp180-220	L-CA	T200, Ly5	L-CA	+	+
L-SPG	gp95	LIO	gp9	W3/13	±	+
Miscellaneous molecules						
CD2	gp50	T11, 9.6 LFA-2	ND	OX34	–	±
CD3	gp25, gp20, p20	T3, Leu4	T3	ND	–	±
CD5	gp67	TI; Leu1	Ly-1	OX19	–	+
LFA-1	gp180;gp90	LFA-1	LFA-1 Ly 15	ND	+	+
OX44	gp40-50	ND	ND	OX44	+	±

Cells expressed on						
3	4	5	6	Other	Comment	Ref.
+	+	+	+	None	Most T cells express the α:β TcR	103,111
+	+	+	+	Most cell excluding brain	Recognised with Ag by T cells	121,122 126
–	–	–	±	Dendritic, macrophage, thymic epithelium	as above	130,135
+	–	–	–	Leukemias	MHC Class I-like	121
ND	+	+	ND	ND	Linked to MHC	121
+	–	–	±	Brain, fibroblast, mouse T cells	Not on human blood cells	21
+	–	–	±	B cells, neurons, endothelium, dendritic cells	Detect in human/mouse by northern blots	22,183
–	–	–	–	Leukemias, Langerhan cells	MHC Class I-like, relationship to Qa/TL unclear	17a
+	+	–	±	Macrophage, dendritic cells	Ab block T cell response	13,150
+	–	+	±	NK cells (rat)	Ab block CTL reactions	172,178 181,182
+	+	+	+	None	Subset specific Ab; Ab inhibit diverse functions	206,219
+	+	+	+	Plasma cells, brain, stem cells, polymorphs	Mucin-like protein	27
+	+	+	+	Fetal thymus, NK cells	Ab blocks E-rosettes	13,232, 236
+	+	+	+	Cross reacts with Purkinje cells	Associated with TcR, Ab mitogenic	12,235
+	+	+	+	2% B cells, B lymphomas	Ab augments T responses	240,242
+	+	+	+	ND	Ab inhibit adhesion α chain interferon like	246,249, 256
±	+	+	+	B cells, macrophages dendritic cells	Marker of prothymocytes, functional thymocytes	74

(Table 2 *continues*)

Table 2 (*continued*)

Molecules	Molecular nature	Commonly used names: Human	Mouse	Rat	1	2
OX52	gp120; gp90	ND	ND	OX52	–	+
RT6	p25; p28	ND	ND	RT6.2 (Pta)	–	–
TAP	gp15-18	ND	Ly-6	ND	ND	–
Blast markers						
Transferrin receptor	2xgp95	T9, 5E9, B3/25	R17	OX26	±	–
IL-2 receptor	gp50	TAC	PC61, 3C7	ART18, OX39	–	±
4F2	gp80; gp40	4F2	RL73	ND	ND	ND
VLA-1	gp210; gp130	VLA-1	ND	ND	–	–
VLA-2	gp160; gp130	VLA-2	ND	ND	–	–
OX40	gp45	ND	ND	OX40	–	–

Molecules listed are well characterized and functionally or structurally prominent. Glycoproteins are grouped on the basis of their appearance on blast cells, their structural relationship with immunoglobulins, their carbohydrate content, and proteins where a structural relationship with other proteins is still uncertain. References listed contain the best structural information regarding the lymphocyte surface molecule in question (see Ref. 28 for further references). Cell types are as follows: 1) bone marrow, 2) cortical thymocytes, 3) medullary thymocytes, 4) T helper/inducer cells, 5) T cytotoxic/suppressor cells, 6) activated T cells.

[a]The OX2 antigen has been detected in Northern blot analysis in mouse and in human by Southern blot analysis and by sequencing the gene (185).

C. Sequence Determination of Lymphocyte Molecules as an Extension to the Monoclonal Antibody Approach

Monoclonal antibodies have also been employed as tools in a number of strategies to determine the primary structure of proteins expressed in lymphocytes. Monoclonal antibody affinity columns can be used to purify lymphocyte surface proteins, which are then sequenced by the conventional protein chemistry procedures of sequencing overlapping peptides (21). However, full protein sequence

Cells expressed on						
3	4	5	6	Other	Comment	Ref.
+	+	+	+	None	T cell specific marker	304
–	±	±	ND	ND	Attached to membrane via Fatty acid linkage	257a, 257b
+	+	±	+	Activated B cells	Mitogenic for T cells, attached to membrane via fatty acid linkage	17b, 17c
–	–	–	+	Fetal liver, Normal tissues, Brain endothelium	Labels leukemic cells	24,62, 277
–	–	–	+	Fetal thymus, B blasts	Ligand stimulates T cell growth	267,274
ND	–	–	±	Monocytes, kidney tubules	Ab blocks monocyte induction, 4F2 is Na^+ exchanger	309,310
–	–	–	+	ND	Appear on long term T cell lines	269
–	–	–	+	ND		269
–	–	–	±	None	T blast-specific Augments T cell responses	233

determination is now rarely used and virtually all sequencing is now done at the nucleic acid level. Messenger RNA from cells that express the molecule of interest is copied into complementary DNA (cDNA) with reverse transcriptase, and this is then cloned into a plasmid or phage vector, which is then incorporated into bacteria and expanded as a bacterial colony. The inserted DNA from a relevant plasmid is then sequenced. The main problem with this approach is in detecting the relevant clones (Table 3).

One approach commonly employed in detecting the correct clones is to use synthetic oligonucleotide probes constructed from the partial amino acid sequence of an immunoaffinity purified protein (22). Antibodies in the form of antisera or monoclonal antibodies can be used to select epitopes of the correct protein, which have been cloned and expressed in *Escherichia coli*, using λ phage expression vectors (23). Genes encoding lymphocyte cell surface proteins can be isolated by cotransfection of herpes simplex virus thymidine kinase gene (HSV-TK)

Table 3 Methods Used to Determine the Primary Amino Acid Sequence of Lymphocyte Cell-Surface Molecules

Approach	Molecule	Ref.
Amino acid sequencing	Thy-1 (rat)[a]	190
	Thy-1 (mouse)[a]	21
	HLA Dr α chain	311
	HLA-A2; HLA-B7	312
Radiosequencing	H-2K^b	122
Limited protein sequence; cloned with synthetic oligonucleotides	CD3 (T3) δ chain	236
	L-CA	219
	OX2 antigen	22
	Transferrin receptor	285
	Insulin receptor	313
	IL-2 receptor	274,275
	CD5 (T1/Leu-1)	245a
Polysome immunoprecipitation-subtractive hybridization	Transferrin receptor	284
Positive selection hybridization	β_2-microglobulin	314
	RT1B A_α	239
	H-2K^d	315
	HLA-DR$_\beta$	316
Epitope selection of λ clones with antisera	MEL-14	90,91
	CD3 (T3) ε chain	23
	CD3 (T3) γ chain	236a
	CD2 (T11)	234a
Expression of genes in transfected L cells	CD4 (T4)	150
	CD8 (T8)	177
	CD8 (T8)	178
	Transferrin receptor	24
Subtracted library approach	T cell receptor (α, β, γ chains)	25,112, 113

The techniques currently employed to determine the primary amino acid sequence of lymphocyte cell-surface molecules are depicted.

[a]The sequence of Thy-1 was determined after purification from rat or mouse brain cells. The amino acid composition of the Thy-1 protein from brain or thymocytes is identical.

and whole chromosomal DNA into mouse LTK^- fibroblast cells, which are subsequently selected during two sequential steps consisting of hypoxanthine/aminopterin/thymidine (HAT) treatment and then sorting on the FACS (24). Finally, subtracted library techniques can be used to select cDNA clones encoding the correct sequences (25). It should be noted that the final three procedures require confirmation that the selected cDNA clone or gene is correct by independent criteria, such as in vitro translation, or by northern or southern blotting.

III. LYMPHOID CELL TYPES AND THEIR FUNCTIONS

A. Characterization of Lymphoid Lineages and Lymphocyte Antigens Using Antibodies

The use of monoclonal antibodies has revealed multiple lymphoid subsets and the complicated nature of lymphoid differentiation. Three clear conclusions have resulted from these studies. First, marker antigens seem to be expressed, turned off, and then expressed again in a particular differentiation pathway—jumping antigens (26). One example of this is the leukocyte sialoglycoprotein (L-SGP) recognized by the W3/13 antibody in the rat (27). It is expressed on bone marrow stem cells and is not expressed by B cells, but its expression is switched on in plasma cells (27). Second, there are few antigens whose expression is confined to only one differentiation lineage. The only three concrete examples are surface immunoglobulin on B cells and the T-cell antigen receptor and CD3 (T3) on T cells. Third, in some cases homologous molecules are not necessarily expressed on the same cell types in different species. The Thy-1 molecule is expressed on thymocytes but not T cells in rat, whereas in mouse both thymocytes and T cells express Thy-1. In human, Thy-1 is expressed neither by thymocytes or T cells, though it appears to be conserved on fibroblasts and neurons in all species (28). It is therefore not clear whether certain molecules are required for normal lymphocyte function or whether more than one molecule can perform the same function so that a different molecule enables the maintenance of cellular function.

B. Hemopoietic Stem Cells: General Characteristics

It is usual to describe hemopoietic populations as being composed of stem cells, progenitor cells, and morphologically identifiable but still immature cells. Each succeeding population expands in size, and the whole population is generated from relatively few ancestral cells (29).

All hemopoietic cells originate from multipotential stem cells that possess the capacity for self-renewal and a capacity to give rise to differentiated progenitor cells (30). Progenitors differ from stem cells in that they are irreversibly committed to differentiation in a particular lineage and have less capability for self-renewal.

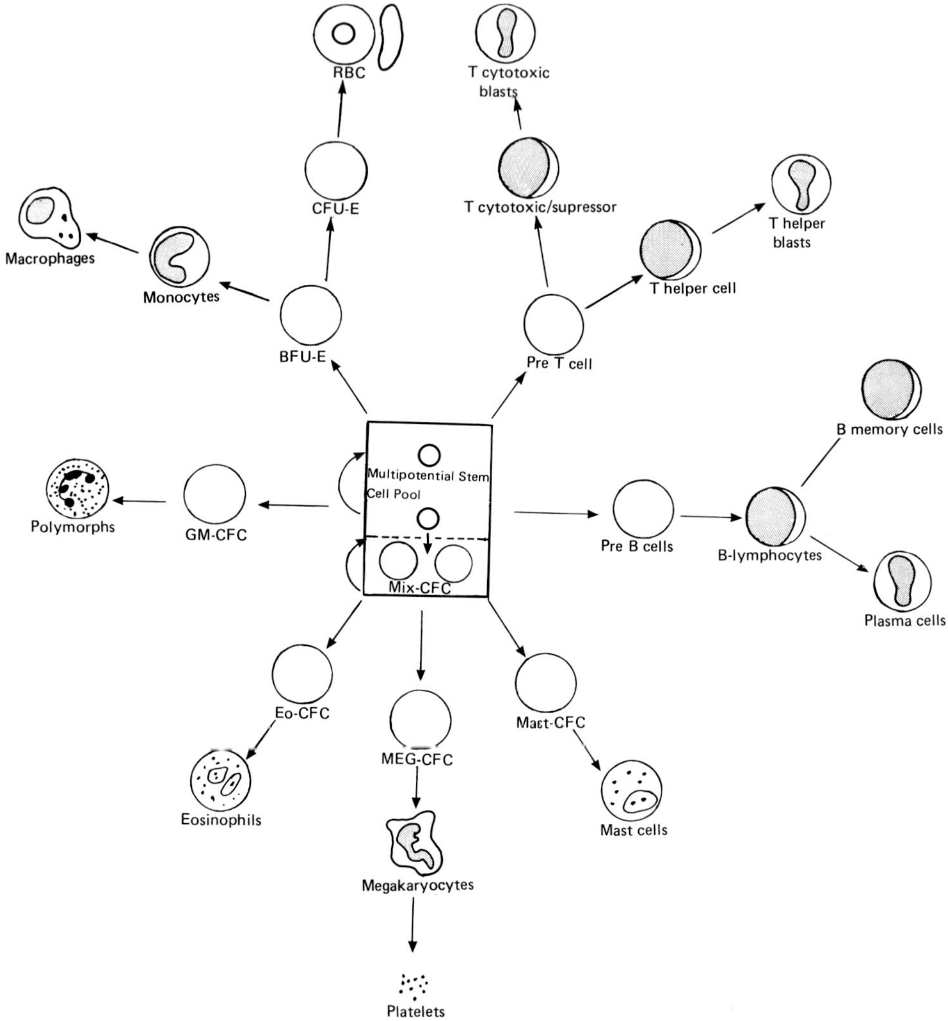

Figure 2 Hemopoietic cells in each lineage are shown. CFU-S I form blast cell colonies, CFU-S II (Mix-CFC or Multi-CFC) form mixed colonies, usually containing erythroid cells (29,50). All other colony forming cells give rise to restricted differentiation lineages. Self-generating stem cells give rise to committed progenitor (colony forming) cells restricted to one differentiation lineage, or two in the case of granulocyte-macrophage and possibly B- and T-lymphocyte progenitors. Some macrophages, mast cells, and B and T lymphocytes retain substantial proliferative capacity and also form colonies in vitro. Evidence for the existence of committed T-lymphocyte stem cells and the proliferative status of pluripotent stem cells is described in the text.

In the embryo, stem cells are found initially in the yolk sac and then in the fetal liver. In adult animals, stem cells with the ability to generate both myeloid and lymphoid progeny are located in the bone marrow, with a small population in the spleen and an even smaller one in the plasma (29,31).

A schematic representation of the differentiation pathways of hemopoietic cells appears in Figure 2. A complete list would include natural killer cells, tissue macrophages, and dendritic cells.

C. Assays of Hemopoiesis

The first in vitro assays for generating granulocytes and macrophages were described by Pluznick and Sachs (32) and Bradley and Metcalf (33). After 7-10 days in culture, the progenitor cells are recognized by their ability to give rise to discrete colonies of cells in agar. Certain cells are capable of giving rise to colonies that contain only granulocytes (G-CFC), while others are capable of giving colonies exclusively containing macrophages (M-CFC). A cell that gives rise to colonies containing both cell types is called a GM-CFC. These colony-forming cells are collectively referred to as CFU-C and are present at a frequency of approximately 500^{-1} in bone marrow cell suspensions (32).

Subsequently, other hemopoietic colony-forming cells have been grown to recognizable stages of differentiation as colonies in vitro (see Fig. 2) including: erythroid cells (BFU-E/CFU-E); eosinophils (Eo-CFC); megakaryocytes (MEG-CFC); B lymphocytes (Pre-B cells); mast cells (mast-CFC), and multipotential stem cells (mix-CFC) (29). Erythroid colonies can be subdivided by their sensitivity to erythropoietin and time of appearance in culture (29).

Culture systems have also been developed that allow the progenitors to grow on a monolayer of cells providing essential growth factors (33). This culture system has allowed the study and isolation of growth and differentiation factors that maintain progenitor cells (29,34). Most hemopoietic cell types including pre-B cells can be maintained in these cultures (29).

Rat lymphoid progenitors have been grown by Hayashi et al. (35), who reported maintaining a terminal deoxynucleotidyl transferase (Tdt) positive rat bone marrow colony for longer than 9 months. On the basis of cell-surface markers and appearance, this colony was determined to be a restricted primitive lymphoid stem cell. It is not clear, however, if it is committed to either the T- or B-cell lineage. The apparent difficulty in growing T lymphocyte stem cells may reflect the need for the specialized thymic environment.

The CFU-S assay, which measures repopulation by injected bone marrow cells in irradiated recipients, was developed by Till and McCulloch (36). The repopulation of the hemopoietic system is manifested as splenic nodules (CFU-S). A linear relationship exists between the number of cells injected and the number of resulting nodules (36). It has been shown using radiation-induced anomalies that all the cells within the CFU-S arise from one stem cell (37,38). It has also been shown that the CFU-S that form at 7 days represent a population of cells capable of transient repopulation, whereas those that form at 14 days are representative of stable repopulating CFU-S (39). It is not clear however, whether 7-day colonies have limited proliferative potential and are to be regarded as progenitors, while the later colonies contain true stem cells that take 14 days to become visible. Alternatively, 7-day colonies may represent stem cells in an inappropriate microenvironment to form long-lived colonies.

Evidence suggests the CFU-S assay measures a pluripotent stem cell because repopulation is long-term, isolated CFU-S from spleen are capable of secondary repopulation, and dissected CFU-S contain mixed cell types (39).

Chimera assays have also been employed to study and measure hemopoietic stem cells in vivo in sublethally irradiated hosts. In CBA mice, a translocation called T6, which is visible in cells undergoing meiosis, has been used to score chimeras (40). The disadvantage of this assay is that it must be scored at metaphase. This analysis selects cells in a state of activation, which is rare for most mature blood cells (see below). Other intracellular markers include hemoglobin alleles in mice for analysis of the erythroid lineage (41) and glucose phosphate isomerase for lymphocytes (29).

The most useful chimera assays utilize polymorphic cell-surface antigens that can be easily detected with antibodies and that do not result in killing the cells under analysis. In the earlier assays, von Boehmer et al. (42) generated MHC-incompatible chimeras, while Kadish and Basch (43) used the Thy-1 allotype in mice to produce MHC-compatible chimeras. Hunt and Fowler (44) bred rats with both T- and B-cell alloantigenic markers which were used to analyze lymphopoietic precursors (Fig. 3).

The Hunt and Fowler (44) assay relies on the ability of relatively few cells to permanently reconstitute both the B- and T-lymphoid compartments of a recipient rat, and assays stem cells that should include common ancestral stem cells for lymphopoiesis and hemopoiesis (44,45). The assumption that this assay measures a primitive stem cell is based on the fact that the assay measures long-term repopulation, and results using this assay have been corroborated using the conventional CFU-S assay. In this assay, bone marrow or fetal liver cell from rats of a strain doubly congenic for surface alloantigenic markers of B cells (immunoglobulin κ chain allotype) (26) and T cells (peripheral T-cell alloantigen, RT6: Pta) (46) is transferred to irradiated recipients of the congenic partner. A constant dose of host-type marrow is simultaneously injected into each recipient to promote survival after irradiation and to act as a reference for the genetically marked test cells. Cells from the marked bone marrow, or another source of lymphopoietic progenitors, can be fractionated on the basis of cell-surface markers using monoclonal antibodies. The fractionated populations are injected separately and 4 weeks later lymph node biopsies are performed and the cells are stained with the B- and T-cell allotypic antibody reagents in order to define the degree

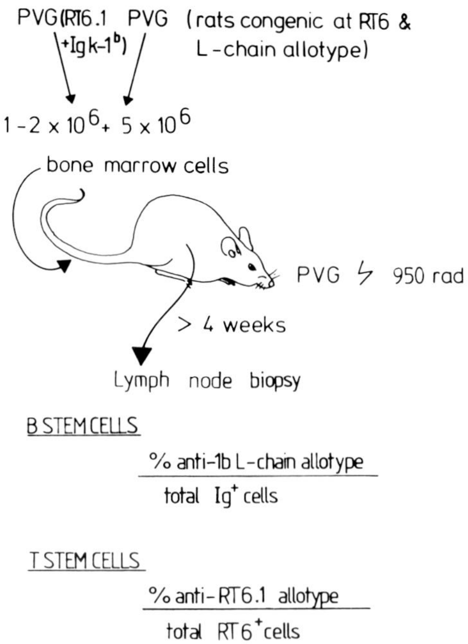

Figure 3 Donor cells carry the appropriate genetic marker (Igκ-1 for B-cell assay, RT6 for T-cell assay) and are congenic with the recipient. These cells may either be unseparated cells from bone marrow or fetal liver cells, or they may be injected after labeling with antibody to surface markers and separation on a fluorescence-activated cell sorter. They compete with a fixed number of unmarked young adult bone marrow cells in irradiated PVG hosts. With unseparated bone marrow as the "test" inoculum, the chimerism eventually measured among T and B lymphocytes in the lymph nodes reflects the proportion of the two kinds of marrow injected. This chimerism is stable for at least 1 year. Fetal liver "test" inoculums may overgrow the reference bone marrow indicating a higher repopulation potency (44,54).

of chimerism given by the marked inoculum. This assay has been used to determine the phenotype of rat B and T stem cells (Table 4) and can also be used quantitatively in the purification of stem cells to determine the overall recovery of repopulating activity. The major disadvantage of this assay is that the analysis of each experiment is slow and can only be done a month after it is started.

D. Purification of the Pluripotent Stem Cell

If stem cells could be purified, then their behavior in tissue culture could be directly visualized and conditions that might stimulate cell division and differentiation investigated. Pure stem cells could also be very useful for quick screening

Table 4 The Phenotype of Rat Hemopoietic Stem Cells

Marker	Assay	Tissue tested	Result	Ref.
RT1A (MHC Class I)	CFU-S	Bone marrow	+	317
RT1B and RT1D (MHC Class II)	CFU-S / B-cell chimera	Bone marrow	–	31
L-CA common epitope (OX1)	CFU-S	Bone marrow	+	300
L-CA (OX22 epitope)	B- and T-cell chimerism	Bone marrow	–	318
Surface immunoglobulin	B-cell chimerism	Bone marrow	–	31
RT6 (Pta)	B- and T-cell chimerism	Bone marrow	–	317
CD8 (OX8)	CFU-S B- and T-cell chimerism	Bone marrow	–	317
CD4 (W3/25)	CFU-S B- and T-cell chimerism	Bone marrow	–	317
CD5 (OX19)	B- and T-cell chimerism	Bone marrow	–	317
Thy-1	CFU-S T- and B-cell chimerism	Bone marrow	+	45,319
Thy-1	CFU-S, GM-CFC G-CFC, M-CFC	Bone marrow	++ (top 10% bright cells)	47

Thy-1	B- and T-cell chimerism	Fetal liver	+	45
W3/13 (L-SGP)	B- and T-cell chimerism	Bone marrow	+ B-cell chimerism low T-cell chimerism	26
W3/13 (L-SGP)	B- and T-cell chimerism	Neonatal spleen	+	300
W3/13 (L-SGP)	B- and T-cell chimerism	Fetal liver	+	300
MRC OX26 (transferrin receptor)	B and T chimerism	Bone marrow	–	54
MRC OX26 (transferrin receptor)	B and T chimerism	Fetal liver (17 day)	–	54
W3/15	CFU-S	Bone marrow	±	300
W3/15	B and T chimerism	Fetal liver	±	300
MRC OX2	B-cell chimerism	Bone marrow	–	317
Terminal deoxynucleotide transferase	CFU-C (prelymphoid)	Bone marrow	+	35,46a
Low angle light scatter	CFU-S	Bone marrow	medium to large	47
Steroid sensitivity	CFU-S	Bone marrow	– (insensitive)	47
93-3	Band T chimerism	Fetal liver	±	46b

The phenotype of the rat pluripotent hemopoietic stem cell is described. Assays used to analyze the stem cell phenotype are indicated along with cell types tested and experimental results.

of new monoclonal antibodies, some possibly specific for stem cells, which could be applied to separating leukemic cells from bone marrow before retransplantation.

The frequency of rat CFU-S in bone marrow is less than one in three hundred (47). A 320-fold purification of rat CFU-S has been achieved by a combination of size, cortisone resistance, and sorting on the FACS for cells expressing a high level of Thy-1 (47). The cells capable of giving rise to CFU-S were shown to lie between the size of lymphocyte and myeloid progenitors, in the upper tenth percentile for expression of the Thy-1 antigen, and to be cortisone resistant. It was speculated that 80% of the purified population were able to give rise to CFU-S.

Visser et al. (48) have obtained a 120-fold enrichment of mouse CFU-S activity by separating mouse bone marrow over a metrizamide gradient, sorting for wheat germ agglutinin-fluorescein isothiocyanate (WGA-FITC) positive cells on the FACS, followed by removal of the WGA-FITC with N-acetyl-D-glucosamine and sorting a second time for high H-2K expressing cells. Of the enriched population, 65% of the cells were able to give rise to CFU-S and 32% could be induced to form myeloid progeny in vitro. Thus some progress has been made in the stem cell purification, but the cell recovery is extremely low and this has hampered direct molecular analysis of these cells.

E. Phase of the Cell Cycle Occupied by the Pluripotent Stem Cell

The pluripotent hemopoietic stem cell, once activated, must commit itself to differentiation or proliferation (49). Stem cells are capable of extensive proliferation (50), but most stem cell activity in an animal is not significantly destroyed by exposure to high specific activity ^{3}H-thymidine or hydroxyurea which kill dividing cells. However, stem cells become sensitive to these treatments during marrow regeneration after transplantation (51-53). These results suggest that most pluripotent stem cells are not active in cell division in a normal animal, but that they enter the cell cycle during hemopoietic stress. Further support for this conclusion derives from the fact that a lethally irradiated rat can be rescued from hemopoietic cell death by the intravenous injection of 400^{-1} of a donor rat's total bone marrow. Thus pluripotent stem cells are present in large excess in normal marrow.

The transferrin receptor is presumably expressed by all proliferating cells and, as such, may be a useful marker in fractionating progenitors of the pluripotent stem cells from the pluripotent stem cell itself. This possibility has been addressed by FACS sorting adult rat bone marrow on the basis of expression of the transferrin receptor recognized by the MRC OX26 mouse monoclonal antibody (54). The sorted populations were individually assayed for their ability to give rise to B or T lymphocytes in the assay devised by Hunt and Fowler (44) (Fig. 3). It was concluded that all lymphopoietic stem cell activity was in the MRC OX26 negative fraction. These data corroborate results in the mouse showing that CFU-S are insensitive to killing by anti-transferrin receptor antibody conjugated with ricin (55). Thus, the conclusion that most primitive stem cells do not express transferrin receptor is in accord with the data discussed above showing that the stem cells are resistant to metabolities that kill dividing cells.

Expression of transferrin receptor on committed progenitors however, has not been clearly assessed. Sieff et al. (56) found that human erythroid progenitors do express the transferrin receptor, whereas Miller et al. (57) found the opposite result for mouse erythroid progenitors. The reason for this discrepancy is not known, but may be due to the detection method used to measure the expression of transferrin receptor; Sieff et al. (56) sorted the bone marrow on the FACS, while Miller et al. (57) prepared subpopulations by rosette depletion. Differences in in vitro culture conditions may also account for the conflicting results.

Rat fetal liver stem cells at 17 days of ontogeny have also been analyzed for expression of transferrin receptor (MRC OX26 antigen) (54). It was determined that although 95% of fetal liver cells express the transferrin receptor, the lymphopoietic stem cells reside in the transferrin receptor negative population. Therefore, the removal of transferrin receptor expressing cells from 17-day fetal liver, for example, by rosette depletion may be a useful first step enrichment for the purification of stem cells (54).

One practical application that might arise from the failure of anti-transferrin receptor monoclonal antibodies to label pluripotent stem cells is that these antibodies might be used in vitro to deplete leukemic cells, which are usually transferrin receptor positive (58), from bone marrow preparations (59). Such bone marrow preparations may then be used to restore the hemopoietic system of the patients, from which the bone marrow was obtained, following treatment with intensive radiotherapy or chemotherapy (55,60). To provide a more effective depletion system, anti-transferrin receptor antibodies may be used together with other antibodies that also label leukemic cells but do not bind to stem cells. The use of ricin A-chain or other toxin conjugated anti-transferrin receptor antibodies in vivo, even if specifically toxic, would be unacceptable because a large number of dividing and some nondividing cell types express the transferrin receptor (54,61,62).

F. Committed Lymphoid Stem Cells

Evidence of the existence of a committed stem cell for T lymphocytes comes from the experiments of Abramson et al. (63). Chromosome abnormalities were induced by radiation, and in some cases these were found in a high proportion of lectin-stimulated T-cell blasts but not in dividing cells of the other lineages. This suggested the existence of a progenitor cell in the T-lymphocyte lineage that was capable of considerable renewal, although the objection has been raised that the chromosomal marker may itself have caused the commitment (64).

Randomly integrated retrovirus vectors have also been used as unique clonal markers to analyze the origin of mouse bone marrow, thymocytes, and spleen cells from transfected bone marrow repopulated anemic W/W^v mutant mice (65). The existence of pluripotential stem cells capable of producing both myeloid and lymphoid progeny as well as more committed stem cells apparently restricted to either the myeloid or lymphoid lineages were inferred by Southern blot analyses. Obviously, this procedure allows analysis of nondividing cells but again, the site of integration of the vector could, in principle, have caused the commitment to the myeloid or lymphoid lineages (66).

The lymphopoietic chimera assay devised by Hunt and Fowler (44) has allowed the identification of a candidate committed rat T-lymphocyte stem cell. This has been accomplished by separation of bone marrow populations using the W3/13 antibody, which recognizes the leukocyte-sialoglycoprotein (L-SGP) (see Table 1 and Table 2). In the rat bone marrow this antibody stains 40% of the cells brightly (mostly neutrophils) and 20% weakly, while in fetal liver 40% of cells are stained. Bright, dim, and negative W3/13 antibody binding bone marrow and fetal liver populations were sorted on the FACS. In fetal liver, all stem cell activity for B and T lymphocytes was in the bright fraction, and in bone marrow this was also true for cells giving rise to B lymphocytes. In contrast, T-lymphocyte chimeras could be derived from both the W3/13 bright and dim bone marrow population, and this established that the W3/13 dim population contains a committed stem cell for T lymphocytes (26). It has not, however, been conclusively proven whether the W3/13^{dim} committed T-lymphocyte stem cell is pre- or postthymic.

IV. T-CELL DIFFERENTIATION IN THE THYMUS

The thymus is an essential organ for the development of T lymphocytes (67). Conventional wisdom suggests that it is at this site that T cells become tolerant to self antigens and restricted by self-MHC molecules (68,69). Anatomically, each lobe of the thymus is divided into an outer cortex region, which constitutes about 85% of the organ, and an inner medulla region (70). The lymphoid cells in the thymus derive from precursors in the bone marrow, and the organ is a site of extensive cell proliferation. However, only a small proportion of the cells in the thymus contribute to the mature T-lymphocyte pool, and most thymocytes are believed to be "dead-end" cells that die in the thymus itself (71).

In the human, rat and mouse four thymocyte subsets have been described on the basis of the CD4 and CD8 markers. The $CD4^-$ $CD8^-$ subset defines the prothymocyte (2%) of total population thought to give rise to other thymocyte subsets (71-73). The CD4+ CD8+ population is the largest subset and defines the majority of thymocytes that are unable to respond to proliferative or differentiation signals. Two other populations, CD4¯ CD8+ and CD4+ CD8¯, define the subsets of thymocytes corresponding to the peripheral T cells. In addition, in the human, the CD1 (T6) marker defines the majority of nonfunctional thymocytes, the CD2 (T11) marker is present on all the thymocytes, and the CD3 (T3) marker defines the functional thymocytes (72). Studies on T-cell receptor β chain rearrangement shows that the CD4+, CD8+ thymocytes rearrange the β chain gene but do not express it, whereas the mature phenotyped cells both rearrange and express the β chain of the receptor. The appearance of the T-cell receptor β chain on the surface corresponds to the appearance of the CD3 (T3) marker (72). In the mouse, DNA rearrangement and the expression of the T-cell receptor β chain mRNA and the expression of the CD3 δ chain mRNA in CD4-CD8-thymocytes precede DNA rearrangement and expression of the T-cell receptor α chain mRNA (73). Furthermore, it is not until α chain rearrangement takes place in CD4+ CD8+ thymocytes that the T-cell receptor complex is expressed on the cell surface (73). This situation may mimic B-cell development where heavy chain rearrangement and mRNA expression precedes light chain rearrangement, mRNA expression, and the appearance of immunoglobulin on the cell surface.

The OX44 antigen is a molecule with an apparent molecular weight of 40 Kd which is found on all rat leukocytes with the notable exception of 88% of thymocytes (74). The OX44+ population of thymocytes resides mainly in the medulla while some scattered cells appear in the cortex. The OX44+ thymocyte population is exclusively capable of responding to ConA and producing IL-2 (74). This population of thymocytes mediate functions that are characteristic of most undifferentiated thymocytes as well as thymic cells that are most like mature cells. On the other hand, the OX44¯ cells fail to proliferate in the MLC or ConA response even when provided a source of IL-2 and irradiated T helper cells. Therefore, the OX44+ cells may include all cells that are on the differentiation pathway to become immunocompetent, whereas the OX44¯ compartment represents cells which fail to respond to a differentiation signal and are bound to die in situ (74). Furthermore, the OX44+ cells reside within the RT1A (MHC class I) bearing thymocytes, which are also expressed on all leukocytes except CD4+ CD8+ cells, whose RT1A are weak or negative. It may be that cells fated to die in the thymus switch-off OX44 expression and then RT1A expression (74).

A highly sensitive and quantitative intrathymic adoptive transfer system for detecting thymocyte precursor cells in rats and mice has been devised by Goldschneider et al. (75). In this assay the generation of donor-origin thymocytes is analyzed on the FACS after injection of test cells directly into the thymus of

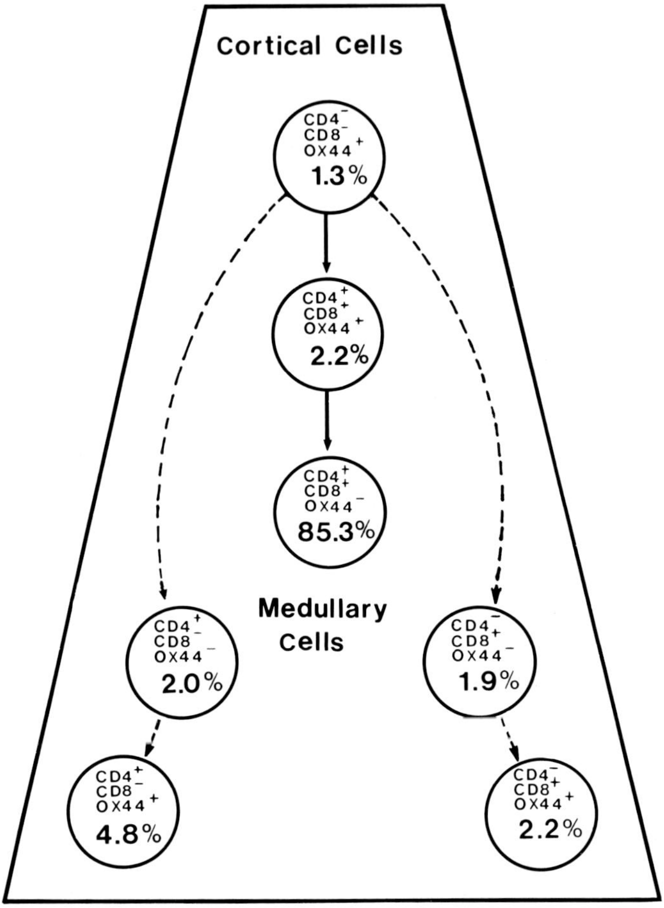

Figure 4 A possible differentiation pathway for rat T lymphocytes within the thymus. The percentages refer to the frequency of a particular subset within each compartment. The thymus contains 2% $OX22^+$ cells but their full phenotype has not been determined. The pathway of differentiation taken by the prothymocyte within the thymus is not clear, and its relationship with medullary cells has not been established. The OX44 antigen is expressed by 12% of rat thymocytes and includes prothymocytes and all thymocytes capable of responding in the ConA response and in the MLR (74). The human and mouse data suggest similar subsets based on the CD4 and CD8 markers, however, the OX44 marker has not been detected in either species. In mouse and human a clear distinction can be detected between peanut agglutinin positive cortical cell and negative mature medullary cells; this separation is not as clearcut in the rat (207). The terminal deoxynucleotide transferase enzyme in all species appears to be present in cortical cells but not in medullary cells (35).

sublethally irradiated histocompatible L-CA congenic rat or mouse recipients. This assay has the advantages of being both independent of cell migration and specific for T-lineage precursor cells.

The Goldschneider assay has been used to analyze the seven thymocyte subsets defined in the rat using the CD4, CD8, and OX44 markers (Fig. 4). It is the $OX44^+$ $CD4^-$ $CD8^-$ (2%) thymocytes that are capable of proliferating and giving rise to the other thymocyte subsets, while the $OX44^-$ (88%) thymic subset is unable to repopulate the thymus. Therefore, $CD4^-$ $CD8^-$ $OX44^+$ cells constitute the much-studied double negative prothymocytes, while the $CD4^+$ $CD8^-$ $OX44^+$ and $CD4^-$ $CD8^+$ $OX44^+$ cells correspond to the mature phenotype T cells. In contrast, the $CD4^+$ $CD8^+$ $OX44^+$, $CD4^+$ $CD8^+$ $OX44^-$, $CD4^+$ $CD8^-$ $OX44^-$, and $CD4^-$ $CD8^+$ $OX44^-$ subsets are potentially intermediates or end cells in thymic differentiation of T cells (74).

V. MOLECULES INVOLVED IN RECIRCULATION OF PERIPHERAL LYMPHOCYTES AND POSITIONING IN LYMPHOID TISSUES

A. Recirculation of Lymphocytes

A key feature of lymphocyte function is that, unlike other body cells, small lymphocytes recirculate from blood to lymph (76,77). Recirculation is likely to be of great functional importance in allowing memory cells to be disseminated from a site of antigen stimulation to other parts of the body. Lymphocytes migrate from blood into lymph nodes, particularly specialized regions of the vasculature termed postcapillary venules where the cells pass between the high-walled endothelial (HEV) cells into the node. This traffic is selective for lymphocytes (78,79). In the spleen the lymphocytes migrate from the anastomozing capillaries at the marginal sinus, which forms the border between the red and white pulp (80). Ultimately, B and T cells exit the lymph nodes by the efferent lymphatics and enter the lymph to be returned to the blood and continue to cycle. Cell emigration from the spleen appears to take place via blood vessels.

B. Positioning in Peripheral Lymphoid Organs

Though B and T lymphocytes enter at the same region within the spleen or lymph nodes, they segregate to different areas. Within peripheral lymphoid organs, lymphocyte subsets can be identified with specific monoclonal antibodies (81) or by isotope labeling (82). In the lymph nodes, B lymphocytes are present mainly in the follicles and outer cortex, while T lymphocytes occupy the paracortex; plasma cells and macrophages are abundant in the medulla (81). In the spleen, B cells reside in the follicles, while T cells reside in the periarteriolar sheath (80, 83).

C. Candidate Molecules Involved in Lymphocyte Recirculation and Positioning

Recirculation is likely to involve recognition of endothelial cells by lymphocytes, which results from interactions of cell-surface molecules. This view is supported by the fact that limited digestion of rat lymphocytes by trypsin destroys the ability of these cells to recirculate (84). Similarly, the removal of the carbohydrate from lymphocytes (85) or from HEVs (86) appears to inhibit lymphocyte adhesion to HEVs.

Fatty acids extracted in organic solvents from many tissues inhibit lymphocyte-HEV adhesion (87). This suggests that glycolipids on the HEV surface may also be recognized by lymphocytes.

Several proteins have been associated with homing or HEV binding by lymphocytes, but the relationship between these molecules has not been determined. One specific molecule that may be involved is the mouse lymphocyte cell-surface protein defined by monoclonal antibody MEL-14, which has an apparent molecular weight of 80 Kd (88). An antibody against MEL-14 inhibits lymphocyte attachment to HEVs in lymph node cryostat sections. The MEL-14 protein has also been associated with mannose-6-phosphate binding activity (89). The MEL-14 protein has been purified and shown by radiosequencing to possess two N-termini. One N-terminal sequence corresponds to ubiquitin, a modification previously found only in cytoplasmic and nuclear proteins (90,91). A cDNA encoding MEL-14 has been isolated from a expression library using antisera raised against the MEL-14 protein. The cDNA sequence also encodes ubiquitin (91). These findings may indicate a common processing pathway for other proteins (79).

A rat molecule with an apparent molecular weight of 45-50 Kd (with multiple higher nolecular weight bands) has been identified on peripheral rat lymphocyte (92). An antibody (A.11) against this protein inhibits adhesion of lymphocytes to lymph node HEVs. Yet another antibody (1B.2) binds to a rat lymphocyte-surface protein with an apparent molecular weight of 80 Kd (apparently not MEL-14) and inhibits lymphocyte adhesion to Peyer's patch HEVs (93). Thus there may be specialized homing molecules for recognition of particular lymphoid organs.

VI. IMPORTANT MARKER MOLECULES OF THYMOCYTES AND T LYMPHOCYTES

In this section individual marker antigens of thymocytes/T lymphocytes will be considered. Many of these antigens provide markers for identifying functional T-lymphocyte subsets and for several the primary amino acid sequence has been determined (see Table 3). Lymphocyte cell-surface glycoproteins are categorized in several different groups, which are made for convenience. The groups include

1) molecules where a primary sequence relationship has been established with immunoglobulins (immunoglobulin superfamily), 2) molecules that are heavily glycosylated, 3) miscellaneous marker molecules—those that are not heavily glycosylated or where structural homologies have not been established, and 4) marker molecules of T-cell activation. It is clear, however, that many antigens fall into more than one category; for example, Thy-1 is both Ig-like and heavily glycosylated.

A. Molecules with Immunoglobulin Homology

It is now evident that a group of cell-surface proteins show considerable primary sequence homology to immunoglobulins and contain immunoglobulin-like domains (Fig. 5). Though certain rules have been established for determining their evolutionary relationship (94), at present an understanding of the co-evolution of these proteins is lacking (95,96).

All immunoglobulin-like molecules with known functions are involved in recognition interactions, i.e., T-cell receptor, poly-Ig receptor, N-CAM, immunoglobulins, and MHC Class I and Class II molecules. Furthermore, it is clear from the functions of antibody combining sites that the Ig-fold provides a framework upon which variation in loops of sequence can occur to give differences in recognition specificity (94,97). This idea may also be true for the difference in specificity of the other Ig-related molecules in cell-cell recognition or ligand binding (95).

1. T-Cell Antigen Receptor

T cells recognize antigens presented at the surface of target cells. Unlike B cells, this recognition predominantly takes place in the context of the products of the major histocompatibility complex—MHC restriction (98). The activation of functional T cells with cytotoxic or immunoregulating functions is dependent on this dual recognition (99-101). Antigen and probably MHC recognition by T lymphocytes is mediated by a cell-surface molecule—the T-cell antigen receptor (102). It is a two-chain molecule and, like immunoglobulin, it has a variable antigen interacting segment, a constant region, and a hydrophobic segment that enables it to integrate in the membrane (103,104).

Progress in the detection of the T-cell receptor did not occur until 1983, when several groups produced monoclonal antibodies that recognize a molecule which is a disulphide-linked dimer glycoprotein chain of around 43 Kd and 49 Kd. These antibodies were originally identified as being specific for particular T-cell clones or hybridomas and having the property of being mitogenic or blocking antigen-specific activation. The antibodies reacting with different clones all precipitated molecules with similar overall properties, and the clonotype specificity is apparently due to the fact that the antibodies react with the combining sites of the

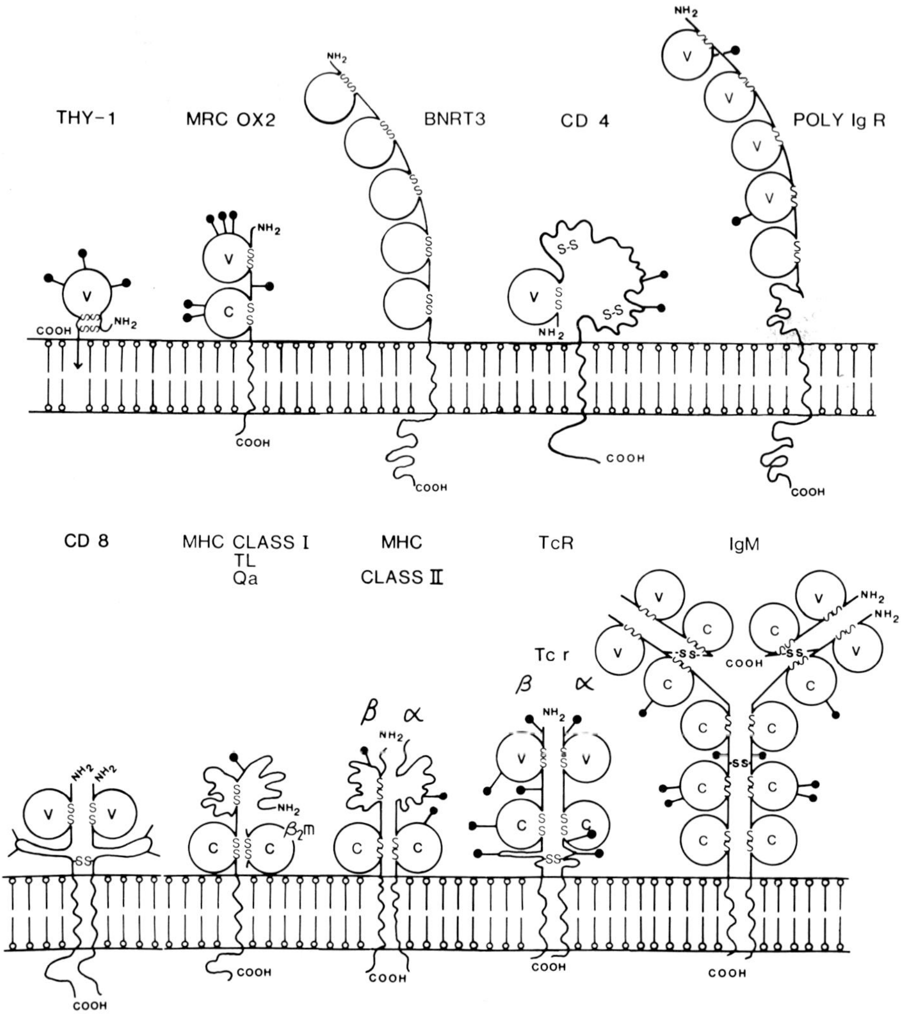

Figure 5 Circles marked V are like an IgV domain, while those marked C are more like IgC domains. Possible intrachain disulfide bonds are shown by vertical double S, interchain bonds are shown by horizontal SS, and N-linked carbohydrate structures are depicted as pinpoints. The poly Ig receptor, N-CAM and the BNRT3 molecule are the only members not found in either thymocytes, B cells, or T cells (320,321,322). (*Figure courtesy of Dr. A. F. Williams.*)

molecules, which differ between the T-cell clones (105-107). Monoclonal antibodies have subsequently been produced that react with either an allotypic determinant on the T-cell receptor or with a family of expressed V regions (108, 109), and antisera have been raised in rabbits immunized with the purified molecule that recognized all T-cell receptors (110). More recently, a monoclonal antibody has been produced which appears to recognize all human T-cell receptors, but only when associated with the CD3 complex (111).

Sequences for the T-cell receptor chains were first obtained from cDNA clones identified on the basis that they were T-cell specific and showed genetic rearrangement during T-cell differentiation (25,112-115). Subsequently, these sequences were shown to be identical to protein sequences from the structures identified with monoclonal antibodies (116,117). Both the α (49 kD) and β (43 kD) chains appear to have homology to immunoglobulins and have a carboxy-terminal constant region and an amino-terminal variable region (Figure 5). Evidence suggests that the variability of the putative T-cell receptor antigen binding region arises from a large combination of variable (V), diversity (D), and joining (J) segments but not from point mutations, which contribute to immunoglobulin variable region diversity (104). Furthermore, the data now suggest that the same antigen receptor genes are expressed by T cytotoxic and T helper cells (104).

Using the nucleic acid approach, a third cDNA sequence called γ has been cloned (113). The gene for the γ chain shows rearrangement during T-cell differentiation but compared to the α and β chains has few V-gene segments and is yet to be identified as a protein (113,118,119). No information is yet available for the rat T-cell receptor.

The phenomena of MHC restriction in which nominal antigen and MHC antigen appear to be co-recognized has not thus far been illuminated by the structural studies on the T-cell receptor. The combining site of the T-cell receptor looks like an immunoglobulin Fab, and there is no well-established precedent in studies on antibody binding for dual recognition of two determinants by one receptor (see below) (97,120).

2. MHC Class I Molecules

MHC class I antigens, called H-2 in mouse, RT*1A* in rat and HLA in human, were first detected as the target antigens for graft rejection. The most important finding relating to class I antigen function is the phenomenon of H-2 restriction, originally observed for the H-2K and H-2D locus products (99). T cells were found to recognize viral antigen in association with self MHC class I antigen. Most cells in higher vertebrates appear to express conventional class I molecules; one notable exception is brain cells, but immunological stimuli can readily induce expression on virtually all cells in the central nervous system.

The classical transplantation antigens (H-2K, D, and L in the mouse) are cell-surface glycoproteins which span the membrane (121). They comprise a glycosylated heavy chain of 44-47 kD that is noncovalently linked to β_2 microglobulin (11.5 kD) that is not encoded by the MHC region.

Structural analyses of class I antigens suggest that they can be divided into three extracellular domains of 90 amino acids each ($\alpha_1, \alpha_2, \alpha_3$). They also contain a transmembrane segment of approximately 25 amino acids and a cytoplasmic domain of 30-40 amino acids (122). The extracellular domain closest to the membrane (α_3) appears to be associated with β_2 microglobulin (123), and both of these molecules share structural and sequence homology with immunoglobulin constant domains (94).

A remarkable feature of the MHC class I antigens is the very high degree of polymorphism they display, which is mostly confined to the α_1 and α_2 domains. About 50 different alleles have been identified at the K and D loci, respectively (124), and no single allele is predominantly expressed. It is also the α_1 and α_2 domains that carry the alloantigenic determinants (125).

In addition to the products of H-2K, L, and D loci, two products have been identified, Qa and Tla, which are coded for by genes located on the telomeric side of the mouse MHC. These proteins have a similar structure to other H-2 products, but their particular functions are not known (121).

A mouse H-2 K^d probe has been used to isolate two partial RT*1A* cDNAs from a NEDH rat insulinoma library (126). One cDNA RT*1A*-1 encodes the α_3 domain, transmembrane segment, the cytoplasmic tail, and the 3' noncoding region of a molecule, which has considerable homology to the K^d protein: 84% in the α_3 domain. However, the exact identity of this molecule has not been determined.

The second cDNA clone, RT*1A*-2, encodes a protein containing part of the MHC class I α_2 domain, the entire α_3 domain up to the transmembrane segment (126). At this point there is a premature stop codon, which was later confirmed in the genomic sequence of a Wistar rat. The RT*1A* mRNA is present in the insulinoma and testis, but not in kidney or liver. In addition, the genomic sequence did not contain a polyadenylation site, which suggests that it is a transcribed pseudogene (126).

Recent functional studies imply that MHC class I molecules can themselves interact directly with amphipathic influenza hemagglutinin (127) and nuclear protein peptides (128,129). This direct interaction may be the molecular basis for MHC restriction at the level of the target or antigen presenting cell.

3. MHC Class II Molecules (Ia)

MHC Class II antigens (Ia) are also highly polymorphic and genetically linked to the class I antigens to form the major histocompatibility complex (124). The only known role for these molecules is that they are recognized together with nominal antigen in the activation of T helper cells and some T cytotoxic cells and confer immune response (Ir) gene effects (130,131). MHC class II molecules have recently been shown to have a measurable affinity for peptides (132), and T cells appear to recognize an antigen-Ia complex (133,134).

Ia antigens are present on thymic epithelium, macrophages, dendritic cells, B cells, and can be induced by interferon-γ on a variety of other tissues (135). The rat *RT1-B* region codes for the MHC class II molecules referred to as A, while the RT1-D region encodes the MHC class II molecules referred to as E. Each class II molecule is composed of two glycosylated polypeptides, which are strongly associated by noncovalent forces to form a two-chain structure (7). The large chain is referred to as α with an M_r of 32-36 kD, while the smaller one is called β with an M_r of 25-30 kD.

Monoclonal antibodies have been produced against rat I-A and I-E gene products (136,137), which inhibit the MLC (138). The rat Aα chain has been cloned and sequenced (139). It shows considerable homology with human HLA-DQα (85%) and mouse H-2 I-Aα (91%) chains. The transmembrane region is the most conserved between rat and man; there is 91% homology, while there is 100% homology between mouse and rat. The cytoplasmic domain is the least homologous, with 86% homology between mouse and rat and 73% homology between rat and human. Overall, rat *RT1-B* Aα, mouse H-2 I-Aα, and human HLA-DQα chains are more homologous to each other than to the chains of the H-2 I-Eα or HLA-DRα molecules. This suggests that class II Aα and Eα genes diverged prior to the divergence of mammals (139).

The gene encoding the Aβ chain has been isolated using a HLA-DQβ chain cDNA as a probe (140). The Aβ gene has a high degree of sequence conservation in both exons and introns with H-2 I-Aβ and HLA-DQβ chains. This indicates that constraints on the divergence of Class II gene introns may exist to facilitate gene conversion between Class II genes.

The cDNA encoding the Eβ has subsequently been isolated with a fragment of Aβ gene (141). The Eβ chain shows considerable sequence homology to H-2 I-Eβ and HLA-DRβ chains. Comparison of the predicted amino acid sequence of mouse, human, and rat Eβ and Aβ chains shows that 105 out of 278 residues are identical (38%) in all six β chains. Analyses of silent and replacement substitutions suggest that class II β chains have evolved at different rates in different species. The products of a third MHC class II loci equivalent to the human DP (SB) have not been identified in the rat and it is not yet possible to determine the extent of polymorphism which exists in the sequence of the rat α and β chains.

4. The CD4 Marker of T Helper Cells

The CD4 marker is found on rat thymocytes, macrophages, dendritic cells, and the T helper/inducer subset of T cells, which is complementary to the $CD8^+$ bearing T-cell subset (reviewed by 142). This population was originally identified in the mouse by Cantor and Boyse (143) as the Lyt $1^+,2^-,3^-$ population.

The molecular weight of the CD4 molecule is 46-58 kD in human (144-146), mouse (147), and rat (148). There seems to be little heterogeneity within the CD4 molecule based on two-dimensional peptide maps of four human $CD4^+$ clones with different antigens/MHC specificities (144). However, there is some polymorphism within the CD4 molecules of unrelated individuals. This possibility was raised by the finding that the OKT4A epitope is absent from T cells of some individuals, whereas the other epitopes of the CD4 molecule are still present (149), and by amino acid sequence differences between outbred and inbred rats (150).

The complete amino acid sequence of the CD4 antigen has been established in rat (150), human (151), and also in mouse (151a). The human molecule is reported to be 435 amino acids long, contains one N-terminal immunoglobulin-like domain, a possible joining (J) segment, a third extracellular domain, an integral membrane segment homologous to MHC class II molecules, and a highly charged cytoplasmic domain (Fig. 5). The N-terminal amino acid sequence of rat CD4 establishes the coding region to be two amino acids downstream from the putative N-terminal amino acid in the human CD4 protein, and overall the rat molecule is 430 amino acids long. The human molecule contains two possible N-linked glycosylation sites, while the rat molecule contains four possible N-linked sites. There is 58% homology at the amino acid level between the human and rat molecules. The transmembrane segment is the most conserved; between rat and man there is 77% homology. One of the interesting features of the CD4 molecule is the presence of segments outside the first immunoglobulin-like domain that contain sequences flanking the Cys residues, which are highly conserved within the immunoglobulin superfamily. In contrast to other immunoglobulin-like molecules, the sequences likely to form two immunoglobulin-folds mediated by two disulfide bridges are in fact 42 and 46 residues apart—some 30 residues shorter than in a classical variable domain immunoglobulin-fold and approximately 15 residues shorter than a constant domain immunoglobulin-fold. Presumably a modified β strand formation would accomodate and stabilize the smaller domains. The mouse CD4 molecule has similar structural features (151a). It may be possible, therefore, that the CD4 molecule contains truncated or half-domains. The disulfide bonds within the CD4 (L3T4) molecule have been established (151b) and are consistant with the existence of half-domains. Half-domains may be of significance in searching for a primordial immunoglobulin-like molecule.

It is now clear that human and rat macrophages express the CD4 antigen. Barclay (152) showed that rat peritoneal and lymph node macrophages are labeled by anti-CD4 (W3/25) antibody, and Steininger et al. (153) showed that Kupffer cells in rat liver and dendritic cells in a variety of tissues are also CD4 (W3/25) positive. A similar study in the human by Wood et al. (154) showed that monocytes, macrophages, and Langerhans cells expressed the CD4 epitopes, recognized by the Leu 3 and OKT4A antibodies. The T4A, B, C, and D epitopes of CD4 were found on human blood monocytes and a human monocyte cell line, U937, by Moscicki et al. (155). Furthermore, it has been established that the CD4 molecule from rat macrophages (nude and normal rats), T cell, and thymocytes have identical molecular weights (13); this has been recently confirmed in the human (156). Evidence exists that mouse macrophages do not express CD4 (156a). The implications of this data on the function of CD4 are not yet clear.

The W3/25 anti-rat CD4 antibody and its $F(ab')_2$ fragment inhibit the MLC without killing the cells involved (8). This inhibition takes place at the level of the responding $CD4^+$ cells. When it was shown that macrophages also expressed the CD4 (W3/25) antigen (152), the W3/25 antibody inhibition studies were repeated using mouse accessory cells that do not bind the W3/25 antibody to exclude the possible involvement of accessory cells (8). These xenogenic cells were used to present alloantigen in the MLC to rat lymphocytes depleted of accessory cells. Again the W3/25 antibody inhibition was shown to take place at the level of the responding T helper cells (157). The W3/25 antibody does not, however, block the ConA response. The interpretation is that the CD4 (W3/25) molecule is intimately involved in the response of T helper cells to antigen. The W3/25 antibody has also been shown to inhibit the formation of "clusters" between rat dendritic cells and T helper cells in the secondary MLC (138). It is interesting that the only other antibody capable of this inhibition is the MRC OX6 antibody, which reacts with rat MHC class II antigens. Finally, the W3/25 antibody blocks in vitro activation of myelin basic protein reactive T cells (158).

In the mouse, inhibition of killing before the lethal hit stage of CTL directed against MHC class II-bearing targets can be inhibited by anti-CD4 (L3T4) antibody (147). It also blocks the MLC and IL-2 release (159). There is clonal heterogeneity of $CD4^+$ mouse CTL in the degree of inhibition that can be achieved with anti-CD4 (L3T4) antibody. It has been interpreted that anti-CD4 (L3T4) inhibitions correlate with the degree to which CTL cross-kill irrelevant MHC class II bearing target cells (159). Anti-CD4 (L3T4) antibodies may also block antigen presentation of soluble antigen to $CD4^+$ hybridomas, but this is unconvincing (159). Watts et al. (160) have shown that anti-CD4 (L3T4) antibody blocks presentation of antigen plus pure Ia in planar membrane to inducer $CD4^+$ clones.

Functional studies of the $CD4^+$ subset of human T cells have shown that it provides helper/inducer activity to T-T, T-B, and T-accessory cell interactions (161,162). The CD4 $(T4)^+$ population proliferates in the MLC, and only a minor component of cytotoxic effector cells reside in the CD4 $(T4)^+$ subset (72). The $CD4^+$ cytotoxic T cells are directed against Class II MHC antigens, whereas the $CD8^+$ CTL are directed against the Class I MHC antigens. These findings and data in the murine system (see above) implies that $CD4^+$ and $CD8^+$ cells have receptors for different classes of MHC antigens (163,164) and led to the hypothesis that the CD8 and CD4 molecules may themselves recognize class I and class II antigens, respectively (165).

In antibody inhibition studies, human $CD4^+$ CTL can be inhibited by 80% with anti-CD4 antibody (72). Other results show that CTL activity can be restored by lectin even in the presence of anti-CD4 antibodies (72). Antibodies against CD4 are also able to block proliferation in the MLC (166). The CD4 molecule appears to be phosphorylated and modulated from the cell surface in response to antigen or PMA (166a). Therefore, CD4 may be involved in the recognition events or as a receptor for an unknown ligand rather than in the lytic activity of T cells.

An attempt has been made to examine whether the CD4 molecule can interact with the nonpolymorphic domain of MHC class II molecules. Golding et al. (167) have shown that the recognition of MHC class I/class II hybrid molecules in transfected L cells can be inhibited by anti-mouse CD4 (L3T4) antibody. This hybrid molecule contains the polymorphic domains of MHC class II A_β^k molecule and the conserved α_3 domain of MHC class I H-2D^d molecules, which, at least partially, associates with β_2 microglobulin. The interpretation is that the CD4 molecule does not recognize the nonpolymorphic domain of MHC class II molecules. Furthermore, recent data in the human suggests that CD4 and CD8 more likely function as negative signal receptors, not as MHC receptors (168). It seems clear that the molecular function of CD4 still awaits elucidation.

One interesting functional involvement of CD4 is that anti-CD4 antibodies in human block human immunodeficiency virus (HIV) infections, which cause acquired immune deficiency syndrome (AIDS), and this finding may account for the specific tropism of this virus for $CD4^+$ cells (169,170). It also appears that the direct interaction of CD4 with HIV proteins can be detected by co-immunoprecipitation with anti-CD4 (T4) antibodies (171). As discussed above, it has been established that human and rat macrophages express the CD4 molecule. In this light it would be interesting to know if human macrophages are infected by HIV in a manner similar to $CD4^+$ T cells. Two CD4 mRNA transcripts (3.7 Kb and 2.7 Kb) have also been found in mouse and human brain (151a,171a). This result may explain the neurotropic qualities of HIV (171a). It is not clear, however, which cells in the brain express the CD4 protein.

5. The Cytotoxic/Suppressor Marker CD8

The CD8 antigen is expressed on thymocytes and defines the cytotoxic/suppressor subset in human, mouse, and rat, which was previously identified with alloantibodies as the mouse Lyt $1^-,2^+,3^+$ T-cell subset (143,148). In the rat it is also expressed by the majority of natural killer cells, but in the human this does not appear to be the case (142).

In the rat, anti-CD8 (OX8) antibody blocks the generation of cytotoxic T lymphocytes in the MLC (172). However, the antibody has no effect on proliferation in the MLC of the T cytotoxic/suppressor cells. It should be noted that one difference between rat and human $CD8^+$ T cytotoxic/suppressor cells is that rat $CD8^+$ cells do not proliferate in the MLC without help from $CD4^+$ T cells, while in the human $CD8^+$ cells can proliferate on their own (142). The generation of rat cytotoxic T cells in the MLC is blocked by anti-CD8 (OX8) $F(ab')_2$ and requires the interaction of the responder cells with antibody during the first 24 hr of the MLC, indicating that it is the early stage of activation that is most affected (172). Furthermore, anti-rat CD8 (OX8) antibody does not block the effector lytic stage of CTL in ^{51}Cr release assays (173,174) and has no effect on NK killing (172). The results obtained suggest that the anti-CD8 (MRC OX8) antibody may interfere with the ability of the $CD8^+$ cytotoxic T cell to respond to a differentiation signal.

Antibodies against CD8 in both mouse and human block MHC class I restricted T cell-mediated cytotoxicity in the effector assay (72,175). As with the anti-CD4 inhibition of cytotoxicity, the amount of inhibition using anti-CD8 (Lyt-2) varies considerably depending upon the particular cytotoxic T cells used in the assay (175). In some instances, with putative "high-affinity" cytotoxic effector cells, there is no inhibition at all. Anti-CD8 (Lyt-2) also inhibits the generation of cytotoxic T cells (176), but this has not been reported for anti-CD8 (T8) antibodies. However, anti-CD8 (T8) antibodies block cytotoxicity against MHC class I targets by T-cell clones (72). Therefore, there are some differences between the effects of anti-CD8 antibodies in the three species, possibly arising from the relationship between the active site of the molecule and the epitope recognized by the different antibodies. However, these functional affects have implicated CD8 in a recognition function (see Section VI.A.4).

The molecular nature of CD8 has been defined in mouse, man, and rat. In both rodent species the antigen is a heterodimer with an M_r of 33 and 36 kD, but in human the antigen can consist solely of a homodimer structure with an M_r of 34 kD (reviewed by 94), although it is conceivable that a second chain exists in the human as well. The human antigen was cloned (177,178) and shown to encode 210 amino acids, which contain a segment like an immunoglobulin-V domain plus a short segment like an immunoglobulin hinge sequence prior to the transmembrane segment, which connects to a small cytoplasmic domain (Fig. 5). The equivalent sequences were then determined for mouse and rat, and the same features were identified (179-181). On the basis of sequence homologies it appears that the cloned human molecule is equivalent to the rodent Lyt-2 chain (181)

The CD8 Lyt-2 equivalent chains are notable for their variation between species. First, there is the differences in chain composition noted above; second there is the fact that the human, mouse, and rat sequences have, respectively, 0, 3, and 1 potential sites for N-glycosylation, and finally, the CD8 immunoglobulin-like domain outside the cell is only 40% homologous between human and rodent (181).

The Lyt-3 chain of the rat CD8 heterodimer has recently been cloned (182). It has only 21% homology to the rat Lyt-2 chain. Like the Lyt-2 chain the Lyt-3 chain also contains a N-terminal immunoglobulin-like domain and an immunoglobulin hinge-like region. There is also a segment that corresponds to an immunoglobulin joining region sequence, and it will be interesting to determine if this is encoded by a separate intron, as it is in immunoglobulin and the T-cell receptor genes. This may help to establish a closer evolutionary link between Lyt-3 and the antigen receptor molecules of lymphocytes.

Another important finding is that the Lyt-3 chain in rat is 187 amino acids long compared to the rat Lyt-2 chain which is 210 amino acids long. Furthermore, the Lyt-3 chain has three potential N-linked carbohydrate attachment sites compared to one in the rat Lyt-2 chain. This may help to clarify the discrepancy between the apparent molecular weights of mouse and the rat Lyt2 and Lyt3 chains (182). The rat Lyt-3 chain is larger (37 kD) than the rat Lyt2 chain (32 kD) because of the presence of two more glycosylation sites, whereas in the mouse the situation is probably reversed because of the presence of three sites for N-linked sugars in the Lyt-2 chain (38 kD). However, the sequence and thus the number of N-linked carbohydrates has not been determined for the mouse Lyt-3 chain (30 kD). It will be important to determine if the human has a Lyt-3 equivalent that may so far have eluded description.

6. The OX2 Antigen

The OX2 antigen is a rat cell-surface glycoprotein of 41-47 kD found on neurons, cortical thymocytes, B cells, follicular dendritic cells, endothelium, and activated T cells (152,182-184). The amino acid composition of the brain and thymocytes forms are indistinguishable (183). The full amino acid sequence of the OX2 protein has been deduced from a rat thymocyte cDNA clone (22). The OX2 molecule is 202 amino acids long and contains two immunoglobulin-like domains. The OX2 looks like a T-cell receptor β chain or Ig light chain, both of which contain a V- and a C-type domain (Fig. 5). The OX2 antigen also contains an integral membrane segment (22). The antibody against the OX2 antigen (MRC OX2) does not inhibit lymphocyte function, and the biological role of the molecule is not known. Homologues of the OX2 molecule have been detected in human and mouse by Northern and Southern blot analysis (185).

7. The Thy-1 Molecule

The Thy-1 molecule was first described as the theta (θ) alloantigen on mouse thymocytes and T lymphocytes (186). Thy-1 was later found to be expressed on mouse and human neurons and fibroblasts (28). In the rat, Thy-1 is a 111 amino acid major glycoprotein, which has an M_r of 25 kD and is found on the surface of neurons, thymocytes, fibroblasts, denervated muscle, and hemopoietic stem cells and on activated T cells (45,152,184,187,188). There are one million molecules of Thy-1 per rat thymocyte, and it may be the most abundant molecule on the cells on which it is found (28). It is structurally like a single Ig-V domain (Fig. 5) and contains 30% carbohydrate by weight (Fig. 6) (21,189,190). One unusual feature of this protein is that it contains no sequence likely to span the lipid bilayer (21,189,190). Instead, it has been established that a glycophospholipid group is attached to the carboxy-terminus of residue Cys 111 (191), which can be cleaved from the cell surface with phospholipase C (192). The

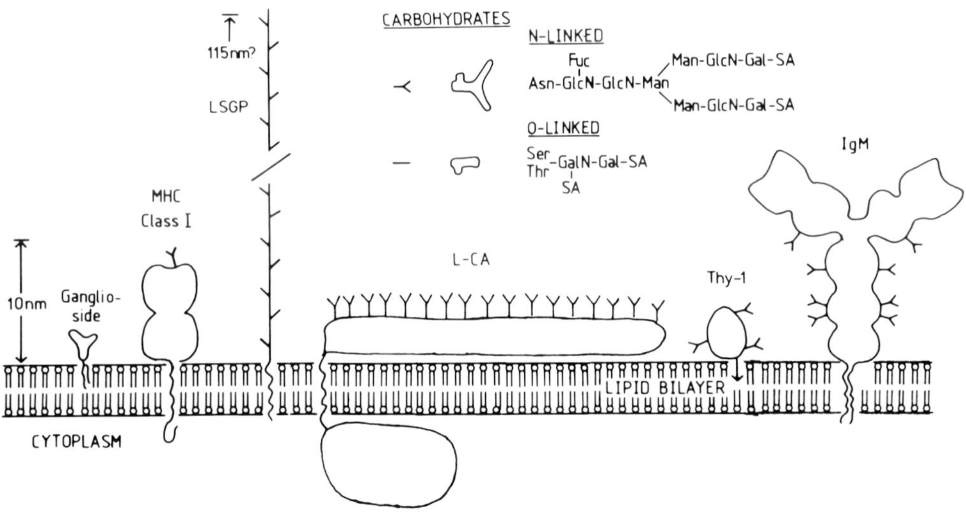

Figure 6 Many of the best characterized lymphocyte cell-surface glycoproteins are illustrated. The number of polypeptides are not shown (see Table 2), but the number of N-linked carbohydrates is indicated for L-CA, Thy-1, and class II proteins. Possible O-linked structures are not well established for these antigens but are indicated on the L-SGP structure. The carbohydrates could not be drawn to scale on the models, but are shown to the scale of their greatest cross-sectional area in the upper left-hand part of the figure. MHC class I molecules would appear similar to MHC class II proteins. (*Figure courtesy of Drs. A. F. Williams and A. N. Barclay.*)

Thy-1 cDNA (193) predicts an extra 31 amino acids after Cys 111, and it is assumed that these must be cleaved from the molecule when the nonprotein tail is attached. Though the linkage has not been established, the Thy-1 tail contains ethanolamine, phosphate, mannose, galactosamine, glucosamine, stearic acid, myoinositol, two unknown fatty acids, and probably glycerol (191). The major cell surface glycoproteins of *Trypanosoma* (194) and *Leishmania* (195) have a similar structure, which enables them to integrate into the plasma membrane (see Section VI.C.5).

The other interesting feature of the Thy-1 molecule is that the brain and thymocyte forms have different carbohydrate structures (196), although the polypeptide is the same (21). In addition, two forms of the thymocyte form can be distinguished by their ability or inability to bind lentil lectin (197). The carbohydrate therefore may be involved in the function of the Thy-1 molecule (Fig. 6).

No function has been assigned to this molecule although in the mouse anti-Thy-1 antibodies are mitogenic for T cells (198), and this also appears to be the case when the mouse Thy-1 gene is expressed in human T cells (199).

B. Heavily Glycosylated Molecules

Most cell-surface proteins are glycosylated. At present there are no clear ideas regarding the function of carbohydrate moieties on glycolipids or glycoproteins. However, carbohydrates may be involved in the maintenance of protein conformation and solubility, in proteolytic processing and stabilization of the polypeptide against uncontrolled proteolysis, in intracellular sorting and transport of glycoproteins, and in embryonic development and differentiation (200,201).

1. Leukocyte-Common Antigen

The leukocyte-common antigen (L-CA) includes a family of high molecular weight glycoproteins found, as major molecules, on the surface of lymphoid and myeloid cells but not other tissues (202-204) (Fig. 6). The L-CA molecules show heterogeneity with respect to molecular weight (205,206). For example, on SDS-PAGE analysis, rat thymocyte L-CA is a single band of 180 kD; rat peripheral T cells have four bands of 180 kD, 190 kD, 200 kD, and 220 kD; and rat B cells have one broad band of 240 kD (206). The L-CAs from different cell types have different carbohydrate structures (Fig. 6) (207,208), but this may not wholly account for the observed difference in molecular weight (209).

The L-CA molecule is polymorphic within a species, and allotypes have been defined which include the rat ART-1 or LY-1 allotypes (210-212) and the mouse Ly-5 allotypes (204,213).

The L-CA molecule also shows considerable heterogeneity with respect to antigenic determinants (9,206). Some xenogenic monoclonal antibodies recognize all the L-CA forms, but others are restricted to binding L-CA exclusively expressed

Table 5 Markers and Functions of Rat T-Cell Subsets

	T helper for B-cell response		T helper for T-cell response		T cytotoxic/suppressor	
Peripheral T lymphoid compartment	20%	$CD4^+$ $CD8^-$ MRC $OX22^-$	60%	$CD4^+$ $CD8^-$ MRC $OX22^+$	16%	$CD4^-$ $CD8^+$ MRC $OX22^+$
T helper for T cytotoxic cells	(±)		+		–	
In vivo T helpers for B cells	+		(±)		–	
In vitro T helper for B cells	+		(±)		–	
T cytotoxic precursors specific for Class I^+ targets	–		–		+	
T cell suppression	–		–		+	
Mix lymphocyte culture	a		+		b	
GvH lymph node reaction	–		+		–	
GvH disease	–		+		+	
Con A proliferation	–		+		–	
IL-2 production	–		+		–	
Induction of Ia in epithelium		+[c]			+	
Allograft rejection		+			+[d]	
T cytotoxic precursors specific for Class II^+ targets		+			–	

The markers and functions of peripheral rat T lymphocytes are summarized. The OX22 epitope is found on the L-CA molecule and this marker has also been detected in human but not in mouse. The manifestations of T-cell functions takes place after antigen stimulation and the phenotype of the T cells activated in vitro and in vivo includes some $CD4^+$ $CD8^+$ cells while those T cells activated by antigen in vitro also include $CD4^+$ Ia^+ and $CD8^+$ Ia^+ cells. (See Sections VI.D.4 and VI.D.5).

[a,b]Cells with the $CD4^+$ $CD8^-$ $OX22^-$ phenotype show little response in the MLC but it is not known if they will proliferate when provided help by the $CD4^+$ $CD8^-$ $CD22^+$ population, as is the case when $CD4^+$ $CD8^-$ $OX22^+$ cells are added to the $CD4^-$ $CD8^+$ $OX22^+$ cells, which ordinarily would not respond in the MLC by themselves.

[c]The OX22 phenotype of the $CD4^+$ $CD8^-$ cells that induce Ia expression on epithelial cells during graft-versus-host disease has not been determined.

[d]$CD4^-$ $OX8^+$ cells play a role in skin allograft rejection in the rat but they may not be essential for rejection to occur (see Refs. 9,142,215).

on specific cell types (206). The common epitopes have been useful in recognizing leukocytes in various tissues (214).

The OX22 antigen of rat L-CA has a restricted distribution and has allowed the identification of two functionally distinct subsets of rat T helper cells (Table 5) (9). The $CD4^+$ $CD8^-$ $OX22^+$ cells in vitro provide help for cytotoxic T-cell responses, proliferate during ConA mitogenesis and the MLC, and produce IL-2 (215). The $CD4^+$ $CD8^-$ $OX22^+$ T cells mediate the graft-versus-host reaction in vivo. On the other hand, the $CD4^+$ $CD8^-$ $OX22^-$ T cells provide help for B-cell responses in vitro and in vivo (215).

The human F-8-11-13 antigen has a similar distribution as that of the rat OX22 antigen and also defines a subset of the L-CA molecule (216). However, functional data using this antibody is lacking for the human.

A large part of the L-CA molecule appears to be on the inside of the cell (217) (Fig. 6). Furthermore, the L-CA molecule appears to be attached to the cytoskeleton via the fodrin molecule, and this may allow L-CA to participate in transmembrane signaling (218).

The partial amino acid sequence of the L-CA molecule has been obtained, which has enabled the isolation of a rat thymocyte cDNA clone that encodes most of the L-CA molecule, with the exception of the N-terminal region (219). The sequence contains only one segment that is hydrophobic enough to cross the membrane and includes a possible cytoplasmic phosphorylation site. It also contains a region of internal homology. B-cell and thymocyte L-CA mRNA are identical at the 3' end, but there is a size difference on Northern blot analysis. This suggests that the N-terminal regions may differ in the many forms of L-CA. In summary, the molecular weight heterogeneity of the L-CA molecule may be due to either differences in glycosylation and/or to alternate mRNA splicing mechanisms that generate differences in N-terminal amino acid sequence (219).

L-CA may mediate an important leukocyte-specific function. In antibody blocking studies, anti-L-CA antibodies block NK cytolysis (220), the generation of CTL (221), cytolysis by T cells (222), and B-cell differentiation (223).

2. Leukocyte Sialoglycoprotein (L-SGP)

The leukocyte sialoglycoprotein of rats is found on thymocytes, T but not B lymphocytes, bone marrow cells, hemopoietic stem cells, neutrophils, and brain cells (6,26). It is also found on plasma and myeloma cells (27). The L-SGP molecule is 95 kD and is heavily glycosylated. It was first of structural interest because the thymocyte form did not bind to lentil lectin which recognizes mannose, a core component of N-linked carbohydrate. Also, the removal of sialic acid resulted in an apparent increase of size on SDS-PAGE analysis (207). Brown et al.(27) purified L-SGP from rat thymocytes, which have approximately 70,000 molecules of L-SGP per cell and showed that L-SGP contains O-linked sugars and is 60% w/w carbohydrate. However, it contained no mannose or glucosamine, which indicates the absence of N-linked sugars. The protein itself does not contain Cys or Trp but has a high ratio of Ser, Thr, and Pro. Based on this structural information, the L-SGP molecule is expected to be related to glycophorin, the major sialoglycoprotein of human erythrocytes (27). The molecule, because of its high O-linked carbohydrate content, may be extended in structure (Fig. 6) and may contribute to the negative charge of rodent T lymphocytes (224). These peculiar features may affect the ease with which the L-SGP expressing membrane can align with that of another cell and thus be important in dictating the physical constraints in cell interactions (27). The W3/13 antibody that binds to rat L-SGP does not perturb any assayable lymphocyte function.

Molecules with characteristics similar to those of rat L-SGP have been detected in mouse and human (27,225,226). Wiskott-Aldrich syndrome patients have been shown to lack the human L-SGP homologue on their lymphocytes. This lesion may be responsible for some, if not all, of the manifestations of the syndrome (227).

C. Miscellaneous Marker Molecules

1. CD2 (The E-Rosette Receptor/LFA-2)

The human T-lymphocyte E-rosette receptor (CD2) is found on thymocytes, peripheral T lymphocytes, and natural killer cells (228). It was so named because some anti-CD2 antibodies inhibit the spontaneous formation of rosettes between human T cells and sheep red blood cells (229,230). Subsequently, CD2-derived peptides have been shown to inhibit E-rosette formation (230a). The CD2 molecule is a single, heavily glycosylated polypeptide chain of 50 kD (231). Two different CD2 epitopes have been detected on resting T cells—$T11_1$ and $T11_2$. Antibodies against $T11_1$ but not $T11_2$ inhibit sheep red blood cell rosette formation (228). MLC and lectin activated T-cell blasts express an additional CD2 epitope which is a T-blast specific marker—$T11_3$ (228). The CD2 molecule may be important in T-cell activation because antibodies against $T11_2$ and $T11_3$ added at the same time to resting T cells or thymocytes induce a mitogenic response (228,232).

There does not appear to be an identified CD2 homologue in the mouse, but in the rat the OX34 antigen (M_r 50-54 kD) has been identified as the rat CD2 homologue (233,234). It is found on T cells, NK cells, and 98% of thymocytes but not B cells or peritoneal macrophages but does appear on macrophages in the red spleen pulp (13,233). cDNAs encoding both the rat and human CD2 proteins have been identified (234, 234a). Notable features of the molecule include its large (125 amino acid) cytoplasmic domain and slight homology to members of the immunoglobulin superfamily (234a). CD2, like CD4, may contain a half immunoglobulin domain (234).

It is possible that the T-blast antigen OX40 (see below) is a determinant on the rat equivalent of the CD2 molecule, and the OX40 and OX34 determinants are found on the same molecule of activated rat T cells. This has now been tested (233) and is not the case since the antigens can be independently immunoprecipitated. Therefore, OX34 and OX40 antigens are not related in a similar fashion to the $T11_1$, $T11_2$, and $T11_3$ determinants (228).

2. The CD3 Complex (T3)

CD3 is an antigen expressed on the majority of thymocytes and all peripheral T cells in the human (15). The CD3 molecule appears to be composed of at least three protein chains, δ, ϵ, γ, of 19 kD, 20 kD, and 25 kD, respectively. The ϵ chain is not glycosylated, whereas the other two chains are (23). The γ chain is associated with the T-cell receptor, and this molecule may be essential for T-cell antigen receptor function (235). The δ, ϵ, and γ chains have been cloned in human (23,236,236a), and the δ chain has been cloned in mouse (18). The 20 kD δ chain has an extracellular domain of 79 amino acids with two N-linked oligosaccharides, one transmembrane segment, and an intracellular domain of 44 residues (236). The 19 kD ϵ chain contains two hydrophilic domains with no potential N-linked glycosylation sites (23). The 25 kD γ chain has an 89-amino-acid hydrophilic extracellular domain with two N-linked glycosylation sites. It also contains a hydrophobic segment and an intracellular domain of 44 residues (236a). The δ and ϵ chains contain regions of homology to each other, although the strongest homology is between the δ and the γ chains, which may have arisen by gene duplication 200 million years ago. They also appear to possess sequence homologies with immunoglobulin domains that were not identified in the original analysis of the two sequences (234). Secondary structure predictions and the assignment of the disulfide bonds within the three chains may definitively identify them as members of the immunoglobulin superfamily.

Anti-CD3 antibodies in very low concentrations are mitogenic for T cells (72). Furthermore, it appears that only anti-CD3 IgG_{2a} antibodies mediate this mitogenesis and that it is dependent on accessory cells which allow cross-linking of the CD3/T cell receptor complex (237). Antibodies against CD3 in higher concentration also inhibit CTL killing (238), and cause a calcium flux which has been associated with T cell activation (239). At present the rat CD3 complex has not been identified.

3. The CD5 Antigen

The CD5 molecule is 67 kD in mouse, rat, and human and is expressed on thymocytes, T cells, and 2% of B cells (229,240,241). It was initially detected as the mouse Lyt-1 alloantigen (242), which was incorrectly considered a marker of T helper/inducer cells. It may have an important functional role in T-cell activation and differentiation (240,243). Although a mouse anti-rat CD5 antibody

(MRC OX19) is not mitogenic by itself, when included in in vitro functional assays, it increases the proliferation of T cells stimulated with lectins or in the MLC (240). T-cell proliferation requires interleukin-2 (244), which is produced by the $CD4^+$ T-helper subset in the rat (245). The increased proliferation induced by anti-CD5 antibody is correlated with a higher level of IL-2 production. Anti-CD5 (OX19) antibody also inhibits the generation of cytotoxic T cells but not the CTL lytic phase (240). Although the mechanism of action of this antibody is unknown, it has been suggested that it mimics a component that regulates the production of IL-2, or it may block the action of a suppressor factor or cell that would normally limit proliferation (240).

The functional effects of anti-CD5 antibodies have not been reported in the human, but augmentation of T-cell response has been recorded in the mouse (176). The cDNA clone encoding the human CD5 protein (471 amino acids) reveals that the molecule contains a 347-amino-acid extracellular domain, a transmembrane segment, and a 93-amino-acid intracellular segment. The CD5 protein contains five potential N-linked glycosylation sites but only two N-terminal sites are used. The extracellular segment is probably composed of two structurally related domains. No significant sequence homology has been found between CD5 and other proteins but the overall structure and functional information are consistent with CD5 being a receptor for an unknown ligand.

4. LFA-1 (Lymphocyte Function-Associated Antigen-1)

The LFA-1 protein has been identified as a heterodimer of 190 kD (α chain) and 95 kD (β chain) and is present on the surface of all human and mouse leukocytes (246,247). The α and β chains are noncovalently associated in a 1:1 ratio (α:β chain) on the cell surface (248). The immunoaffinity purified α chain of mouse LFA-1 has considerable N-terminal sequence homology to members of the interferon group of peptide hormones (249).

LFA-1 belongs to a family of cell-surface molecules that all share the same β chain (95 kD) but have different α chains (150-190 kD). This family includes the mouse Mac1 and the human OKM1/Mac1 molecules, which have an α chain of 170 kD and are associated with the complement receptor-3 (CR3) functions of macrophages and monocytes (248,250). In the human, a third member of this family has been identified, which is designated p150,95 (244). Another molecule, OX42, which is probably a fourth member of this family, has been identified in the rat (251).

Most antibodies against mouse LFA-1 appear to partially block T-cell proliferation to soluble antigen and alloantigen as well as CTL responses (246,247,252, 253). In addition, one monoclonal antibody H155-78 potentiates these responses, while another H15-266 has no functional effects (253). Furthermore, the different functional effects of these antibodies can be directly related to their reactivity with particular antigenic domains on the LFA-1 molecule (253,254). Antibodies against the human LFA-1 molecule have functional effects similar to those in the mouse (255). A deficiency in β-chain expression has been associated with susceptibility to infections in humans (256). Overall, these diverse involvements have implicated the LFA-1 molecule in mediating nonspecific adhesion between T cells and target cells (253,254,257).

5. RT6 Alloantigen

The RT6 rat alloantigen, formerly designated Pta, AgF, ART, or RTLy-2 (257a) exists in at least two allelic forms, RT6.1 and RT6.2. RT6 expression is restricted to approximately 85% of peripheral T cells. The RT6.2 protein appears to be a noncovalently linked heterodimer composed of 21 kD and 24 kD (nonreduced) polypeptide chains (257a). This molecule is extraordinary for two reasons. First, it does not bind to lectin columns, incorporate radiolabeled sugars, reduce in molecular weight after treatment with endoglycosidase-F, O-glycanase, or mild alkaline hydrolysis (257a). These results suggest that it is not glycosylated and point to similarities with the CD3 ϵ chain (see above). Second, like Thy-1, it appears to be anchored to the plasma membrane via a fatty acid linkage which is cleavable with phospholipase-C (257b). It is important to determine the primary structure of the RT6.2 chains and to analyze the intracellular pathway of biosynthesis and processing of this molecule.

D. Functional Markers of T-Cell Activation: The Fidelity of Marker Molecules

The sequence of events leading to activation of T cells by antigen has been difficult to study because the number of T cells that will respond to any given antigen is small. The stimulation of lymphocytes with polyclonal mitogen or alloantigen in vitro is thought to be the experimental equivalent of antigen specific activation of lymphocytes (258). Since more cells respond, polyclonal activation has been more amenable to study. At a molecular level, T-cell stimulation is characterized by a change in membrane permeability resulting in a pH shift (259) and an increase in transmembrane transport of Ca^{+2}, glucose, and amino acids (239, 260). This is followed by synthesis of RNA and protein (258). Proteins which are synthesized at this time include growth factors, their receptors, and cell surface proteins possibly involved in cellular interactions (261). These molecular events precede DNA synthesis and cell division (262).

The majority of antigens expressed only on activation of lymphocytes are not T-cell specific membrane proteins (Table 2) (262,269). For example, the receptors for insulin (264) and transferrin (265) are absent from resting T and B lymphocytes but are expressed on activated lymphocytes and other cell types as well. MHC class II molecules (Ia) normally absent from resting T cells appear after mitogen or allogenic stimulation (266) but are constitutively expressed on many other cell types (135). Furthermore, the interleukin-2 receptor (267), which was initially thought to be exclusively expressed on activated T cells (244), has been found on mitogen-activated B cells and thymocytes (263), although the receptors on B cells may not be functional (268). The activated human T-cell marker, VLA-1, which has an M_r of 210/130 kD, may be T-cell specific but a complete distribution has not been undertaken (269). The $T11_3$ (228) and T200A (270) antigens are exclusively expressed on activated T cells, but these antigens (epitopes) exist as part of modified molecules which are themselves present in a different form, CD2 and L-CA, respectively, on unstimulated T cells (see above). Thus, although there are some phenotypic differences already noted between resting and activated T cells, more markers are needed. These markers would be useful in identifying T cells responding to antigen stimulation in vivo and in vitro.

1. The OX40 Antigen: A T-Cell Specific Activation Marker in Rat

The OX40 antigen has an apparent molecular weight of 45-50 kD. An exhaustive study has been done on its distribution, and it appears to be a specific marker of activated rat T cells. There is no definite correlation between the OX40 antigen and cell-surface antigens in other species, and since it can be immunoprecipitated separately from the OX34 protein, the equivalent of the human E-rosette receptor CD2, it is not the $T11_3$ epitope of the CD2 molecule expressed on activated T cells (233) (see Section VI.C.1). An antibody against the OX40 antigen (MRC OX40) variably augments T-cell proliferation in the MLC and Con A responses, and the OX40 antigen is a candidate for involvement in a function specific to activated T cells (233).

2. The IL-2 Receptor

The antibodies ART-18 and MRC OX39 react with the rat IL-2 receptor and, like the anti-human IL-2 receptor antibody Tac and anti-mouse IL-2 receptor antibodies, e.g., PC61 and 3C7, inhibit IL-2 binding to T cell blasts (263,271-273). MRC OX39 and ART-18 do not bind to resting lymphocytes but inhibit rat T-lymphocyte blast proliferation in response to IL-2 (233,267). The MRC OX39 antibody partially cross-reacts with the mouse IL-2 receptor (233).

The IL-2 receptor in rat, mouse, and human is a glycosylated protein of 50-60 kD (233,271,272). The cDNAs for the human (274,275) and mouse receptors have been cloned (276) and both code for single 251 amino acid peptide chains which are 61% homologous to one another. The molecule contains a single hydrophobic segment, which allows the molecule to span the lipid bilayer. It has no apparent homology to other sequenced proteins or oncogenes (274).

3. The Transferrin Receptor

The expression of transferrin receptors at a cell surface has also been associated with cell growth and cell division (265). Monoclonal antibodies against transferrin receptors invariably label tissue culture cell lines and many normal dividing cells, whereas nondividing cells are often not detectably labeled (54,277,278). The uptake of transferrin is a well-characterized pathway for iron to enter cells, and in some cases may be obligatory for cell growth, since it has been shown for one cell line that division is inhibited by a monoclonal antibody that blocks binding of transferrin to its receptor (279).

The human, mouse, and rat transferrin receptors are disulfide-linked dimers of glycoproteins of about 95 kD (54,279-281). The receptor is posttranslationally modified with phosphate (280), a fatty-acyl group (282), and three N-linked carbohydrate attachments (283). The transferrin receptor has been cloned in human (24,284) and mouse (285). In human it is 760 amino acids long and it does not contain an N-terminal signal sequence. There is a 670-amino-acid C-terminal extracellular domain, a 28-amino-acid transmembrane segment (leader sequences), and a 62-amino-acid N-terminal cytoplasmic domain. Thus the receptor is inverted in the membrane in relation to most cell surface proteins.

4. Ia Antigens

The MRC OX6 (Ia) antigen appeared on 26-58% of activated rat T cells (184, 286a). The percentage of Ia+ cells increases when the T cells are cultured (286) and Ia antigens are expressed on both the rat T helper and T cytotoxic/suppressor cell subsets (184,286a). The presence of Ia molecules on T cells has previously been regarded as a marker of T-cell activation in man (262) and mouse (287). Furthermore, this molecule is not normally acquired from B cells or accessory cells (288), and mRNA for mouse Ia molecules has been detected in mouse T-cell clones (289). It has been hypothesized that Ia is expressed on T cells so that after the initial antigen triggering in association with antigen presenting cells, they may be able to present antigen to themselves (289,290). In this way, T cells would bypass the antigen-triggering mechanism involving accessory cells. No definitive study has shown that T cells express Ia in vivo, therefore the expression seen in vitro may be an aberration.

5. Blast Cells Positive for CD4 (W3/25) and CD8 (MRC OX8) Antigen

A population of CD4+ CD8+ rat lymphocytes has been detected in experiments using rat T cells activated by Con A or in the MLC (184,286a). This double labeled population can arise from purified CD4+ (W3/25) cells, and in this case it is clear that the CD8 (OX8) antigen could not be acquired passively from another source (291).

Under physiological conditions, Blue et al. (292) have shown that about 2% of resting T cells express both CD4 (T4) and CD8 (T8), and Spickett and Mason (293) showed that during an anti-dinitrophenyl immune response there was a consistent population of double labeled cells. There is also a report that cyclosporin induces a double labeled population of T cells in allografted rats (294). 5-Azacytidine, an inhibitor of DNA methylation is capable of inducing CD4 in cloned human CD8+ T cells (294a). Furthermore, cloned cell lines have been reported to constitutively express both CD4 (T4) and CD8 (T8) (295), but the role of these cells will await tests to determine whether they have a unique function.

VII. CONCLUSION

This review has summarized the structure, function (where it is known), and distribution of many rat lymphoid cell-surface proteins and put this information in the context of information available for other species. Knowledge of this kind is providing a foundation for understanding lymphoid differentiation and lymphocyte cell-surface functions. Despite this, there remains a need for approaches that allow the determination of molecular functions. This is difficult since it involves complex biological phenomena. One approach, discussed throughout this review, is to study any in vitro functional reaction involving cells that bear the antigen and see if the assay is perturbed by antibodies against the antigen in question. This has yielded some significant results. Alternatively, expression of a particular cell-surface protein in a cell not normally expressing the protein may yet prove to be a useful approach (199). Finally, the emerging technique of transfection with antisense DNA to test the consequences of suppressing a particular protein's expression may be useful (296).

These are crude approaches and ultimately the aim would be to reconstruct an immunological system from its components, for example, to show interactions between recognition molecules by measuring associations during ultracentrifugation or by another type of binding test. If this could be achieved, the particular segments that determine the specificity of the interactions could be directly examined. Eventually a clearer picture of lymphocyte cell-surface functions should emerge.

ACKNOWLEDGMENTS

I would like to thank all of my former colleagues at the Medical Research Council, Cellular Immunology Unit in Oxford for their continued help and encouragement. I am grateful to Drs. H-G. Burgert, S. V. Hunt, D. W. Mason, and A. F. Williams for their critical reading of the manuscript, and to Claudine Ravussin and Mary Sanders for their tremendous technical assistance. This review has been supported by the Wellcome Trust and by the Medical Research Council of Canada.

NOTES ADDED IN PROOF

Table 1. New monoclonal antibodies against rat T and B lymphocytes have been described. [F. G. M. Kroese, A. S. Wubbena, D. Opstelten, G. J. Deenen, E. H. Swander, L. D. Leij, H. Vos, S. Poppema, J. Volberda, and P. Nieuwenhuis, B lymphocyte differentiation in the rat: Production and characterization of monoclonal antibodies to B lineage-associated antigens. *Eur. J. Immunol., 17*: 921-928 (1987).] [P. Joling, F. J. Tielen, L. M. B. Vaessen, J. M. A. Huijbrejts, and J. Rozing, New markers on T cell subpopulations defined by monoclonal antibodies, *Transplant. Proc., 17*: 1857-1860 (1985).]

VI.A.1. The T cell receptor γ (gamma) (44 kD) gene product in association with a novel δ (delta) (40 kD) chain has been detected on WT-31$^-$,CD3$^+$,CD4$^-$,CD8$^-$ human T cells and on CD4$^-$,CD8$^-$ mouse thymocytes. The δ chain has not been characterized in detail but is possibly encoded by a new T-cell-receptor gene located within the murine α locus (5' to the $J_\alpha C_\alpha$ regions). This gene is expressed early in T-cell differentiation and has the potential to be deleted by α gene rearrangement during T-cell ontogeny. [E. L. Reinherz, T cell receptors—Who needs more? *Nature, 325*: 660-663 (1987). Y. Chein, M. Iwashima, K. B. Kaplan, J. F. Elliott, and M. M. Davis, A new T cell receptor gene located within the alpha locus and expressed early in differentiation, *Nature, 327*: 677-682 (1987).]

VI.A.2. Several RT1 class I and class II genes have been cloned and transfected into fibroblasts in order to identify their gene products. [A. G. Diamond, J. M. Windle, G. W. Butcher, A. Winoto, L. Hood, and J. C. Howard, Identification and expression of genes encoding rat class I and class II major histocompatibility complex molecules from two genomic libraries, *Transplant. Proc., 17*: 1808-1811 (1985).]

VI.A.2. Refer to Butcher and Howard (1985) for a detailed description of the rat MHC complex-RT1. [G. W. Butcher and J. C. Howard, The MHC of the laboratory rat, *Rattus norvegicus*, in *The Handbook of Experimental Immunology* (D. M. Weir, ed.), 4th Edition, Chapter 101, Blackwell Scientific Publications Ltd., Oxford, 1985.]

VI.A.6. The OX2 gene has been cloned in human (185). Between human and rat there is 75% homology at the protein level and a putative Ig-J segment is found on the same exon as the Ig-V-like region. This finding diminishes the possibility that OX2 is an ancestor of the T-cell receptor or immunoglobulin genes. The gene encoding the OX2 proteins in human is on chromosome 3, and OX2 mRNA has been detected in human brain and B cells but not in thymoma cell lines (185).

VI.B.1. The molecular-weight heterogeneity of CD45 (L-CA) has been traced to alternative splicing at the 5' end of the CD45 (L-CA) mRNA. This mechanism results in different numbers of possible N-linked carbohydrate attachment sites in the mature forms of the CD45 (L-CA) mRNA. [S. S. Ralph, M. L. Thomas, C. C. Morton, and I. S. Trowbridge, Structural variations of human T200 glycoprotein (leukocyte-common antigens), *EMBO J., 6*: 1251-1257 (1987). A. W. Barclay, D. I. Jackson, A. C. Willis, and A. F. Williams, Lymphocyte heterogeneity in the rat leukocyte-common antigen (T200) is due to differences in polypeptide sequences near the NH_2-terminus, *EMBO J., 6*: 1259-1264 (1987).]

VI.B.2. The monoclonal antibody L10 which binds to the human L-SPG molecule is mitogenic for peripheral T cells. [S. J. Mentzer, E. Remold-O'Donnell, M. A. V. Crimmins, B. E. Bierer, F. S. Rosen, and S. J. Burakoff, Sialophorin, a surface sialoglyco-protein defective in the Wiskott-Aldrich syndrome, is involved in human T lymphocyte proliferation, *J. Exp. Med., 165*: 1383-1392 (1987).]

VI.C.1. Purified CD2 can directly bind LFA-3 (gp45). This demonstrates that LFA-3 is a ligand for CD2. [P. Selvaraj, M. L. Plunkett, M. Dustin, M. E. Sanders,

S. Shaw, and T. A. Springer, The T lymphocyte glycoprotein CD2 binds the surface ligand LFA-3, *Nature, 326*: 400-402 (1987).]

VI.C.2. A monoclonal antibody reactive with the murine CD3 antigen has been generated in hamsters. [O. Leo, M. Foo, D. H. Sachs, L. E. Samelson, and J. A. Bluestone, Identification of a monoclonal antibody specific for a murine T3 polypeptide, *Proc. Natl. Acad. Sci. USA, 84*: 1374-1378 (1987).]

VI.C.4. The β (beta) chain of CD11 (LFA-1) has been cloned and reveals considerable homology to Band III of integrin and to the β chains of the chicken fibronectin receptor and luminin receptor. These extracellular matrix molecules recognize the tripeptide Arg-Gly-Asp (RGD), but this has not been demonstrated for CD11 (LFA-1). [T. G. Kishimoto, K. O'Connor, A. Lee, T. M. Roberts, and T. A. Springer, Cloning of the β subunit of the leukocyte adhesion proteins: Homology to an extracellular matrix receptor defines a novel supergene family, *Cell, 48*: 681-690 (1987).]

REFERENCES

1. A. F. Williams, Surface antigens of lymphocytes: Markers and molecules, *Biochem. Soc. Symp., 45*: 27-50 (1980).
2. E. A. Boyse, and L. J. Old, Some aspects of normal and abnormal cell surface genetics, *Ann. Rev. Genet., 3*: 269-290 (1969).
3. A. F. Williams, and G. R. Woollett, Monoclonal antibodies: Their applications in exploring molecules and cells, *Biochem. Soc. Trans., 13*: 1-3 (1985).
4. G. Köhler, and C. Milstein, Derivation of specific antibody-producing tissue culture and tumour lines by cell fusion, *Eur. J. Immunol., 6*: 511-519 (1976).
5. G. Galfré, and C. Milstein, Preparation of monoclonal antibodies; strategies and procedures, *Methods in Enzymol., 73*: 3-46 (1981).
6. A. F. Williams, G. Galfré, and C. Milstein, Analysis of cell surfaces by xenogeneic myeloma-hybrid antibodies: Differentiation antigens of rat lymphocytes, *Cell, 12*: 663-673 (1977).
7. W. R. McMaster, and A. F. Williams, Monoclonal antibodies to Ia antigens from rat thymus: Cross reaction with mouse and human and use in purification of rat Ia glycoproteins, *Immunol. Rev., 47*: 117-137 (1979).
8. M. Webb, D. W. Mason, and A. F. Williams, Inhibition of the mixed lymphocyte response with a monoclonal antibody specific for a rat T lymphocyte subset, *Nature, 282*: 841-843 (1979).
9. G. P. Spickett, M. R. Brandon, D. W. Mason, A. F. Williams, and G. R. Woollett, MRC OX22, a monoclonal antibody that labels a new subset of T lymphocytes and reacts with the high molecular weight form of the leukocyte-common antigen, *J. Exp. Med., 158*: 795-810 (1983).
10. D. P. Lane, and W. K. Hoeffler, SV40 large T shares an antigenic determinant with a cellular protein of molecular weight 68,000, *Nature, 288*: 167-170 (1980).
11. R. Dulbecco, M. Unger, M. Bologna, H. Battifora, P. Syka, and S. Okada,

Cross-reactivity between Thy-1 and a component of intermediate filaments demonstrated using a monoclonal antibody, *Nature, 292*: 772-774 (1981).
12. J. A. Garson, P. C. L. Beverley, H. B. Coakhas, and E. I. Harper, Monoclonal antibodies against human T lymphocytes label Purkinje neurones of many species, *Nature, 298*: 375-377 (1982).
13. W. A. Jefferies, J. R. Green, and A. F. Williams, Authentic T helper CD4 (W3/25) antigen on rat peritoneal macrophages, *J. Exp. Med., 162*: 117-127 (1985).
14. M. Pierres, personal communication.
15. A. Bernard, L. Boumsell, J. Dausset, C. Milstein, and S. F. Schlossman (eds.), *Human Leukocyte Markers Detected by Monoclonal Antibodies–Leucocyte Typing*, Springer-Verlag, Heidelberg, 1984.
16. J. P. Alison, and L. L. Lanier, Identification of antigen receptor-associated structures on murine T cells, *Nature, 314*: 107-109 (1985).
17. H. C. Oettgen, C. L. Pettey, W. L. Maloy, and C. Terhorst, A T3-like protein complex associated with the antigen receptor on murine T cells, *Nature, 320*: 272-275 (1986).
17a. L. H. Martin, F. Calabi, and C. Milstein, Isolation of CD1 genes: A family of major histocompatibility complex-related differentiation antigens, *Proc. Natl. Acad. Sci. USA, 83*: 9154-9158 (1986).
17b. E. T. H. Yeh, H. Reiser, B. Benacerraf, and K. L. Rook, Expression of T cell-activating protein in peripheral lymphocyte subsets, *Proc. Natl. Acad. Sci. USA, 83*: 7424-7428 (1986).
17c. H. Reiser, H. Oettgen, E. T. H. Yeh, C. Terhorst, M. G. Low, B. Benacerraf, and K. L. Rook, Structural characterisation of the TAP molecule: A phosphatidylinositol-linked glycoprotein distinct from the T cell receptor/T3 complex and Thy-1, *Cell, 47*: 365-370 (1986).
18. P. Van den Elsen, B. A. Shepley, M. Cho, and C. Terhorst, Isolation and characterization of a cDNA clone encoding the murine homologue of the human 20K T3/T-cell receptor glycoprotein, *Nature, 314*: 542-544 (1985).
19. C. Morimoto, N. L. Letvin, A. W. Boyd, M. Hagan, H. M. Brown, M. M. Kornacki, and S. F. Schlossman, The isolation and characterization of the human helper inducer T cell subset, *J. Immunol., 134*: 3752-3769 (1985).
20. F. Sanchez-Madrid, P. Szklut, and T. A. Springer, Stable hamster-mouse hybridomas producing IgG and IgM hamster monoclonal antibodies of defined specificity, *J. Immunol., 130*: 309-312 (1983).
21. A. F. Williams, and J. Gagnon, Neuronal cell Thy-1-homology with immunoglobulins, *Science, 216*: 696-703 (1982).
22. M. J. Clark, J. Gagnon, A. F. Williams, and A. N. Barclay, MRC OX-2 antigen: A lymphoid/neuronal membrane glycoprotein with a structure like a single immunoglobulin light chain, *EMBO J., 4*: 113-118 (1985).
23. D. P. Gold, J. M. Puck, C. L. Pettey, M. Cho, J. Goligan, J. N. Woody, and C. Terhorst, Isolation of cDNA clones encoding the 20 K non-glycosylated polypeptide chain of the human T cell receptor /T3 complex, *Nature, 321*: 431-434 (1986).
24. L. C. Kühn, A. McClelland, and F. H. Ruddle, Gene transfer expression and molecular cloning of the human transferrin receptor gene, *Cell, 37*: 95-103 (1984).

25. S. M. Hedrick, E. A. Nielson, J. Kavalar, D. I. Cohen, and M. M. Davis, Sequence relationships between putative T cell receptor polypeptides and immunoglobulins, *Nature, 308*: 153-158 (1984).
26. M. J. S. Dyer, and S. V. Hunt, Committed T lymphocyte stem cells of rats characterization by surface W3/13 antigen and radiosensitivity, *J. Exp. Med., 154*: 1164-1177 (1981).
27. W. R. A. Brown, A. N. Barclay, C. A. Sunderland, and A. F. Williams, Identification of a glycophorin-like molecule at the cell surface of rat thymocytes, *Nature, 289*: 456-460 (1981).
28. A. F. Williams, and A. N. Barclay, in *Handbook of Experimental Immunology* (D. M. Weir and L. A. Herzenberg, eds.), 4th edn. chapter 25, Blackwell Scientific Publications Ltd, Oxford, 1985.
29. D. Metcalf, *The Hemopoietic Colony Stimulating Factors,* Elsevier Science Publishers B.V., Amsterdam, 1984.
30. D. Metcalf, and M. A. S. Moore, in *Haemopoietic Cells.* Frontiers of Biology *24* (A. Neuberger and E. L. Tatum, eds.), North-Holland Publishing Co., Amsterdam and London, 1970.
31. S. V. Hunt, Surface antigens characterizing lymphopoietic stem cells in rats, *Haematology and Blood Transfusion, 25*: 193-203 (1980).
32. D. H. Pluznick, and L. Sachs, The cloning of normal "mast" cells in tissue culture, *J. Cell Comp. Physiol., 66*: 319-324 (1965).
33. T. R. Bradley, and D. Metcalf, The growth of mouse bone marrow cells *in vitro, Aust. J. Exp. Biol. Med. Sci., 44*: 287-299 (1966).
34. T. M. Dexter, Hemopoietic growth factors, *TIBS, 11*: 207-211 (1986).
35. J. Hayashi, C. S. Medlock, and I. Goldschneider, A selective culture system for generating terminal deoxynucleotidyl transferase-positive (TdT^+) lymphoid precursor cells *in vitro, J. Exp. Med., 160*: 1622-1639 (1984).
36. J. E. Till, and E. A. McCulloch, A direct measurement of the radiation sensitivity of normal mouse bone marrow cells, *Radiation Res., 14*: 213-222 (1961).
37. A. J. Becker, E. A. McCulloch, and J. E. Till, Cytological demonstration of the clonal nature of spleen colonies derived from transplanted mouse marrow cells, *Nature, 197*: 452-454 (1963).
38. A. M. Wu, J. E. Till, L. Siminovitch, and E. A. McCulloch, CFU_S, thymus and LN can be members of one clone, *J. Exp. Med., 127*: 455-463 (1968).
39. M. C. Magli, N. N. Iscove, and N. Odartchenko, Transient nature of early hemopoietic spleen colonies, *Nature, 295*: 527-529 (1982).
40. H. S. Micklem, C. E. Ford, E. P. Evans, and J. Gray, Interrelationships of myeloid and lymphoid cells: Studies with chromosome marked cells transfused into lethally irradiated mice, *Proc. Roy. Soc. Lond. B., 165*: 68-102 (1966).
41. D. E. Harrison, Competitive repopulation: A new assay for long-term stem cell functional capacity, *Blood, 55*: 77-81 (1980).
42. H. Von Boehmer, J. Sprent, and M. Nabholz, Tolerance to histocompatibility determinants in tetraparental bone marrow chimeras, *J. Exp. Med., 141*: 322-334 (1975).

43. J. L. Kadish, and R. S. Basch, Hemopoietic thymocyte precursors. I. Assay and kinetics of the appearance of progeny, *J. Exp. Med., 143*: 1082-1093 (1976).
44. S. V. Hunt, and M. H. Fowler, A repopulation assay for B and T lymphocyte stem cells employing radiation chimeras, *Cell Tissue Kinetics, 14*: 445-464 (1981).
45. S. V. Hunt, The presence of Thy-1 on the surface of rat lymphoid stem cells and colony-forming units, *Eur. J. Immunol., 9*: 853-859 (1979).
46. Workshop discussion, Standardized nomenclature for the rat T-cell alloantigens; report to the committee. *Transplantation Proceedings, 15*: 1683-1685 (1983).
46a. D. Opstelten, G. J. Deenen, J. Rozing, and S. V. Hunt, B lymphocyte-associated antigens on terminal deoxynucleotidyl transferase-positive cells and Pre-B cells in bone marrow of the rat, *J. Immunol., 137*: 76-84 (1986).
46b. K. Crook, S. D. M. Highnam, and S. V. Hunt, Use of the leukocyte-common (RT7) alloantigen in monitoring enrichment of fetal liver lymphopoietic stem cells, *Transplantation Proceedings,* in press.
47. I. Goldschneider, D. Metcalf, F. Battye, and T. Mandel, Analysis of rat haemopoietic cells on the fluorescence-activated cell sorter. I. Isolation of pluripotent hemopoietic stem cells and granulocyte-macrophage progenitor cells, *J. Exp. Med., 152*: 419-437 (1980).
48. J. W. M. Visser, J. G. J. Bauman, A. H. Mulder, J. F. Eliason, and A. M. de Leeuw, Isolation of murine pluripotent hemopoietic stem cells, *J. Exp. Med., 59*: 1576-1590 (1984).
49. L. E. Botnick, E. C. Hannon, and S. Hellman, Nature of the hemopoietic stem cell compartment and its proliferative potential, *Blood Cells, 5*: 195-210 (1979).
50. J. E. Till, and E. A. McCulloch, Hemopoietic stem cell differentiation, *Biochemica et Biophysica Acta, 605*: 431-459 (1980).
51. A. J. Becker, E. A. McCulloch, L. Siminovitch, and J. E. Till, The effect of differing demands for blood cell production on DNA synthesis by hemopoietic colony forming cells of mice, *Blood, 26*: 296-301 (1965).
52. F. Vassort, M. Winterhofer, E. Frindel, and M. Tubiana, Kinetic parameters of bone marrow stem cells using *in vivo* suicide by tritiated thymidine and by hydroxyurea, *Blood, 41*: 489-496 (1973).
53. E. A. M. Ross, N. Anderson, and H. S. Micklem, Serial depletion and regeneration of the murine haemopoietic system, *J. Exp. Med., 155*: 432-444 (1982).
54. W. A. Jefferies, M. R. Brandon, A. F. Williams, and S. V. Hunt, Analysis of lymphopoietic stem cells with a monoclonal antibody to the rat transferrin receptor, *Immunology, 54*: 333-341 (1985).
55. J. Lesley, D. L. Domingo, R. Schulte, and I. S. Trowbridge, Effect of an anti-transferrin receptor-ricin A conjugate on bone marrow stem and progenitor cells treated *in vitro, Cell Research, 150*: 400-415 (1984).
56. C. Sieff, D. Bicknell, G. Caine, J. Robinson, G. Lam, and M. F. Greaves, Changes in cell surface antigen expression during hemopoietic differentiation, *Blood, 60*: 703-713 (1982).

57. B. A. Miller, G. Antognetti, and T. A. Springer, Identification of cell surface antigens present on murine hemopoietic stem cells, *J. Immunol., 134*: 3286-3290 (1985).
58. S. Kvaöly, R. Langholm, O. Kaalhus, T. Michaelson, S. Funderud, A. F. Abramson, and T. Godal, Transferrin receptor and B-lymphoblast antigen—their relationship to DNA synthesis, histology and survival in B-cell lymphomas, *Int. J. Cancer, 33*: 173-177 (1984).
59. I. S. Trowbridge, and D. L. Domingo, Prospects for the clinical use of cytotoxic monoclonal antibody conjugates in the treatment of cancer, *Cancer Surveys, 1*: 554-556 (1982).
60. D. W. Mason, P. E. Thorpe, and W. C. J. Ross, Elimination of leukaemia cells from rodent bone marrow *in vitro* with antibody-ricins conjugates; implications for autologous marrow transplantation in man, *Cancer Surveys, 1*: 389-415 (1982).
61. K. C. Gatter, G. Brown, I. S. Trowbridge, R. Woolston, and D. Y. Mason, Transferrin receptors in human tissues; their distribution and possible clinical relevance, *J. Clinic. Pathol., 36*: 539-545 (1983).
62. W. A. Jefferies, M. R. Brandon, S. V. Hunt, A. F. Williams, K. C. Gatter, and D. Y. Mason, Transferrin receptor on endothelium of brain capillaries, *Nature, 312*: 162-163 (1984).
63. S. Abramson, R. G. Miller, and R. A. Phillips, The identification in adult bone marrow of pluripotent and restricted stem cells of the myeloid and lymphoid systems, *J. Exp. Med., 145*: 1567-1569 (1977).
64. R. A. Phillips, in Differentiation of Normal and Neoplastic Hemopoietic Cells (B. Clarkson, P. A. Marks, and J. E. Till) *Cold Spring Harbor Conference on Cell Proliferation, 5*: 109-140 (1978).
65. J. E. Dick, M. C. Magli, D. Huszar, R. A. Phillips, and A. Bernstein, Introduction of a selectable gene into primitive stem cells capable of long-term reconstitution of the hemopoietic system of W/W^v mice, *Cell, 42*: 71-79 (1985).
66. A. Schnieke, K. Harbers, and R. Jaenisch, Embryonic lethal mutation in mice induced by retrovirus insertion into the $\alpha 1$ (I) collagen gene, *Nature, 304*: 315-310 (1983).
67. J. F. A. P. Miller, Effect of neonatal thymectomy on the immunological responsive of the mouse, *Proc. Roy. Soc. Lond. B., 156*: 415-430 (1962).
68. R. M. Zinkernagel, G. N. Callahan, A. Althage, S. Cooper, P. A. Klein, and J. Klein, On the thymus in the differentiation of "H-2 Self Recognition" by T cells: Evidence for Dual Recognition? *J. Exp. Med., 147*: 882-896 (1978).
69. A. Singer, and R. J. Hodes, Mechanisms of T cell-B cell interaction, *Ann. Rev. Immunol., 1*: 211-241 (1983).
70. R. Scollay, Intrathymic events in the differentiation of T lymphocytes: A continuing enigma, *Immunology Today, 4*: 282-286 (1983).
71. R. Scollay, and K. Shortman, Identification of early stages of T lymphocyte development in the thymus cortex and medulla, *J. Immunol., 134*: 3632-3642 (1985).

72. H. D. Royer, T. J. Campen, D. Ramarli, H. C. Chang, O. Acuto, and E. L. Reinherz, Molecular aspects of human T lymphocyte antigen recognition, *Transplantation, 39*: 571-582 (1985).
73. L. E. Samelson, T. Lindstem, B. J. Fowlkes, P. van den Elsen, C. Terhorst, M. M. Davis, R. N. Germain, and R. H. Schwartz, Expression of genes of the T-cell antigen receptor complex in precursors thymocytes, *Nature, 315*: 765-768 (1985).
74. D. J. Paterson, J. R. Green, W. A. Jefferies, M. P. Klavec, and A. F. Williams, The MRC OX44 antigen marks a functionally relevant subset among rat thymocytes, *J. Exp. Med., 165*: 1-13 (1987).
75. I. Goldschneider, K. L. Komschlies, and D. L. Greiner, Studies of thymocytopoiesis in rats and mice. 1. Kinetics of appearance of thymocytes using a direct intrathymic adoptive transfer assay for thymocyte precursors, *J. Exp. Med., 163*: 1-17 (1986).
76. J. L. Gowans, and E. J. Knight, The route of recirculation of lymphocytes in the rat, *Proc. R. Soc. Lond. B. Biol. Sci., 159*: 257-282 (1964).
77. P. B. Carter, and H. Bazin, in *The Laboratory Rat. Volume II, Research Applications* (H. J. Baker, J. R. Lindsey, and S. H. Weisbroth, eds.), Academic Press, New York, 1980.
78. J. M. Harlan, Leukocyte-endothelial interactions, *Blood, 65*: 513-525 (1985).
79. M. Gallatin, T. P. St. John, M. Siegelman, R. Reichert, E. C. Butcher, and I. L. Weissman, Lymphocyte homing receptors, *Cell, 44*: 673-680 (1986).
80. P. Nieuwenhius, and W. L. Ford, Comparative migration of B and T lymphocytes in the rat spleen and lymph nodes, *Cell Immunol., 23*: 254-267 (1976).
81. A. N. Barclay, The organization of B and T lymphocytes in lymph nodes, *Immunol. Today, 3*: 330 331 (1982).
82. J. C. Howard, The life span and recirculation of marrow-derived small lymphocytes from the rat thoracic duct, *J. Exp. Med., 135*: 185-199 (1972).
83. W. Van Ewijk, and P. Nieuwenhius, Compartments, domains and migration pathways of lymphoid cells in the splenic pulp, *Experientia, 41*: 199-208 (1985).
84. W. L. Ford, M. Sedgley, S. M. Sparshott, and M. E. Smith, The migration of lymphocytes across specialized vascular endothelium. II. The contrasting consequences of treating lymphocytes with trypsin or neuraminidase, *Cell Tissue Kinet., 9*: 351-361 (1976).
85. R. J. Hooghe, N. Schaaf-Lafontaine, E. L. Hooghe-Peters, F. Van der Plaetse, L. de Saint-Georges, P. Dorlings, and M. Janowski, Integrity of glycoprotein complex sugars is required for homing but not for several other membrane-mediated functions, *Cell Biochem. and Function, 2*: 102-105 (1984).
86. S. D. Rosen, M. S. Singer, and T. A. Yednock, Involvement of sialic acid on endothelial cells in organ-specific lymphocyte recirculation, *Science, 228*: 1005-1007 (1985).
87. D. D. True, M. S. Singer, L. M. Stoolman, and S. D. Rosen, Interactions of acidic glycolipids with a lymphocyte homing receptor, *J. Cell Biol., 101*: 234a (1985).
88. W. M. Gallatin, I. L. Weissman, and E. C. Butcher, A cell-surface molecule involved in organ-specific homing of lymphocytes, *Nature, 304*: 30-34 (1983).

89. T. A. Yednock, E. C. Butcher, L. M. Stoolman, and S. D. Rosen, Lymphocyte homing receptor: Relationship between the Mel-14 antigen and a cell surface lectin, *J. Cell Biol., 101*: 233a (1985).
90. M. Siegelman, M. W. Bond, W. M. Gallatin, T. St. John, H. T. Smith, V. A. Fried, and L. L. Weissman, Cell surface molecule associated with lymphocyte homing is a ubiquitinated branched-chain glycoprotein, *Science, 231*: 823-832 (1986).
91. T. St. John, W. M. Gallatin, M. Siegelman, H. T. Smith, V. A. Fried, and I. L. Weissman, Expression cloning of a lymphocyte homing receptor cDNA: Ubiquitin is the reactive species, *Science, 231*: 845-849 (1986).
92. R. A. Rasmussen, Y.-H. Chin, J. J. Woodruff, and T. G. Easton, Lymphocyte recognition of lymph node high endothelium. VII. Cell surface proteins involved in adhesion defined by monoclonal anti-$HEBF_{LN}$ (A.11) antibody, *J. Immunol., 135*: 19-24 (1985).
93. Y.-H. Chin, R. A. Rasmussen, J. J. Woodruff, and T. G. Easton, A monoclonal anti-$HEBF_{PP}$ antibody with specificity for lymphocyte surface molecules mediating adhesion to peyer's patch high endothelium of the rat, *J. Immunol., 136*: 2556-2561 (1986).
94. A. F. Williams, Molecules in the immunoglobulin superfamily, *Immunology Today, 5*: 219-221 (1984).
95. A. F. Williams, Immunoglobulin-related domains for cell surface recognition, *Nature, 314*: 579-580 (1985).
96. L. Hood, M. Kronenberg, and T. Hunkapillar, T cell antigen receptors and the immunoglobulin supergene family, *Cell, 40*: 225-229 (1985).
97. J. Novotny, S. Tonegawa, H. Saito, D. M. Kranz, and H. N. Eisen, Secondary, tertiary and quaternary structure of T-cell-specific immunoglobulin-like polypeptide chains, *Proc. Natl. Acad. Sci. USA, 83*: 742-746 (1986).
98. J. Klein, *Biology of the Mouse Histo-Compatibility-2 Complex*, Springer Verlag, New York, 1975.
99. R. M. Zinkernagel, and P. C. Doherty, H-2 compatibility requirement for T cell mediated lysis of target infected with lymphocytic choriomeningitis virus: Different cytotoxic T cell specificities are associated with structures coded in H-2K or H-2D, *J. Exp. Med., 141*: 1427-1436 (1975).
100. J.-C. Cerottini, H. D. Engers, H. R. MacDonald, and K. T. Brunner, Generation of cytotoxic T lymphocytes *in vitro, J. Exp. Med., 140*: 703-717 (1974).
101. H. R. MacDonald, H. D. Enger, J.-C. Cerrotini, and K. T. Brunner, Generation of cytotoxic T lymphocytes *in vitro, J. Exp. Med., 140*: 718-730 (1974).
102. J. C. Jensenius, and A. F. Williams, The T lymphocyte antigen receptor-paradigm lost, *Nature, 300*: 583 588 (1982).
103. M. M. Davis, Molecular genetics of the T cell-receptor beta chain, *Ann. Rev. Immunol., 3*: 537-560 (1985).
104. M. K. L. Collins, and M. J. Owen, The T cell antigen receptor, review article, *Biochem. J., 230*: 281-291 (1985).

105. J. P. Allison, B. W. McIntyre, and D. Bloch, Tumour-specific antigen of murine T-lymphoma defined with monoclonal antibody, *J. Immunol., 129*: 2293-2300 (1982).
106. J. White, K. M. Haskins, P. Marrack, and J. Kappler, Use of I region restricted, antigen-specific T cell hybridomas to produce idiotypically specific anti-receptor antibodies, *J. Immunol., 130*: 1033-1037 (1983).
107. S. C. Meuer, O. Acuto, R. E. Hussy, J. C. Hodgdon, K. A. Fitzgerald, S. F. Schlossman, and E. L. Reinherz, Clonotypic structure involved in antigen specific human T cell function: Relationship to the T3 molecular complex, *J. Exp. Med., 157*: 705-719 (1983).
108. K. Haskin, J. Kappler, and P. Marrack, The major histocompatibility complex-restricted antigen receptor on T cells, *Ann. Rev. Immunol., 2*: 51-66 (1984).
109. U. D. Staerz, H. G. Rammensee, J. D. Benedetto, and M. J. Bevan, Characterization of a murine monoclonal antibody specific for an allotypic determinant on T cell antigen receptor, *J. Immunol., 134*: 3994-4000 (1985).
110. M. Fabbi, O. Acuto, A. Bensussam, C. B. Poole, and E. L. Reinherz, Production and characterization of antibody probes directed at constant regions of the α and β subunit of the human T cell receptor, *Eur. J. Immunol., 15*: 821-827 (1985).
111. H. Spits, J. Borst, W. Tax, P. J. A. Capel, C. Terhorst, and J. E. deVries, Characteristics of a monoclonal antibody (WT-31) that recognizes a common epitope on the human T cell receptor for antigen, *J. Immunol., 135*: 1922-1928 (1985).
112. Y. Yanagi, Y. Yoshikai, K. Leggett, S. P. Clark, I. Alexsander, and T. W. Mak, A human T cell specific cDNA clone encodes a protein having extensive homology to immunoglobulin chains, *Nature, 308*: 145-149 (1984).
113. H. Saito, D. M. Krantz, Y. Takagaki, A. C. Hayday, H. N. Eisen, and S. Tonegawa, Complete primary structure of a heterodimeric T-cell receptor deduced from cDNA sequences, *Nature, 309*: 757-764 (1984).
114. Y.-H., Chien, D. M. Becker, Lindsten, M. Okamura, D. I. Cohen, and M. M. Davis, A third type of murine T-cell receptor gene, *Nature, 312*: 31-35 (1984).
115. H. Saito, D. M. Krantz, Y. Takagaki, A. C. Hayday, H. N. Eisen, and S. Tonegawa, A third rearranged and expressed gene in a clone of cytotoxic T lymphocytes, *Nature, 312*: 36-41 (1984).
116. M. Fabbi, O. Acuto, J. E. Smart, and E. L. Reinherz, Homology of T1α-subunit of a T-cell antigen-MHC receptor with immunoglobulin, *Nature, 312*: 269-271 (1984).
117. C. H. Hannum, J. W. Kappler, I. S. Trowbridge, P. Marrack, and J. H. Freed, Immunoglobulin-like nature of the α-chain of a human T-cell antigen/MHC receptor, *Nature, 312*: 65-67 (1984).
118. A. C. Hayday, H. Saito, S. D. Gillies, D. M. Kranz, G. Tanigawa, H. N. Eisen, and S. Tonegawa, Structure, organization and somatic rearrangement of T cell gamma genes, *Cell, 40*: 259-269 (1985).

119. T. Quertermous, C. Murre, D. Dialynas, A. D. Duby, J. L. Strominger, T. A. Waldman, and J. G. Seidman, Human T-cell γ chain genes: Organization, diversity, and rearrangement, *Science, 231*: 252-255 (1986).
120. R. F. Siliciano, A. D. Keegan, R. E. Dintzis, H. M. Dintzis, and H. S. Shin, The interaction of normal antigen with T cell antigen receptors. 1. Specific binding of multivalent nominal antigen to cytolytic T cell clones, *J. Immunol., 135*: 906-914 (1985).
121. M. Steinmetz, Structure, function and evolution of the major histocompatibility complex of the mouse, *TIBS, 9*: 224-226 (1984).
122. J. E. Coligan, T. J. Kindt, H. Uehara, J. Martinko, and S. G. Nathenson, Primary structure of a murine transplantation antigen, *Nature, 291*: 35-39 (1981).
123. J. McCluskey, R. N. Germain, and D. H. Margulies, Cell surface expression of an *in vitro* recombinant class II/class I major histocompatibility complex gene product, *Cell, 40*: 247-257 (1985).
124. J. Klein, The major histocompatibility complex of the mouse, *Science, 206*: 516-521 (1979).
125. B. Arnold, U. Horstmann, W. Kuon, H. G. Burgert, G. J. Hämmerling, and S. Kvist, Alloreactive cytolytic T-cell clones preferentially recognize conformational determinants on histocompatibility antigens: Analysis with genetically engineered hybrid antigens, *Proc. Natl. Acad. Sci. USA, 82*: 7030-7034 (1985).
126. W. Kastern, Characterisation of two class I major histocompatibility rat cDNA clones, one of which contains a premature termination codon, *Gene, 34*: 227-233 (1985).
127. C. DeLisi, and J. A. Berzofsky, T-cell antigenic sites tend to be amphipathic structures, *Proc. Natl. Acad. Sci. USA, 82*: 7048-7052 (1985).
128. A. R. M. Townsend, F. M. Gotch, and J. Davey, Cytotoxic T cells recognize fragments of the influenza nucleoprotein, *Cell, 42*: 457-467 (1985).
129. A. R. M. Townsend, J. Rothbard, F. M. Gotch, G. Bahadur, D. Wraith, and A. J. McMichael, The epitopes of influenza nucleoprotein recognized by cytotoxic T-lymphocytes can be defined with short peptides, *Cell, 44*: 959-968 (1986).
130. J. Klein, and V. Hauptfeld, Ia antigens: Their serology, molecular relationship and their role in allograft reactions, *Transplant Rev., 30*: 83-100 (1976).
131. B. Benacerraf, and H. O. McDevitt, Histocompatibility-linked immune response genes, *Science, 175*: 273-279 (1972).
132. B. P. Babbit, P. M. Allen, G. Matsueda, E. Haber, and E. R. Unanue, Binding of immunogenic peptides to Ia histocompatibility molecules, *Nature, 317*: 359-361 (1985).
133. J. D. Ashwell, and R. H. Schwartz, T-cell recognition of antigen and the Ia molecule as a ternary complex, *Nature, 320*: 176-179 (1986).
134. T. H. Watts, H. E. Gaub, and H. M. McConnell, T-cell-mediated association of peptide antigen and major histocompatibility complex protein detected by energy transfer in an evanescent wave-field, *Nature, 320*: 179-181 (1986).

135. D. W. Mason, and A. N. Barclay, Constitutive and inducible expression of Ia antigens, *Immunobiol., 168*: 167-171 (1984).
136. T. Fukumoto, W. R. McMaster, and A. F. Williams, Mouse monoclonal antibodies against rat major histocompatibility antigens. Two Ia antigens and the expression of Ia and class I antigens in rat thymus, *Eur. J. Immunol., 12*: 237-243 (1982).
137. W. R. MacMaster, A monoclonal antibody which detects a polymorphic Ia antigenic determinant reacts with the beta polypeptide chain, *Immunogenetics, 13*: 347-350 (1981).
138. J. Green, and R. Jotte, Interactions between T helper cells and dendritic cells during the rat mixed lymphocyte reaction, *J. Exp. Med., 162*: 1546-1560 (1985).
139. A. E. Wallis, and W. R. McMaster, Sequence of a cDNA coding for a rat class II A alpha chain: Extensive DNA and protein sequence identity to H-2 A alpha and HLA-DCI alpha chains, *Immunogenetics, 19*: 53-62 (1984).
140. S. J. Eccles, and W. R. McMaster, DNA sequence analysis of a rat RTI class II A beta gene, *Immunogenetics, 22*: 653-663 (1985).
141. K. A. Robertson, and W. R. McMaster, Complete structure of a rat RTI E beta chain: Extensive conservation of MHC class II beta chains, *J. Immunol., 135*: 4095-4099 (1985).
142. D. W. Mason, R. P. Arthur, M. J. Dallman, J. R. Green, G. P. Spickett, and M. L. Thomas, Functional T cell subsets defined by monoclonal antibodies, *Immunol. Rev., 74*: 57-82 (1983).
143. H. Cantor, and E. A. Boyse, Functional subclasses of T lymphocytes bearing different L antigens, *J. Exp. Med., 141*: 1376 1389 (1975).
144. P. H. sayre, and E. L. Reinherz, Structural invariance of T4 molecules from T cell clones of different antigen and major histocompatibility complex specificities, *Eur. J. Immunol., 15*: 291-295 (1985).
145. C. Terhorst, A. Van Agthoven, E. Reinherz, and S. Schlossman, Biochemical analysis of human T lymphocyte differentiation antigens T4 and T5, *Science, 209*: 520-521 (1980).
146. F. Phan-Dinh-Tuy, P. Niaudet, and J. F. Bach, Molecular identification of human T lymphocyte antigens defined by the OKT5 and OKT8 monoclonal antibodies, *Mol. Immunol., 19*: 1649-1654 (1982).
147. D. P. Dialynas, Z. S. Quan, K. A. Wall, A. Pierres, J. Quintans, M. R. Loken, M. Pierres, and F. W. Fitch, Characterization of the murine T cell surface molecule, designated L3T4, identified by monoclonal antibody GK1.5: Similarity of L3T4 to the human Leu3/T4 molecules, *J. Immunol., 131*: 2445-2451 (1983).
148. M. L. Thomas, and J. R. Green, Molecular nature of the W3/25 and MRC OX-8 marker antigens for rat T lymphocytes: Comparisons with mouse and human antigens, *Eur. J. Immunol., 13*: 855-858 (1983).
149. R. A. Karol, J. Eng, D. K. Dennison, E. Farris, and D. M. Marcus, Hereditary abnormalities of the OKT4 human lymphocyte epitope in two families, *J. Clin. Immunol., 4*: 71-78 (1984).

150. S. J. Clark, W. A. Jefferies, A. N. Barclay, J. Gagnon, and A. F. Williams, Peptide and nucleotide sequences of rat CD4 (W3/25) antigen: Evidence for derivation from a structure with four immunoglobulin-related domains, *Proc. Natl. Acad. Sci. USA, 84*: 1649-1653 (1987).

151. P. J. Maddon, D. R. Littman, M. Godfrey, D. E. Maddon, L. Chess, and R. Axe, The isolation and nucleotide sequence of a cDNA encoding the T cell surface protein T4: A new member of the immunoglobulin gene family, *Cell, 42*: 93-104 (1985).

151a. B. Tourvielle, S. D. Gorman, E. H. Field, T. Hunkapiller, and J. R. Parnes, Isolation and sequence of L3T4 complementary DNA clones: Expression in T cells and brain, *Science 234*: 610-614 (1986).

151b. B. J. Classon, J. Tsagaratos, I. F. C. McKenzie, and I. D. Walker, Partial primary structure of the T4 antigens of mouse and sheep: Assignment of intrachain disulphide bonds, *Proc. Natl. Acad. Sci. USA, 83*: 4499-4503 (1986).

152. A. N. Barclay, The localization of populations of lymphocytes defined by monoclonal antibodies in rat lymphoid tissues, *Immunology, 42*: 593-600 (1981).

153. B. Steininger, J. Klempnauer, and K. Wonigeit, Phenotype and histological distribution of interstitial dendritic cells in the rat pancreas, *Transplantation, 38*: 169-175 (1984).

154. G. S. Wood, N. L. Warner, and R. A. Warnke, Anti-Leu-3/T4 antibodies react with cells of monocyte/macrophage and Langerhans lineage, *J. Immunol., 131*: 212-216 (1983).

155. R. H. Moscicki, E. P. Amento, S. M. Krane, J. T. Kurnick, and R. B. Colvin, Modulation of surface antigens of a human monocyte cell line, U937, during incubation with T lymphocyte-conditioned medium: Detection of T4 antigen and its presence on normal blood monocytes, *J. Immunol., 131*: 743-748 (1983).

156. S. J. Stewart, J. Fujimoto, and R. Levy, Human T lymphocytes and monocytes bear the same Leu-3 (T4) antigen, *J. Immunol., 136*: 3773-3778 (1986).

156a. P. R. Crocker, W. A. Jefferies, S. J. Clark, L. P. Chung, and S. Gordon, Species heterogeneity in macrophage expression of the CD4 antigen, *J. Exp. Med.,* in press.

157. D. W. Mason, C. W. Pugh, and M. Webb, The rat mixed lymphocyte reaction: Roles of a dendritic cell in intestinal lymph and T-cell subsets defined by monoclonal antibodies, *Immunology, 44*: 75-87 (1981).

158. S. W. Brostoff, and D. W. Mason, Experimental allergic encephalomyelitis: Successful treatment *in vivo* with a monoclonal antibody that recognizes T helper cells, *J. Immunol., 133*: 1938-1942 (1984).

159. D. Wilde, P. Marrack, J. Kappler, D. P. Dialynas, and F. W. Fitch, Evidence implicating L3T4 in class II MHC antigen-specific proliferation, release of lymphokines, and binding by cloned murine helper T lymphocyte lines, *J. Immunol., 131*: 2178-2183 (1983).

160. T. H. Watts, A. A. Brian, J. W. Kappler, P. Marrack, and H. M. McConnell, Antigen presentation by supported planar membranes containing affinity-purified I-A^d, *Proc. Natl. Acad. Sci. USA, 81*: 7564-7568 (1984).

161. E. L. Reinherz, P. C. Kung, G. Goldstein, and S. F. Schlossman, Separation of functional subsets of human T cells by a monoclonal antibody, *Proc. Natl. Acad. Sci. USA, 76*: 4061-4065 (1979).
162. E. L. Reinherz, R. E. Hussey, and S. F. Schlossman, A monoclonal antibody blocking human T cell function, *Eur. J. Immunol., 10*: 758-762 (1980).
163. W. E. Biddison, P. E. Rao, M. A. Talle, G. Goldstein, and S. Shaw, Possible involvement of the OKT4 molecule in T cell recognition of class II HLA antigens, *J. Exp. Med., 156*: 1065-1076 (1982).
164. A. M. Krensky, C. Clayberger, C. S. Reiss, J. L. Strominger, and S. J. Burakoff, Specificity of OKT4$^+$ cytotoxic T lymphocyte clones, *J. Immunol., 129*: 2001-2003 (1982).
165. S. L. Swain, Significance of lyt phenotypes: Lyt2 antibodies block activities of T cells that recognize class I major histocompatibility complex antigens regardless of their function, *Proc. Natl. Acad. Sci. USA, 78*: 7101-7105 (1981).
166. E.G. Engleman, C.J. Benike, C. Matzler, P.A. Gatenby, and R.L. Evans, Blocking of human T lymphocyte functions by anti-Leu-2 and anti-Leu-3 antibodies: Differential inhibition of proliferation and suppression, *J. Immunol., 130*: 2623-2628 (1983).
166a. R. B. Acres, P. J. Conlon, D. Y. Mochizuki, and B. Gallis, Rapid phosphorylation and modulation of the T4 antigen on cloned helper T cells induced by phorbol myristate acetate or antigen, *J. Biol. Chem., 261*: 16210-16214 (1986).
167. H. Golding, J. McCluskey, Z. T. I. Munitz, R. N. Germain, D. H. Margulies, and A. Singer, T cell recognition of a chimaeric class II/class I MHC molecule and the role of L3T4, *Nature, 317*: 425-427 (1985).
168. B. Fleischer, H. Schrezenmeier, and H. Wagner, Function of the CD4 and CD8 molecules on human cytotoxic T lymphocytes: Regulation of T cell triggering, *J. Immunol., 136*: 1625-1628 (1986).
169. A. G. Dalgleish, P. C. L. Beverley, P. R. Clapham, D. H. Crawford, M. F. Greaves, and R. A. Weiss, The CD4 (T4) antigen is an essential component of the receptor for the AIDS retrovirus, *Nature, 312*: 763-766 (1984).
170. D. Klatzmann, E. Champagne, S. Chamaret, J. Gruest, D. Guetard, T. Heroend, J. C. Gluckman, and L. Montagnier, T lymphocyte T4 molecule behaves as the receptor for human retrovirus LAV, *Nature, 310*: 767-768 (1984).
171. J. S. McDougal, M. S. Kennedy, J. M. Sligh, S. P. Cort, A. Mawle, and J. K. A. Nicholson, Binding of HTLV-III/LAV to T4$^+$T cells by a complex of the 11OK viral protein and the T4 molecule, *Science, 231*: 382-385 (1986).
171a. P.J. Maddon, A.G. Dalgleish, J.S. McDougal, P.R. Clapham, R.A. Weiss, and R. Axel, The T4 gene encodes the AIDS virus receptor and is expressed in the immune system and the brain, *Cell, 47*: 333-348 (1986).
172. J. R. Green, Generation of cytotoxic T cells in the rat mixed lymphocyte reaction is blocked by monoclonal antibody MRC OX-8, *Immunology, 52*: 253-260 (1984).

173. J. S. Rosenberg, S. C. Gilman, and J. D. Feldman, Regulation of rat B cell responses by T cell subsets and interleukin-2, *J. Immunol., 129*: 996-1001 (1982).
174. S. C. Gilman, J. S. Rosenberg, and J. D. Feldman, Membrane phenotype of the rat cytotoxic T lymphocyte, *J. Immunol., 129*: 1012-1016 (1982).
175. H. R. MacDonald, A. L. Glasebrook, C. Bron, A. Kelso, and J. C. Cerottini, Clonal heterogeneity in the functional requirement for Lyt-2.3 molecules on cytotoxic T lymphocytes (CTL): Possible implications for the affinity of CTL antigens receptors, *Immunol. Rev., 68*: 89-115 (1982).
176. N. Hollander, E. Pillemer, and I. L. Weissman, Effects of Lyt antibodies on T cell functions: Augmentation by anti-Lyt-1 as opposed to inhibition by anti-Lyt-2, *Proc. Natl. Acad. Sci. USA, 78*: 1148-1151 (1981).
177. D. R. Littman, Y. Thomas, P. J. Maddon, L. Chess, and R. Axel, The isolation and sequence of the gene encoding T8: A molecule defining functional classes of T lymphocytes, *Cell, 40*: 237-246 (1985).
178. V. P. Sukhatni, K. C. Sizer, A. C. Vollmer, T. Hunkapiller, and J. R. Parnes, The T cell differentiation antigen Leu-2/T8 is homologous to immunoglobulin and T cell receptor variable regions, *Cell, 40*: 591-597 (1985).
179. H. Nakauchi, G. P. Nolan, C. Hsu, H. S. Huang, P. Kavathas, and L. A. Herzenberg, Molecular cloning of Lyt-2, a membrane glycoprotein marking a subset of mouse T lymphocytes: Molecular homology to its human counterpart, Leu-2/T8, and to immunoglobulin variable regions, *Proc. Natl. Acad. Sci. USA, 82*: 5126-5130 (1985).
180. R. Zamoyska, A. C. Vollmer, K. C. Sizer, C. W. Liaw, and J. R. Parnes, Two Lyt-2 polypeptides arise from a single gene by alternative splicing patterns of mRNA, *Cell, 43*: 153-163 (1985).
181. P. J. Johnson, J. Gagnon, A. N. Barclay, and A. G. Williams, Purification, chain separation, and sequence of the MRC OX-8 antigen, a marker of rat cytotoxic T lymphocytes, *The EMBO Journal, 4*: 2539-2545 (1985).
182. P. J. Johnson, and A. F. Williams, Striking similarities between antigen receptor J pieces and sequence in the second chain of the murine CD8 antigen, *Nature, 323*: 74-76 (1986).
183. A. N. Barclay, and H. A. Ward, Purification and chemical characterization of membrane glycoproteins from rat thymocyte and brain, recognized by monoclonal antibody MRC OX2, *Eur. J. Biochem., 129*: 447-458 (1982).
184. W. A. Jefferies, Lymphocyte surface glycoproteins, D.Phil. thesis, University of Oxford, Oxford, 1985.
185. G. McGaughan, M. J. Clark, and A. N. Barclay, Characterization of the human homolog of the rat MACOX-2 membrane glycoprotein, *Immunogenetics, 25*: 329-335 (1987).
186. A. E. Reif, and J. M. V. Allen, The AKR thymic antigen and its distribution in leukemias and nervous tissues, *J. Exp. Med., 120*: 413-433 (1964).
187. I. L. Goldschneider, K. Gordon, and R. J. Morris, Demonstration of Thy-1 antigen on pluripotent hemopoietic stem cells in rat, *J. Exp. Med., 148*: 1351-1366 (1978).
188. C. M. Booth, M. C. Brown, R. J. Keynes, and A. N. Barclay, Muscles of adult rats and mice re-express the Thy-1 glycoprotein on denervation, *Brain Research, 308*: 380-384 (1984).

189. F. E. Cohen, J. Novotny, M. J. E. Sternberg, D. G. Campbell, and A. F. Williams, Analysis of structural similarities between brain Thy-1 antigen and immunoglobulin domains, *Biochem. J., 195*: 31-40 (1981).
190. D. G. Campbell, J. Gagnon, K. B. M. Reid, and A. F. Williams, Rat brain Thy-1 glycoprotein, *Biochem. J., 195*: 15-30 (1981).
191. A. G. D. Tse, A. N. Barclay, A. Watts, and A. F. Williams, A glycophospholipid tail at the carboxyl terminus of the Thy-1 glycoprotein of neurons and thymocytes, *Science, 230*: 1003-1008 (1985).
192. M. G. Low, and P. W. Kincade, Phosphatidylinositol is the membrane-anchoring domain of the Thy-1 glycoprotein, *Nature, 318*: 62-64 (1985).
193. T. Seki, T. Moriuchi, H. C. Chang, R. Denome, and J. Silver, Structural organization of the rat Thy-1 gene, *Nature, 313*: 485-487 (1985).
194. J. D. Bangs, D. Herreld, J. L. Krakow, G. W. Hart, and P. T. Englund, Rapid processing of the carboxyl terminus of a trypanosome variant surface glycoprotein, *Proc. Natl. Acad. Sci. USA, 82*: 3207-3211 (1985).
195. R. Etgas, J. Bouvier, and C. Bordier, The major surface protein of Leishmania promastigotes is anchored in the membrane by a myristic acid-labeled phospholipid, *EMBO Journal, 5*: 597-601 (1986).
196. A. N. Barclay, M. Letarte-Muirhead, A. F. Williams, and R. Faulkes, Chemical characterization of the Thy-1 glycoproteins from the membranes of rat thymocytes and brain, *Nature, 263*: 563-567 (1976).
197. M. Letarte-Muirhead, A. N. Barclay, and A. F. Williams, Purification of the Thy-1 molecule, a major stem cell surface glycoprotein of rat thymocytes, *Biochem. J., 151*: 685-697 (1975).
198. H. R. MacDonald, C. Bron, M. Rousseaux, C. Horvath, and J. C. Cerottini, Production and characterization of monoclonal anti-Thy 1 antibodies that stimulate lymphokine production by cytolytic T cell clones, *Eur. J. Immunol., 15*: 495-501 (1985).
199. K. C. Gunter, A. Kroczek, E. M. Shevach, and R. N. Germain, Functional expression of the murine Thy 1.2 gene in transfected human T cells, *J. Ex. Med., 163*: 285-300 (1986).
200. J. R. L. Pink, Changes in T lymphocyte glycoprotein structures associated with differentiation, in *Contemporary Topics in Molecular Immunology 9, 89* (F. P. Inman and T. J. Kindt, eds.), Plenum Press, New York, 1984.
201. K. Olden, B. A. Bernard, M. J. Humphries, T. K. Yeo, K. T. Yeo, S. L. White, S. A. Newton, H. C. Bauer, and J. B. Parent, Function of glycoprotein glycans, *TIBS, 10*: 78-82 (1985).
202. I. S. Trowbridge, P. Ralph, and M. J. Bevan, Differences in the surface proteins of mouse B and T cells, *Proc. Natl. Acad. Sci. USA, 72*: 157-161 (1975).
203. J. W. Fabre, and A. Williams, Quantitative serological analysis of a rabbit anti-rat lymphocyte serum and preliminary biochemical characterization of the major antigen recognized, *Transplantation, 23*: 349-359 (1977).
204. M. P. Scheid, and D. Triglia, Further description of the Ly-5 system, *Immunogenetics, 9*: 423-433 (1979).

205. R. Standring, W. R. McMaster, C. A. Sunderland, and A. F. Williams, The predominant heavily glycosylated glycoproteins at the surface of rat lymphoid cells are differentiation antigens, *Eur. J. Immunol., 8*: 832-839 (1978).
206. G. R. Woollett, A. W. Barclay, P. Puklavec, and A. F. Williams, Molecular and antigenic heterogeneity of the rat leucocyte-common antigen from thymocytes and T and B lymphocytes, *Eur. J. Immunol., 15*: 168-173 (1985).
207. W. R. A. Brown, and A. F. Williams, Lymphocyte cell surface glycoproteins which bind to soybean and peanut lectins, *Immunology, 46*: 713-726 (1982).
208. R. A. Childs, R. Dalchau, P. Scudder, E. F. Hounsell, J. W. Fabre, and T. Feizi, Evidence for the occurrence of O-glycosydically linked oligosaccharides of poly-N-acetyllactosamine on the human leucocyte common antigen, *Biochem. Biophys. Res. Commun., 110*: 424-431 (1983).
209. J. S. Tung, M. C. Deere, and E. A. Boyse, Evidence that Ly-5 product of T and B cells differ in protein structure, *Immunogenetics, 19*: 149-154 (1984).
210. D. M. Lubaroff, An alloantigenic marker on rat thymus and thymus-derived cells, *Transplant. Proc., 5*: 115-118 (1973).
211. J. W. Fabre, and P. J. Morris, The definition of a lymphocyte-specific alloantigen system in the rat (Ly-1), *Tissue Antigens, 4*: 238-246 (1974).
212. P. B. Carter, and C. A. Sunderland, Biochemical identification of rat ART-1 and Ly-1 alloantigens, *Immunogenetics, 10*: 583-593 (1980).
213. M. B. Omary, I. S. Trowbridge, and M. P. Scheid, The T200 cell surface glycoprotein of the mouse: Polymorphism defined by the Ly-5 system of alloantigens, *J. Exp. Med., 151*: 1311-1316 (1980).
214. K. C. Gatter, Z. Abdulaziz, P. Beverley, J. R. F. Corvalen, C. Ford, E. B. Lane, M. Mota, J. R. G. Nash, K. Pulford, H. Stein, J. Taylor-Papdimitriou, C. Woodhouse, and D. Y. Mason, Use of monoclonal antibodies for the histopathological diagnosis of human malignancy, *J. Clin. Pathol., 35*: 1253-1267 (1982).
215. R. P. Arthur, and D. Mason, T cells that help B cell responses to soluble antigen are distinguishable from those producing interleukin-2 on mitogenic or allogenic stimulation, *J. Exp. Med., 163*: 774-786 (1986).
216. R. Dalchau, and J. W. Fabre, Studies on the distribution among T lymphocytes of the high molecular form of the leukocyte-common antigen, in *Human Leukocyte Markers Detected by Monoclonal Antibodies. Leukocyte Typing* (A. Bernard, J. Baumsell, J. Dausset, C. Milstein, and S. Schlossman, eds.), Springer-Verlag, Heidelberg, 1984.
217. R. Hyman, I. Trowbridge, V. Stallings, and J. Trotter, Revertant expressing a structural variant of T200 glycoprotein, *Immunogenetics, 15*: 413-420 (1982).
218. L. Y. W. Bourguignon, S. J. Suchard, M. L. Nagpal, and J. R. Glenney, A T-lymphoma transmembrane glycoprotein (gp 180) is linked to the cytoskeletal protein, Fodrin, *J. Cell Biology, 101*: 477-487 (1985).

219. M. L. Thomas, A. N. Barclay, J. Gagnon, and A. F. Williams, Evidence from cDNA clones that the rat leukocyte-common antigen (T200) spans the lipid bilayer and contains a cytoplasmic domain of 80,000 M_r, *Cell, 41*: 8393 (1985).
220. R. L. Sparrow, and I. F. C. McKenzie, A function for human T200 in natural killer cytolysis, *Transplantation, 36*: 166-171 (1983).
221. J. A. Harp, B. S. Davis, and S. T. Ewald, Inhibition of T cell responses to alloantigens and polyclonal mitogen by Ly-5 antisera, *J. Immunol., 133*: 10-15 (1984).
222. L. Lefrançois, and M. J. Bevan, Functional modification of cytotoxic T-lymphocyte T200 glycoprotein recognized by monoclonal antibodies, *Nature, 314*: 449-452 (1985).
223. H. Yakura, F. W. Shen, E. Bourcet, and E. A. Boyse, On the function of Ly-5 in the regulation of antigen-driven B cell differentiation. Comparison and contrast with Lyb-2, *J. Exp. Med., 157*: 1077-1088 (1983).
224. S. Nordling, L. C. Anderson, and P. Häyry, Thymus-dependent and thymus-independent lymphocyte separation: Relation to exposed sialic acid on cell surface, *Science, 178*: 1001-1002 (1972).
225. B. Axelson, S. Hammarstrom, E. S. Robertson, P. Aman, P. Perlmann, and H. Mellstedt, The large sialoglycoprotein of human lymphocytes. I. Distribution on T and B lineage cells as revealed by a monospecific chicken antibody, *Eur. J. Immunol., 15*: 417-426 (1985).
226. B. Axelson, S. Hammarstrom, J. Finne, and P. Perlmann, The large sialoglycoprotein of human lymphocytes. III. Biochemical features, *Eur. J. Immunol., 15*: 427-433 (1985).
227. E. Remold-O'Donnell, D. M. Kenney, R. Parkman, L. Cairns, B. Savage, and F. S. Rosen, Characterization of a human lymphocyte surface sialoglycoprotein that is defective in Wiskott-Aldrich syndrome, *J. Exp. Med., 159*: 1705-1723 (1984).
228. S. C. Meuer, R. E. Hussey, M. Fabbi, D. Fox, O. Acuto, K. A. Fitzgerald, J. C. Hodgdon, J. P. Protentis, S. F. schlossman, and E. L. Reinherz, An alternative pathway of T-cell activation: A functional role for the 50 kd T11 sheep erythrocyte receptor protein, *Cell, 36*: 897-906 (1984).
229. F. D. Howard, J. A. Ledbetter, J. Wong, C. P. Bieber, E. B. Stinson, and L. A. Herzenberg, A human T lymphocyte differentiation marker defined by monoclonal antibodies that block E-rosette formation, *J. Immunol., 126*: 2117-2121 (1981).
230. M. Kamoun, P. J. Martin, J. A. Hansen, M. A. Brown, A. W. Siadak, and R. C. Nowinski, Identification of a human T lymphocyte surface protein associated with the E rosette receptor, *J. Exp. Med., 153*: 207-212 (1981).
230a. M. L. Plunkett, and T. A. Springer, Purification and characterization of the lymphocyte function-associated-2 (LFA-2) molecule, *J. Immunol., 136*: 4181-4187 (1986).
231. J. A. Hansen, P. J. Martin, and R. C. Nowinski, Monoclonal antibodies identifying a novel T-cell antigen and Ia antigens of human lymphocytes, *Immunogenetics, 10*: 247-260 (1980).

232. D. A. Fox, R. E. Hussey, A. K. Fitzgerald, A. Bensussan, J. F. Daley, S. F. Schlossman, and E. L. Reinherz, Activation of human thymocytes via the 50 kd T11 sheep erythrocyte binding protein induces the expression of interleukin 2 receptor on both $T3^+$ and $T3^-$ populations, *J. Immunol., 134*: 330-335 (1985).
233. D. J. Paterson, W. A. Jefferies, J. R. Green, M. R. Brandon, P. Corthesy, M. Puklavec, and A. F. Williams, Antigens on activated rat T lymphocytes including a molecule of 50,000 M_r detected only on CD4 positive T blasts, submitted.
234. A. F. Williams, A. N. Barclay, S. J. Clark, D. J. Paterson, and A. C. Willis, Similarities in sequences and cellular expression between rat CD2 and CD4 antigens, *J. Exp. Med., 165*: 368-380 (1987).
234a. W. A. Sewell, M. H. Brown, J. Dunne, M. J. Owen, and M. J. Crumpton, Molecular cloning of the human T-lymphocyte surface CD2 (T11) antigen, *Proc. Natl. Acad. Sci. USA, 83*: 8718-8722 (1986).
235. M. B. Brenner, I. S. Trowbridge, and J. L. Strominger, Cross linking of human T cell receptors proteins: Association between the T cell idiotype subtype and the T3 glycoprotein heavy subunit, *Cell, 40*: 183-190 (1985).
236. P. Van den Elsen, B. A. Shepley, J. Borst, J. E. Coligan, A. F. Markham, S. Orkin, and C. Terhorst, Isolation of cDNA clones encoding the 20 K T3 glycoprotein of human T cell receptor complex, *Nature, 312*: 413-418 (1984).
236a. G. W. Krissansen, M. J. Owen, W. Verbi, and M. J. Crumpton, Primary structure of the T3 γ subunit of the T3/T cell antigen receptor complex deduced from cDNA sequences: Evolution of the T3 γ and δ subunits, *EMBO Journal, 5*:1799-1808 (1986).
237. W. J. M. Tax, H. W. Willems, P. P. M. Reekers, P. J. A. Chapel, and R. A. P. Koene, Polymorphism in mitogenic effect of IgG1 monoclonal antibodies against T3 antigen on human T cells, *Nature, 304*: 445-447 (1983).
238. S. C. Meuer, O. Acuto, T. Hercend, S. F. Schlossman, E. L. Reinherz, The human T cell receptor, *Ann. Rev. Immunol., 2*: 23-50 (1984).
239. K. O'Flynn, E. D. Zanders, J. R. Lamb, P. C. L. Beverley, D. L. Wallace, P. E. R. Tathan, W. J. M. Tax, and D. C. Lynch, Investigation of early T cell activation. Analysis of the effect of specific antigen, interleukin-2 and monoclonal antibodies on intracellular free calcium concentration, *Eur. J. Immunol., 15*: 7-11 (1985).
240. M. J. Dallman, M. L. Thomas, and J. R. Green, MRC OX19 monoclonal antibody that labels rat T lymphocytes and *in vitro* proliferative responses, *Eur. J. Immunol., 14*: 260-267 (1984).
241. Y. Ishii, A. Matsuura, H. Yuasa, H. Narita, T. Takami, and K. Kikuchi, Two distinct antigenic markers for rat thymus and T cells defined by monoclonal antibodies, *Immunology, 48*: 743-754 (1983).
242. J. Ledbetter, and L. A. Herzenberg, Xenogeneic monoclonal antibodies to mouse lymphoid differentiation antigens, *Immunol. Rev., 47*: 63-90 (1979).

243. J. A. Ledbetter, R. L. Evans, M. Lipinski, C. Cunningham-Rundles, R. A. Good, and L. A. Herzenberg, Evolutionary conservation of surface molecules that distinguish T lymphocyte helper-inducer and T cytotoxic-suppressor subpopulations in mouse and man, *J. Exp. Med., 153*: 310-323 (1981).
244. K. A. Smith, Interleukin 2, *Ann. Rev. Immunol., 2*: 319-333 (1984).
245. D. A. Cantrell, R. A. Robins, and R. W. Baldsin, Rat lymphocyte subsets: Cellular requirements for the generation of T cell growth factor, *Cell. Immunol., 70*: 367-375 (1982).
245a. N. H. Jones, M. L. Clabby, D. P. Dialynas, H.-J. S. Huang, L. A. Herzenberg, and J. L. Strominger, Isolation and complementary DNA clones encoding the human lymphocyte glycoprotein T1/Leu-1, *Nature, 323*: 346-349 (1986).
246. F. Snachez-Madrid, A. M. Krensky, C. F. Ware, E. Robbins, J. L. Strominger, S. J. Burakoff, and T. A. Springer, Three distinct antigens associated with human T-lymphocyte-mediated cytolysis: LFA-1, LFA-2, LFA-3, *Proc. Natl. Acad. Sci. USA, 79*: 7489-7493 (1982).
247. M. Pierres, C. Goridis, and P. Goldstein, Inhibition of murine T cell-mediated cytolysis and T cell proliferation by a rat monoclonal antibody immunoprecipitating two lymphoid cell surface polypeptides of 94,000 and 180,000 molecular weight, *Eur. J. Immunol., 12*: 60-69 (1982).
248. F. Sanchez-Madrid, J. Nagy, P. Robbins, and T. A. Springer, A human leukocyte differentiation antigen family with a distinct alpha subunits and a common beta subunit: The lymphocyte function-antigen (LFA-1), the C3 bicomplement receptor (OKm1/Mac-1) and the gp150, 95 molecule, *J. Exp. Med., 158*: 1785-1802 (1983).
249. T. A. Springer, D. B. Teplow, and W. J. Dreyer, Sequence homology of the LFA-1 and Mac-1 leukocyte adhesion glycoproteins and unexpected relation to leukocyte interferon, *Nature, 314*: 540-542 (1985).
250. D. I. Beller, T. A. springer, and R. D. Schreiber, Anti-Mac-1 selectively inhibits the mouse and human type 3 complement receptor, *J. Exp. Med., 156*: 1000-1009 (1980).
251. A. R. Robinson, T. M. White, and D. W. Mason, Macrophage heterogeneity in the rat as delineated by two monoclonal antibodies MRC OX41 and MRC OX42, the latter recognising complement receptor type 3, *Immunology, 57*: 239-247 (1986).
252. P. Goldstein, C. Goridis, A. M. Schmitt-Verhulst, B. Hayot, A. Pierres, A. van Agthoven, Y. Kaufmann, Z, Eshhar, and M. Pierres, Lymphoid cell surface interaction structures detected using cytolysis-inhibiting monoclonal antibodies, *Immunol. Rev., 68*: 5-56 (1982).
253. S. Pont, P. Naquet, S. Marchetto, A. Regnier-Vigouroux, D. Blanc, A. Pierres, and M. Pierres, Identification of 5 topographic domains of the mouse LFA-1 molecule: Subunit assignment and functional involvement in lymphoic cells interactions, *J. Immunol., 136*: 3750-3759 (1986).
254. F. Sanchez-Madrid, S. Simon, S. Thompson, and T. A. Springer, Mapping of antigenic and functional epitopes on the alpha and beta subunits of two related glycoproteins involved in cell interactions, LFA-1 and Mac1, *J. Exp. Med., 158*: 586-602 (1983).

255. C. F. Ware, F. Sanchez-Madrid, A. M. Krensky, S. J. Burakoff, J. L. Strominger, and T. A. Springer, Human lymphocyte function associated antigen-1 (LFA-1): Identification of multiple antigenic epitopes and their relationship to CTL-mediated cytotoxicity, *J. Immunol., 131*: 1182-1188 (1983).

256. A. M. Krensky, S. J. Mentzer, C. Clayberger, D. C. Anderson, F. C. Schmalstie, S. J. Burakoff, and T. A. Springer, Heritable lymphocyte function-associated antigen-1 deficiency: Abnormalities of cytotoxicity and proliferation associated with abnormal expression of LFA-1, *J. Immunol., 135*: 3102-3108 (1985).

257. H. Spits, W. Van Schooten, H. Keizer, G. Van Seventer, M. Van de Rijn, C. Terhorst, and J. E. De Vries, Alloantigen recognition is preceded by nonspecific adhesion of cytotoxic T cells and target cells, *Science, 232*: 403-405 (1986).

257a. H.-G. Thiele, F. Koch, A. Hamann, and R. Arndt, Biochemical characterization of the T-cell alloantigen RT-6.2, *Immunology, 59*: 195-201 (1986).

257b. F. Koch, H.-G. Thiele, and M. G. Low, Release of the rat T cell alloantigen RT-6.2 from cell membranes by phosphotidylinositol-specific phospholipase C, *J. Exp. Med., 164*: 1338-1343 (1986).

258. J. M. Williams, H. M. Shapiro, E. L. Milford, and T. B. Strom, Multiparameter flow cytometric analysis of lymphocyte subpopulation activation in lectin-stimulated cultures, *J. Immunol., 128*: 2676-2681 (1982).

259. D. F. Gerson, H. Kiefer, and W. Eufe, Intracellular pH of mitogen-stimulated lymphocytes, *Science, 216*: 1009-1010 (1982).

260. H. J. Wedner, and C. W. Parker, Lymphocyte activation, *Prog. Allergy, 20*: 195-300 (1976).

261. J. R. Apgar, and P. Cresswell, Expression of cell surface lectins on activated human lymphoid cells, *Eur. J. Immunol., 12*: 570-576 (1982).

262. T. Cotner, J. M. Williams, L. Christenson, H. M. Shapiro, T. B. Strom, and J. Strominger, Simultaneous flow cytometric analysis of human T cell activation antigen expression and DNA content, *J. Exp. Med., 157*: 461-472 (1983).

263. J. W. Lowenthal, P. Corthésy, C. Tougne, R. Less, H. R. McDonald, and M. Nabholz, High and low affinity IL2 receptors: Analysis by IL2 dissociation rate and reactivity with monoclonal anti-receptor antibody PC61, *J. Immun., 135*: 3988-3994 (1985).

264. J. H. Helderman, T. C. Reynolds, and T. B. Strom, The insulin receptor as a universal marker of activated lymphocytes, *Eur. J. Immunol., 8*: 589-595 (1978).

265. J. W. Larrick, and P. J. Cresswell, Modulation of cell surface iron transferrin receptors by cellular density and state of activation, *Supramol. Struct., 11*: 579-586 (1979).

266. R. L. Evans, H. Lazaurus, A. C. Penta, and S. F. Schlossman, Two functionally distinct subpopulations of human T cells that collaborate in the generation of cytotoxic cells responsible for cell mediated lympholysis, *J. Immunol., 120*: 1423-1428 (1978).

267. H. Osawa, and T. Diamantstein, The characteristics of a monoclonal antibody that binds specifically to rat T lymphoblasts and inhibits IL2 receptor function, *J. Immunol., 130*: 51-55 (1983).
268. R. Ceredig, J. W. Lowenthal, M. Nabholz, and H. R. MacDonald, Expression of interleukin-2 receptors as a differentiation marker on intrathymic stem cells, *Nature, 314*: 98-100 (1985).
269. M. E. Hamler, J. G. Jacobsen, M. B. Brenner, D. Mann, and J. L. Strominger, VLA-1: A T cell surface antigen which defines a novel late stage of human T cell activation, *Eur. J. Immunol., 15*: 502-508 (1985).
270. M. Sarmiento, M. R. Loken, I. S. Trowbridge, R. L. Coffman, and F. W. Fitch, High molecular weight lymphocyte surface proteins are structurally related and are expressed on different cell populations at different times during lymphocyte maturation and differentiation, *J. Immunol., 128*: 1676-1684 (1982).
271. H. Osawa, and T. Diamentstein, Partial characterization of the putative rat interleukin-2 receptor, *Eur. J. Immunol., 14*: 374-376 (1984).
272. W. J. Leonard, J. M. Depper, T. Uchiyama, K. A. Smith, T. A. Waldman, and W. C. Green, A monoclonal antibody that appears to recognize the receptor for human T-cell growth factor; partial characterization of the receptor, *Nature, 300*: 267-269 (1982).
273. G. Oretga, R. Robb, E. Shevach, and T. Malek, The murine IL-2 receptor. I. Monoclonal antibodies that define distinct functional epitopes on activated T cells and react with activated B cells, *J. Immunol., 133*: 1970-1975 (1984).
274. W. J. Leonard, J. M. Depper, G. R. Crabtree, S. Rudikoff, J. Pumphrey, R. J. Robb, M. Krönke, P. B. Svetlik, N. J. Peffer, T. A. Waldman, and W. C. Green, Molecular cloning and expression of cDNAs for the human interleukin-2 receptor, *Nature, 311*: 626-631 (1984).
275. T. Nikaido, A. Shimizu, N. Ishida, H. Sabe, K. Teshigawara, M. Maeda, T. Uchiyama, J. Yodoi, and T. Honjo, Molecular cloning of cDNA encoding human interleukin-2 receptor, *Nature, 311*: 631-635 (1984).
276. J. Miller, T. R. Malek, W. J. Leonard, W. C. Green, E. M. Shevach, and R. N. Germain, Nucleotide sequence and expression of a mouse interleukin-2 receptor cDNA, *J. Immunol., 134*: 4212-4217 (1985).
277. I. S. Trowbridge, and M. B. Omary, Human cell surface glycoprotein related to cell proliferation is the receptor for transferrin, *Proc. Natl. Acad. Sci. USA, 78*: 3039-3043 (1981).
278. R. Sutherland, D. Delia, C. Schneider, R. Newman, J. Kemshead, and M. Greaves, Ubiquitous, cell surface glycoprotein on tumor cells is proliferation-associated receptor for transferrin, *Proc. Natl. Acad. Sci. USA, 78*: 4515-4519 (1981).
279. I. S. Trowbridge, and F. Lopez, Monoclonal antibody to transferrin receptor blocks transferrin binding and inhibits human tumor cell growth *in vitro, Proc. Natl. Acad. Sci. USA, 79*: 1175-1179 (1982).
280. C. Schneider, R. Sutherland, R. Newman, and M. Greaves, Structural features of the cell surface receptor for transferrin that is recognized by the monoclonal antibody OKT9, *J. Biol. Chem., 257*: 8516-8522 (1982).

281. I. S. Trowbridge, J. Lesley, and R. Schulte, Murine cell surface transferrin receptor: Studies with an anti-receptor monoclonal antibody, *J. Cell Phy., 112*: 403-410 (1982).
282. M. B. Omary, and I. S. Trowbridge, Biosynthesis of the human transferrin receptor in cultured cells, *J. Biol. Chem., 256*: 12888-92 (1981).
283. R. Newman, C. Schneider, R. Sutherland, L. Vodinelich, and M. Greaves, The transferrin receptor, *TIBS, 7*: 397-400 (1982).
284. C. Schneider, M. J. Owen, D. Banville, and J. G. Williams, Primary structure of human transferrin receptor deduced from the mRNA sequence, *Nature, 311*: 675-678 (1984).
285. P. A. Stearne, G. A. Pietersz, and J. W. Goding, cDNA cloning of the murine transferrin receptor: Sequence of trans-membrane and adjacent regions, *Journal of Immunology, 134*: 3474-3479 (1985).
286. J. R. Green, personal communication.
286a. J. Bevan, and P. M. Chisholm, Co-expression of CD4 and CD8 molecules and *de nova* expression of MHC Class II antigens on activated rat T cells, *Immunology, 59*: 621-625 (1986).
287. J. R. Nepom, B. Benacerraf, and R. N. Germain, Acquisition of syngeneic I-A determinants by T cells proliferating in response to poly (Glu^{60} Ala^{30} $Tyr^{10})^1$, *J. Immunol., 127*: 888-892 (1981).
288. D. J. Charron, E. G. Engleman, C. J. Benike, and H. O. McDevitt, Ia antigens on alloreactive T cells in man detected by monoclonal antibodies. Evidence for synthesis of HLA-D/DR molecules of the responder type, *J. Exp. Med., 152*: 127-136 (1980).
289. A. Ben-Nun, W. Strauss, S. A. Leeman, L. E. Cohn, C. Murre, A. Duby, J. G. Seidman, and L. H. Glimcher, An Ia-positive mouse T-cell clone is functional in presenting antigen to other T cells, *Immunogenetics, 22*: 123-130 (1985).
290. J. R. Lamb, and M. Feldman, Essential requirement for major histocompatibility complex recognition in T cell tolerance induction, *Nature, 308*: 72-74 (1984).
291. J. Fujimoto, S. J. Stewart, and R. Levy, Immunochemical analysis of the released Leu-2 (T8) molecule, *J. Exp. Med., 160*: 116-124 (1984).
292. M. L. Blue, J. F. Daley, H. Levine, and S. F. Schlossman, Coexpression of T4 and T8 on peripheral blood T cells demonstrated by two-color fluorescence flow cytometry, *J. Immunol., 134*: 2281-2286 (1985).
293. G. P. Spickett, and D. W. Mason, Demonstration of the stability of the membrane phenotype of T helper cells after priming and boosting with a hapten-carrier conjugate, *Eur. J. Immunol., 13*: 785-788 (1983).
294. U. Godden, J. Herbert, R. D. Stewart, and B. Roser, A novel cell type carrying both T_h and $T_{c/s}$ markers in the blood of cyclosporine-treated, allografted rats, *Transplantation, 39*: 624-628 (1985).
294a. B. Richardson, L. Kahn, E. J. Lovett, and J. Hudson, Effect of an inhibitor of DNA methylation on T cells, *J. Immunol., 137*: 35-39 (1986).
295. M. C. Mingari, G. Melioli, A. Moretta, G. Pontaleo, and L. Moretta, Surface markers of cloned human T cells with helper or suppressor activity

on pokeweed mitogen-driven B cell differentiation, *Eur. J. Immunol., 12*: 900-903 (1982).
296. J. G. Izant, and H. Weintraub, Inhibition of thymidine kinase gene expression by anti-sense RNA: A molecular approach to genetic analysis, *Cell, 36*: 1007-1015 (1984).
297. C. A. Sunderland, W. R. McMaster, and A. F. Williams, Purification with monoclonal antibody of a predominant leukocyte-common antigen and glycoprotein from rat thymocytes, *Eur. J. Immunol., 9*: 155-159 (1979).
298. D. W. Mason, and A. F. Williams, The kinetics of antibody binding to membrane antigens in solution and at the cell surface, *Biochem. J., 187*: 1-20 (1980).
299. R. J. Brideau, P. B. Carter, W. R. McMaster, D. W. Mason, and A. F. Williams, Two subsets of rat T lymphocytes defined with monoclonal antibodies, *Eur. J. Immunol., 10*: 609-615 (1980).
300. M. J. S. Dyer, D.Phil. thesis, University of Oxford, Oxford, 1980.
301. L.-M. Hsiung, A. N. Barclay, M. R. Brandon, E. Sim, and R. R. Porter, Purification of human C3b inactivator by monoclonal antibody affinity chromatography, *Biochem. J., 203*: 293-298 (1982).
302. A. P. Robinson, T. M. White, and D. W. Mason, MRC OX43: A monoclonal antibody which reacts with all vascular endothelium in the rat except that of brain capillaries, *Immunology, 57*: 231-237 (1986).
303. J. Arvieux, W. A. Jefferies, D. Paterson, A. F. Williams, and J. R. Green, Monoclonal antibodies against a new rat leukocyte antigen block antigen-induced T cell responses via an effect on macrophages, *Immunology, 58*: 337-342 (1986).
304. A. P. Robinson, M. Puklavec, and D. W. Mason, MRC OX52: A new rat T-cell antigen, *Immunology, 57*: 527-531 (1986).
305. C. J. Barnstable, W. F. Bodmer, G. Brown, G. Galfre, C. Milstein, A. F. Williams, and A. Ziegler, Production of monoclonal antibodies to group A erythrocyte, HLA and other human cell surface antigens—new tools for genetic analysis, *Cell, 14*: 9-20 (1978).
306. A. Matsuura, Y. Ishii, H. Iwaki, and K. Kikuchi, A novel cell-surface antigen expressed on most leukocytes and a minor cortisone-resistant population of thymocytes in rat: Characterisation by monoclonal antibodies, *Microbiol. Immunol., 29*: 873-881 (1985).
307. C. D. Dijkstra, E. A. Dopp, P. Joling, and G. Kraal, The heterogeneity of mononuclear phagocytes in lymphoid organs: Distinct macrophage subpopulations in the rat recognised by monoclonal antibodies ED1, ED2, and ED3, *Immunology, 54*: 589-599 (1985).
308. T. Uede, H. Kohda, H. Yuasa, H. Osawa, T. Diamantstein, J. Yodoi, Y. Ishii, and K. Kikuchi, 5C6-F4, a novel 100,000-dalton rat lymphocyte activation antigen defined by monoclonal antibody, *J. Immunol., 136*: 3968-3976 (1986).
309. B. F. Haynes, M. E. Hemler, D. L. Mann, E. M. Eisenbarth, G. S. Shelhamler, J. Mostowski, H. S. Thomas, J. L. Strominger, and A. S. Fauci, Characterisation of a monoclonal antibody (4F2) which binds to human monocytes

and to a subset of activated lymphocytes, *J. Immunol., 126*: 1409-1414 (1981).

310. M. Michalak, E. J. Quackenbush, and M. Letarte, Inhibition of Na^+/Ca^{+2} exchanger activity in cardiac and skeletal muscle sarcoleminal vescicles by monoclonal antibody 42D7, *J. Biol. Chem., 261*: 92-95 (1986).
311. H. Kratzin, C.-Y. Yang, H. Gotze, E. Pauly, S. Kolbel, G. Egert, F. P. Thinnes, P. Wernet, P. Altevogt, and N. Hilschmann, Primärstruktur menschlicher histokompatibilitätsantigene der Klasse II. *Hoppe-Seyler's Z. Physiol. Chem., 362*: 1665-1669 (1981).
312. H. T. Orr, J. A. Lopez de Castro, D. Lancet, and J. L. Strominger, Complete amino acid sequence of a papain-solubilized human histocompatibility antigen, HLA-B7.2. Sequence determination and search for homologies, *Biochemistry, 18*: 5711-5720 (1979).
313. A. Ullrich, J. R. Bell, E. Y. Chen, R. Herrera, L. M. Petruzzelli, T. J. Dull, A. Gray, L. Coussens, Y.-C. Liao, M. Tsubokawa, A. Mason, P. H. Seeburg, C. Grunfeld, O. M. Rosen, and J. Ramachandran, Human insulin receptor and its relationship to the tyrosine kinase family of oncogenes, *Nature, 313*: 756-761 (1985).
314. J. R. Parnes, B. Velan, A. Felsenfeld, L. Ramanthan, U. Ferrini, E. Appella, and J. G. Seidman, Mouse β2-microglobulin cDNA clones corresponding to rare mRNAs, *Proc. Natl. Acad. Sci. USA, 78*: 2253-2257 (1981).
315. S. Kvist, F. Bregegere, L. Rask, B. Cami, H. Garoff, H. Daniel, K. Wiman, D. Larhammar, J. P. Abastado, G. Gachelin, P. A. Peterson, B. Dobberstein, and P. Kourilsky, cDNA clone coding for part of a mouse H-2d major histocompatibility antigen, *Proc. Natl. Acad. Sci. USA, 78*: 2772-2776 (1981).
316. K. Wiman, D. Larhammar, L. Claesson, K. Gustaffson, L. Schenning, P. Bill, J. Bohme, M. Denaro, B. Dobberstein, U. Hammerling, S. Kvist, B. Serveius, J. Sundelin, P. Peterson, and L. Lask, Isolation and identification of a cDNA clone corresponding to an HLA-DR antigen chain, *Proc. Natl. Acad. Sci. USA, 79*: 1703-1707 (1982).
317. S. V. Hunt, unpublished observations.
318. S. D. M. Highnam, Rat haemopoietic stem cells, D.Phil. thesis, University of Oxford, Oxford, 1983.
319. I. Goldschneider, L. K. Gordon, and R. J. Morris, Demonstration of Thy-1 antigen on pluripotent stem cells in the rat, *J. Exp. Med., 148*: 1351-1366 (1978).
320. K. E. Mostov, M. Freidlander, and G. Blobel, The receptor for transepithelial transport of IgA and IgM contains multiple immunoglobulin-like domains, *Nature, 308*: 37-43 (1984).
321. J. J. Hemperly, B. A. Murray, G. M. Edelman, B. A. Cunningham, Sequence of a cDNA clone encoding the polysialic acid-rich and cytoplasmic domains of the neural cell adhesion molecule N-CAM, *Proc. Natl. Acad. Sci. USA, 83*: 3037-3041 (1986).
322. C. Lai, M. A. Brow, G. Sutcliffe, and R. Milner, in preparation.

7
Differentiation Antigens on Lymphoid Cells of the Guinea Pig

REINHARD BURGER and HUBERT SCHAEFER
Institute for Immunology, University of Heidelberg, Heidelberg, Federal Republic of Germany

I. INTRODUCTION

The guinea pig is a classical animal species used in immunological research. It has a number of advantages compared to other species. Several immune phenomena were initially described in the guinea pig. For instance, the first Ir gene was discovered in this species and major contributions to the analysis of Ir-gene/Ia-antigen function were made subsequently (for review see Refs. 1,2). The guinea pig possesses a marked reactivity for delayed type hypersensitivity, such as contact dermatitis and other cell-mediated immune reactions. In vitro assay systems for these reactions are well established. In addition, it provides a useful model for a number of autoimmune diseases, such as experimental allergic encephalomyelitis, thyroiditis, or autoimmune orchitis. Finally, humoral immune mechanisms underlying allergic reactions, anaphylaxis, and other complement-dependent phenomena can be analyzed in great detail in this animal species.

Studies of cell-mediated immune reactions have been greatly facilitated by the availability of specific cell-surface antigens which mark various cell populations in the murine and human immune systems. Such cell-surface markers have provided an important tool for elucidating the organization of the immune system. They also permitted the identification of functionally distinct subpopulations of lymphocytes, analyses of their effector function, of their interaction and regulatory mechanisms. In the murine system the presence of alloantigenic determinants on surface proteins permitted the production of alloantisera. They were directed to individual membrane components and allowed the identification and characterization of cell-specifically expressed, polymorphic "differentiation antigens." The consequent application of the hybridoma technique in the last several years has allowed major progress in this field. Numerous reports revealed by the use of monoclonal antibodies (mAb) that a few of the membrane proteins detected by mAb are not only useful markers but also functional molecules directly or indirectly involved in cellular interaction or activation processes (3-5).

In contrast to the substantial amount of literature on markers of human and murine lymphoid cells, there are only a few reports on differentiation antigens of the guinea pig. A detailed characterization was achieved only with a few of these proteins. In most cases their analogy to human or murine differentiation antigens has not been established.

There are several obvious reasons for the paucity of reports on guinea pig lymphoid differentiation antigens: a) Only a few immunologically characterized inbred guinea pigs strains are available (6). b) The extended gestation period (60-70 days) in this species and the small litter size are handicaps for establishing inbred or congenic lines, which limits the chance for production of defined alloantisera. In fact, up to now, no guinea pig alloantiserum detecting a differentiation antigen on lymphoid cells has been obtained by cross-immunization with cells of allogeneic strains. c) The bigger body size of the guinea pig results in higher costs for keeping the animals. d) To our knowledge, there are no established guinea pig T-cell leukemia lines that have been immunologically well-characterized. In humans T-cell leukemia cell lines have been used effectively as immunogens to develop mAb against various differentiation antigens. e) A number of in vitro assay systems for T-cell functions have been successfully developed in the guinea pig, but several principal assays, such as those for cytotoxic T cells and for suppressor T cells, are not yet available. Recently, guinea pig T-cell clones were described and used for functional assays (7-9). However, the establishment of functionally stable T-cell clones, and their propagation in long-term cultures have met with difficulties.

In this chapter we attempt to summarize what is currently known about cell-surface markers of guinea pig lymphoid cells, with emphasis on markers defined by monoclonal antibodies. Markers defined by conventional antisera or by other techniques will also be discussed.

II. DIFFERENTIATION ANTIGENS OF T LYMPHOCYTES

A. Conventional Markers

1. Rabbit Red Blood Cell Receptors

Guinea pig T lymphocytes have the capacity for spontaneous rosette formation with untreated rabbit erythrocytes (10-12). Rosette formation is useful for quantitation of T lymphocytes in heterogenous cell populations. It has been reported that natural antibodies to guinea pig T cells might be involved in the rosetting phenomenon in guinea pigs since antisera to rabbit Ig allotypes can block the rosetting (11). Such natural antibodies might physiologically be present in rabbit sera and subsequently be absorbed to the erythrocyte surface. However, there are no other reports confirming this assumption. It is not known whether the guinea pig T-cell surface protein involved in the rosetting is homologous to the human T11 protein which mediates rosette formation with sheep red blood cells. The T11 protein recently aroused considerable interest when its involvement in T-cell triggering via the so-called alternative pathway of T-cell activation was discovered (13).

2. Heteroantisera to T-Cell Membrane Components

Several attempts have been made to raise conventional antisera to guinea pig T cells in rabbits (14,15). After extensive absorption procedures with a B-cell leukemia line L2C, these antisera reacted with T cells and still had the capacity to block rosette formation with rabbit erythrocytes, confirming the T-cell specific expression of the E-rosette receptor protein. T-cell transfer experiments were performed after treatment with anti-T-cell antiserum and complement. T cell subpopulations capable of transferring delayed type hypersensitivity reactions (contact sensitivity, reactivity to DNP-derivatives, PPD reactivity) into untreated recipient animals differed in their sensitivity to the antiserum treatment. Similar to these in vivo studies, treatment with anti-T-cell serum and complement varied in its effect on in vitro T-cell functions, depending on the antigens used (reactive DNP sensitizers, DNP-PPD) and on the parameter studied (lymphokine production, blast transformation) (14,16).

Guinea Pig Thy1 Antigen. The murine Thy1 antigen is expressed predominantly on thymocytes, T cells, and brain. The corresponding guinea pig homologue is not yet clearly identified (see also below). Rabbit antisera to guinea pig brain do react with T cells after absorption with L2C B-cell leukemia (14). However, it remains to be demonstrated whether the molecule detected is the genuine guinea pig Thy1.

Guinea Pig Lyt-1 Antigen. Rabbit antisera to in vitro antigen-primed T cells had mitogenic activity on T cells primed to the corresponding antigen but not on T cells derived from animals with a different MHC haplotype or T cells with a different antigen specificity (17). Two molecular species were identified by these antisera (MW 70,000 and MW 98,000). The smaller protein resembles antigenically immunoglobulin and a contribution to T-cell recognition processes has been discussed. Subsequent detailed analysis of the smaller protein revealed that it might represent the guinea pig homologue of the murine Lyt-1 or the human Leu-1 antigen (18). The single-chain protein (its MW now determined 75,000; p 75) exhibited charge heterogeneity which was not affected by neuraminidase treatment, and it was synthesized by thymocytes, spleen cells, and lymph node cells. Activated T cells and also L2C leukemia cells synthesized the antigen, whereas normal B cells or macrophages did not. Thus, the biochemical characteristics and the cellular distribution (Lyt-1 is also expressed on some B-cell lymphomas) support the hypothesis that the guinea pig Lyt-1 homologue is recognized by these antisera.

Unfortunately, no monoclonal antibody to this protein has been obtained so far (with the possible exception of mAb 8BEG described below). Several monoclonal antibodies to mouse Lyt-1 protein failed to react with the guinea pig protein.

Guinea Pig TL and Qa-2 Antigens. The thymus-leukemia (TL) alloantigen and the Qa-2 alloantigen of mice are organ-specific differentiation antigens. The genes for these proteins are located in the mouse to the right of the H-2 complex (MHC). The TL antigen is expressed on thymocytes of certain strains of mice and on leukemia cell lines. The Qa-2 is present on thymocytes and lymphocytes in the peripheral lymphoid organs. Like the conventional MHC class I products, both proteins consist of a heavy chain (MW 44,000) associated with a smaller β2-microglobulin (β2M; MW 11,800). Antisera to the β2M and to the presumptive TL end Qa-2 antigens in guinea pigs were prepared (20) and sequential immunoprecipitation experiments have been performed. These experiments permitted the identification of the guinea pig homologues of the mouse TL and Qa-2 proteins. (21). In contrast to the mouse no evidence was within three inbred guinea pig strains (strain 2, strain 13, and strain DHCBA) obtained for polymorphism of the guinea pig TL antigen (22). Monoclonal antibodies to the guinea pig TL- or Qa-2 antigens are not available so far.

3. Fc-IgG and Fc-IgM Receptors

In the prehybridoma era the presence or absence of receptors for the Fc-portion of IgG or IgM was used for classifying T-cell subsets. Similar to human T cells, two subpopulations of guinea pig T lymphocytes, Tμ and Tγ, were identified and they differed in their tissue distribution (12). However, no association with functionally distinct T-cell subpopulations was achieved. However, with the availability of monoclonal antibodies the analytical approach employing the Fc-receptors is obviously no longer justified.

4. Alkaline Phosphatase

In a number of studies endogenous alkaline phosphatase activity detected in lymphocytes was shown to be a useful marker to distinguish various maturations steps of guinea pig T lymphocytes (24-28). The activity detected in cortical thymocytes whereas only little or no alkaline phosphatase activity is found in medullary thymocytes or peripheral T cells. A monoclonal antibody to this enzyme which could replace the enzyme histocytochemistry is not available so far.

B. T-Cell Antigens Defined by Monoclonal Antibodies

The advantages of monoclonal antibodies for the detection and analysis of differentiation antigens have been frequently discussed (29,30). Monoclonal antibodies represent the reagent of choice to define new cell-surface antigens and provide a tool for functional analysis. A number of T-cell specific surface molecules of guinea pig lymphocytes have been identified by the use of monoclonal antibodies. These newly identified cell-surface components are useful markers and are of value for serological assays and for immunohistological studies. However, only a few of them have been associated with functionally defined T-cell subpopulations. These markers are discussed separately.

In order to generate monoclonal antibodies, the following methods were used in most studies. Mice were immunized with normal or activated T cells and the hybridomas obtained after fusion were screened for T-cell specific reactivity by means of indirect binding assays. Antibody binding was determined using either single cell suspensions in combination with enzyme- or ^{125}I-labeled detection reagents or, alternatively, by immunohistological methods using tissue sections. T-cell specificity was determined in several studies by using the B-cell leukemia line L2C as a non-T-cell control. However, it turned out that this strategy was not strict and selective enough. Several T-cell specific antibodies selected by this strategy turned out to react also with normal, nonmalignant B cells or other lymphoid cells. Therefore, the L2C leukemia cells obviously do not express a normal set of B-cell or leukocyte differentiation antigens. It should also be mentioned that the L2C leukemia is derived from the inbred guinea pig strain 2. Therefore, antibodies to alloantigenic determinants of Ia antigens that are absent in strain 2 do not react with L2C cells in this screening system and appear erroneously to be T-cell specific. In fact, such antibodies were identified in several studies (31-33). Double staining with an anti-B-cell reagent should be performed to exclude such errors in an initial stage of antibody screening. FACS analysis is obviously a method to be used preferentially. Immunohistochemical techniques provide additional information about tissue distribution of antigens defined by mAb (31).

1. T-Cell Markers with Unknown Functions

Antibodies defining pan-T-cell markers and antibodies reactive with T-cell subpopulations were described by several laboratories.

mAb 8B E6. This antibody was obtained by immunization with purified T cells (32). It reacts with 80% of lymph node cells, 45% of spleen cells, and 10% of thymocytes, but fails to react with bone marrow cells or granulocytes. Normal surface Ig positive B cells do not bear this antigen as shown by double staining. The antigen is weakly expressed on the EN-L2C B cell leukemia, but surprisingly not on an Ia-negative variant of this cell line, BZ-L2C. It reacts primarily with medullary thymocytes (28). In immunoprecipitation the antibody detects a polypeptide with an apparent MW 68,000 and a second polypeptide with 57,000, which might represent either a precursor polypeptide or a degradation product. Since the 8B E6-reactive antigen resembles the murine Lyt-1 and the human CD-5 (OKT-1 or Leu-1) antigens in its molecular weight and tissue distribution, it has been suggested that it represents the Lyt-1 or CD-5 homologous protein of the guinea pig (32).

Treatment with mAb 8BE6 and complement eliminates T cells from a mixed cell population. Another antibody, mAb 5C C2, was reported to possess properties similar to 8B E6 (34) but has weak reactivity against B lymphocytes (35).

mAb 5C D2 and 11 AE3. Both antibodies were obtained by methods as described with antibody 8B E6 and were used for analysis of T lymphocyte development in the guinea pig (28). They react with 60-70% of lymph node cells, 40-50% of spleen cells, and do not react with thymocytes or with B cells (surface Ig positive cells). MAb 5CD2 reacts weakly with medullary thymocytes. These two antibodies as well as mAb 8B E6 and also alkaline phosphatase activity have been shown to be useful markers for defining maturation states of T cells (28). The function and biochemical properties of the reactive antigens are not known.

mAb CT5. This mouse antibody, similar to the aforementioned antibodies, probably recognizes a pan-T-cell marker and labels the majority of peripheral T cells and thymocytes. It was obtained by immunization with purified T cells (31). It also reacts with EN-L2C cells but not with normal B cells. Biochemical data on the antigen are not available.

mAb CT6. Antibody CT6 (31) reacts with the majority of cortical thymocytes but with only a small proportion of medullary thymocytes. It reacts with about 20% of peripheral T cells. The distribution of CT6 positive cells in lymphoid structures of the guinea pig resembles the distribution of CD8 positive T cells in man, i.e., the cytotoxic/suppressor T-cell subpopulation. There are, however, no functional or biochemical data available to support this assumption.

mAb154. This rat monoclonal antibody as well as several other antibodies (see below) were obtained by immunization of rats with membrane fragments of guinea pig T cells followed by booster injections with Ag188-protein (see below) that had been partially purified by immunoadsorption (33). This antibody recognizes antigen on most, if not all, T cells and thymocytes. It shows strong reactivity with T-cell-dependent areas of lymph nodes as revealed by immunoperoxidase staining. It reacts in Western blot analysis with a broad band of an apparent molecular weight 30,000. This protein may represent the guinea pig Thy1 homologue.

2. T-Cell Markers of Functional Relevance

In the human and the mouse several T-cell specific antigens have been shown to be closely involved in T-cell function. It appears that the selective expression of these serologically defined antigens in the T-cell membrane results from the requirement for these proteins in the specialized functions performed by T lymphocytes.

mAb CT7. This antibody resembles mAb CT5 (31; see above) and probably recognizes a pan-T-cell antigen. It reacts with most peripheral T cells and labels the majority of cortical and medullary thymocytes. This antibody has the capacity to inhibit T cell proliferation to soluble protein antigens in vitro. Biochemical data on the antigen are not available. A similarity to Ag188 will be discussed later.

mAb 5C3 to an interleukin 2 receptor-associated protein expressed on activated T cells. The antibody 5C3 was identified by its capacity to inhibit efficiently T-cell proliferation of alloreactive T-cell clones in vitro (36,37). It differs from the other T-cell markers described above in that the recognized antigen is expressed only on activated T cells, not on resting T cells. Expression occurs independently of the nature of activation, and alloantigens, soluble protein antigens, or mitogens provide an appropriate stimulus. This antibody had an inhibitory effect in an interleukin 2 (IL2) assay where Con A-activated guinea pig T-cell blasts are cultured with IL2-containing guinea pig culture supernatant or partially purified human IL2. However, the following results suggest that the antibody is not directed against the guinea pig IL2 receptor. a) This antibody 5C3 failed to interfere with the binding of radiolabeled (human) IL2 to guinea pig T-cell blasts and did not inhibit subsequent degradation of the bound IL2. b) Culturing the cells in the presence of the antibody 5C3 resulted in antigen modulation and the cells no longer expressed the antigen. The 5C3-antigen-negative cells had an unimpaired capacity for binding of IL2 compared to 5C3-positive cells. However, the 5C3-negative cells failed to respond to IL-2 and no proliferation occurred. Upon subsequent stimulation with mitogen and reexpression of the 5C3-reactive protein on the 5C3-negative cells, their capacity to proliferate to IL2 was restored (37). Therefore, this antibody seems to be directed to a protein associated with the guinea pig IL2 receptor but does not directly contribute to IL2 binding. The 5C3 membrane protein obviously plays an indirect but nevertheless essential role in IL2-dependent T-cell proliferation. It might contribute in signal transduction upon binding of IL2 to IL2 receptor. Binding of the monoclonal antibody 5C3 blocks this critical signal in IL2-dependent proliferation. Biochemical properties of the antigen remain to be examined. An homologous protein in the human or mouse system is not known.

mAb 188 to a protein involved in T-cell recognition or activation. Among the various markers of guinea pig T cells, the antigen defined by mAb 188 has probably—together with the 5C3 antigen—been analyzed in most detail (33,38,39). The antibody was obtained by immunization with purified T cells. The 188-reactive antigen (Ag188) represents a pan-T-cell marker. This protein is present on the majority (70-90%) of peripheral T lymphocytes of inbred strain 2 and strain 13 guinea pigs and of outbred animals. About 10-20% of thymocytes bear the antigen. It is absent on L2C leukemia cells, granulocytes, macrophages, thrombocytes, or erythrocytes. mAb188 exhibits marked inhibitory effect on the T-cell proliferative response to antigen, mitogen, or alloantigen (MLR). The antigen is obviously involved in an early phase of T-cell activation. Maximal inhibition (up to 85%) requires the presence of the antibody from the beginning of the culture. Addition of the antibody after 24 hr of culture no longer provides the inhibitory effect, suggesting that once the cells are triggered, binding of the antibody per se is not sufficient for inhibition. mAb 188 has no mitogenic activity. Biochemical analysis of the immunoprecipitated protein in two-dimensional gels reveals a two-chain structure. The protein consists of two noncovalently associated polypeptide chains (α chain; MW 43,000, β chain 39,000). Both subunits displayed a marked charge heterogeneity. Among the various T-cell markers a similar structure is known for the human or murine T-cell receptor with the exception that T-cell receptor proteins possess a disulfide bridge between the two chains. Based on the functional data it has been suggested that the Ab188 might be directed against a determinant which is present on the nonvariant region of the guinea pig T-cell receptor, i.e., a determinant which is expressed independent of the specificity of a given T cell (39).

Alloreactive T-cell clones derived from secondary MLR (strain 13 vs. strain 2) were analyzed in order to test this hypothesis (39). Long-term T-cell lines still expressed Ag188 and their specific proliferative response was inhibited by the mAb 188. In addition, cytotoxic activity of these strain 13 T-cell lines against strain 2 target cells (Con A-activated T-cell blasts) was inhibited. In contrast, lectin-dependent cellular cytotoxicity remained unaffected. mAb188 also inhibited one of the earliest detectable biochemical events, namely calcium-influx (39).

In summary, these data indicate that mAb188 interferes with a structural T-cell surface protein involved in T-cell recognition or in an initial step of T-cell activation. Structural comparison, e.g., by peptide mapping, of the Ag188 obtained from different T-cell clones should reveal whether the protein exhibits clonotypic variability. This would prove or, alternatively, exclude whether the mAb188 recognizes the T-cell antigen receptor or another structurally and functionally related protein involved in T-cell activation.

mAb155. This rat monoclonal antibody, obtained as described for Ab154 (33), defines a T-cell subpopulation. It reacts with 40-45% of lymph node T cells, and weakly with more than 50% of thymocytes but not with the L2C B-cell leukemia, macrophages, or bone marrow cells. Antibody-containing culture supernatant strongly inhibits the antigen- or mitogen-induced T-cell proliferation and the MLR. Biochemical data are not available.

mAb159. mAb159 obtained from the same fusion as mAb155 reacts with 60-70% of T cells and a small proportion of thymocytes (less than 10%). It does not inhibit but enhances T-cell proliferation. In Western blot analysis mAb159 reacts with two polypeptide chains with an apparent MW 85,000 and 90,000.

mAb 167. This antibody was obtained by using a method similar to that used for the generation of mAb188 (see above). It defines a pan-T-cell marker. The antibody exhibits intensive binding to T dependent areas of lymph nodes as demonstrated by immunofluorescence or immunoperoxidase staining techniques. mAb-167 does not inhibit antigen- or mitogen-induced T-cell proliferation, rather it is able to induce T-cell proliferation. After incubation of purified lymph node T cells with mAb167 and subsequent cross-linking of the antibody with a rabbit anti-mouse Ig reagent, the cells respond with vigorous proliferation (Schaefer and

Burger, unpublished observation). Co-stimulation with phorbol myristate acetate is required in this system. This cell-surface antigen might be involved in T-cell triggering, similar to the CD2 (T11) antigen of human T cells (13), and the monoclonal antibody might replace the physiological ligand. However, immunoprecipitation technique has so far failed to identify the cell-surface protein.

III. LEUKOCYTE ANTIGENS NOT RESTRICTED TO T LYMPHOCYTES

Several antigens are not restricted in their expression to a particular subpopulation of lymphoid cells but, in contrast, are detected on several distinct lymphocyte populations, or even on all leukocytes.

A. mAb 5AB2: A Lymphocyte Marker

A useful marker for lymphocytes is provided by mAb 5AB2. This antibody reacts with T and B lymphocytes but not with macrophages or other cells. It was obtained by immunization with purified T cells (32). Detailed characterization using FACS analysis revealed that it reacted with 100% of thymocytes and purified T cells, 90% of lymph node cells, and 80% of spleen cells. It failed to react with an Ia-bearing B-cell leukemia line EN-L2C or granulocytes. Forty percent of bone marrow cells expressed the antigen. Two-color immunofluorescence analysis confirmed that almost all B cells (surface Ig-positive cells) expressed the antigen. T cells, however, express this antigen at a higher density than B cells as revealed by cytofluorometry. The antigen consists of two subunits with apparent MW 60,000 and 35,000 under reducing conditions, and migrates as a larger complex of an apparent MW of more than 250,000 under nonreducing conditions. This antibody is a useful reagent in the preparation of macrophages free of contaminating T or B cells. Treatment of lymphoid cells with this antibody and complement abolishes the proliferative capacity, but it does not affect the ability of macrophages for antigen presentation.

B. mAb CT1 to CT4, CT8

These antibodies were obtained by immunization of mice with guinea pig T cells. They react with all T cells and most small B-lymphocytes. They do not react, however, with B cells in the germinal center (31).

C. Ab160 and Ab201

These rat antibodies were obtained similarly to Ab154 (see above) and recognize leukocyte markers, which are expressed on T cells as well as on other leukocytes including the L2C B-cell leukemia cells (33). Ab201 shows very intense reactivity. These antibodies do not react with erythrocytes or thrombocytes. Antibody 160 inhibits T-cell proliferation. It does not react in Western blot analysis, whereas Ab201 recognizes a protein with an apparent MW 205,000. It might well represent the guinea pig analogue of the L-CA antigen (leucocyte common antigen; T200) described in the human, mouse, and rat (40,41).

IV. B-LYMPHOCYTE DIFFERENTIATION ANTIGENS

There have been no reports on B-cell specific cell-surface antigens except on the conventional cell-surface markers, such as surface immunoglobulin, Fc receptors, or complement receptors in guinea pigs. The monoclonal antibody 31 D2, however, provides a useful reagent for detection and quantification of B cells in this species.

A. mAb 31 D2

Antibody 31 D2 was obtained in our own laboratory (Burger and Shevach, manuscript in preparation) by immunization with the Ia-bearing B-cell leukemia line EN-L2C. It reacted with EN-L2C, its Ia-negative variant BZ-L2C, and spleen cells but not with purified T cells and thymocytes. It was analyzed in detail because this reactivity pattern indicated that it reacts with a B-cell differentiation antigen. Immunoprecipitation after lactoperoxidase-mediated surface labeling of EN-L2C cells with ^{125}I revealed high molecular weight material at the top of the gel under nonreducing conditions. After reduction two polypeptide chains were detectable with apparent MW about 70,000 and 22,000. These molecular characteristics correspond to the properties of the μ heavy chain and IgM light chains.

Ouchterlony analysis confirmed that this antibody reacts with IgM. This monoclonal antibody produced a precipitin line against purified pentameric serum IgM, but not against monomeric IgM obtained by treatment with 2-mercaptoethanol. No precipitation line was observed with IgG. This reactivity for IgM but not for IgG was also confirmed by ELISA. Ab 31 D2 shows cross-reactivity with rabbit IgM but not with human IgM. The antibody provides a useful reagent to detect surface IgM positive cells and IgM producing cells (28,42). It gives intensive staining B cells in germinal centers but not on T dependent areas of lymph nodes. The antibody has no mitogenic effect on lymphocytes.

B. B-Cell Antigen 7420

A xenoantiserum to a human B-lymphocyte antigen was produced in the rabbit. It recognized a B-cell antigen distinct from HLA-DR antigens, surface immunoglobulin, or Fc-receptor (43). This antiserum reacted with peripheral blood lymphocytes from several species, including the guinea pig. It obviously defines an alloantigen because only two out of four guinea pigs were reactive. In two animals

12 and 25% of blood lymphocytes were positive, whereas no positive cells were detected in the two remaining animals. The functional and biochemical properties of this antigen are unknown.

V. MACROPHAGE DIFFERENTIATION ANTIGENS

Mononuclear phagocytes display heterogenous properties. They exhibit a variety of functions contributing to host defense and inflammation and play a central role in the induction of the immune response. The local environment and inflammatory or microbial agents influence the functional state. Monoclonal antibodies to cell-surface antigens are obviously a preferential tool for identifying different stages of differentiation, maturation, or, alternatively, of activation because qualitative and quantitative variations in the expression of cell-surface molecules often occur in the course of various cellular events. Monoclonal antibodies should be particularly helpful for the distinction of subpopulations of macrophages that might differ in their functional state, e.g., in their ability to respond to exogenous or endogenous stimuli, in their secretory pattern, or in their capacity to act as accessory cells.

A number of monoclonal antibodies to guinea pig macrophages have been obtained: One macrophage specific antibody (44) was used mainly for analysis of mycobacterial granuloma and studies of the central nervous system (45,46). We described a series of 10 different monoclonal antibodies to guinea pig macrophages which permitted the distinction of monocyte/macrophage differentiation antigens and activation processes (47). All antibodies were obtained by immunization of mice with oil-induced peritoneal macrophages. Screening was carried out by using immunofluorescence, immunoperoxidase, or ^{125}I-radiolabeling techniques, and the reactivity pattern against a variety of macrophage and lymphoid cell populations was determined.

A. mAb "Anti-macrophage"

This antibody reacts with most macrophages (44). It binds to the majority (74%) of oil-induced peritoneal macrophages, a small percentage (1-9%) of lymph node cells, and 1% of thymocytes. It does not react with EN-L2C cells, hepatocytes, or fibroblasts. Immunoperoxidase staining revealed that this antibody labeled macrophages in various tissues. It reacted with Kupffer cells of the liver, alveolar macrophages, and macrophages in lymph nodes. Resting microglia in the brain also reacted with this antibody, supporting their classification as a member of the mononuclear phagocyte series. In contrast, skin Langerhans cells were not stained, suggesting that these cells may belong to a separate line of differentiation within the antigen-presenting cell populations (45). However, apparent nonreactivity could also be a consequence of quantitative differences in expression of the antigens.

In BCG-induced granuloma, epitheloid cells expressed in macrophage antigen but not Ia antigens. In contrast, granuloma induced by Mycobacterium leprae contained macrophages bearing Ia antigen in addition to the macrophage antigen (44). This antibody permitted preparative sorting of the granuloma cells using a FACS. The isolated cells were shown to possess a markedly reduced capacity for antigen presentation compared to peritoneal macrophages (46). Such studies are obviously helpful for the understanding of differentiation processes that take place during granuloma formation, in particular of the relationship between tissue macrophages, and epitheloid cells and of the contribution of each cell population to this process.

B. Macrophage Markers Associated with Maturation and Activation

A series of 10 antibodies to oil-induced adherent macrophages was produced (47). Antibodies reactive with macrophages but nonreactive with EN-L2C cells and thymocytes were further characterized. Most of these antibodies (8 out of 10) did not react with granulocytes or with erythrocytes, lymph node T cells, thrombocytes, connective tissue, or endothelial cells of the liver. Kupffer cells were intensively stained. These antibodies permit the identification of differentiation antigens associated with cells in the monocyte/macrophage lineage. They provide therefore useful reagents for the detection of macrophages in different tissues. The macrophage-specific antigens can be divided into three groups based on the reactivity pattern of the monoclonal antibodies. None of the antibodies recognized antigens that are involved in presentation of antigen, mitogen, or alloantigen, since no inhibitory effect was observed in respective proliferation assays by the addition of the antibodies. The physiological function of these membrane proteins remains to be elucidated, although their selective distribution on cells of the monocyte/macrophage lineage suggests a participation in the specialized functions of these cells. Nothing is known so far about the biochemical properties of the antigens.

1. mAb342, 322, and 249 Defining "Lineage Antigens" of Mononuclear Phagocytes

These three antibodies reacted with antigens expressed continuously during maturation of monocytes to macrophages and also after cell activation ("lineage antigens"). MAb342 reacts with about 90% of the cells in the monocyte/macrophage series. mAb249 differs from the Ab342 in that it also reacts with thrombocytes.

2. Markers of Mature Macrophages (mAb305, 320, 321, and 344)

Monocytes differentiate into mature macrophages and acquire new surface characteristics. These four antibodies are directed to macrophage markers, which are not expressed on blood monocytes. Tissue macrophages and also elicited or activated macrophages bear these antigens.

3. Markers Expressed on Macrophage Subpopulations or on Activated Macrophages (mAb253, 310, and 257)

The antigens defined by these antibodies are absent in monocytes or residential (wash-out) peritoneal macrophages. In contrast, oil-elicited and, with the exception of mAb257, PPD-activated macrophages (BCG immunization followed by PPD injection) bear these antigens. Ab257 reacts only with elicited cells. MAb253 reacts also with thrombocytes. The three antibodies reacted with discrete macrophage subpopulations. The antigens were inducible on monocytes or residential macrophages by appropriate stimulation in vivo or in vitro, e.g., incubation with phorbol myristate acetate or platelet activating factor.

Antibodies 249 and 344 were employed for flow-cytometric studies in order to compare the antigen expression to other cell-surface markers (48). Simultaneous three-parameter measurements for Fc-receptor, cell volume, and relative antigen density measured by indirect immunofluorescence were performed. The antigen pattern was qualitatively similar in residential and oil-induced macrophages, but quantitative differences were observed. Generally, the antigen density was decreased on oil-induced macrophages. Incubation of oil-induced macrophages with poly-inosinic-polycytidylic acid (poly I:C) caused an increase in density of several antigens, whereas incubation with lipopolysaccharide caused no significant alterations.

VI. EXPRESSION OF THE MHC PRODUCTS ON LYMPHOID CELLS

The "GPLA complex" represents the MHC of the guinea pig (1,2). It includes the B and S antigens, which are the guinea pig MHC class I products equivalent to the H-2D/K antigens or the human HLA-A/B/C antigens. The Ia antigens of the guinea pig (MHC class II products) are also associated with an invariant chain (49) and show selective expression on the various lymphoid cells in contrast to the ubiquitous MHC class I antigens. Ia expression in the guinea pig is different from other species in that resting, nonactivated T cells and also thymocytes bear Ia antigens (see below). These analyses of Ia expression were facilitated by the use of anti-Ia monoclonal antibodies (50,51). Meanwhile, several other antibodies recognizing additional alloantigenic Ia determinants were described (31,33). In addition some antibodies to human Ia antigens were found to cross-react with guinea pig Ia antigens. These antibodies detect apparently evolutionarily conserved epitopes of Ia antigens, which may contribute to Ia-antigen function such as antigen presentation (52).

Ia antigens were detected on lymphoid cells with appropriate alloantisera but were absent on a number of nonlymphoid cell lines. B cells and the EN-L2C B-cell leukemia express Ia antigens in a relatively high density. A subpopulation (15-25%) of purified macrophages bears Ia antigens. Purified Kupffer cells, Langerhans cells, and a transplantable granulocytic leukemia were also shown to bear Ia antigen.

A. Expression of Ia Antigens on Nonactivated T Cells and Thymocytes

In the murine and human species Ia antigens are expressed on only a minor subpopulation of T cells. However, Ia antigens in these two species can be readily demonstrated on activated T cells after appropriate stimulation with mitogens, antigens, or alloantigens (53-55). In contrast, in the guinea pig Ia antigens can be easily demonstrated on normal peripheral T cells utilizing alloantisera in cytotoxicity tests as well as with absorption and immunochemical techniques (56,57). Monoclonal antibodies permitted a more quantitative determination by combination with cytofluorometric analysis using a FACS (58). The majority (70-90%) of resting peritoneal exudate cells, lymph node T cells, and also about 80% of thymocytes expressed Ia antigens. The density of Ia antigens on T cells was about 5-10% of that found on the EN-L2C B-cell leukemia. Thymocytes bore less Ia antigen than T cells. The Ia-bearing T cells and thymocytes were shown to be at least partially identical with T-cell populations bearing the T-cell differentiation antigens described in the previous sections, confirming the Ia expression on T cells. One monoclonal antibody, 25E3 which had previously been shown by serological analysis to react exclusively with an alloantigenic Ia determinant of one inbred strain (strain 2), displayed an unusual pattern of reactivity with thymocytes. It reacted with thymocytes but not with mature T cells or B cells of another inbred strain (strain 13). The significance of the expression of "wrong" Ia determinants remains unclear. It might have some association with differentiation processes in the thymus.

B. Expression of the Complement Component C4 (MHC Class III Product) on T Lymphocytes

Genes controlling several complement components are located within the MHC in a number of species. In contrast to the genetic linkage, there was no indication that any functional association exists between the MHC-linked complement components and other products of the MHC that play a major role in antigen recognition by the T cell and in cellular interaction. Studies in the human system lead to the hypothesis that membrane-associated C4 might play a role in the afferent phase of the immune response. This assumption was based on the demonstration of C4 on the surface of human lymphoid cells and also on the finding that xenoantisera to C4 significantly inhibited the mixed lymphocyte reaction and the proliferative response to phytohemagglutinin (59). Attempts were made to reproduce and extend these observations in the guinea pig system (60). Various monospecific antisera to C4 had no inhibitory effect on the mixed leukocyte reaction or on the T-cell proliferative response to mitogens or soluble protein antigens. In addition, T lymphocytes from genetically C4-deficient guinea pigs responded to the same extent as lymphocytes from a normal strain with the same MHC haplotype indicating a normal capacity of T cells from C4-deficient animals for recognition of antigen or mitogen and for proliferation. These findings argue strongly against a general role of C4 in T-lymphocyte activation. The finding in the human remains therefore controversial.

VII. LYMPHOCYTE MARKERS EXPRESSED ON NONLYMPHOID CELLS

A. Differentiation Antigens of Natural Killer Cells

In the literature several reports give evidence for the sharing of antigenic determinants between lymphocytes and elements of the nervous system. Monoclonal antibodies recognizing markers of human natural killer cells have been described. One of those antibodies, anti-Leu-7, specifically binds to both central and peripheral nervous tissue in man, especially to myelin sheaths (61,62). This antibody also reacts with the guinea pig spinal cord, especially with the white matter. Immunohistochemical techniques reveal the staining of the surface of interfascicular oligodendroglia and the small myelin sheaths. However, no evidence is available as to whether the recognized antigen is also expressed on guinea pig natural killer cells. Analysis in appropriate systems remains to be performed.

B. T-Lymphocyte Markers Expressed on Purkinje Neurones

Some T-lymphocyte markers were found to be expressed on defined elements of the nervous system. The monoclonal antibodies UCHT 1 and Leu-4 are pan-T-cell markers (63), but they have been shown to react with Purkinje cells in human central nervous tissue (64). The antibody UCHT 1 also reacted with guinea pig Purkinje cells. However, it failed to react with spleen cells, indicating that the antigen is not expressed on guinea pig T cells. Therefore, this antibody apparently does not provide an additional marker for guinea pig T cells. However, additional serological analysis with defined T-cell populations might be required.

VIII. CONCLUDING REMARKS

This review summarizes the present state of differentiation antigens or "markers" of guinea pig lymphoid cells. It is obvious that, in contrast to the situation a few years ago, there are a number of suitable markers available, which are mainly defined by monoclonal antibodies (see Table 1). One of the major areas of application of these reagents was to our surprise the field of neurological research. Experimental allergic encephalomyelitis, which is induced readily in strain 13, served as an experimental model (28,34,35,65-68). In several reports monoclonal antibodies permitted detailed analysis of the cellular composition in the nervous tissue at various stages of the disease. They allowed the definition of discrete stages and of the migratory changes of the various cell populations. These studies obviously help to elucidate the role and contribution of the various cell populations in the

Table 1 Overview of Differentiation Antigens Defined by Monoclonal Antibodies on Guinea Pig Lymphoid Cells

mAb	Reactivity pattern	Molecular characteristics	Functional role	Possible homology	Ref.
T-cell markers, function unknown:					
8B E6	mature T, some thym., EN-L2C	68K, 57K	?	CD5 (OKT1/Leu 1); Lyt 1	32
5C C2	T, B	?	?	?	35
5C D2	mature T	?	?	?	28
11 A E 3	mature T	?	?	?	28
CT5	pan T (T, thym.), EN-L2C	?	?	?	31
CT6	T-subpopulation, cortical thym.	?	?	CD8	31
154	pan T (T, thym.)	25-30K	?	Thy 1?	33
T-cell markers, functionally relevant:					
CT 7	pan T (T, thym.)	?	Inhibition of T proliferation	?	31
5C 3	activated T	?	IL2-receptor assoc. protein	?	36,37
188	pan T, some thym.	43K, 39K	Ag-recognition or T activation	T cell receptor ?	33,38,39
155	T-subpopulation, thym.	?	Inhibition of T proliferation	?	33
159	T-subpopulation, some thym.	85K, 90K	Enhancement of T prolifera-tion	?	33
167	pan T (T, thym.)	?	Enhancement of T prolifera-tion	?	33,38
Leukocyte markers:					
5 AB2	T, thym, B	60K, 35K	?	?	32
CT1-CT4, CT8	T, B	?	?	?	31

160	leucocytes	?	Inhibition of T proliferation	?	33
201	leucocytes	205K	Inhibition of T proliferation	L-CA (T200)	33
B-lymphocyte marker:					
31 D2	B, EN-L2C, μ-chain	70K, 22K	surface IgM	surface IgM	in prep.
Macrophage markers:					
Anti-Mph	Mph	?	?	?	44
249	Monocytes, Mph, thromb.	?	?	?	47
322	Monocytes, Mph	?	?	?	47
342	Monocytes, Mph	?	?	?	47
305,320,321,344	mature Mph	?	?	?	47
310	Mph-subpopulation,	?	?	?	47
	elicited and activated Mph	?	?	?	
257	Mph subpopulation,	?	?	?	47
	elicited Mph, thromb.	?	?	?	
253	Mph-subpopulation, elicited and activated Mph, thromb.	?	?	?	47

T = T lymphocytes; B = B lymphocytes; thym. = thymocytes; EN-L2C = Ia-positive B-cell leukemia; thromb. = thrombocytes; Mph = macrophages; k = kilodaltons.

development of the clinical symptoms. One antibody (8BEG) was applied successfully for treatment of chronic experimental allergic encephalomyelitis (69).

Another important application was the ontogenetic analysis of T-cell development and maturation processes in the thymus (28). A series of appropriate monoclonal reagents helped to define the localization of thymocyte or T-cell subpopulations and permitted identification of certain stages of development.

In the guinea pig, there are definitely fewer marker proteins defined than in the mouse or human system. Unfortunately, among the monoclonal antibodies available and tested as above only a small number seems to react with the membrane proteins homologous to the classical lymphocyte markers of man or mouse. There is no well-defined (i.e., serologically, functionally, *and* biochemically defined) antibody available against the CD3, CD4, or CD8 antigens, and further work is obviously required. In contrast, some of the antibodies to guinea pig differentiation antigens might define "new" antigens not yet recognized in other species.

ACKNOWLEDGMENTS

Work from the authors' laboratory described in this article was supported by Deutsche Forschungsgemeinschaft, Bu 400/1 and Bu 400/2, and by the Sonderforschungsbereich 107. We thank Ms. Bodensohn and Ms. Schubert for assistance in preparation of the manuscript.

ABBREVIATIONS

FACS	fluorescence activated cell sorter.
GPLA	guinea pig leukocyte antigen-complex.
LNL	lymph node T lymphocytes.
MHC	major histocompatibility complex.
β2M	β2-microglobulin.
MLR	mixed leukocyte reaction.
mAb	monoclonal antibody.
PEC	peritoneal exudate cells.
PEL	peritoneal exudate T lymphocytes.

REFERENCES

1. E. M. Shevach, The guinea pig I-region. A functional analysis of Ia-Ir association. *Springer Semin. Immunopathol., 1*: 207 (1978).
2. R. Burger and E. M. Shevach in *Ia antigens* (S. Ferrone and C. S. David, eds.), CRC Press, Boca Raton, Florida, 1982.
3. E. L. Reinherz and S. F. Schlossman, The differentiation and function of human T cells. *Cell, 19*: 821 (1980).

4. J. A. Bluestone and R. J. Hodes, Cell surface molecules involved in T cell functions. *Immunol. Today, 4*: 256 (1983).
5. A. M. Krensky and C. Clayberger, Diagnostic and therapeutic implication of T cell surface antigens. *Transplantation, 29*: 339 (1985).
6. Inbred and genetically defined strains of laboratory animals. Part 2, Data book of the Federation of American Societies for Experimental Biology.
7. T. R. Malek, R. B. Clark, and E. M. Shevach, Alloreactive T cells from individual soft agar colonies specific for guinea pig Ia antigens. I. Production and initial characterization. *J. Immunol., 127*: 616 (1981).
8. T. R. Malek and E. M. Shevach, Alloreactive T cells from individual soft agar colonies specific for guinea pig Ia antigens. II. Cellular and molecular requirements for optimal proliferative responses. *J. Immunol., 127*: 2113 (1981).
9. L. Schrod, H. Schaefer, and R. Burger, Characterization of a T lymphocyte membrane protein involved in T cell function: Its contribution to T cell recognition or cellular interaction. *Immunology, 57*: 533 (1986).
10. M. J. Stadecker, G. Bishop, and H. H. Wortis, Rosette formation by guinea pig thymocytes and thymus derived lymphocytes with rabbit red blood cells. *J. Immunol., 111*: 1834 (1973).
11. H. P. Godfrey, A. F. Geczy, P. G. H. Gell, and B. Rubin, Induction of specific anti-guinea pig T cell sera in rabbits. *J. Immunol. Methods, 9*: 211 (1976).
12. S. Kataoka, K. Itoh, I. Kurane, and K. Kumagai, Detection of guinea pig Tμ and Tγ cells by a double rosette assay. *J. Immunol. Methods, 51*: 89 (1982).
13. S. C. Meuer, R. E. Hussey, M. Fabbi, D. Fox, O. Acuto, K. A. Fitzgerald, J. C. Hodgdon, J. P. Protentis, S. F. Schlossman, and E. L. Reinherz, An alternative pathway of T cell activation: A functional role of the 50kd T11 sheep erythrocyte receptor protein. *Cell, 36*: 897 (1984).
14. H. P. Godfrey, Differences in sensitivity to a cytotoxic anti-thymus-derived lymphocyte serum of cells mediating delayed-onset reactions in guinea pigs to hapten-protein conjugates and contactants. *Cell. Immunol., 22*: 28 (1976).
15. E. Shevach, I. Green, L. Ellman, and J. Maillard, Heterologous antiserum to thymus-derived cells in the guinea-pig. *Nature New Biology, 235*: 19 (1972).
16. H. P. Godfrey and C. Koch, Ability of an anti-T-cell serum to dissociate two features of cellular hypersensitivity in the guinea-pig. *Immunology, 40*: 247 (1980).
17. D. W. Thomas, S. K. Meltz, Y. Hahn, and B. D. Schwartz, Biologic activity of rabbit antisera directed against in vitro stimulated guinea pig T lymphocytes. *J. Immunol., 123*: 1565, (1979).
18. H. Quill, M. D. Hoffman, D. W. Thomas, and B. D. Schwartz, Characterization of a 75.000 mol. wt. glycoprotein synthesized by guinea-pig T-lymphocytes: A possible homologue of Lyt-1 antigen. *Mol. Immunol., 19*: 1587 (1982).
19. J. Klein, *Biology of the Mouse Histocompatibility-2-Complex*, Springer, Berlin, 1975.
20. R. Cigén, Structural difference between the two forms of guinea-pig β_2-microglobulin and their occurrence in inbred guinea-pig strains. *Mol. Immunol., 22*: 1039 (1985).

21. B. D. Schwartz, R. Cigén, I. Berggard, and E. M. Shevach, Guinea pig homologues of TL and Qa-2 antigens. *J. Immunol., 121*: 835 (1978).
22. R. S. Surratt, L. N. K. Fuge Abruzzini, M. P. Zacheis, R. Cigén, and B. D. Schwartz, Structural identity of the TL antigen homologues derived from strain 2 and strain 13 guinea pigs. *J. Immunol., 131*: 1344 (1983).
23. G. Stingl, W. J. Pichler, and E. M. Shevach, T-Zell-Subpopulationen im Merrschweinchen. *Wiener klin. Wochenschrift, 90*: 741 (1978).
24. O. Ruuskanen and K. Kouvalainen, The fate of thymocytes: A study of kinetics of thymocytes using high alkaline phosphatase activity as an endogenous label. *Scand. J. Haemat., 9*: 174 (1972).
25. O. Ruuskanen and K. Kouvalainen, Differentiation of thymus and thymocytes: A study in foetal guinea-pigs using alkaline phosphatase as a label of thymocytes. *Immunology, 26*: 187 (1974).
26. O. J. Ruuskanen, L. J. Pelliniemi, and K. E. Kouvalinen, Alkaline phosphatase in differentiating guinea pig thymocytes: An ultra-cytochemical study. *J. Immunol., 114*: 1611 (1975).
27. O. Ruuskanen, Subpopulations of guinea pig thymocytes: Different distribution patterns of alkaline phosphatase positive and negative autologous thymocytes. *Cell. Immunol., 15*: 246 (1975).
28. J. M. Elias, J. Chiba, E. M. Shevach, and H. P. Godfrey, Guinea pig T lymphocyte development analyzed by enzyme histocytochemistry, monoclonal antibodies, and flow cytometry. *Laboratory Invest., 52*: 270 (1985).
29. S. Ferrone and M. P. Dierich (eds.), *Handbook of Monoclonal Antibodies*, Noyes Publication, Park Ridge, 1985.
30. A. J. McMichael and I. W. Fabre (eds.), *Monoclonal Antibodies in Clinical Medicine*. Academic Press, London, 1982.
31. B. T. G. Tan, F. Ekelaar, J. Luirink, G. Rimmelzwaan, A. J. R. de Jonge, and R. J. Scheper, Production of monoclonal antibodies defining guinea pig T-cell surface markers and a strain 13 Ia-like antigen: The value of immunohistological screening. *Hybridoma, 4*: 115 (1985).
32. J. Chiba, T. M. Chused, W. M. Leiserson, S. E. Zweig, and E. M. Shevach, Production and characterization of monoclonal antibodies to guinea pig lymphoid differentiation antigens. *J. Immunol. Methods, 63*: 247 (1983).
33. R. Burger, L. Schrod, and H. Schafer, Functionally relevant membrane proteins of human and guinea pig T lymphocytes. *Mol. Immunol.*, in press.
34. U. Traugott, E. Shevach, J. Chiba, S. H. Stone, and C. R. Raine, Acute experimental autoimmune encephalomyelitis: T- and B-cell distribution within the target organ. *Cell. Immunol., 70*: 345 (1982).
35. R. A. Sobel, B. W. Blanchette, A. K. Bhan, and R. B. Colvin, The immunopathology of experimental allergic encephalomyelitis. I. Quantitative analysis of inflammatory cells in situ. *J. Immunol., 132*: 2392 (1984).
36. T. R. Malek, R. J. Robb, and E. M. Shevach, Identification of a membrane antigen that is distinct from the interleukin 2 receptor and that may be required for interleukin 2-driven proliferative responses. *J. Immunol., 130*: 747 (1983).

37. T. R. Malek and E. M. Shevach, Interleukin 2-driven T lymphocyte proliferation is dependent upon a surface antigen distinct from the interleukin 2 receptor: Requirements for inhibition of T-cell proliferation by monoclonal antibody 5C3. *Cell. Immunol., 84*: 85 (1984).
38. R. Burger, K. Reske, U. Mauer, D. von Steldern, and M. Husman, Identification and characterization of gp TFA-1, a guinea pig T cell surface antigen associated with T cell function. *J. Immunol., 131*: 1350 (1983).
39. L. Schrod, H. Schaefer, and R. Burger, Characterization of a T-lymphocyte membrane protein involved in T-cell function: Its contribution to T-cell recognition or cellular interaction. *Immunology, 57*: 533 (1986).
40. R. Dalchau, J. Kirkley, and J. W. Fabre, Monoclonal antibody to a human leukocyte-specific membrane glycoprotein probably homologous to the leukocyte-common (L-C) antigen of the rat. *Eur. J. Immunol., 10*: 737 (1980).
41. M. L. Thomas, A. N. Barclay, J. Gagnon, and A. F. Williams, Evidence from cDNA clones that the rat leukocyte-common antigen (T200) spans the lipid bilayer and contains a cytoplasmic domain of 80,000 M_r. *Cell, 41*: 83 (1985).
42. E. C. Bottger, T. Hoffman, U. Hadding, and D. Bitter-Suermann, Guinea pigs with inherited deficiencies of complement components C2 or C4 have characteristics of immune-complex disease. *J. Clin. Invest.*, in press.
43. E. Berntorp, I. Turesson, and O. Zettervall, Cellular expression of the non-HLA-DR B-cell antigen 7420: Studies on non-lymphoid cells and on lymphocytes from different species. *Scand. J. Immunol., 13*: 461 (1981).
44. R. C. Mathew, I. Katayama, S. K. Gupta, J. Curtis, and J. L. Turk, Analysis of cells of the mononuclear phagocyte series in experimental mycobacterial granulomas by monoclonal antibodies. *Infec. Immun., 39*: 344 (1983).
45. R. C. Mathew, S. K. Gupta, I. Katayama, J. Curtis, and J. L. Turk, Macrophage specific antigen is expressed by resting microglia in the CNS but not by Langerhans cells in the skin. *J. Pathol., 141*: 435 (1983).
46. S. Gupta, J. Curtis, and J. L. Turk, Accessory cell function of cells of the mononuclear phagocyte system isolated from mycobacterial granulomas. *Cell. Immunol., 91*: 425 (1985).
47. U. Mauer-Gross, D. von Steldern, U. Hadding, D. Bitter-Suermann, and R. Burger, Cell surface antigens on the guinea-pig macrophage: Identification by monoclonal antibodies and association with the activation state. *Immunology, 55*: 519 (1985).
48. A. Raffael, G. Valet, U. Mauer-Gross, and R. Burger, Flow-cytometric studies of cell surface antigens on guinea pig macrophages: Analysis with 12 different monoclonal antibodies, submitted for publication.
49. H. Quill and B. D. Schwarts, Invariant proteins associated with guinea-pig Ia antigens. *Mol. Immunol., 20*: 1333 (1983).
50. R. Burger, L. Clement, J. Schroer, J. Chiba, and E. M. Shevach, Monoclonal antibodies to guinea pig Ia antigens. I. Production, serologic, and immunochemical characterization. *J. Immunol., 126*: 32 (1981).
51. R. Burger and E. M. Shevach, Monoclonal antibodies to guinea pig Ia antigens. II. Effect on alloantigen-, antigen-, and mitogen-induced T lymphocyte proliferation in vitro. *J. Exp. Med., 152*: 1011 (1980).

52. S. E. Zweig, S. Ferrone, and E. M. Shevach, Monoclonal antibodies directed against human Ia antigens detect an evolutionary conserved epitope on guinea pig Ia antigens with unique functional properties. *J. Leukocyte Biol., 35*: 101 (1984).
53. C. S. David, T. Meo, J. McCormick, and D. Shreffler, Expression of individual Ia specificities on T and B cells. I. Studies with mitogen-induced blast cells. *J. Exp. Med., 143*: 218 (1976).
54. H. S. Ko, S. M. Fu, R. J. Winchester, D. T. Yu, and H. G. Kunkel, Ia determinants on stimulated human T lymphocytes. Occurrence on mitogen- and antigen-activated T cells. *J. Exp. Med., 150*: 246 (1979).
55. E. L. Reinherz, P. C. Kung, J. M. Pesando, J. Rik, G. Goldstein, and S. F. Schlossman, Ia determinants on human T-cell subsets defined by monoclonal antibody. Activation stimuli required for expression. *J. Exp. Med., 150*: 1472 (1979).
56. B. D. Schwartz, W. E. Paul, and E. M. Shevach, Guinea pig Ia antigens: Functional significance and chemical characterization. *Transplant. Rev., 30*: 1974 (1976).
57. E. M. Shevach, D. L. Rosenstreich, and I. Green, The distribution of histocompatibility antigens on T and B cells in the guinea pig. *Transplantation, 16*: 126 (1973).
58. R. Burger, I. Scher, S. Sharrow, and E. M. Shevach, Non-activated guinea pig T lymphocytes and thymocytes express Ia antigens: FACs analysis with alloantibodies and monoclonal antibodies. *Immunology, 51*: 93 (1984).
59. S. Ferrone, M. A. Pellegrino, and N. R. Cooper, Expression of C4 on human lymphoid cells and possible involvement in immune recognition. *Science, 193*: 53 (1976).
60. R. Burger and E. M. Shevach, Evaluation of the role of C4 in the cellular immune response in vitro. *J. Immunol., 122*: 2388 (1979).
61. S. Schuller-Petrovic, W. Gebhart, H. Lassmann, H. Rumpold, and D. Kraft, A shared antigen determinant between natural killer cells and nervous tissue. *Nature, 306*: 179 (1983).
62. W. Gebhart, S. Schuller-Petrovic, H. Lassmann, and D. Kraft, NK-Zellen und Nervensystem. *Wiener klin. Wochenschrift, 95*: 828 (1983).
63. P. C. L. Beverly and R. E. Callard, Distinctive functional characteristics of human "T" lymphocytes defined by E rosetting or a monoclonal anti-T cell antibody. *Eur. J. Immunol., 11*: 329 (1981).
64. J. A. Garson, P. C. L. Beverly, H. B. Coakham, and E. I. Harper, Monoclonal antibodies against human T lymphocytes label Purkinje neurones of many species. *Nature, 298*: 375 (1982).
65. R. A. Sobel, B. W. Blanchette, A. K. Bhan, and R. B. Colvin, The immunopathology of experimental allergic encephalomyelitis. II. Endothelial cell Ia increases prior to inflammatory cell infiltration. *J. Immunol., 132*: 2402 (1984).
66. A. J. Suckling, P. W. Baron, U. Mauer, R. Burger, and M. G. Rumsby, Quantitative analysis of the cellular constituents of the cerebrospinal fluid in the

chronic relapsing experimental allergic encephalomyelitis. *J. Neuroimmunol., 11*: 57 (1986).
67. U. Traugott, E. Shevach, J. Chiba, J. H. Stone, and C. S. Raine, Autoimmune encephalomyelitis: Simultaneous identification of T and B cells in the target organ. *Science, 214*: 1251 (1981).
68. A. V. Antoniou, D. Parker, J. L. Turk, B. T. G. Tan, and R. J. Scheper, Immunocytochemical identification and quantitation of mononuclear cells in the meninges during the development of chronic relapsing experimental allergic encephalomyelitis (CREAE) in the guinea pig. *Cell. Immunol., 97*: 386 (1986).
69. R. A. Sobel and R. B. Colvin, Treatment of chronic experimental allergic encephalomyelitis (CEAE) in guinea pigs (GP) with an anti-T cell monoclonal antibody (Mab). *Neurology, 35*: 169 (Suppl 1) (Abstract) (1985).

8
Antigens that Distinguish Lymphocyte Subsets in the Syrian Hamster

PAMELA L. WITTE
University of Texas Health Science Center, Dallas, Texas

JOAN STEIN-STREILEIN
University of Miami School of Medicine, Miami, Florida

I. INTRODUCTION

As a model for experimental immunology, the Syrian or golden hamsters (*Mesocricetus auratus*) possess a number of features that make them unique among common laboratory animals. The species was domesticated relatively recently from an initial breeding stock of three hamsters captured in 1930. Even at that time, it was recognized that hamsters were exceptional models for parasitic diseases, such as leishmaniasis. Later, immunological studies focused on the rejection (or then anomalous lack of rejection) of transplanted tumor and skin allografts (reviewed in Refs. 1,2). Several "classical" inbred lines were derived from the original three parents (MHA, CB, LSH, LHC, and PD4) by R.E. Billingham and colleagues (2). Other inbred lines from more recent captures of breeding stocks have been developed. With these lines, a major histocompatibility complex (MHC), Hm-1, was defined by W. Duncan, T. Phillips, and J.W. Streilein (3-5).

The definition of the hamster MHC uncovered many perplexities, which predictably spilled over to the issues of immune function in this species (6). Using serologic methods, Streilein and co-workers found that, while polymorphism existed at a class II locus [at least 6 Ia-alleles have been defined (4)], no polymorphism appeared to exist at a class I locus (7,8). Lymphocytes themselves may be used to detect polymorphism where serology often fails, and further experiments were designed to test the MHC restriction of cytotoxic cells from hamsters that were infected with vaccinia, LCM virus, and Sendai virus. These studies corroborated the previous conclusions; lymph node and spleen cells from virus-immune hamsters were quite capable of killing target cells from Hm-1 disparate strains in an apparent unrestricted manner (9). Although the effector cells demonstrated antigen specificity, they were not T cells, as anticipated (10,11). Rather, the cytolytic immune response depended predominantly on natural killer cells and antibody-dependent cell-mediated cytotoxicity (ADCC) (12). Others had similar results with Pichinde and herpes simplex viruses (13,14) and with SV-40 transformed tumor cells (15).

Based on the earlier supposition of Zinkernagel and Doherty (16) that an advantage for survival of viral epizootics is bestowed on those species with expanded MHC polymorphism [and the breadth of antigens detected by T-cell populations (17)], Nelles and Streilein proposed that hamster T cells may have limited functional diversity, and perhaps limited development, of certain T-cell subpopulations. Those that mediate cytolysis and suppression, in particular, were lacking functionally (10,12,18) as measured by established immunological protocols and assays.

Lymphocyte subpopulations of discrete function have been defined most productively by the detection of unique cell-surface antigens. We addressed the dilemma of lymphocyte diversity in the hamster by generating a panel of monoclonal antibody reagents against MHC antigens and other molecules present on T lymphocytes, B lymphocytes, NK-cells, and other hematopoietic cells. Table 1 and Figure 1 summarize the tissue distribution and the existing biochemical identity of the cell-surface molecules detected with these monoclonal antibodies. In addition, Table 1 includes a synopsis of well-defined polyclonal reagents and cross-reactive monoclonal antibodies that have been useful in studies of hamster lymphocyte function.

II. HAMSTER B- AND T-LYMPHOCYTE SUBSETS DEFINED BY MONOCLONAL REAGENTS

A. The Distribution of Thy 1 Antigen on Hamster Cells

The Thy 1 antigen was one of the first and proved to be one of the most useful of mouse lympho-hemopoietic "markers." Because molecules homologous with mouse and rat Thy 1 have been detected on tissues from lower vertebrates and invertebrates as well as mammals (33,34), one might suppose that this cell-surface molecule performs some highly necessary and evolutionarily conserved function. Perhaps in nervous tissue this is true, since Thy 1 homologues have been found in the brains of all species tested (33). However, the expression of the Thy 1 antigen on lymphocytes varies among mammalian species (20,35-38), which suggests that the molecule may play different roles on different cells.

The distribution of Thy 1 on lymphocytes of the Syrian hamster was found to deviate from patterns described in mouse, rat, human, or dog (20). Highly absorbed goat anti-hamster thymocyte serum, the activity of which could be further absorbed

Table 1 Cross-reactive and Hamster-Specific Antibody Reagents

Designation		Subclass	Tissue distribution	Comments	Refs.
Cross-reactive to hamster					
Anti-Thy 1.2	HO-13-4	IgM	Thymocytes; peripheral T cells and B cells; natural killer cells	Negative cells include GD-36, PLA-1, plaque-forming cells	11,19-21
Asialo GM-1	Polyclonal (rabbit)	–	Natural killer cells		22-23
Anti-IE^k	14.4.4	IgG_2a	B cells; some thymocytes; thymic epithelial cells; GD-36; PLA-1	Precipitates 29-39,000 MW Ia-like dimer from lymph node	24-25
Monoclonal antibodies to hamster lymphocytes					
Anti-Ia	S11, S12, S34 P51 28	IgG_1 IgM IgG_2a	B cells, macrophages, Langerhans cells, some thymocytes, thymic epithelial cells; GD-36; PLA-1	Precipitates 29-39,000 MW Ia-like complex	25-26 47
Anti-T cell	20 110	IgM IgG_1	>90% of peripheral T cells; medullary thymocytes; <5% of bone marrow	Negative cells include B cells, GD-36, PLA-1, SA-7	26-27
	38	IgG_2a	Subset of peripheral T cells; 80% of thymocytes; <5% bone marrow	Present on cytotoxic T cells	26-27

(Table 1 *continues*)

Table 1 (*continued*)

Designation		Subclass	Tissue distribution	Comments	Refs.
Monoclonal antibodies to unknown hemopoietic antigens					
	25 P12	IgG IgM	>90% of thymocytes and lymph node cells; subset of spleen cells	Negative cells include GD-36, PLA-1, SA-7	26
	WIV3	IgG_1	>90% of thymocytes and lymph node cells; GD-36, PLA-1	Negative cells include SA-7	26
	106 WIII6	IgG_1 IgG_1	>90% of thymocytes and lymph node cells; GD-36, PLA-1, SA-7		
	17	IgG_1	99% of thymocytes and lymph node cells; SA-7	Negative cells include GD-36, PLA-1	26
Anti-NK cell	3G1.4 3D7.5	IgG_2a IgG_2a	Pulmonary NK cells; subset of spleen and lymph node NK cells; subset of T cells	Blocks NK lysis	28
Anti-macrophage	7C2G6 10A312F	IgG_2b IgG_1	Pulmonary macrophages	Blocks phagocytosis	29

GD-36 (30) and PLA-1 (31) are B-cell lymphomas. SA-7 (32) is a lymphoma of unknown lineage.

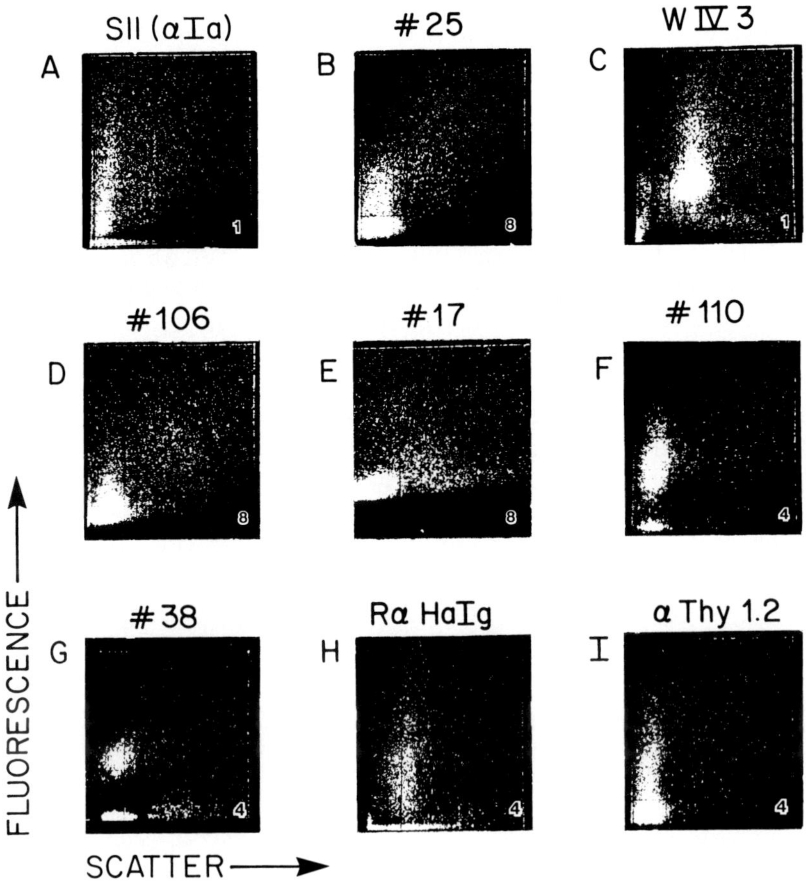

Figure 1 FACS-generated dot plots of lymph node cells stained with antibodies to hamster lymphocyte antigens. Shown are immunofluorescence patterns of several antibodies described in Table 1. Each represents a unique tissue distribution on normal lymphocytes or lymphoma cell lines. Fluorescence amplification settings are recorded in the lower right corner (gain 1-8; 8 is the most amplified). Fluoresceinated goat anti-mouse IgG (heavy chain specific) was used to reveal positive cells in panels A-G. Biotinylated anti-Thy 1.2 and fluorescein-conjugated avidin were used in panel I. Note that rabbit anti-hamster Ig (panel H) is not at saturating conditions here; at saturation, the intensity is comparable to mAb S11.

with hamster or mouse brain tissue, and a cross-reactive mouse monoclonal antibody to the Thy 1.2 alloantigen [(39) clone HO-13-4] bound to the vast majority of lymph node and spleen cells as well as thymocytes (10,11,20). Early studies noted that most T-cell responses to mitogen or alloantigen were removed by treatment with either of these reagents plus complement (10,11,19). B-lymphocyte functions were not effectively depleted. Such studies suggested that the hamster Thy 1 homologue adequately distinguished hamster T cells from other lymphocytes and that the T-cell compartment was unusually large. Yet, when hamster lymph node or splenic lymphocytes were stained with anti-Thy 1.2 or anti-immunoglobulin, flow cytofluorometry analysis clearly demonstrated an overlap in the frequency of cells detectable by either reagent alone (20). Minimally, 60% of sIg-positive cells also expressed Thy 1, and the amount of Thy 1 antigen that could be detected on the surface of peripheral sIg-positive cells was much greater than that found on peripheral T cells (Figure 2).

Thy 1-2-bearing cells were enriched from lymph nodes and subjected to several analyses to ascertain their identify (20). First, lymphocyte proliferation to B-cell stimuli, lipopolysaccharide or rabbit anti-Ig, was greater in the Thy 1-selected sub-

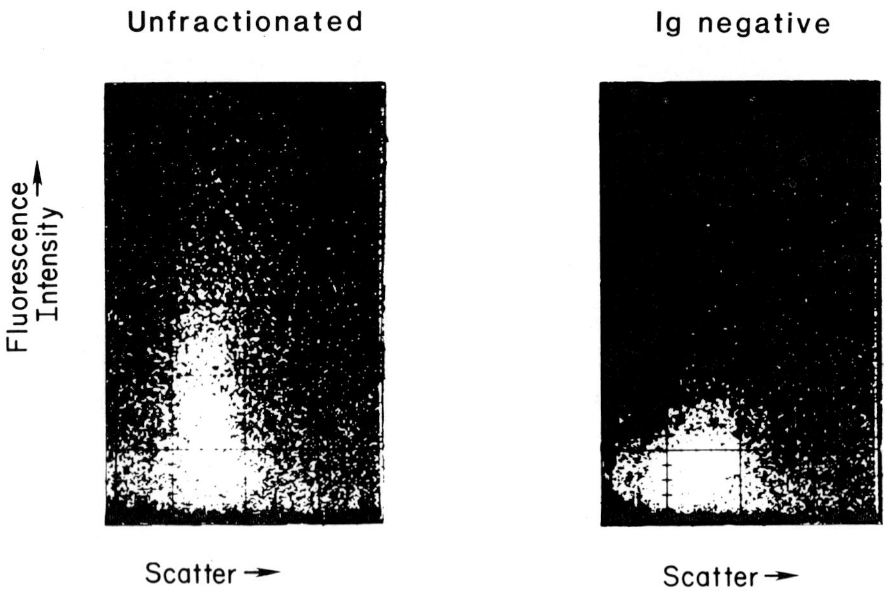

Figure 2 FACS-generated dot plots of LSH hamster lymph noae cells stained with biotin-labeled anti-Thy 1.2 and fluoresceinated avidin. In panel B, surface Ig-bearing cells have been depleted by incubation on anti-Ig-coated plates. [Reproduced from *J. Immunol., 131*:2903 (1983)].

population than with unselected cells. Second, those cells that simultaneously expressed surface Ig and Thy 1 were stripped of immunoglobulin by incubating with rabbit anti-hamster Ig. Cell-surface immunoglobulin was reexpressed within 24 hours by a proportion of cells expected if all Thy 1, sIg-positive cells were B cells (20).

It is interesting to compare the distribution of Thy 1 in the hamster and rat, as these are the only species described to date that possess Thy 1-positive B cells. In the rat, Thy 1 expression appears to be developmentally controlled (40). Immature forms of both T and B cells display Thy 1, whereas most mature, peripheral cells in the adult animal lack the antigen (35,40). An analogous scheme for hamster is not simply applied. Nelles et al. (19) previously observed that plaque forming cells against sheep erythrocytes were not removed by this Thy 1.2 reagent, and a hamster IgG1-bearing B-cell lymphoma, GD-36, and a plasmacytoma, PLA-1, also lacked Thy 1 expression. Cumulatively, these results implied that a major subset of hamster B-lineage cells, as well as all T cells, display the Thy 1 homologue, but Thy 1 expression disappears on antigen-activated or plasmocyte stages of the B lineage. The low frequency of positive cells in hamster bone marrow (11,20) further indicated that B-lineage cells that are early in the developmental pathway may not express Thy 1. Thus, it is likely that the Thy 1 homologue is expressed only on specific stages of the hamster B-lymphocyte lineage (Table 2). The pattern of Thy 1 expression on hamster cells is, therefore, unique to this species.

Extensive interspecies cross-reactivity has been observed with most heterologous anti-brain sera, even after absorption to remove nonlymphoid specific determinants. However, it was somewhat surprising to find that an anti-allotype specific monoclonal antibody reacted with appropriate tissue (brain and thymocytes) from a distant species. This observation indicates that the hamster Thy 1 polypeptide bears the Thy 1.2 allele. We have found that anti-Thy 1.1 antibodies do not bind to hamster lymphocytes. Other monoclonal antibodies (rat anti-mouse) to the Thy 1.2 allele bind only weakly (Witte, unpublished observations). The anti-Thy 1.2 used in the above studies has some cross-reactivity on Thy 1.1 thymocytes

Table 2 Summary of Thy 1 Expression on Hamster Lymphocytes

Differentiation stage	T lineage	B lineage
Immature	++	–[a]
Mature (resting)	+	++
Postactivation	+	–

[a]Assumed from the low frequency of Thy 1^+ cells in bone marrow.

but not lymph node cells. As this pattern is similar to one other monoclonal anti-Thy 1.2 (41), a slightly different epitope may be detected by clone HO-13-4 than by most anti-Thy 1.2 reagents. By anti-Thy 1 affinity chromatography, predominant bands of 26 Kd from mouse thymocytes and 28 Kd from hamster thymocytes were eluted at high pH (Witte, Streilein, and Spurgeon, unpublished observations). This strongly suggests that the anti-Thy 1.2, clone HO-13-4, recognizes the hamster Thy 1 homologue.

The precise cellular function of this widely distributed and conserved molecule is as yet unknown. Murine Thy 1 is anchored to the cell membrane via an uncommon association with a lipid domain rather than an intramembrane peptide, and the molecule is easily released from the surface of mouse T lymphocytes by phosphatidylinositol-specific phospholipase C (42). Evidence that activation kinetics are altered by either enzyme treatment (43) or by monoclonal anti-Thy 1 antibodies (44) suggests that the Thy 1 glycoprotein may act as a signal transducer (44). It will be important to compare the effects of such agents on Thy 1-positive B cells, T cells, and natural cytotoxic cells (see Section III) of the hamster.

B. The Distribution of Ia-like Molecules on Hamster Cells

Because some cell-surface products of the MHC in mouse and man can be used to discriminate lymphocyte subpopulations, the utility of the approach was explored in hamsters. Of the molecules encoded by genes within the MHC, class II molecules (murine Ia-like) have been especially useful in this regard because they are restricted in expression to certain subpopulations of lymphocytes and to a few nonlymphoid cell types.

Class II-like molecules have been described in hamster using polyspecific alloantisera, generated between classical inbred strains and partially inbred stocks acquired 16 years ago (5,7), and using cross-reactive murine alloantisera with activity to the Ia.7 determinants (45). Both types of reagents immunoprecipitate similar, but distinctly different, sets of cell-surface molecules of 29,000 and 39,000 molecular weight. Both sets of molecules co-precipitate with a third invariant chain that is typical of class II molecules in other species (24). One of the molecular sets is precipitated by a cross-reactive monoclonal antibody, clone 14.4.4, which is against the mouse Ia.7 specificity (anti-I-E^k). The hamster glycoproteins are possibly the I-E homologues (24). When analyzed by two-dimensional PAGE, a completely different set of Ia-like molecules is identified after immunoprecipitation with several hamster alloantisera, exemplified by MIT anti-MHA serum (24). Whether the molecules recognized by MIT anti-MHA represent the hamster equivalent of mouse I-A subregion glycoproteins or other different Ia-like molecules expressed on the surface of hamster lymphocytes is not yet known.

A panel of monoclonal anti-hamster Ia antibodies are described in Table 1. Each antibody precipitates from lymph node cells a 29-39,000 MW dimer by gel electrophoresis under reducing conditions. One of the first antibodies generated, S11, was used in further studies to determine if it bound to overlapping determinants of the known hamster Ia-like molecules or new determinants (25). The specificity of S11 was compared with the alloantiserum MIT anti-MHA and with the cross-reactive 14.4.4 monoclonal antibody by sequential immunoprecipitation. Whereas preclearing the lysate with MIT anti-MHA serum completely removed S11-specific determinants, molecules precipitated by 14.4.4 were not removed by preclearing with S11 (Figure 3). Therefore, the hamster specific monoclonal anti-Ia S11 detected a complex including that identified by the hamster alloantisera.

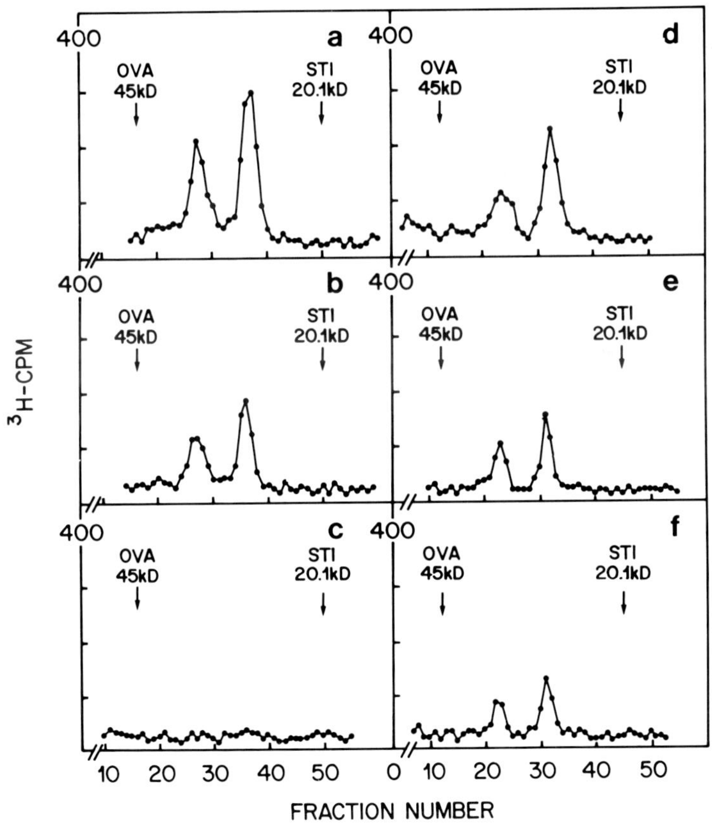

Figure 3 Hamster Ia antigens immunoprecipitated with monoclonal antibodies S11 (left column) and 14.4.4 (right column). Lymph node cells were labeled with ^{3}H-leucine and analyzed by SDS-PAGE. Panels a and d represent untreated lysates; panels b and e, lysates precleared with irrelevant ascites; and panels c and f, lysates precleared with S11 ascites. [Reproduced from *J. Immunol.*, *130*:2282 (1983).]

The tissue distribution of the two Ia-like molecular complexes was investigated by flow cytofluorometry using S11 and 14.4.4 (25). Similar to other mammals, the distribution of Ia on hamster cells is restricted to lymphoreticular cells (7,25). On spleen and lymph node cells, the two monoclonal antibodies bound to subgroups of cells, but these populations almost entirely overlapped. The subset of lymphocytes which displayed S11 and 14.4.4 determinants were largely B cells bearing surface IgM. Moreover, depletion or enrichment of S11-positive cells on antibody-coated dishes also removed or enriched a similar number of B cells. This indicated that among hamster lymphocytes, most, if not all, B cells bear Ia antigens and can be distinguished from T cells and other lymphoid cells with these anti-Ia reagents (25). These monoclonal antibodies have been extremely helpful in separating T and B lymphocytes for many studies.

In addition to B cells, Ia-like molecules have been found in very low levels on 20-30% of hamster thymocytes (25). Among nonlymphoid cells, hamster lung and peritoneal macrophages are known to express Ia (46), epidermal Langerhans cells are detected with monoclonal anti-hamster Ia (47), and thymic reticular epithelial cells display a pattern of Ia expression indistinguishable from that of murine thymus (Hoot and Witte, unpublished observations).

C. Monoclonal Antibodies that Distinguish Subsets of T-Cells

Most T-cell reactions to antigenic stimuli have been analyzed to some extent in the Syrian hamster. Similar to other mammalian species, the antigen-challenged hamster gives immune responses that depend on an intact thymus (10,48-50). In vivo alloantigen responses, such as acute skin graft rejection, delayed-type hypersensitivity reactions, and graft-versus-host reactions, are easily detected (51,52). Contact hypersensitivity to derivatizing haptens has been demonstrated (53,54), and this sensitivity can be transferred to naive recipients with immune lymphoid cells (55). Hamster T lymphocytes also proliferate vigorously in vitro to allogeneic or mitogenic stimuli. Clearly, hamster T cells respond as expected to most nonpathogen experimental agents. In contrast, experiments designed specifically to identify cytotoxic and suppressor functions mediated by hamster T cells have often met with difficulty.

In light of the monomorphism of hamster class I molecules and drawing from the conclusions of Swain (56) and Krensky et al. (57) that the phenotypic subsets of T cells are correlated primarily with the class of MHC antigen which they detect, a reasonable postulate (6,10) was that hamsters would have poorly developed responses requiring class I restriction (i.e., cytotoxic and some suppressor activity). All the responses cited above could be mediated by a single T-cell population, one analogous to the helper subset of mouse, rat, and man. However, other mechanisms, such as aberrant maturation or suppression of T-cell activity, might explain the apparent lack of certain T-cell functions in the hamster.

Because hybridoma antibodies have been produced successfully to functional T-cell subsets in many other species, we used this approach to ascertain if more than one T-cell population existed in the hamster. This was accomplished by selecting anti-lymphocyte hybridoma antibodies for differential tissue expression and for association with lymphocyte function.

1. Tissue Distribution of Anti-T-Cell Monoclonal Antibodies

Monoclonal antibodies 38, 20, and 110 (Table 1 and Figure 1) detected cell-surface antigens expressed by discrete subpopulations of hamster lymphocytes (26). The identities of these subpopulations were further resolved by removing Ia-positive cells (B cells) and enriching Ia-negative cells (T cells). Sixty percent of unselected lymph node cells were identified by mAb 110, and these were greatly enriched, to greater than 90% positive, by depleting B cells. Likewise, the percentage of lymph node cells that bound mAb 38 increased from 23 to 30% by removing Ia-positive lymph node cells. Isolated B cells did not bear these antigens. mAb 20 (IgM isotype) bound to a subset of peripheral and thymic lymphocytes with frequency similar to 110. Moreover, preincubation with 20 blocked the subsequent binding of 110, suggesting that the two antibodies bound to the same cell population and perhaps to the same molecule (Witte, unpublished observations). Complement-mediated lysis with mAb 20 effectively removed T-cells from the lymph node cell population; anti-Ia plus complement abolished B-cell activity. Both 20 and 110, therefore, detected most, and perhaps all, peripheral T cells.

2. Functional Dichotomy Defined with mAb 38

Monoclonal antibody 38 divided peripheral T cells into two subpopulations, 38^+ and 38^-. Many T-cell functions have been tested with 38-depleted cells and with 38^+ cells isolated by cell sorting, and the results of these experiments are summarized in Table 3. Proliferation to Con A or PHA was negligibly affected by removing 38^+ lymph node cells, if equivalent numbers of 38^- lymph node cells were analyzed. The response to alloantigenic stimulus also was not significantly changed by lysing 38^+ lymph node cells. Because class II, but not class I, hamster MHC antigens are allogeneic between the stimulating and responding cells, proliferation most likely occurred as a consequence of the Ia-like disparity. The 38^- lymph node cells were comprised, at least in part, of T cells analogous to $L3T4^+$ mouse T cells.

This conclusion was supported by other experiments. Like mouse effector T cells of Lyt 2-negative phenotype, 38^- lymph node cells elicited vigorous graft-versus-host reaction as measured by the popliteal lymph node hypertrophy assay (Table 4). Whether depleted of 38^+ cells or not, equivalent numbers of hapten-sensitized (to DNFB) lymph node cells were able to adoptively transfer a typical 48-hour contact hypersensitivity response to naive hamsters (Figure 4). Depletion of the subset that expressed 38-antigen seemed to alter the responses so little as to appear nonparticipating.

Table 3 Functional Abilities of T-Cell Subsets Distinguished by mAb 38

Function	38^- T cells	38^+ T cells
Proliferation to:		
Con A	+++	+
Con A + IL 2	+++	+++
Alloantigen	++	+
Contact hypersensitivity	+++	ND
Graft-vs.-host response	+++	ND
IL2 production	+++	±
IL2 receptor expression	+++	ND
Delayed-type hypersensitivity	+++	ND
Antigen-specific cytotoxicity	–	+++

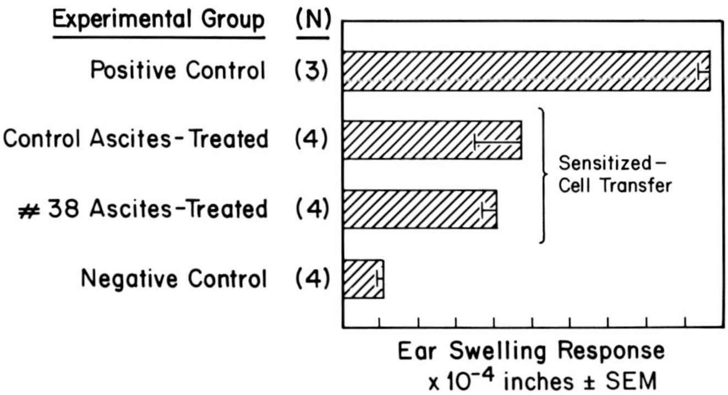

Figure 4 Adoptive transfer of contact hypersensitivity to DNFB. Lymph node cells (one donor equivalent) from DNFB-immune donors were inoculated intravenously into irradiated (250R) syngeneic recipients. The ears of recipients were challenged 1 hour later with dilute DNFB. Positive control animals were skin-painted with 0.5% DNFB and ear-challenged 5 days later with dilute DNFB. The ear swelling of normal animals challenged with dilute DNFB served as negative control. Presented is the mean ear swelling response (48 hours) ± SEM of four animals.

Table 4 Graft-Versus-Host Response by 38^- LSH Lymph Node Cells

Treatment of donor cells	F_1 host #	Weight (mg) of popliteal LN[a]		
		LSH donor LNC	F_1 donor LNC	SI
Control-treated	1	39.72	6.13	6.5
	2	31.48	6.85	4.6
	3	37.43	5.84	6.4
	4	24.92	5.85	4.2
			Mean SI = 5.4 ± 1.2[b]	
mAb38-treated	1	43.62	6.07	7.1
	2	77.37	8.67	8.9
	3	66.00	6.75	9.7
	4	103.86	18.53	5.6
			Mean SI = 7.8 ± 1.8[b]	

[a](MIT x LSH)F_1 female hamsters received 8 x 10^6 viable LSH lymph node cells in the right footpad. The contralateral footpad received 8 x 10^6 untreated F_1 lymph node cells.
[b]Average stimulation index (SI) ± SD.

To determine directly the responsive capabilities of the 38⁺ peripheral T-cell population, 38⁺ lymph node cells were labeled by indirect immunofluorescence and sorted with the fluorescence-activated cell sorter. The sorted cells were incubated with varying concentrations of Con A in the presence of adherent peritoneal cells to assure that a source of accessory cells was not limiting. Under these conditions, 38⁺ lymph node cells gave weak responses compared to stained, unsorted lymph node cells (Figure 5).

Several investigators have reported that Con A will induce proliferation of almost all mature mouse T cells if the correct environment is provided in vitro (58-60). Part of this environment is a nonlimiting source of interleukin 2 (IL 2). In the mouse, Lyt 2⁺ T cells require the presence of IL 2 or Lyt 2⁻ T cells for optimal proliferation to exogenous stimuli. We tested the assertion that IL 2 was the limiting factor in the proliferation of 38⁺ cells to Con A. 38⁺ lymph node cells gave greatly enhanced proliferation to mitogen if the cells were stimulated in the presence of exogenous IL 2 (Figure 5), up to 40 times greater than the enhancement of unsorted cells incubated with IL 2. The proliferation of 38⁺ lymph node cells to Con A in the presence of IL 2 implied that 38⁺ lymphocytes were fully functional T cells and that T-cell growth factor (TCGF) production was a limiting element in the proliferation of the 38⁺ subpopulation but not in the unsorted population.

A clear functional dichotomy was apparent between 38⁺ and 38⁻ T cells in the ability to produce IL 2. The IL 2 component of rodent TCGF is conserved in

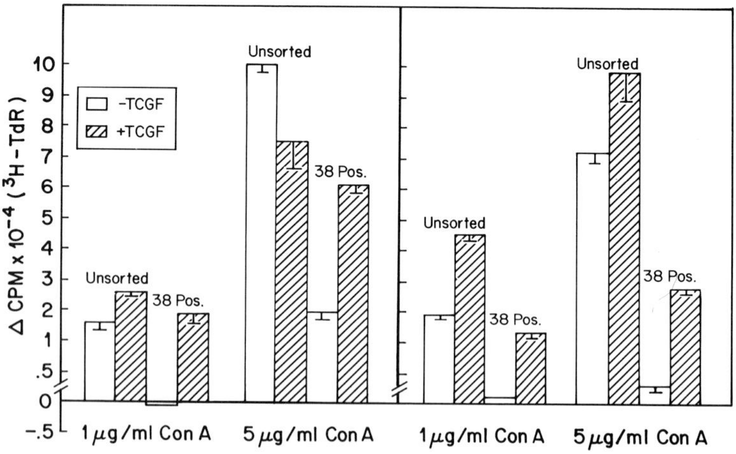

Figure 5 Proliferative response of FACS-sorted 38⁺ lymph node cells and thymocytes to Con A with or without addition of TCGF. Fifty thousand cells per well were tested and harvested at 72 hours. Each bar represents the mean cpm ± SD of four wells. Left, lymph node cells; right, thymocytes. [Modified from *J. Immunol., 134*: 2908 (1985).]

function; rat Con A-induced TCGF will support a mouse IL 2-dependent T-cell line (61). Supernatants from LSH hamster lymph node cells induced with Con A or alloantigenic stimulation also will support the mouse T-cell line, HT-2. The detectable amount of hamster IL 2 increased with time in the supernatants from unselected lymph node cells stimulated with Con A, and the kinetics and units of IL 2 produced were not altered by depletion of 38^+ cells. Moreover, isolated 38^+ lymph node cells produced only low levels of detectable IL 2; thus, their inability to respond to proliferative stimuli correlated with the lack of IL 2 produced. In comparison with mouse T cells, the hamster 38^+ subset was most like the Lyt 2^+ subset because IL 2-producers are infrequent, whereas IL 2-producing T cells are very frequent among the Lyt 2^- T cells (60,62,63). In most functions tested, 38^- T cells proved to be analogous to mouse Lyt 2^- T helper cells.

3. IL 2 Production by Hamster T Cells

Curiously, these studies did reveal a striking difference between hamster and mouse T cells. The proliferative response (determined by ^{3}H-TdR uptake) to Con A generally peaks at 48 hours and wanes thereafter with stimulated mouse cells. One reason for the decline is thought to reflect the availability of IL 2, most of which is eventually absorbed by IL 2 receptor-bearing cells (64). Proliferation of hamster T cells, stimulated by Con A, also peaks by 48 hours, but a decline in thymidine incorporation is not seen until after 96-120 hours of culture. Growth arrest may be entirely due to depletion of nutrients in the medium because detectable IL 2 levels remain high throughout the incubation period (Table 5). This phenomenon

Table 5 Proliferation and IL2 Production by Hamster Lymph Node Cells Stimulated with Con A

	△CPM ^{3}H-TdR			
Treatment	48 hr	72 hr	96 hr	
Normal mouse Ig + complement	157382	125734	132203	
mAb 38 + complement	137536	151068	130062	
	Units of IL2 in supernatant			
	24 hr	48 hr	72 hr	96 hr
Normal mouse Ig + complement	0.25	0.59	0.82	0.84
mAb 38 + complement	0.33	0.65	0.77	0.78

IL 2 is shown in arbitrary units as compared to the proliferation of HT-2 cells with a standard rat TCGF.

was also noted with alloantigen-stimulated T cells but not with LPS-stimulated cells.

The previous data implied that at least one population of hamster T cells required the presence of IL 2 for proliferation, and by inference these cells must express IL 2 receptors. We tested the expression of IL 2 receptors on unselected and 38^- lymph node cells by their ability to absorb hamster IL2 (64) after stimulation with Con A for 24-72 hours. Surprisingly, equal numbers of hamster (LSH) or mouse (B10.S) Con A-blast cells showed very different absorption efficiency. Neither unselected nor 38^- hamster blasts removed all the IL 2 activity (Table 6) whereas an equal number of mouse Con A blasts entirely depleted the ability of the conditioned medium to sustain proliferation of the IL 2-dependent line.

Several explanations might be posed. First, exhaustively washing the hamster blast cells may not remove all the IL 2 on the surface and thus block their absorbing capacity. Second, the hamster IL 2 receptor may not have the same up-regulated kinetics found with mouse and human T cells (65). Third, the hamster may possess only low-affinity IL 2 receptors (65). Fourth, another stimulatory activity may be present and absorbed by mouse Con A blasts but not by hamster Con A blasts. Several previous studies suggested that some hamster immune responses, once initiated, continued virtually unchecked, as if suppression or down-regulatory mechanisms were sluggish (18). Others noted that the proliferation stimulated by Con-A induced supernatants is genetically controlled and varies considerably with cells from different hamster strains (66). Our findings suggest that the regulation of IL 2 production and receptor expression may offer explanation for the previous results, and, again, incongruities have been found in the immune response patterns of hamsters and other rodents.

Table 6 Ability of Hamster Con A-Induced Blast Cells to Absorb IL2

Source of IL2		cpm of HT-2 cells
Experiment 1		
Unabsorbed supernatant		50551
Absorbed with mouse (B10.S) blasts–	72 hr	232
Absorbed with hamster (LSH) blasts–	24 hr	17126
	48 hr	12457
	72 hr	18937
Experiment 2		
Unabsorbed supernatant		39489
Control-treated blasts–	72 hr	14510
38^- blasts–	24 hr	10689
	48 hr	13497
	72 hr	13300

Standard Con A-induced hamster TCGF was incubated (4°C, 1 hr) with 30 x 10^6 hamster or mouse T-cell blasts at various times after culture with Con A.

4. Cytotoxic T Cells Distinguished by mAb 38

There were many indications that 38$^+$ hamster T cells were similar to mouse Lyt 2$^+$ cells and therefore should include killer cells if they existed in the hamster. However, intraperitoneal inoculation with several different viruses yielded enhanced natural killer activity and ADCC-mediated cytolysis, but T killer cells were not found in spleen and lymph nodes (10-12). Intratracheal inoculation of influenza virus, on the other hand, gave rise to virus-specific killer cells within 6 days (22,67,68), as well as cells that mediated a delayed-type hypersensitivity response when transferred to naive recipients (22). We used this model to determine if the effector cells were T cells and if the participating lymphocyte subsets could be discriminated with our monoclonal antibodies.

Approximately 31% of influenza-immune lung cells were identifiable T cells (mAb 20$^+$) and 22% were 38$^+$. When lung cells were treated with mAb 20 and complement, all virus-specific cytolytic and DTH activities were lost, demonstrating that the mediators were of the T lineage. Furthermore, lung cells depleted of 38$^+$ cells were also deprived of antigen-specific killer cell function. mAb 38, however, did not alter the ability of the immune cells to elicit a DTH response. Neither monoclonal antibody depleted nonspecific cytolysis due to natural killer cells (22,26,28).

In summary, hamster-specific mAbs, 20, 38, and 110 detect differentiation antigens found on T cells. mAbs 20 and 110 identify most peripheral T-lymphocytes, and mAb 38 divides these into two phenotypically and functionally discrete subpopulations.

One reasonable extrapolation from the above results is that the 38 marker may also distinguish class I and II restricted T-cell subsets. A direct test of class I restriction is, of course, difficult in the hamster, but it is unlikely that the influenza-specific cytotoxic T cells were restricted by class II molecules because the SA-7 target cells do not bear Ia antigens (26). However, in mixed lymphocyte culture, isolated 38$^+$ LNC did proliferate above background in the presence of F1-stimulating cells. This proliferation was always one-third to one-fourth that of unselected LNC, and addition of exogenous IL 2 enhanced the response (Table 7). A gene locus such as MIs has not yet been uncovered in the hamster. Because the only known MHC disparity between the responding and stimulating hamster cells used here are class II-like products, it must be considered that mAb 38 discriminates hamster T cells by function and not by MHC restriction alone.

D. Development of Hamster T-Lymphocyte Subpopulations

The generation of T-cell diversity and the generation of an effective antigen receptor repertoire are pivotal issues in the dilemma of hamster T-cell heterogeneity. Among the hypotheses that might explain the apparent limited function of cytotoxic T cells is the suggestion that a maturational aberration exists in the T cells of this species. Because the development of the thymic structure and the progression of T lymphocytes through the thymus appears to be highly conserved in ver-

Table 7 Proliferation of 38^{+} LNC to Allogeneic Stimulus

Stimulator	Responder[a]		Δcpm experimental[c] (control ± SD)	SI	% Specific increase with IL2[d]
(MITxLSH)F_1 LNC	*Unsorted LNC*	−IL2	1280 (114 ± 25)	12.2	
		+IL2[b]	1327 (415 ± 32)	4.2	−19.8%
(MITxLSH)F_1 LNC	*38-positive LNC*	−IL2	333 (93 ± 26)	4.5	
		+IL2	931 (372 ± 67)	3.5	+95.0%

[a]Fifty thousand cells/well, plated with adherent accessory cells, were harvested at 72 hours.
[b]Semipurified rat IL2 was purchased from Collaborative Research, Inc., and used at a final dilution of 1:100.
[c]Δcpm experimental = (cpm LSH LNC + F_1 LNC) − (cpm LSH LNC + LSH LNC).
[d]Percent specific increase in proliferation with IL2 added =

$$\frac{(\Delta\text{cpm experimental} + \text{IL2} - \Delta\text{cpm syngeneic stimulators} \pm \text{IL2})}{\Delta\text{cpm experimental IL2}} \times 100 - 100\%$$

tebrates, the processes of development and selection may be very similar and comparisons may be informative from species to species. We have used several conserved characteristics to follow development and ontogeny of hamster T-cell subsets distinguished by mAbs 110 and 38.

In many diverse species, including mouse and man, a seemingly redundant chorus of thymic markers hails to one point—the mass of cortical thymocytes differs vastly from medullary thymocytes. This forms the first line of phenotypic heterogeneity among developing T cells. In the hamster, mAbs 110 and 20 distinguished at least some medullary thymocytes from cortical thymocytes. This was shown by immunofluorescence on frozen sections of hamster thymus; mAb 110 bound only to medullary thymocytes (27). Taken as a whole, 110^+ thymocytes were also more resistant to cortisone treatment than were 110^- thymocytes (Table 8). Moreover, a majority of 110^- thymocytes were small in size and contained terminal deoxynucleotidyl transferase (TdT), whereas, 110^+ cells were medium sized (by flow cytometry) and virtually lacked the TdT enzyme. These criteria, which distinguish most cortical and medullary cells in mammals and birds, demonstrated that the hamster thymus was similar to that in other species.

As in mouse, rat, and man, further delineation occurred with markers of peripheral T-cell subsets. mAb 38 divided both 110^- and 110^+ cells into two subgroups, implying that the dichotomy of hamster T cells marked by our mAbs occurred in the thymus. Therefore, four subsets of thymocytes have been identified: 110^-38^+, 110^-38^-, 110^+38^-, and 110^+38^+. The largest subset 110^-38^+ was greater than 80% TdT positive and consisted of relatively cortisone-sensitive cells, which indicated that these are likely cortical thymocytes. The 110^-38^- subpopulation, on the other hand, was heterogeneous, and a small proportion of these were large thymocytes which contained nuclear TdT, a pattern characteristic of early subcapsular thymocytes. The remaining 90% of 110^-38^- cells were distinct in size (medium by light-scatter properties) and were relatively cortisone resistant. We believe that many of the 110^-38^- thymocytes may be found in the medulla of neonatal and adult hamsters and may be the immediate precursors of 110^+38^- peripheral T cells (27).

Although the expression of the 110 antigen marked peripheral T cells and was limited to medullary cells of the thymus, acquisition of the 110 antigen was not a hallmark of initial function, because 110^- thymocytes responded to mitogens and alloantigen. In postnatal hamsters, extremely few 110^+ cells were found in the thymic medulla until about 10 days after birth, although thymocytes from newborn animals are responsive to Con A. Selected 38^+ adult thymocytes were similar to their peripheral counterparts in dependence on exogneous IL 2 for proliferation. Thus, the functional dichotomy of peripheral T cells reflected an early separation of the subsets within or before entering the thymus (27).

How then does the schematic development of hamster T cells compare with murine and human models? Ultimately, one must beware that we draw from the

Table 8 Summary of the Maturational Characteristics of Four Thymocyte Subpopulations

Cell-surface phenotype	Expression of TdT	Cortisone sensitivity	Anatomical location	Presumed maturation status
110^-38^+	Majority of cells	Relatively sensitive	Cortex	Less
110^-38^+	None	Relatively resistant	Medulla	More
110^+38^-	None	Relatively resistant	Medulla	More
110^-38^-	Minority of cells	Relatively resistant	Medulla and cortex	Heterogeneous

same "thought collective" (69), but the hypothetical pathway proposed for hamster T-cell development (27 and Figure 6) is quite similar to that proposed recently by Scollay and Shortman (70) for the mouse. Either scheme derives from the interpretations of many investigators over the last several years (see Refs. 71-74 for brief reviews): The major thymic subsets are the progeny of a common thymic progenitor; minor thymic populations are likely to be points on a developmental continuum of the two major subsets; the two major subsets (helper and cytotoxic in the hamster) develop in segregated microenvironments within the thymus; peripheral T cells that migrate back to the thymus become a distinct medullary subpopulation.

It is now apparent that the hamster, for all its unusual characteristics in MHC genetics and T-cell function, is not significantly deviant in the development of those T lymphocytes. However, many interesting questions can be asked in this species because of the monomorphic MHC class I antigens, very short gestation time (only 16 days), and unique T-cell markers available. For instance, a critical issue is the actual extent of T-cell antigen receptor repertoire specificities. This might be approached by determining what xenogeneic MHC specificities hamster T cells can respond to or become tolerant to (75). Although environmental antigens are not thought to play a major role in T-cell development in the thymus, the hamster may present another view as the thymus is not fully formed ultrastructurally until 1 week after birth (76). Finally, a distinct subset of medullary cells, which share at least one characteristic with peripheral T cells, appears postnatally at a particular time in thymic ontogeny. The markers 110 and 20, therefore, may allow an analysis of the possible function of these T cells in the thymus.

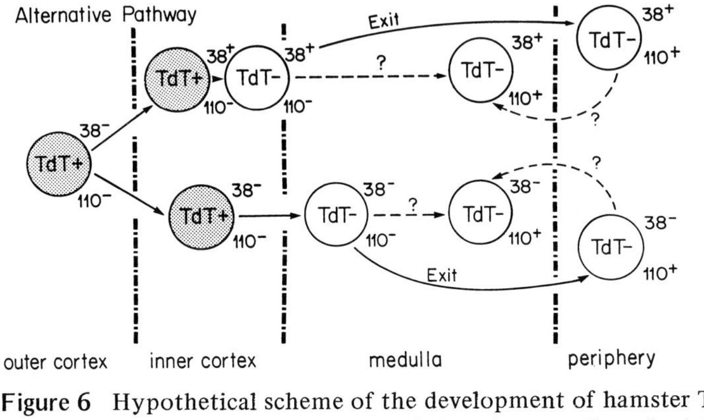

Figure 6 Hypothetical scheme of the development of hamster T-cell subsets in the thymus. This scheme is presented, based on studies of adult and neonatal tissues, as an alternative model to the conventional "straight-through" scheme. [Modified from *J. Immunol., 137*:45 (1986).]

III. ANTIBODIES THAT DISTINGUISH NATURAL KILLER CELLS

Historically, the natural killer (NK) cell and antibody-dependent cytotoxic cell (ADCC) were defined by functional properties (77,78). Recent information identifies these functions as properties of the same cells. Several surface markers have been identified on human and mouse NK cells, but only few are precise markers because their distribution is not restricted to the NK cell (79,80). However, some of these antibodies have been useful in defining NK-cell function because, while the antigenic determinant is expressed on many cell populations, not all cell types are susceptible to lysis by the antibody and complement.

An example of this kind of reagent is anti-asialo GM1 antibody, directed against a neutral glycosphingolipid, which is expressed by a variety of cells. Asialo GM1 is present on mouse thymocytes, some peripheral T cells, activated peritoneal macrophages, pulmonary macrophages, and NK cells (81-83). Prior incubation of mouse or hamster effector cell populations with rabbit anti-asialo GM1 (RAGM1) and complement removed NK activity and not cytotoxic T-cell or macrophage activity (23,81,84). Thus, RAGM1 antiserum is functionally specific for NK cells despite its wide distribution on bone marrow-derived cells. We have used this antibody in conjunction with anti-hamster T-cell mAbs 20 and 38 to demonstrate that effector cells that developed during a pulmonary influenza infection in hamsters were cytotoxic T lymphocytes and not NK cells (22). The RAGM1 is also useful for depletion of NK cells from hamsters or mice when given intravenously or intratracheally as well as by in vitro treatment. Cytotoxic macrophage activity was not affected by in vivo or in vitro administration of the antibody (23). Using RAGM1 in vivo to make NK-deficient hamsters (and mice), we demonstrated that NK cells contribute to the early defenses of the animals to influenza virus infections. Survival was significantly altered, and recoverable virus from lung was greatly increased in NK-deficient hamsters (and mice). A note of caution should be mentioned, however, as one group has reported that cytotoxic T-cell function is affected if the antibody is given at late stages of infection (85).

Another antigen that is similarly expressed by hamster and mouse NK cells is Thy 1. In the mouse it is known that there is a subpopulation of NK cells that express Thy 1.2 antigens (86,87). Yang and co-workers (11) demonstrated that in the hamster neither natural cytotoxic cells nor vaccinia-induced killer (K) cells express significant levels of Thy 1.2 homologue. However, later reports from this group of investigators showed that the Thy 1.2 homologue could be induced on hamster NK cells by co-culture technique and that nonspecific cytotoxicity was also apparent in the Thy 1.2 positive, nonadherent fraction of peritoneal exudate cells from vaccinia-infected hamsters (21). In our laboratory (Stein-Streilein) we were consistently able to eliminate the NK activity to SA-7 targets from lung and splenic mononuclear cell populations with anti-Thy 1.2 (Table 9) or RAGM1 (data not shown) plus complement. Pretreatment of the effector cells with complement

Table 9 Effect of Monoclonal Anti-Thy 1.2 Treatment on Lysis of SA7 NK Targets

	% Cytotoxicity[a] E:T ratio		
Tissue treatment	50:1	25:1	12.5:1
Experiment 1			
Lung + C[b]	14.3	12.8	12.6
Lung + C + anti-Thy 1.2	2.6	1.5	-0.1
Spleen + C	28.3	11.1	2.8
Spleen + C + anti-Thy 1.2	5.3	4.5	-1.0
Experiment 2			
Lung + C	12.5	27.1	24.8
Lung + C + anti-Thy 1.2	4.1	-0.4	12.6
Spleen + C	32.5	21.8	9.9
Spleen + C + anti-Thy 1.2	4.4	4.0	5.0
Experiment 3			
Lung + C	62.5	59.4	56.4
mAb20 + C	58.4	63.5	57.2
Anti-Thy 1.2 + C	8.2	6.7	5.4
Spleen + C	70.4	68.6	58.3
mAb20 + C	69.6	70.5	61.0
Anti-Thy 1.2 + C	7.1	7.0	5.1

[a]SEM was less than 5 in all cases.
[b]C, baby rabbit complement.

and anti-hamster T-cell mAb 20 had no effect on the lysis of the NK target. It is not known if RAGM1 treatment removes NK activity to vaccinia virus-infected BHK cells.

A major unresolved issue in the study of NK cells is the specificity of the effector-target cell interaction. A common approach is to analyze monoclonal antibodies which will block the lytic function of NK cells. At the very least, such reagents could be instructive as to the nature of the recognition and lytic process performed by these cells. RAGM1 will not block NK activity. Since the hamster utilizes its NK cells effectively, we theorized that this species is a good candidate from which to harvest NK cells and make monoclonal antibodies.

Monoclonal antibodies were made by standard procedures (88). Because we were particularly interested in NK-cell activity in the lung and in the potential compartmentalization of this activity (86,87), we used nylon-wool nonadherent mononuclear cells isolated from collagenase-treated hamster lungs as a source of NK antigens. Hybridomas were selected by positive reaction to nylon-wool nonadherent lung mononuclear cells and by negative reaction with RAGM1-depleted populations in an ELISA assay. Our efforts resulted in two hybridomas, 3G1.4 and 3D7.5 (both produce mouse IgG2a antibodies). These mAbs lysed NK cells and removed all NK activity from lung cell suspensions in the presence of complement. In addition, the mAbs were able to block NK activity after incubation of the effector cell population without complement. 3G1.4 and 3D7.5 blocked NK activity against both Yac-1 (mouse lymphoma target) and SA-7 cells, and the continued presence of antibody during the cytotoxic assay was not necessary to mediate this inhibition.

The antibodies removed all the NK activity from an isolated mononuclear cell population from the lung but only partially depleted NK activity in spleen, peripheral lymph node, and bone marrow cell suspensions. Moreover, intravenous administration of either antibody depleted NK activity in the lung and not in other lymphoid tissues. [Unlike the mouse, NK activity in the hamster is high in peripheral lymph nodes and bone marrow (23,89).] MAb 3G1.4 appears to be a murine autoantibody which similarly binds to mouse lung NK cells.

The molecules recognized by 3D7.5 and 3G1.4 are distributed on T cells as well as NK cells (Table 10). Lung cells detected by mAbs 20 and 28 (anti-Ia) are partially overlapping with 3D7.5$^+$ and 3G1.4$^+$ cells. Previous studies showed that mAbs 20 and 28 did not lyse NK cells (22). Functional studies have demonstrated that prior incubation with 3G1.4 and complement removed antigen-specific cytotoxic T-cell activity, and that 3D7.5 removed immune DTH activity to influenza virus. mAbs 3D7.5 and 3G1.4 obviously do not recognize the same epitope, since each is displayed on a separate T effector-cell subset, but both may be expressed on the same NK-cell population. In conjugate binding and single cell cytotoxic assays, we observed that these mAbs did not block conjugate formation but did inhibit lysis of the target cell. Thus, these antibodies define molecules that are not involved in NK target-cell recognition but are involved in lysis and have broad distribution on other lymphocyte lineages. Two molecular families have been defined on human and mouse cells by monoclonal antibodies that detect lymphoid and

Table 10 Cell-Surface Phenotype of Hamster Lymphocyte Subpopulations in the Lung

Cell type	RAGM1	Thy-1	#20	#28	#38	3G1.4	3D7.5
Natural killer cells	+	±	–	–	–	+	+
Cytotoxic T lymphocyte	–	+	+	?	+	+	–
Delayed-type hypersensitivity T lymphocyte	–	+	+	?	–	–	+

myeloid cells, and the anti-hamster NK antibodies may detect analogous molecules. Several of these reagents to T200 (common leukocyte antigens) and LFA-1 cell-surface glycoproteins will inhibit the NK target-cell binding and lysis (90,91). T200, in particular, is a likely candidate because of its display of heterogeneous epitopes on certain hemopoietic cells. Another molecule known to be present on both differentiated T cells and NK cells is the IL 2 receptor. One report (92) suggested a role for IL 2 in the function of NK cells; however, more studies are needed. The biochemical identification and functional role of the antigens detected by 3D7.5 and 3G1.4 on T cells is under investigation.

IV. THE ROLE OF REGIONAL IMMUNITY IN THE GENERATION OF EFFECTOR-CELL SUBSETS

In 1964, Gowans and Knight performed an important series of experiments. Using thoracic duct drainage, they discovered that recirculating lymphocytes passing through the lymph are not homogeneous (93). In particular, a subpopulation of IgA-bearing B cells did not migrate freely throughout the body but localized in the gastrointestinal tract. Based on these and related observations, the idea emerged that a segment of the immune system is dedicated to antigenic challenges that occur chiefly within the gastrointestinal tract. Subsequently, it was suggested that there might be integrated immunity for all mucosal surfaces (94). Such a common mucosal organ would include the respiratory tract, mammary gland, and conjunctiva.

The concept of regional immunity may embody many separate organ systems that respond to local antigenic challenge with little or no contribution from either systemic or mucosa-derived regulation or effector cells (23,95,96). It is now well accepted that lymphocyte populations vary from organ to organ. That is to say, there might be a 4:5 ratio of T to B cells in the spleen and a 7:3 ratio in the lymph nodes. The relative proportions of T-cell subpopulations, such as the T4:T8 ratio among human blood mononuclear cells, can be used to define certain disease states. One would expect that the T4:T8 composition would differ between lymphoid tissues. In the B lineage, the segregation of functional potential and anatomical location has been shown quite remarkably for subsets which produce certain immunoglobulin isotypes and subsets which secrete autoantibodies (97,98).

Before our studies of influenza virus infection in hamsters, little evidence existed to support the notion that hamsters mounted cytotoxic T-cell responses to any antigenic confrontation. Two other groups did characterize immune effector cells as T cells based on antigen specificity and time course of the response (67,68). Notably, both these studies were done with a respiratory virus, parainfluenza III virus. A clear definition of cytotoxic T-lymphocyte mediators was not possible at that time, because reliable reagents were not yet available and tests of MHC restriction were difficult.

While we could easily induce a cytotoxic T-cell response in the hamster lung to influenza virus, we were unable to induce a CTL response to the virus if it was inoculated by systemic routes. The ability to induce the development of cytotoxic T lymphocytes in the lungs and not in systemic lymphoid tissue by intratracheal inoculation and parenteral immunization, respectively, suggests that the potential or outcome of the immune response is not uniform throughout the body (22). Corroborative evidence also comes from a different system. O'Hara and Duncan (99) found that CTL precursors to xenoantigens were actually suppressed in hamster lymph node and spleen and were revealed only by special culture technique. Any of several interesting possibilities may explain the apparent disproportionate generation of anti-virus CTL in lung versus peripheral lymphoid tissues: (a) Hamster CTL may have a limited antigen specific repertoire and influenza virus happens to be part of that repertoire; (b) Antigen-specific CTL clones may be regionally distributed; and (c) The ability to develop CTL to virus may be dependent on local immunoregulatory events within each regional sphere of immunity. In this regard, the lung milieu may provide an effective environment for the maturation of CTL because there is an apparent absence of suppression of this response in the respiratory tract.

It is important to remember that not all lymphocytes migrate freely through the lymphatics and thoracic duct. For example, NK cells have access to tissues only through the blood vasculature (100,101). The potential exists for these effector cells to remain within the local organ and to remain responsive to the local regulation. In addition, cells migrating through the thoracic duct could circulate to specialized areas in a fashion similar to that described for the gut but within a small subloop unrelated to the common mucosal loop. The lung, defined as the lowest part of the respiratory tract, loses its mucosal lining as it prepares for gas exchange (102). Antigen presented to the lung must be transported to the hilar lymph nodes (or BALT) where primary immune responses take place. It would not be unreasonable to suggest that cells then return to the lung through specialized receptors on the high endothelial venules. Just as the mesenteric lymph node is involved in gut immunity and contains a unique distribution of lymphocytes such as T helper lymphocytes for IgA-producing B cells (98,103), regional lymph nodes might contain unique selection of various lymphocytes. Such a selection could include T-cell clones for respiratory viruses and not for gastrointestinal viruses.

Support for regional immunity also comes from the NK literature. We have shown that NK cells can be regulated locally (95). Intratracheal inoculation of influenza can selectively augment pulmonary NK activity in the absence of any systemic effect. In addition, in vivo administration of RAGM1 antiserum selectively depletes NK activity in the lung (23). Wiltrout and co-workers have demonstrated regional NK activity in the liver (104).

It is not surprising, then, that raising monoclonal antibodies to NK cells from the lung would produce specificities which distinguish lung NK cells from those in spleen, lymph node, and bone marrow. This emphasizes the possible heterogeneity of NK populations derived from various tissues and may reflect different activation or maturational points of a single lineage. Alternatively, our results may depict stable heterogeneity of NK cell subsets in different anatomical compartments. Because the comprehension of regional immunity is important to the understanding and treatment of various diseases, antibodies that distinguish cells within or trafficking to regional spheres of immunity should facilitate research in this area.

V. SUMMARY

All inbred strains of the Syrian hamster express monomorphic class I MHC molecules. This unusual characteristic has been linked to the apparent lack of cytotoxic and suppressor T-cell function in this species. We have used cell-surface phenotype, as discriminated with monoclonal and polyclonal antibody reagents, to identify subpopulations of T, B, and NK cells. Class II (Ia-like) antigens can be used to distinguish unstimulated T and B cells. In contrast to mouse cells, both T and B lymphocytes of the hamster express the Thy 1 antigen. Two monoclonal antibodies, 110 and 20, appear to bind to T cells exclusively, and another antibody, 38, divides T cells into two subsets. With these reagents we identified a subset of antigen-specific cytotoxic T cells (38^+) in the hamster. T cells which do not express the 38 antigen mediate delayed-type hypersensitivity response and helper cell function. By following the ontogeny of T-cell subsets in the hamster thymus, we found that T-cell development proceeds in a pattern comparable to other rodents, but it is extended well into neonatal life. The two functionally distinct, peripheral T-cell subsets form early in thymic development. Two other monoclonal antibodies have been prepared against pulmonary NK cells–3G1.4 and 3D7.5. Both block the lysis of NK-sensitive targets. These antibodies also bind to discrete T-cell subpopulations.

Yet to be explained is the apparent anomalous behavior of cytotoxic T lymphocytes to many viral antigens. Among the explanations considered are that the hamster possesses a limited antigen receptor repertoire, aberrant differentiation of the cytotoxic-cell subset, or regulation or suppression of these T cells occurs. Deficiencies in the development of CTL precursors is probably not at fault, because this subset is readily generated in virus-challenged lung tissue. Although we cannot discard the idea that hamster CTL are unresponsive to numerous antigens, we have entertained the notion that local regulatory networks suppress or expose certain functional subsets in different lymphoid tissues. In this regard, we demonstrated that CTL activity is augmented in the lung after exposure to antigen, whereas NK cells are the lytic effectors in peripheral lymph nodes and spleen. Certainly many questions remain unanswered about immunity in this curious species. The lack of class I MHC polymorphism, the possible link of this situation with the T-cell antigen receptor repertoire, the short gestation time and neonatal thymic development, and the apparent differential regulation of T cells in various tissues make Syrian hamsters a very interesting comparison to mouse, rat, and man.

ACKNOWLEDGMENTS

The generation of anti-hamster MHC and T-cell monoclonal antibodies was accomplished as partial fulfillment for the Ph.D. degree by P. Witte in the laboratory of Dr. J. Wayne Streilein. Dr. Streilein's support and insight were invaluable to this work. The anti-hamster NK-cell monoclonal antibodies were prepared by Ms. Judy Guffee. We thank Dr. Sabra Sullivan for expertise in the contact hypersensitivity experiments.

REFERENCES

1. G. Yerganian, History and cytogenetics of hamster, *Prog. Exp. Tumor Res., 16*: 2 (1972).
2. R. E. Billingham, Concerning the laboratory career of *Mesocricetus auratus* with special reference to transplantation, *Fed. Proc. 37*: 2024 (1978).
3. W. R. Duncan, and J. W. Streilein, Analysis of the major histocompatibility complex in Syrian hamsters II. Linkage studies, *Transplantation, 25*: 17 (1978).
4. W. R. Duncan, and J. W. Streilein, Genetic analyses of alloreactions between recently wild and classical inbred strains of Syrian hamsters: Evidence in favor of a major histocompatibility complex, *Immunogenetics, 13*: 393 (1981).
5. J. T. Phillips, J. W. Streilein, and W. R. Duncan, The biochemical characterization of Syrian hamster cell-surface antigens I. Analysis of allogeneic differences between recently wild and highly inbred hamsters, *Immunogenetics, 7*: 445 (1978).
6. J. W. Streilein, and W. R. Duncan, On the anomalous nature of the major histocompatibility complex in Syrian hamsters, *Hm-1, Transplantation Proc., 15*: 1540 (1983).
7. J. W. Streilein, J. T. Phillips, J. Stein-Streilein, D. A. Proia, and W. R. Duncan, Biochemical characterization of Syrian hamster cell surface alloantigens III. Hamster alloantisera immunoprecipitate class II-like, but not class I-like molecules, *Transplantation, 32*: 106-110 (1981).
8. A. G. Darden, and J. W. Streilein, Syrian hamster express two monomorphic class I major histocompatibility complex molecules, *Immunogenetics, 20*: 603 (1985).
9. M. J. Nelles, and J. W. Streilein, Immune response to acute virus infection in the Syrian hamster I. Studies on genetic restriction of cell-mediated cytotoxicity, *Immunogenetics, 10*: 185 (1980).
10. M. J. Nelles, and J. W. Streilein, Hamster T-cells participate in MHC alloimmune reactions but do not effect virus-induced cytotoxic activity, *Immunogenetics, 11*: 75 (1980).
11. H. Yang, C. A. Cain, M. C. Woan, and W. A. F. Tompkins, Evaluation of hamster natural cytotoxic cells and vaccinia-induced cytotoxic cells for Thy 1.2 homologue by using a mouse monoclonal anti-Thy 1.2 antibody, *J. Immunol., 129*: 2239 (1982).

12. M. J. Nelles, W. R. Duncan, and J. W. Streilein, Immune response to acute virus infection in the Syrian hamster II. Studies on the identity of virus-induced cytotoxic effector cells, *J. Immunol., 126*: 214 (1981).
13. S. R. Gee, D. A. Clark, and W. E. Rawls, Differences between Syrian hamster strains in natural killer cell activity induced by infection with Pichindi virus, *J. Immunol., 123*: 2618 (1979).
14. R. N. Lausch, N. Patton, and D. Walker, Natural cytotoxicity by hamster lymphoid cells for virus-infected and transformed cells, *Adv. Exp. Med. Biol., 134*: 135 (1981).
15. R. N. Lausch, J. Sofanko, and S. O. Prather, Analysis of sera from SV40-immunized and tumor-bearing hosts for blocking activity and antibody-dependent cellular cytotoxicity, *J. Immunol., 115*: 682 (1975).
16. R. M. Zinkernagel, and P. C. Doherty, H-2 compatibility requirement for T-cell-mediated lysis of target cells infected with lymphocytic choriomeningitis virus: Different cytotoxic T-cell specificities are associated with structures coded for in *H-2*K or *H-2*D, *J. Exp. Med., 141*: 1427 (1975).
17. M. Cohn, The T-cell receptor mediated restrictive recognition of antigen, *Cell, 33*: 657 (1983).
18. D. B. Lause, and J. W. Streilein, Lymphoid cell interactions in allograft immunity. Failure of hamsters to generate suppressor specific immunization, *Transplantation, 26*: 80 (1978).
19. M. J. Nelles, Ph.D. dissertation, University of Texas Health Science Center, Dallas, Texas, 1980.
20. P. W. Witte, and J. W. Streilein, Thy 1 antigen is present on B and T lymphocytes of the Syrian hamster, *J. Immunol., 131*: 2903 (1983).
21. H. Yang, C. A. Cain, and W. A. F. Tompkins, Induction of Thy 1.2 homologue positive and Thy 1.2 negative nonspecific cytotoxic lymphocytes in the hamster, *J. Immunol., 131*: 622 (1983).
22. J. Stein-Streilein, P. L. Witte, J. W. Streilein, and J. Guffee, Local cellular defenses in influenza-infected lungs, *Cell. Immunol., 95*: 234 (1985).
23. J. Stein-Streilein, and J. Guffee, In vivo treatment of mice and hamsters with antibodies to asialo GM1 increases morbidity and mortality to pulmonary influenza infection, *J. Immunol., 136*: 1435 (1986).
24. E. Sung, W. R. Duncan, J. W. Streilein, and P. P. Jones, Detection of two class II α:β:Ii complexes in the Syrian hamster, *Immunogenetics, 16*: 425 (1982).
25. P. L. Witte, and J. W. Streilein, Monoclonal antibodies to hamster class II MHC molecules distinguish T and B cells, *J. Immunol., 130*: 2282 (1983).
26. P. L. Witte, J. Stein-Streilein, and J. E. Streilein, Description of phenotypically distinct T lymphocyte subsets which mediate helper/DTH and cytotoxic functions in the Syrian hamster, *J. Immunol., 134*: 2908 (1985).
27. P. L. Witte, and J. W. Streilein, Development and ontogeny of hamster T-cell subsets, *J. Immunol., 137*: 45 (1986).
28. J. Guffee, and J. Stein-Streilein, Monoclonal antibodies that distinguish pulmonary NK cells harvested from other lymphoid organs, *Fed. Proc.* (abst.), *45*: 1117 (1986).

29. R. J. Parod, J. J. Godleski, and J. D. Brain, Inhibition of immune opsinin-independent phagocytosis by antibody to a pulmonary macrophage cell surface antigen, *J. Immunol., 136*: 2048 (1986).
30. J. E. Coe, and I. Green, B-cell origin of hamster lymphoid tumors induced by simian virus 40, *J. Natl. Cancer Inst., 54*: 269 (1975).
31. M. J. Nelles, R. L. Proia, D. A. Hart, L. Eidels, and J. W. Streilein, Unusual cell surface immunoglobulin on a plasma cell tumor, *Molecular Immunol., 16*: 535 (1979).
32. S. K. Datta, M. T. Gallagher, and J. J. Trentin, Natural cell-mediated cytotoxicity in hamsters, *Int. J. Cancer, 23*: 728 (1979).
33. A. F. Williams, and J. Gagnon, Neuronal cell Thy 1 glycoprotein: Homology with immunoglobulin, *Science, 216*: 696 (1982).
34. M. H. Mansour, and E. L. Cooper, Purification and characterization of *Rana pipiens* brain Thy 1 glycoprotein, *J. Immunol., 132*: 2515 (1984).
35. M. A. Ritter, L. K. Gordon, and I. Goldschneider, Distribution and identity of Thy 1-bearing cells during ontogeny in rat hemopoietic and lymphoid tissues, *J. Immunol., 121*: 2463 (1978).
36. S. V. Hunt, The presence of Thy 1 on the surface of rat lymphoid stem cells and colony-forming units, *Eur. J. Immunol., 9*: 853 (1979).
37. R. Dalchau, and J. W. Fabre, Identification and unusual tissue distribution of the canine and human homologues of Thy 1, *J. Exp. Med., 149*: 576 (1979).
38. J. McKenzie and J. W. Fabre, Human Thy 1: Unusual localization and possible functional significance in lymphoid tissues, *J. Immunol., 126*: 843 (1981).
39. A. Marshak Rothstein, P. Fink, T. Gridley, D. H. Raulet, M. J. Bevan, and M. L. Gefter, Properties and applications of monoclonal antibodies directed against determinants of the Thy 1 locus, *J. Immunol., 122*: 2491 (1979).
40. J. M. Crawford, and I. Goldschneider, Thy 1 antigen and B lymphocyte differentiation in the rat, *J. Immunol., 124*: 969 (1980).
41. H. Auchincloss, Jr., K. Ozato, and D. H. Sachs, A monoclonal antibody detecting unusual Thy 1 determinants, *J. Immunol., 128*: 1584 (1982).
42. R. A. Kroczek, K. C. Gunter, B. Seligmann, and E. M. Shevach, Induction of T cell activation by monoclonal anti-Thy 1 antibodies, *J. Immunol., 136*: 4379 (1986).
43. M. G. Low, and P. W. Kincade, Phosphatidylinositol is the membrane-anchoring domain of the Thy 1 glycoprotein, *Nature, 318*: 62 (1985).
44. J. Stiernberg, M. G. Low, and P. W. Kincade, Activation of surface Thy 1 depleted lymphocytes, *J. Cell. Biochem.* (suppl.), *10c*: 206 (1986).
45. J. T. Phillips, W. R. Duncan, J. Klein, and J. W. Streilein, Immunochemical detection of hamster class II MGC homologues by murine anti-Ia sera. *Immunogenetics, 9*: 477 (1979).
46. J. Stein-Streilein, Allergic contact dermatitis induced by intratracheal administration of hapten, *J. Immunol., 131*: 1748 (1983).
47. S. Sullivan, P. R. Bergstresser, and J. W. Streilein, Intravenously injected, TNP-derivatized, Langerhans cell-enriched epidermal cells induce contact hypersensitivity in Syrian hamsters, *J. Invest. Derm., 84*: 249 (1985).

48. J. L. Cook, A. M. Lewis, and C. H. Kirkpatrick, Age related and thymus dependent rejection of adenovirus 2-transformed cell tumors and immune responsiveness in Syrian hamsters, *Cancer Res., 39*: 4949 (1979).
49. D. P. Byington, and K. P. Johnson, Subacute sclerosing panencephalitis virus in immunosuppressed adult hamsters, *Lab. Invest., 32*: 91 (1975).
50. K. P. Johnson, E. G. Feldman, and D. P. Byington, Effect of neonatal thymectomy on experimental subacute sclerosing panencephalitis in adult hamsters, *Infection and Immunity, 12*: 1464 (1975).
51. W. R. Duncan, and J. W. Streilein, Analysis of the major histocompatibility complex in Syrian hamsters III. Cellular and humoral immunity to alloantigens, *J. Immunol., 118*: 832 (1977).
52. W. R. Duncan, and J. W. Streilein, Analysis of the major histocompatibility complex in Syrian hamsters I. Skin graft rejection, graft-versus-host reaction, mixed lymphocyte reactions, and immune response genes in inbred strains, *Transplantation, 25*: 12 (1978).
53. J. W. Streilein, S. Sullivan, and S. Thompson, Contact hypersensitivity, humoral immunity, and specific unresponsiveness can be induced in Syrian hamsters with simple haptens, *J. Immunol., 124*: 577 (1980).
54. H. C. Maguire, Allergic contact dermatitis in the hamster, *Invest. Dermatol., 75*: 166 (1980).
55. J. W. Streilein, P. L. Witte, K. Burnham, and P. R. Bergstresser, Induction and regulation of contact hypersensitivity in Syrian hamsters, *Adv. Exp. Med. Biol., 134*: 43 (1981).
56. S. L. Swain, T cell subsets and the recognition of MHC class, *Immunol. Rev., 129*: 142 (1983).
57. A. M. Krensky, C. A. Reiss, J. W. Mier, J. L. Strominger, and S. J. Burakoff, Long-term human cytolytic T cell lines allospecific for HLA-Dr6 antigen are $OKT4^+$, *Proc. Natl. Acad. Sci., 79*: 2365 (1982).
58. A. Wilson, W.-F. Chen, R. Scollay, and K. Shortman, Semi-automated limit dilution assay and clonal expansion of all T-cell precursors of cytotoxic lymphocytes, *J. Immunol. Methods, 52*: 283 (1982).
59. W.-F. Chen, A. Wilson, R. Scollay, and K. Shortman, Limit-dilution assay and clonal expansion of all T cells capable of proliferation, *J. Immunol. Methods, 52*: 307 (1982).
60. K. Pfizenmaier, P. Scheurich, W. Daubener, M. Kronke, M. Rollinghoff, and H. Wagner, Quantitative representation of all T cells committed to develop into cytotoxic effector cells and/or interleukin 2 producing helper cells with murine T-lymphocyte subsets, *Eur. J. Immunol., 14*: 33 (1984).
61. P.-A. Guerne, P.-F. Piguer, and P. Vassali, Positively selected Lyt 2^+ and Lyt 2^- mouse T lymphocytes are comparable, after Con A stimulation in release of IL2 and of lymphokines acting on B cells, macrophages, and mast cells but differ in interferon production, *J. Immunol., 130*: 2225 (1983).
62. R. A. Miller, and O. Stutman, Enumeration of IL 2 secreting helper T cells by limiting dilution analysis, and demonstration of unexpectedly high levels of IL 2 production per responding cell, *J. Immunol., 128*: 2258 (1982).

63. S. Gillis, M. M. Ferm, W. Ou, and K. A. Smith, T cell growth factor: Parameters of production and a quantitative microassay for activity, *J. Immunol., 120*: 2027 (1978).
64. J. J. Farrar, W. R. Benjamin, M. L. Hilfiker, M. Howard, W. L. Farrar, J. Fuller-Farrar, The biochemistry, biology, and role of interleukin 2 in the induction of cytotoxic T cells and antibody-forming B cell responses, *Immunol. Rev., 63*: 129 (1982).
65. T. Waldmann, The structure, function, and expression of interleukin-2 receptors on normal and malignant lymphocytes, *Science, 232*: 727 (1986).
66. K. E. Wright, D. A. Clark, and W. E. Rawls, Differences in lymphocyte responsiveness to lymphokines in two inbred strains of Syrian hamster, *J. Immunol., 133*: 286 (1984).
67. F. W. Henderson, Pulmonary cell-mediated cytotoxicity in hamsters with parainfluenza virus type 3 pneumonia, *Am. Rev. Respir. Dis., 120*: 41 (1979).
68. K. A. Kimmel, P. R. Wyde, and W. P. Glezen, Evidence of a T-cell mediated cytotoxic response to parainfluenza virus type 3 pneumonia in hamsters, *J. Reticuloendothelial Soc., 31*: 71 (1982).
69. L. Fleck, *Genesis and Development of a Scientific Fact*, University of Chicago Press, Chicago, 1979.
70. R. Scollay, and K. Shortman, Identification of early stages of T lymphocyte development in the thymus cortex and medulla, *J. Immunol., 134*: 3632 (1985).
71. R. Scollay, and K. Shortman, Thymocyte subpopulations: An experimental review, including flow cytometric cross-correlations between the major murine thymocyte markers, *Thymus, 5*: 245 (1983).
72. R. H. Ceredig, and H. R. MacDonald, Intrathymic differentiation: Some unanswered questions, *Surv. Immunol. Res., 4*: 87 (1985).
73. B. Adkins, C. Mueller, C. Y. Okada, R. A. Reichert, I. L. Weissman, and G. J. Spangrude, Early events in T-cell maturation, *Ann. Rev. Immunol., 5*: 325 (1987).
74. B. J. Fowlkes, and B. J. Mathieson, Intrathymic differentiation: Thymocyte heterogeneity and the characterization of early T-cell precursors, *Surv. Immunol. Res., 4*: 96 (1985).
75. R. O'Hara, Ph.D. dissertation, University of Texas Health Science Center, Dallas, Texas, 1985.
76. P. L. Witte, J. W. Streilein, and W. A. Shannon, Jr., C-type particles in thymic development: A correlation with thymic function, *Adv. Exp. Med. Biol., 134*: 455 (1981).
77. R. B. Herberman, and H. T. Holden, Natural cell mediated immunity, *Adv. Cancer Res., 27*: 305 (1978).
78. J. C. Roder, K. Kane, and R. Kiessling, Natural killer cells, *Prog. Allergy, 28*: 66 (1981).
79. H. Cantor, M. Kasai, F. Shen, L. C. Leclec, and L. Glimcher, Immunogenetic analysis of "natural killer" activity in the mouse, *Immunol. Rev., 44*: 3 (1974).
80. T. Abo, and C. M. Balch, A differentiation antigen of human NK and K cells identified by a monoclonal antibody (HNK-1), *J. Immunol., 127*: 1024 (1981).

81. M. Kasai, M. Iwamore, Y. Nagai, K. Okumura, and T. Tada, A glycolipid on the surface of mouse natural killer cells, *Eur. J. Immunol., 10*: 175 (1980).
82. K. Akagawa, and T. Tokunaga, Appearance of cell surface antigen associated with the activation of peritoneal macrophages in mice, *Microbiol. Immunol., 26*: 831 (1982).
83. K. Akagawa, Y. Maruyama, M. Takano, M. Kasai, and K. Tokunaga, A cell surface antigen expressed on mouse lung macrophages, *Microbiol. Immunol., 25*: 1215 (1981).
84. I. D., Kawase, L. Urdal, C. G. Brooks, and C. S. Henney, Selective depletion of NK cell activity *in vivo* and its effects on growth of NK sensitive and NK resistant tumor cell variants, *Intl. J. Cancer, 29*: 567 (1982).
85. L. Stitz, J. Baenziger, H. Pircher, H. Hengartner, and R. M. Zinkernagel, Effect of rabbit anti-asialo GM1 treatment in vivo or with anti-asialo GM1 plus complement in vitro on cytotoxic T cell activities, *J. Immunol., 136*: 4674 (1986).
86. R. B. Herberman, M. E. Nunn, and H. T. Holden, Low density of Thy-1 antigen on mouse effector cells mediating natural cytotoxicity against tumor cells, *J. Immunol., 121*: 304 (1978).
87. J. Stein-Streilein, M. Bennett, D. Mann, and V. Kuman, Natural killer cells in mouse lung: surface phenotype preference and response to local influenza virus infection, *J. Immunol., 131*: 2699 (1983).
88. G. Kohler, and C. Milstein, Derivation of specific antibody-producing tissue culture and tumor lines by cell fusion, *Eur. J. Immunol., 6*: 15 (1976).
89. J. J. Trentin, and S. K. Datta, Natural killer (NK) cells in hamsters and their modulation in tumorigenesis, *Adv. Exp. Med. Biol., 134*: 153 (1981).
90. R. L. Sparrow, and I. F. C. McKenzie, A function for human T200 in natural killer cytolysis, *Transplantation, 36*: 166 (1983).
91. A. M. Krensky, S. J. Mentzer, C. Clayberger, D. C. Anderson, F. C. Schmalstieg, S. J. Burakoff, and T. A. Springer, Heritable lymphocyte function-associated antigen-1 deficiency: abnormalities of cytotoxicity and proliferation associated with abnormal expression of LFA-1, *J. Immunol., 135*: 3102 (1985).
92. W. Domgiz, and B. M. Stadler, The relationship between human natural killer cells and interleukin 2, in *NK Cells and Other Natural Killer Cells* (R. B. Herberman, ed.), Academic Press, New York, 1982, p. 409.
93. J. L. Gowans, and E. J. Knight, The route of recirculation of lymphocytes in the rat, *Proc. Soc. Lond., 159*: 257 (1964).
94. J. Bienenstock, M. McDermott, D. Befus, and M. O'Neilt, A common mucosal immunological system involving the bronchies, breast, and bowel, *Adv. Exp. Med. Biol., 107*: 53 (1978).
95. D. W. Mann, G. Sonnefeld, and J. Stein-Streilein, Pulmonary compartmentalization of interferon and natural killer cell activity, *Proc. Biol. Exp. Med., 180*: 224 (1985).
96. J. W. Streilein, Skin-associated lymphoid tissues (SALT): Origins and functions, *J. Invest. Dermatol., 80*: 125 (1983).
97. K. Hayakawa, R. R. Hardy, M. Honda, L. A. Herzenberg, A. D. Steinberg, and L. A. Herzenberg, Ly-1 B cells: Functionally distinct lymphocytes that secrete IgM autoantibodies, *Proc. Natl. Acad. Sci., 81*: 2494 (1984).

98. H. Kawanishi, L. E. Saltzman, and W. Strober, Characteristics and regulatory function of immune Con A-induced cloned T-cells obtained from Peyer's patches and spleen: Mechanisms regulating isotype-specific immunoglobulin production by Peyers patch B-cells, *J. Immunol., 129*: 475 (1982).
99. R. M. O'Hara, Jr. and W. R. Duncan, Antigen-specific xenogeneic CTL activity in the Syrian hamster, *J. Immunol., 133*: 1163 (1984).
100. C. W. Reynolds, A. C. Denn III, T. Barlozzori, R. H. Wiltrout, D. A. Reichardt, and R. B. Herberman, Natural killer activity in the rat. IV. Distribution of large granular lymphocytes (LGL) following intravenous and intraperitoneal transfer, *Cell. Immunol., 86*: 371 (1984).
101. B. Rolstad, R. B. Herberman, and C. W. Reynolds, Natural killer activity in the rat. V. The circulation patterns and tissue localization of peripheral blood large granular lymphocytes (LGL), *J. Immunol., 136*: 2800 (1986).
102. M. Whitcomb, *Normal structure and function in "the lung normal and diseased,"* The C. V. Mosby Company, St. Louis, Missouri, 1982, p. 3.
103. R. A. Allardyce, and J. Bienenstock, The mucosal immune system in health and disease with an emphasis on parasitic infection, *Bulletin W.H.O., 62*: 7 (1984).
104. R. H. Wiltrout, B. J. Mathieson, J. E. Talmadge, C. W. Reynolds, S. R. Zhang, R. H. Herberman, and J. R. Ortaldo, Augmentation of organ associated natural killer activity by biological response modifiers: isolation and characterization of large granular lymphocytes from the liver, *J. Exp. Med., 160*: 1431 (1984).

9
Differentiation and Function of Lymphohemopoietic Cells in the Dog

WARREN C. LADIGES
Fred Hutchinson Cancer Research Center and University of Washington, Seattle, Washington

H. JOACHIM DEEG,* JOSEPH A. APRILE, ROBERT F. RAFF, FRIEDRICH SCHUENING, AND RAINER STORB
Fred Hutchinson Cancer Research Center, Seattle, Washington

I. INTRODUCTION

We have chosen to broadly define differentiation and function of canine lymphohemopoietic cells (LHC) to include the canine major histocompatibility complex (DLA). An attempt will be made to correlate specific antigens with comparable systems in mouse and man. Our interest in the functional characteristics of canine LHC is related to their role in bone marrow engraftment, tolerance, and development of graft-versus-host disease (1). Since the DLA complex has been a focus of many of our studies, we will begin our discussion by presenting a brief updated overview.

The genetic organization of DLA appears similar to HLA of man, in that three loci (A, B, and C) code for antigens identified by alloantisera, and a fourth locus or region (D) codes for antigens recognized in the mixed lymphocyte culture (MLC). However, alloantisera specific for antigens analogous to human DR, DP, or DQ molecules have not yet been described.

The Third International Workshop on Canine Immunogenetics, conducted in 1984, confirmed the serological definition for alleles DLA-A2,A3,A9; DLA-B4, B5,B6,B13; DLA-C11(Cw1) and C12(Cw2) as shown in Table 1 (2). Two new specificities (Aw14 and Aw15) were assigned to the DLA-A locus. A third specificity (Cw3) was assigned to the DLA-C locus. Mixed leukocyte culture (MLC) data, using 80 potential homozygous typing cells (HTC), were sorted according

**Present affiliation*: Lombardi Cancer Research Center, Georgetown University, Washington, D.C.

Table 1 DLA Determinants as Defined by the Third International Canine Immunogenetics Workshop[a]

DLA-A	*-B*	*-C*	*-D*
2	4	w1	w1
3	5	w2	w2
9	6	w3	w3
w14	13		w4
w15			w5
			w6
			w7
			w8
			w9
			w10

[a]See Refs. 3 and 4.

to "nonresponses" or "typing responses," which allowed for identification of 10 groups or clusters (3), designated as Dw1 to Dw10 (Table 1).

Class I and class II antigens are descriptive terms originally used for the mouse H-2 system. Typical class I antigens are defined biochemically as dimers of a 45 Kd glycoprotein noncovalently linked to $\beta 2$ microglobulin, which is a 12 Kd glycoprotein. Class II antigens are biochemically defined as glycoprotein dimers consisting of a 28-29 Kd chain and a 33-35 Kd chain, termed β and α, respectively. The term "Ia antigen" has become synonymous with class II antigens in the mouse (4) and will be used interchangeably with class II antigens in the dog.

Apart from serological workshop studies, canine class I antigens have received relatively little attention in the literature. A biochemical study of class I antigens using two-dimensional gel electrophoresis presented evidence of only a single locus coding for class I determinants (5). The development of mAbs to class I antigens might provide additional tools to help establish the validity of this initial finding. A number of class I-specific mAbs generated against man and domestic animals have been shown to cross-react with canine PBMC (Table 2). However, none have been tested biochemically to confirm the identity of the typical class I molecule using canine cell lysate. One mAb, 60.5, specific for HLA-A determinants (P. Beatty, personal communication), cross-reacts in a monomorphic fashion in the dog, but radioimmunoprecipitation studies in our laboratory using SDS-PAGE have not indicated identity of the typical 45 and 12 Kd molecular structure. mAb 60.5 was studied in the functional assays and shown not to interfere with CML, MLC, or mitogen stimulation. mAb H58A, a less-studied mAb specific for bovine class I antigen (6), inhibited all three in vitro functions.

Table 2 Murine Monoclonal Antibodies Generated Against Major Histocompatibility Antigens of Dog or Other Species Reactive with Canine Peripheral Blood Mononuclear Cells

mAb	Ig isotype	Specificity	Comments	Source
60.5	IgG3	class I HLA		Beatty,Seattle
H58a	IgG2	class I BOLA	Inhibits MLC	Davis,Pullman,WA
7.2	IgG2b	class II HLA-DR	Stem cells	Hansen,Seattle
HB10a	IgG2a	class II HLA-DR+DP	Inhibits MLC	Clark,Seattle
$ISCR_3$	IgG2b	class II H-2,DR		Watanabe,NIH
I-3.1	IgM	class II HLA-DP	18% PBMC[a]	Pesando,Seattle
H81-98.21[b]	IgG2a	class II H-2,DR		Pierres,Marseille, France
H40-315.7[b]	IgG2a	class II H-2,DR+DQ		Pierres,Marseille
H74-202.2[b]	IgG2a	class II H-2,DR		Pierres,Marseille
H40-164.3[b]	IgG2a	class II H-2,DR		Pierres,Marseille
7.5.10.1[c]	IgG2b	class II HLA		Doveren,Maastricht, The Netherlands
62.3.34[c]	IgG2b	class II HLA		Doveren,Maastricht, The Netherlands
1.41[c]	IgG	class II HLA	B cells	Doveren,Maastricht, The Netherlands
H76[c]	IgM	class II rat	B cells	Doveren,Maastricht, The Netherlands
c1A[c]	IgG3	class II HLA		Iwaki,Los Angeles
B1F6	IgG2a	class II, canine, DR+DP	blocks MLC	Alejandro,Miami
W3G10	IgM	DLA associated, p39	polymorphic	Ladiges,Seattle

[a]Percent reactivity as determined by indirect cytofluorescence (FACS 440).
[b]mAbs courtesy of Dr. P. Mannoni, Edmonton, Canada.
[c]Studies with these mAbs not performed in our laboratory.

mAbs specific for Ia antigens have been found to identify typical class II antigens in the dog (Table 2). mAb 7.2, specific for a framework determinant of human Ia antigens (7) was used to show that, in contrast to mouse and man, but similar to guinea pig (8) and swine (9), most mature canine T lymphocytes express Ia-like antigens (10). This has been confirmed with additional mAbs specific for Ia-framework determinants, including B1F6 for canine (11), ISCR3 for murine (12), and HB10a for human (E. Clark, personal communication). These antibodies were also examined for their effect on MLC and CML reactivity (13). All antibodies abrogated lysis of target cells when alloantigen-primed CTL were pretreated with mAb and C'. B1F6 and HB10a, both reactive with HLA-DR and HLA-DP positive human lymphoblastoid cells, decreased the MLC response when added to cells on day 0 (Figure 1). ISCR3 and 7.2, reactive with HLA-DR but not with DP-positive lymphoblastoid cells, had no effect on MLC responses. These results suggest that the more broadly reactive mAbs (in man) may be of interest to determine functional relevance of Ia antigens in the dog. An additional mAb, I-3.1 (human Ia framework), which is less reactive with canine T cells and reactive with HLA-DP but not DR-positive lymphoblastoid cells, also did not inhibit MLC. Other

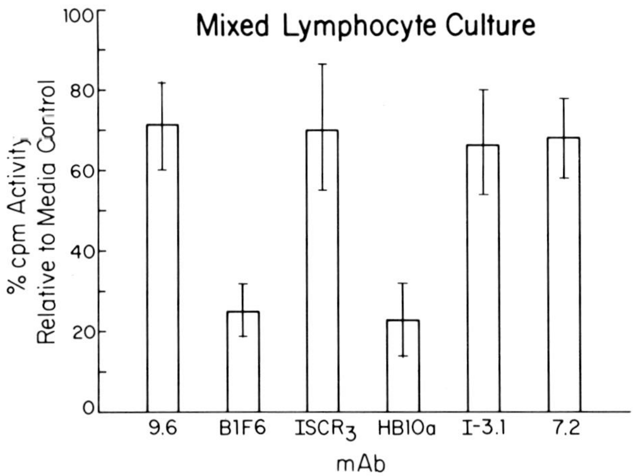

Figure 1 Mixed lymphocyte cultures were treated with mAbs by adding, on day 0 of a 7-day assay, 25 μl mAb to 1 x 10^5 responder cells and 1 x 10^5 stimulator cells suspended in 200 μl media per well (in triplicate). All mAbs except 9.6, specific for human T-cell erythrocyte receptor and nonreactive in the dog (irrelevant control), recognize framework determinants of Ia-like antigens (B1F6 for dog, ISCR3 for mouse and HB10a, I-3.1 and 7.2 for human) and are reactive with canine PBMC. All were used as purified supernatant. Values represent the percent reactivity, compared to media controls, of median cpm from MLC using ten unrelated dogs.

mAbs that identify Ia-like antigens in the dog (Table 2) include H81.98.21, H40-315.7 and 1474.202.2 (14), 7.5.10.1, 62.3.34, 1.41 and H76 (15), and CIA (16). mAb H81.98.21 was found to inhibit canine MLC, while another mAB, H40-164.32 (17), was shown to be a potent inhibitor of canine MLC in our laboratory.

Other studies of the DLA complex have employed effector cells sensitized in vitro against specific DLA determinants. CTL were generated in bulk MLC using PBMC from homozygous dogs matched for DLA-A and -B antigens, but differing for DLA-D alleles (18). These CTL were then assayed in CML against ^{51}Cr-labeled targets derived from a panel of HTC. Target cell lysis patterns showed that target determinants were different from sero-defined specificities and also from those responsible for stimulation in MLC. However, there was a strong association of those determinants with DLA-D locus encoded products based on sharing of specific HTC target determinants by three distinct CTL (Table 3). Another study using the primed lymphocyte test (PLT) also found a correlation with specificities encoded for by genes within the DLA complex (19). PLT cells, generated by priming with HTC and subsequently restimulated with cells phenotypically homozygous for DLA-D locus alleles, were shown to recognize cells from unrelated dogs sharing the same DLA-D allele. Three PLT cells appeared to mutually recognize a supertypic determinant not previously identified by cellular or serological methods (Table 3). Two additional PLT cells showed mutual cross-reactivity, suggesting the existence of a second supertypic determinant, while another PLT cell showed one-way cross-reactivity with one additional DLA-D type. These results indicate that, in dogs, the PLT not only identifies DLA-D determinants but can detect antigenic specificities which differ from those defined by conventional HTC assays (DLA-D) and which may be gene products of an additional closely related MHC locus.

The mAb W3G10, generated in our laboratory against canine PBMC and shown to recognize a polymorphic antigen closely associated with DLA (20), may be of interest in further canine immunogenetic studies. However, W3G10 recognizes a protein structure of approximately 39 Kd (Table 3), which is not a typical class I or class II molecule.

Table 3 DLA-associated Determinants Defined by Effector Cells or mAb

	CTL	PLT	W3G10
DLA locus association	D	D[a]	D
Unique determinants	CML-1 CML-2 CML-3	PLT-1 PLT-2 PLT-3	p39
Segregation pattern	ND[b]	ND	Mendelian

[a]Data could not rule out an association with the B locus.
[b]ND = not done.

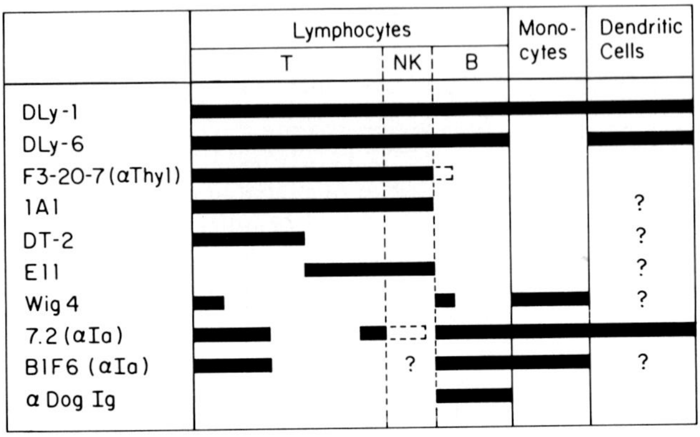

Figure 2 Preliminary assignment of specificities of monoclonal antibodies: DLy-1 recognizes virtually all mononuclear cells; DLy-6 recognizes most PBMC but excludes monocytes; F3-20-7 (provided by Drs. McKenzie and Fabre) is directed at a canine Thy 1-like antigen; 1A1 (provided by Dr. Krawiec) recognizes sIg-negative lymphocytes including NK cells; DT-2 recognizes a large subpopulation of T lymphocytes (presumably helper function), E11 recognizes a small subpopulation of T cells (suppressor/cytotoxic function) and NK cells; Wig4 is directed at monocytes and small subpopulations of T and possibly B lymphocytes but does not recognize NK cells; 7.2 (provided by Dr. Hansen) and B1F6 (provided by Dr. Alejandro) recognize a framework of determinants of Ia-like antigens (DR and DR + DP, respectively, in man); α Dog Ig, polyclonal goat $F(ab')_2$ specific for canine immunoglobulin.

In conclusion, the DLA complex is not as well-defined as comparable mouse and human systems. However, a considerable amount of data is available to indicate that this genetic area encodes equally important determinants in all three species. In addition to DLA-encoded products, other surface antigens on LHC have been described and characterized. We will be discussing these throughout the remainder of the chapter. The subject matter is categorized by morphological cell type with descriptions of surface antigens and relevant functional significance. Knowledge of canine LHC has greatly increased with the use of mAbs, and we currently have developed a panel for routine pheno-typing (Figure 2). It can be seen that LHC subpopulations have been tentatively identified. We begin our discussion with the immature progenitor cells, followed by the leukocytes and their subsets, and we end with a brief description of antigen expression in LHC tumors.

II. PLURIPOTENT STEM AND PROGENITOR CELLS

Pluripotent lympho-hemopoietic stem cells can be defined as cells capable of both self-renewal and pluripotent cellular differentiation throughout the life of an animal (21). These cells were originally identified in the spleen of lethally irradiated mice given syngeneic marrow or spleen grafts. The hemopoietic cell colonies generated were termed colony-forming unit-spleen (CFU-S). No techniques equivalent to the spleen colony assay in mice are available for studies on pluripotent stem cells in dogs. However, focal proliferations of hematopoietic cells have been described in dogs recovering from irradiation (22). The homogeneous nature of these cells has suggested clonal origin. They have been shown to be more differentiated than pluripotent cells and thus represent committed progenitor cells (Figure 3). They were originally termed CFU-C but are currently termed GM-CFC to more adequately reflect their cell lineage. The progenitor cells in the erythroid lineage are referred to as either BFU-E for the less differentiated or CFU-E for the more mature forms. Assays for these cells are routinely performed in the dog (23). T-lymphocyte progenitors (CFU-T) have been studied using a semisolid culture system and Con A and PHA stimulation of whole blood (24).

The study of the antigenic characteristics of stem cells has relevance for evaluating the differentiation of hemopoiesis and also for experimental bone marrow transplantation where removal of certain populations by antibodies is possible.

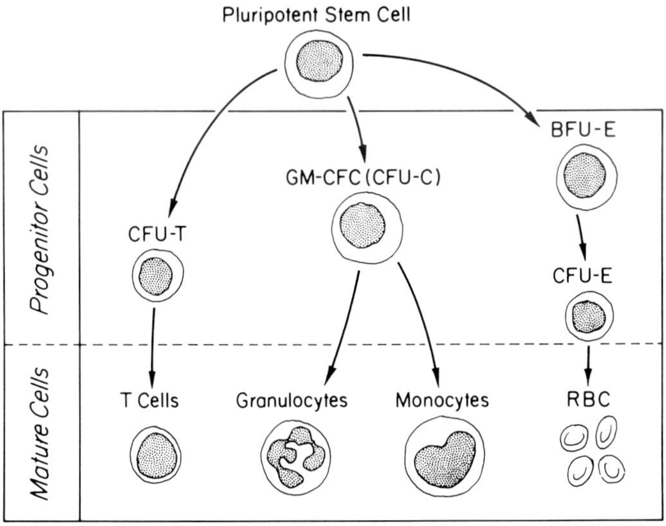

Figure 3 Simplified scheme of lymphohematopoiesis in the dog. There is currently no assay for the pluripotent stem cell. Early erythroid progenitor cells can be detected by BFU-E (burst forming units, erythroid) and later erythroid progenitor cells by CFU-E (colony forming units, erythroid). Granulocyte and monocyte progenitor cells are detected with GM-CFC (granulocyte monocyte colony forming cells) forming cells designated as CFU-C. Finally, T-lymphocyte progenitor cells can be assayed with CFU-T (colony forming units-T).

There is evidence that Ia antigen is expressed on canine marrow stem cells. Hemopoietic stem cell toxicity of mAb 7.2, recognizing Ia-like antigens on canine cells, was tested in an autologous bone marrow transplantation model (25). Dogs were given 9.2 Gy of total body irradiation (TBI) followed by the infusion of autologous marrow cytolytically treated with 7.2 to remove Ia-positive cells. Four dogs received marrow cells separated by density gradient centrifugation and then treated with an excess of antibody 7.2 and two cycles of undiluted rabbit complement. None of these dogs, surviving 17-22 days, had sustained engraftment. Only one dog had detectable residual 7.2 positive cells after treatment. Dogs receiving marrow cells obtained by density gradient centrifugation without additional manipulation or with subsequent treatment with complement engrafted promptly and completely. These data indicate that Ia positive bone marrow cells are essential for the successful engraftment of transplanted marrow in dogs.

III. LEUKOCYTES

A. General

Cell-surface antigens common to canine leukocytes have been characterized with the use of mAbs (Table 4). McAb DLy-1, generated specifically against canine cells, has been extensively characterized (26). The antibody identifies the p213 antigen expressed on resting and activated lymphoid, monocytic and myeloid, but not erythroid cells. DLy-1 + C' blocks GM-CFC and BFU-E, but not CFU-E, suggesting that the mAb may be affecting non-stem cells essential for differentiation. Cytolytic treatment of canine marrow cells with DLy-1 eliminates myeloid cells but not megakaryocytes or erythroid cells. Therefore, DLy-1 appears to recognize a common leukocyte antigen which has a distribution similar to the T200 antigen of humans. Functionally, mitogen- and alloantigen-induced lymphocyte proliferation is abrogated after responding or stimulating PBMC are treated with DLy-1 and C' (Table 5). In addition, DLy-1 recognizes an antigen expressed on mitogen-stimulated lymphoblasts of both T- and B-cell origin. However, the antigen does not appear to be expressed on cytotoxic effector cells per se, since lysis of ^{51}Cr-labeled target cells by MLC-activated CTL is not eliminated after cytolytic treatment with DLy-1.

mAb A5 identifies the p96 antigen expressed on 90-95% PBMC (Thy1-positive as well as Thy1-negative cells), 80-100% puppy thymocytes, 100% thoracic duct lymphocytes, 95% granulocytes, 100% platelets, and 100% MLC lymphoblasts (27). Cytolytic treatment with A5 completely eliminates suppressor cell function of activated T lymphocytes.

Cell-surface antigens common to leukocytes have also been characterized in man with the use of mAbs. mAb 60.3 (Table 4), which identifies a family of common leukocyte antigens designated as CDw18 (28), has been found to cross-react with canine leukocytes. The antigen complex is made up of at least three dimers,

Table 4 Monoclonal Antibodies Generated Against Canine Cells or Cells from Other Species Reactive with Canine Cells

mAb	IgG isotype	Specificity	Antigen	Comments	Source
DLy-1	IgG2b	common leukocyte	p213	T200-like	Wulff,Seattle
A-5	IgG2b	common leukocyte	p96	suppressor cells	Szer,Seattle
6C6	IaG2b	lymphocytes	ND	on medullary but not cortical thymocytes	Krawiec,Minneapolis
DLy-6	IgM	lymphocytes	p60	mature1 cells only	Wulff,Seattle
F3-20-7	IgG1	Thy-1	P24	pan T cell, NK cells	McKenzie and Fabre,Oxford
1A1	IgM	T cells	ND	pan T cell, NK cells, LGL[a]	Krawiec,Minneapolis
DT-2	IgG2a	T-cell subset	P70	helper/inducer cells	Wulff,Seattle
E11	IgG3	T-cell subset	ND	Suppressor cells, CTL	Szer,Seattle
W1D10	IgG1	T-cell subset	p39	Inhibits mitogen activation	Ladiges,Seattle
W1H3	IgG2a	T-cell subset	p26		Ladiges,Seattle
T83[b]	IgG3	T-cell subset	ND	Inhibits MLC	Carreno,Miami
Wig4	IgG1	Monocytes,platelets	p24	Activates C'	Ladiges,Seattle
60.3	IaG2a	leukocytes,human	p97,170,180	51% PBMC[c]	Beatty,Seattle
T811	IgG1	T suppressor, (CD8), human, Tp32	ND	CTL	Rieber,Munich,FRG
9.4	IgG2a	lymphocytes,human, T200	ND	5% PBMC[c]	Martin,Seattle
J2	IgM	activated T cells, malignant B cells, human gp 24	ND	15% PBMC[c]	Pesando,Seattle

(Table 1 *continues*)

Table 4 (*continued*)

mAb	IgG isotype	Specificity	Antigen	Comments	Source
64.1	IaG2a	T cells (CD3), human, p19	ND	~40% PBMC[c]	Martin,Seattle
HB57s (DA4.4)	IgG1	μ heavy chain, human	ND	~20% PBMC[c]	ATCC
5F1	IgM	Monocytes, platelets, human g85	ND	16% PBMC[c]	Bernstein,Seattle
L1B2	IgG2[a]	Monocytes, myeloblasts, human	ND	21% PBMC[c]	Andrews,Seattle
13.1	IgG1	NK cells, human	p47	~15	Newman,Seattle

[a]ND = not done, ATCC = American Type Culture Collection.
[b]We have not studied mAb T83 in our laboratory.
[c]Percent reactivity as determined by indirect cytofluorescence (FACS 440).

Table 5 Cytofluorometric Analysis (FACS) of Reactivity of mAbs DLy-1 and DLy-6 with PBMC Stimulated by PHA for 3 Days or Autologous PBMC or PBMC From an Unrelated Dog in MLC for 7 Days. Fluoresceinated $F(ab')_2$ Fragments of Goat Anti Mouse Were Used as the Second Antibody

PBMC	PBS	DLy-1	DLy-6
No mitogen	–	+++	++
PHA	–	+++	–
Autologous MLC	–	+++	++
Allogeneic MLC	–	+++	–

– = no reactivity; ++ = 40-60% reactivity; +++ = >60% reactivity.

each consisting of a unique α chain, ranging in weight from 135-180,000 daltons, and a common 95,000-dalton β chain. Indirect cytofluorescence (FACS 440) studies in the dog show that the antibody reacts with 51% PBMC, 29% bone marrow cells, and 32% thymocytes. Radioimmunoprecipitation using SDS-PAGE and cell lysates from Con A-stimulated PBMC indicates that 60.3 identifies three antigen bands of 100, 170, and 180 Kd. Its functional significance in the dog has not yet been determined.

B. Lymphocytes

Lymphocytes of the dog have not been characterized as extensively as those of mouse or man. However, use of the dog as a biomedical research model in immunological and transplantation research has necessitated the development of adequate systems to study lymphoid cell subpopulations and their functional significance.

Two mAbs, DLy-6 and 6C6, have been characterized which react with all or most lymphocyte populations (Table 1). mAb DLy-6 identifies the p60 antigen expressed on normal T and B cells in peripheral blood, thoracic duct lymphocytes, and bronchoalveolar lavage fluids (26). This mAb does not react with monocytes or granulocytes except for some eosinophils. The antigen is not expressed on mitogen- (PHA) or alloantigen-stimulated cells (Table 5). Cytolytic treatment with DLy-6 has no effect on GM-CFC, CFU-E, or BFU-E growth. It thus appears that DLy-6 expression is confined to resting lymphocytes and can be used to separate these from activated lymphocytes. Another practical application would be the purification or elimination of lymphocytes from a heterogeneous cell population such as PBMC, lymph node, bone marrow, or bronchoalveolar lavage cells, since the mAb does not react with myeloid or monocytic cells. It has been shown that cytolytic treatment of marrow mononuclear cells with DLy-6 and C' eliminates lymphocytes while sparing nonlymphoid cells (29).

mAb 6C6 has been shown to react with 67% PBMC, 34% lymph node cells, 61% bone marrow cells, 14% thymocytes, and some monocytes (30). It identifies T cells, B cells, and medullary but not cortical thymocytes. Since more mature cells are represented in the thymic medulla, it is interesting to observe the reactivity of the mAb with such a high percentage of bone marrow cells (61%). It does appear that the antigen has a broader range of expression than the DLy-6 antigen. An additional mAb, 9.4 (Table 4), specific for human lymphocytes (Hansen et al., unpublished data) and identifying the T200 antigen (comparable to Ly5 in the mouse) has been found to cross-react with canine PBMC, but has not been further characterized.

1. T Lymphocytes

Approximately 70-79% of human PBMC are T lymphocytes (31), whereas 70-75% of mouse PBMC are T lymphocytes (32). These studies, based on expression of T-cell antigens and unique erythrocyte receptors, when applied to canine lymphocyte populations gave inconsistent findings. Krawkowka and Guyot (33) then showed that the sheep erythrocyte rosetting technique, useful as a marker for human T cells, was not specific for canine T cells. Atkinson et al. (34) demonstrated that only 10-23% of cells in blood, lymph nodes, and bone marrow from normal dogs formed rosettes with human erythrocytes, and only 3% of thymocytes and 1% of thoracic duct cells formed rosettes. In addition, PBMC depleted of rosette-forming cells responded more vigorously to alloantigens in MLC and to the mitogens PHA and Con A than did the population enriched for rosette-positive cells. Nylon-wool nonadherent cells did not form rosettes or express sIg, while a significant number of adherent cells did form rosettes and was sIg positive. The nonadherent population reacted more vigorously to alloantigens in MLC and to PHA than the adherent cells. Clearly the capacity to form rosettes with human red blood cells is not a marker for canine T cells. However, nylon wool separation can be used to obtain T-cell-enriched populations from PBMC.

The use of anti-thymocyte antibody appears to be a more acceptable method of identifying canine T cells. Chandler and Yang (35) identified 74% of PBMC as T cells using a rabbit anti-dog thymycyte serum (ATS) in an indirect fluorescent antibody (FA) technique. Their ATS reacted with 97% of thymic cells. Koyama et al. (36) used rabbit anti-dog ATS in an indirect FA procedure and showed that 53 PBMC from 21 mixed-breed dogs were ATS positive. Treatment of thymus cells with ATS and complement resulted in 99-100% killing of thymocytes. ATS-positive cells were markedly increased (73%) in nylon-wool nonadherent populations. Mitogenic responses to Con A and PHA were eliminated when PBMC were treated with ATS and complement. An additional study compared anti-dog thymocyte globulin (ATG) as a marker for canine T lymphocytes using indirect FA or a rosette assay with staphylococcal protein A (SpA)-coated sheep red blood cells (37). It was shown that 74% PBMC were ATG positive using indirect FA, while 72% were positive with the ATG SpA rosetting assay. In conclusion, polyclonal anti-canine thymocyte antibody can be prepared and shown to identify classical T-lymphocyte populations representing approximately 70% of PBMC in the dog. These levels are comparable to those for T cells in mice and man.

Other types of markers on canine T cells have been studied. Trail and Yang (38) showed that T cells express IgG and IgM Fc receptors. They used an erythrocyte antibody rosette technique employing sheep red blood cells sensitized with canine and rabbit IgM and IgG antibodies and determined that 53% and 18% of peripheral blood T lymphocytes expressed Fc receptors for IgM and IgG respectively. A characteristic staining for nonspecific esterase (NSE) has been suggested as a marker for canine T cells. Since focal paranuclear positivity for NSE has been shown to be a reliable marker for T cells in humans and mice, canine lymphoid tissue sections and cell suspensions were stained for this enzyme (39). The same focal distribution patterns of NSE-positive cells found in humans and mice were displayed in sections of five lymph nodes and 11 puppy thymuses. Focal NSE-positive cells were found in the medullary but not cortical thymus, and in lymph nodes only the thymus-dependent, paracortical zones but not central areas of germinal centers, displayed focal-NSE reactivity. In addition, 56-78% of PBMC and 60-71% of thoracic duct lymphocytes were positive for NSE. It was concluded that focal NSE reactivity is a marker for a canine T-cell subpopulation.

The Thy-1 antigen has been identified and characterized by Dalchau and Fabre (40), who used liver absorbed rabbit anti-dog xenosera assayed on thymus cells to study the tissue distribution. They established homology with purified rat Thy-1 by showing cross-reactivity. They found Thy-1 to be expressed on cells from brain, thymus, kidney, and peripheral lymphoid tissue, all peripheral blood T cells, and virtually all dog thymocytes (Table 6). The Thy-1 antigen was purified from dog

Table 6 Summary of Tissue Distribution of Thy-1 in Mouse, Rat, Dog, and Man

Location	Mouse	Rat	Dog	Man
Brain	+++	+++	+++	+++
Kidney	0	0	+	+
Liver, heart	0	0	0	0
Thymus	+++	+++	+	0
Lymph node	++	0	+	0
Spleen	++	+	+	0
Bone marrow	0	+	+	0
RBC, platelets, serum	0	0	0	0

Reproduced from *The Journal of Experimental Medicine, 149*: 576-591, 1979, by copyright permission of the Rockefeller University Press.

brain using lentil lectin and Sephadex G-200. Further characterization of Thy-1 occurred with development of the mAb F3-20-7 (Table 1), which was shown to identify the p24 antigen by SDS-PAGE (41). This antigen had the same mobility as pure rat Thy-1 and could inhibit an assay shown previously to be directed at canine Thy-1. All thymocytes and peripheral blood and lymph node T cells express Thy-1, while 15% of nucleated bone marrow cells are Thy-1 positive. Thy-1 is present early in the differentiation of the lymphoid series, and conceivably a percentage of newly released B cells are Thy-1-positive. Thy-1 appears early in the bone marrow stage and persists throughout T-cell differentiation. In the mouse it does not appear in bone marrow but is seen on cortical thymocytes and persists throughout T-cell differentiation. In man Thy-1 is not expressed in bone marrow or the bulk of the thymic cortex but is seen only at the periphery of the thymic lobule where newly arrived T-cell precursors lodge.

T-cell populations have been identified with other mAbs (Table 4). mAb 1A1 reacts with 61% PBMC, 73% thymocytes, 9% bone marrow cells, and 37% lymph node cells (42). It was shown not to react with sIg-positive cells as identified by a thalamine-conjugated goat anti-canine IgG, or latex-ingesting monocytes. Reactivity occurred with cells from connective tissue and brain, but not with biopsied tumor cells obtained from dogs with B-cell lymphosarcoma. However, preliminary studies in our laboratory found 20 of 36 sIg-positive lymphomas to be reactive with mAb 1A1, suggesting differential expression on more immature cells. Several other mAbs have been found to react with canine T-cell subpopulations. mAbs W1D10 and W1H3, generated in our laboratory (43), were found not to inhibit alloantigen-stimulated cells. W1D10 does, however, abrogate response to mitogens Con A and PHA. T83, described by Carreno et al. (44), reacts with 32-67% PBMC, inhibits in vitro MLC, and when given in vivo to dogs, results in the disappearance of MLC reactivity for greater than 5 weeks. Another mAb, 64.1 (Table 4) specific for human T cells (45) cross-reacts with canine PBMC, but has not been further characterized.

Helper and Suppressor Function. Helper and suppressor lymphocyte function have been tentatively characterized in the dog using 2 mAbs: DT-2 and E11 (Table 4). Although there are differences in regard to the antigens that are recognized by these antibodies, the respective cell populations appear to be functionally analogous to the CD4 (OKT4) and CD8 (OKT8) specific mAbs in man. A third mAb, T811 (Table 4), specific for the human CD8 antigen, has been shown to cross-react with canine cells having cytotoxic function comparable to that of human cells.

The DT-2 antigen is expressed on small lymphoid cells among PBMC which were shown to be sIg-negative by double-fluorescence FACS analysis (46). DT-2 is also expressed on thoracic duct lymphocytes, lymph node cells, and thymocytes, but not monocytes, bronchoalveolar macrophages, granulocytes, erythrocytes, or platelets. C'-mediated lysis showed the antigen is on the responder population of cells in MLC or mitogen stimulation assays. A co-culture system of thymocytes/

bronchoalveolar macrophages for mitogen stimulation was used to confirm DT-2 antigen expression on T cells but not on monocytes or other accessory cells. Cytolytic treatment with DT-2 abrogated the proliferative ability of thymocytes but not the accessory function of monocytes/macrophages.

mAb E11 identifies an antigen associated with suppressor cells (27). The antigen is expressed on 15-40% normal PBMC, 30-50% of Thy-1-positive PBMC, 70-80% of puppy thymocytes, 10-15% of thoracic duct cells, and 90-100% of MLC lymphoblasts. It is not found on Thy-1-negative PBMC, granulocytes, or platelets. Cytolytic treatment of lymphocytes with E11 eliminates their suppressor ability. E11-positive cells obtained by FACS sorting show potent suppressor function in MLC. Cytolytic treatment of lymphocytes with DT-2 does not eliminate suppressor function, suggesting that E11 and DT-2 separate functionally distinct groups of canine T cells. E11 has also been shown to recognize cytotoxic lymphocytes, further supporting the analogy between E11 positive cells in the dog and CD8 (OKT8) positive cells in humans.

mAb T811, an antihuman Tp32 (CD 8)-specific mAb, cross-reacts with canine lymphoid cells (47). It reacts with 14-17% PBMC, 21-30% of Thy-1-positive cells, 40% thymocytes, 35-45% of alloantigen-activated peripheral lymphocytes, and 100% of PBMC from a dog with T-cell acute leukemia. It is not expressed on peripheral Thy-1-negative cells or bronchoalveolar cells. Cytolytic treatment with T811 eliminates CML reactivity of bulk MLC-generated CTL. However, no significant difference is seen between T811-positive and T811-negative FACS-separated cells in regard to suppressor function when used in suppressor cell assays. The reason for this is not clear. Conceivably, the T811-negative population contains suppressor inducer cells capable of causing responder cells to attain suppressor function.

Cytotoxic Cells. Cytotoxic cells in the mouse express cell-surface antigens termed LyT2 and LyT3. Cytotoxic T cells of man also bear characteristic membrane markers (CD8) analogous to the murine antigens. These cells require priming, usually by alloantigens, to become cytotoxic. In addition, there are other cells not readily classified in regard to their lineage which are cytotoxic, especially to a wide variety of tumor cells, and do not require prior "priming." Such cells have been termed natural killer (NK) cells. These cells are further distinguished from cytotoxic T cells by the fact that CTL function only if the antigen is presented in the context of the appropriate MHC antigen (MHC restriction), while NK cells are not genetically restricted. Both CTL and NK cells have been described in the dog and appear to play significant roles in cellular immune function in this species.

Canine CTL have mostly been characterized by means of the in vitro CML assay (48). MLC-primed effector cells are cytotoxic for the original stimulating cells and other target cells bearing the same or cross-reactive target determinants. The possibility of quantitative and specific analysis of canine CTL now exists with the techniques of limiting dilution analysis and cloning with IL-2 developed by Buurman et al. (49).

Several studies on the nature of the target determinants recognized by canine CTL have shown that they may have some association with class II antigens. Class I antigens or class I associated antigens are classically recognized by CTL in mouse and man. Cellular cytotoxicity toward human class II antigens, however, has been reported (50). In the dog, Buurman et al. (51) showed that PWM-stimulated B lymphoblasts, traditional class II-bearing cells, could serve as effective targets for cytotoxic lysis. Raff et al. (18) used a panel of cytotoxic typing cells to further characterize target determinants. CTL were generated using PBMC from homozygous dogs identical for the DLA-A and -B alleles but differing for DLA-D alleles. Various target cells were then used to study the target cell determinants recognized by these CTL. The results indicate an association of CTL target determinants with DLA D but not DLA A or B. It has also been suggested that canine CTL themselves express Ia antigens (52). Cytolytic treatment with the anti-Ia mAb 7.2 significantly reduced MLC responses and CTL activity of cells treated on either day 0 or day 6 of culture. Additional studies are necessary to determine the relevant significance of class I and class II antigens in the context of antigen recognition by CTL of the dog.

2. NK Cells

In contrast to CTL, which exhibit immunological specificity, NK cells lack classic immunological specificity and can kill cells across organ, strain, and species barriers, i.e., they are not genetically restricted in their activity. A notable characteristic of NK cells is their ability to lyse a wide variety of cell types, especially tumor cell lines (53). It appears that normal cells, such as fibroblasts, thymocytes, and bone marrow cells, are less susceptible to lysis than tumor cells.

Canine NK activity and antibody-dependent cell-mediated cytotoxicity were studied utilizing a canine thyroid adenocarcinoma cell line (CTAC) and a lymphoblastoid cell line (CT-45S), respectively, as cell targets (54). Fractionation of mononuclear cells by Percoll discontinuous gradient centrifugation resulted in a 6 to 7-fold enrichment in large granular lymphocytes (LGL) in parallel with a 2-fold increase in NK activity in low density fractions. Further enrichment in LGL (78%) and NK activity (3-fold increase) was obtained by lytic treatment of low density fractions 2 and 3 with mAb WiG4. NK cells were phenotyped with mAbs and also found to be relatively radioresistant to irradiation (Table 7). The highest NK activity was found in PBMC. These results indicate that canine NK cells have the morphology of LGL, are relatively radioresistant, and express cell-surface antigens suggesting a T-cell lineage. The mAb 13.1 (Table 2), specific for human NK cells (55), has been shown to cross-react with canine cells and may be useful in future studies.

3. B Lymphocytes

The study of canine B cells, compared to characterization of canine T cells, has received relatively little attention. Purification of B cells by density sedimentation

Table 7 Characteristics of Canine NK Cells

Procedure	Results
Method of assay[a]	Cell lysis
Enrichment	Percoll gradient-low density fractions lytic treatment with mAb Wig4
Phenotype[b]	DLy-1$^+$ Dly6$^+$ E11$^+$ DT-2$^-$ Wig4$^-$ Ia$^+$(7.2) 13.1$^+$
Radioresistant	Yes (up to 40 Gy)

[a]A canine thyroid adenocarcinoma cell line (CTAL) and a lymphoblastoid cell line (CT-455) have been used as target cells.
[b]DLy-1 identifies a common leukocyte antigen, DLy-6 is specific for lymphocytes, E11 and DT-2 are specific for suppressor/cytotoxic and helper T cells, respectively, Wig4 reacts mainly with monocytes, 7.2 is specific for a framework Ia antigen, and 13.1 is specific for human NK cells.

of T lymphocytes forming rosettes with SRBC cannot be applied to canine cells since they do not specifically rosette. sIg has been used as a marker for canine B cells and the capacity of sIg-bearing cells to adhere onto nylon wool fibers has been used as a B-cell enrichment technique similar to that in other species. Atkinson et al. (34) found that an average of 46% of adherent PBMC were sIg positive (Table 8). Recently, the use of polymethyl methacrylate beads (Degalan) 150-500 μ in diameter allowed for an enrichment of 70% sIg-positive cells (56). In addition, Degalan bead column-enriched B cells showed a greater viability than nylon-wool column-enriched B cells. Another method of enriching for B cells, performed in our laboratory which appears to be as efficient as Degalan beads, is the use of Sepharose 6MB beads coupled with F(ab')$_2$ fragments of goat antibody IgG (Table 8). It can be seen that a purity of 69% results in a marked decrease in the Con A response compared to the nonadherent population. A panning technique has also been described (57).

The B-lymphocyte population in PBMC has been reported to be between 12 and 50%, as determined by direct immunofluorescence. Chandler and Yang (35) found 18% of PBMC were B cells using similar direct immunofluorescence technique. Bowles et al. (58), in a similar study, found a close correlation between immunoglobulin-bearing cells and those forming erythrocyte antibody complement (EAC) rosettes. Levels were 49 and 46%, respectively. Atkinson et al. (34) showed a similar correlation with PBMC from 24 dogs, but levels were much lower; 17% for EAC rosetting cells and 21% for sIg-positive cells. They also showed that thoracic duct cells, collected as described by Deeg et al. (59), showed 15% EAC rosetting, while only 1% were sIg positive. Therefore, the EAC rosette assay may detect a subpopulation of T cells or at least non-B cells. The mAb HB57S (Table 2), specific for human IgM heavy chain (60), cross-reacts with canine PBMC and may prove useful in additional studies. Doveren et al. (15) reported that two mAbs

Table 8 Comparison of B-Cell Enrichment Techniques

Study	Procedure		% cells SIg+	DT-2	Con A stimulation (CPM)
Ladiges	1 nylon wool	Ad	33	36	ND
	(n = 3)	NonAd	12	66	ND
Atkinson[a]	2 nylon wool	Ad	46±12	ND	18,600
	(n = 8)	NonAd	5±4	ND	22,200
Ladiges	3 Sepharose 6MB[b]	Ad	69±7	ND	9,297
	(n = 3)	NonAd	30±11	ND	28,945
Krumbacher[c]	4 Degalan[d]	Ad	70±8.6	ND	ND
	nylon wool	Ad	29±11	ND	ND
Wulff[e]	5 Panning	Ad	89	ND	30,207
	(n = 5)	NonAd	0	74	38,169

[a]See Ref. 34.
[b]Pharmacia, Upsula, Sweden. The beads were coupled with goat anti-dog IgG.
[c]See Ref. 56.
[d]Polymethyl methacrylate beads (150-500 μ in diameter).
[e]See Ref. 57. Polystyrene petri dishes treated with goat anti-dog immunoglobulin were used.

(1.41 and H76, Table 2), specific for class II antigens, react with sIg-positive lymph node cells and activated T cells but not with resting peripheral blood T cells. It appears that mAb I-3.1 (Table 2) may show similar reactivity, since it is more reactive with sIg-positive Thy-1-negative PBMC. These mAbs may prove invaluable for the study of canine B cells.

Immunoglobulin-secreting cells have been identified among canine PBMC by the protein A hemolytic plaque assay (61). PBMC were assayed for plaque formation either immediately after isolation or after 6 days of culture in fetal calf serum in the presence of PWM. Immediately assayed PBMC produced a mean of 4870 IgG-related, 1610 IgM-related, and 760 IgA-related plaques per 10^6 PBMC. Many of the plaques formed by freshly isolated PBMC, however, appeared to represent release of previously absorbed antibody. In contrast, plaques formed by cultured cells clearly identified immunoglobulin-secreting cells. Prummer et al. (62) found that the addition of bacterial lipopolysaccharide (LPS) to a PWM system for generating plasmacytoid cells (PC) enhanced the formation of PC. It would appear, then, that a system utilizing PWM and LPS would be most efficient for studying the capacity of canine blood cells to generate a humoral immune response.

B-cell antigens similar to those described in man and non-human primates have not been characterized in the dog. Most mAbs specific for the B1 antigen apparently do not cross-react with canine B cells (E. Clark, personal communication).

subpopulations, a number of which have been shown to have functional significance.

Morphological cell types have been shown to express various antigenic determinants. Current data suggest that canine stem cells express Ia antigen based on the failure of autologous engraftment, using marrow cytolytically treated with mAb 7.2 (Ia specific). More mature cells express both unique as well as common antigens. Lymphoid, monocyte, and myeloid cells have been shown to express a common leukocyte antigen identified by mAb DLy-1. Resting but not activated lymphocytes can be depleted from PBMC and bone marrow by cytolytic treatment with the mAb DLy-6, which is specific for resting lymphocytes. Most T cells express the Thy-1 antigen, suggesting it may be useful as a T-cell marker in peripheral blood. Furthermore, T cells can be functionally delineated into a suppressor population (CD8-like) and a helper population (CD4-like) with mAbs E11 and DT-2 respectively. CTL, which express Ia (as well as other antigens identified by McAbs T811, E11, and A5), have been shown to recognize target cells in association with DLA determinants, i.e., they exhibit genetic restriction similar to mouse and man. Nonspecific cytotoxic cells, or NK cells, have also been described in the dog. They have the morphology of large granular lymphocytes, are relatively radioresistant, and express surface antigens suggestive of a T-cell lineage. B cells are currently best identified with polyclonal antisera specific for surface Ig. It has been demonstrated that canine Ig-producing cells can most efficiently be evaluated using a PWM system to which LPS has been added. Additional cell types involved in immunological reactivity include monocytes and dendritic cells (DC). Recent evidence suggests that peripheral blood monocytes cannot act in an accessory cell manner without the presence of DC, while DC can function as accessory cells independently. Both cell types express Ia, but monocytes are DLy-6 negative, whereas DC are DLy-6 positive, suggesting a different cell lineage.

It can be seen, then, that LHC in the dog have been functionally characterized based on differentiation and DLA antigens. A large number of additional mAbs have been shown to react with LHC but have not yet been studied sufficiently to determine the functional significance of the antigens they identify. In addition, further development and characterization of canine LHC cell lines will be extremely helpful in identifying relevant differentiation antigens and may prove useful in a number of in vitro functional studies.

ACKNOWLEDGMENTS

Many of the studies were supported in part by the following grants: CA18221, CA18105, RR-00019, and HL33859 from the National Institutes of Health. The authors would like to thank Steve Anderson and Audeen Wagner for assistance in preparing the manuscript.

ABBREVIATIONS

C'	complement.
CML	cell-mediated lympholysis.
Con A	Concanavalin A.
CTL	cytotoxic T lymphocytes.
FACS	fluorescence-activated cell sorter.
IgG	immunoglobulin G.
IgM	immunoglobulin M.
Kd	kilodalton.
mAb(s)	monoclonal antibody(ies).
MHC	major histocompatibility complex.
MLC	mixed lymphocyte culture.
PBMC	peripheral blood mononuclear cells.
PHA	phytohemagglutinin.
PLT	primed lymphocyte test.
SDS-PAGE	sodium dodecyl sulfate-polyacrylamide gel electrophoresis.
sIg	surface immunoglobulin.

REFERENCES

1. R. Storb, P. L. Weiden, H. J. Deeg, B. Torok-Storb, K. Atkinson, T. C. Graham and E. D. Thomas. Marrow graft studies in dogs, in *Immunobiology of bone marrow transplantation*, (S. Thierfelder, H. Rodt, H. J. Kolb, eds.), Springer-Verlag, Berlin, 1980, pp. 43-52.
2. R. W. Bull, H. M. Vriesendorp, R. Cech, H. Grosse-Wilde, A. M. Bijma, W. L. Ladiges, K. Krumbacher, I. Doxiadis, H. Ejima, J. Templeton, E. D. Albert, R. Storb, and H. J. Deeg, Joint report of the Third International Workshop on Canine Immunogenetics: II. Analysis of the serological typing of cells, *Transplantation 43*: 154-161 (1987).
3. H. J. Deeg, R. F. Raff, H. Grosse-Wilde, A. M. Bijma, W. Buurman, I. Doxiadia, H. J. Kolb, K. Krumbacher, W. Ladiges, K. L. Glosslein, G. Schoch, D. L. Westbroek, R. W. Bull, and R. Storb, Joint report of the Third International Workshop on Canine Immunogenetics: I. Analysis of homozygous typing cells (HTCs), *Transplantation, 41*: 111-117 (1986).
4. J. Klein, The major histocompatibility complex of the mouse, *Science, 203*: 516-521 (1979).
5. M. J. M. van der Feltz and H. L. Ploegh, Immunochemical analysis of glycosylated and nonglycosylated DLA class I antigens, *Immunogenetics, 19*: 95-107 (1984).
6. W. C. Davis, L. E. Perryman, and T. C. McGuire, The identification and analysis of major functional populations of differentiated cells, in *Hybridoma technology in agricultural and veterinary research*, USDA-BARC, Bettsville, MD, 1983.
7. J. A. Hansen, P. J. Martin, and R. C. Nowinski, Monoclonal antibodies identifying a novel T-cell antigen and Ia antigens of human lymphocytes, *Immunogenetics, 10*: 247-260 (1980).

8. R. Burger, J. Scher, S. O. Sherrow, and E. M. Shevach, Non-activated guinea-pig T cells and thymocytes express Ia antigens: FACS analysis with alloantibodies and monoclonal antibodies, *Immunology, 51*: 93-102 (1984).
9. T. R. Thistlewaite, L. R. Pennington, J. K. Lunney, and D. H. Sachs, Immunologic characterization of MHC recombinant swine: Production of SLA class specific antisera and detection of Ia antigens on both B and non-B PBL, *Transplantation, 35*: 394-400 (1983).
10. H. J. Deeg, J. C. Wulff, S. DeRose, G. E. Sale, M. Braun, M. A. Brown, S. C. Springmeyer, P. J. Martin, and R. Storb, Unusual distribution of Ia-like antigens on canine lymphocytes, *Immunogenetics 16*: 445-457 (1982).
11. R. Alejandro, F. L. Shienvold, Z. Latiff, V. Esquenazi, J. Miller, and D. Mintz, Monoclonal antibodies recognizing canine and human Ia-like antigens, *Transplantation, 38*: 542-543 (1984).
12. M. Watanabe, T. Suzuki, M. Taniguchi, and N. Shinohara, Monoclonal anti-Ia murine alloantibodies cross-reactive with the Ia-homologues of other mammalian species including humans, *Transplantation, 36*: 712-718 (1983).
13. W. C. Ladiges, J. Szer, R. F. Raff, E. Severns, H. J. Deeg, and R. Storb, Canine Ia antigens: Assessment of in vitro functions using monoclonal antibodies, *Fed. Proc., 44* (Suppl. 6): 1884 (1985).
14. R. F. C. Doveren, W. A. Buurman, B. Schutte, G. Groenewegen, and C. J. van der Linden, Class II antigens on canine T lymphocytes, *Tissue Antigens, 25*: 255-265 (1985).
15. R. F. C. Doveren, C. J. van der Linden, E. E. M. Sprinken, G. Greonewegen, and W. A. Buurman, Canine HLC-class II antigens on B and T lymphocytes, *Tissue Antigens, 27*: 87-98 (1986).
16. Y. Iwaki, P. I. Terasaki, T. Kinukawa, T. H. Thai, T. Root, and R. Billing, Cross-reactivity between human and canine Ia antigens using a mouse monoclonal antibody (CIA), *Transplantation, 36*: 189-191 (1983).
17. M. Pierres, P. Mercier, M. Madsen, C. Manas, and T. Kristensen, Monoclonal mouse anti-Ia^k and anti-I-E^k antibodies cross-reacting with HLA-DR supertypic and subtypic determinants rather than classical DR allelic specificities, *Tissue Antigens, 19*: 289-300 (1982).
18. R. F. Raff, R. Storb, W. C. Ladiges, and H. J. Deeg, Recognition of target cell determinants associated with DLA-D-locus-encoded antigens by canine cytotoxic lymphocytes, *Transplantation, 40*: 323-328 (1985).
19. W. C. Ladiges, R. F. Raff, S. Brown, H. J. Deeg, and R. Storb, The canine major histocompatibility complex: Supertypic specificities defined by the primed lymphocyte test (PLT), *Immunogenetics, 19*: 359-365 (1984).
20. W. C. Ladiges, R. F. Raff, and R. Storb, A DLA-associated polymorphic determinant defined by the murine monoclonal antibody W3G10, *Fed. Proc. 45*: 501 (1986).
21. D. Metcalf, *Clonal culture of hemopoietic cells: Techniques and applications*, Elsevier, New York, 1984.
22. W. Clavo, T. M. Fliedner, E. Herbst, E. Hugl, and C. Bruch, Regeneration of blood-forming organs after autologous leukocyte transfusion in lethally irradiated dogs: II. Distribution and cellularity of the marrow in irradiated and transfused animals, *Blood, 47*: 593-601 (1976).

23. V. Erickson and B. J. Torok-Storb, Erythroid burst forming units (BFU_E) grown from canine marrow and peripheral blood, *Exp. Hematol., 9*: 468-472 (1981).
24. F. O. Wilson, S. J. Knox, and M. Shifrine, A "whole-blood" technique for the quantitation of canine "T-lymphocyte" progenitors using a semisolid culture system, *Exp. Hematol., 8*: 1031-1039 (1980).
25. J. Szer, H. J. Deeg, F. R. Appelbaum, and R. Storb, Failure of autologous marrow reconstitution after cytolytic treatment of marrow with anti-Ia monoclonal antibody, *Blood, 65*: 819-822 (1985).
26. J. C. Wulff, N. Durkopp, J. Aprile, M.-S. Tsoi, S. C. Springmeyer, H. J. Deeg, and R. Storb, Two monoclonal antibodies (DLy-1 and DLy-6) directed against canine lymphocytes, *Exp. Hematol., 10*: 609-619 (1982).
27. J. Szer, H. J. Deeg, E. Severns, and R. Storb, DLA-D specific suppressor cells characterized by monoclonal antibodies, *Transplantation, 39*: 187-192 (1985).
28. P. G. Beatty, J. A. Ledbetter, P. J. Martin, T. H. Price, and J. A. Hansen, Definition of a common leukocyte cell-surface antigen (Lp95-150) associated with diverse cell-mediated immune functions, *J. Immunol., 131*: 2913-2918 (1983).
29. J. A. Aprile, H. J. Deeg, J. C. Wulff, and R. F. Raff, Purified canine monocytes fail to confer concanavalin A responsiveness to accessory-cell-depleted lymphocytes, *Exp. Hematol., 12*: 45-51 (1984).
30. D. R. Krawiec and C. C. Muscoplat, Development and characterization of a monoclonal antibody (Aby 6C6) that distinguishes medullary from cortical thymocytes, *Am. J. Vet. Res., 45*: 400-505 (1984).
31. G. E. M. Asma, H. R. E. Schmit, and W. Hijmans, The determination of the number of T and B lymphocytes in the blood of children and adults by the direct immunofluorescence technique, *Clin. Exp. Immunol., 29*: 286-294 (1977).
32. M. C. Raff and J. J. T. Owen, Thymus-derived lymphocytes: Their distribution and role in the development of peripheral lymphoid tissues of the mouse, *Eur. J. Immunol., 1*: 27-38 (1971).
33. S. Krakowka and D. J. Guyot, Rosette formation assays in dogs: Lack of specificity of E rosettes for T lymphocytes, *Infect. Immun., 17*: 73-77 (1977).
34. K. Atkinson, H. J. Deeg, R. Storb, P. L. Weiden, L. Gerhard-Miller, B. J. Torok-Storb, M. Seigneuret, and E. D. Thomas, Canine lymphocyte subpopulations, *Exp. Hematol., 8*: 821-829 (1980).
35. J. P. Chandler and T. J. Yang, Identification of canine lymphocyte populations by immunofluorescence surface marker analysis, *Allergy Appl. Immun., 65*: 62-68 (1968).
36. H. Koyama, Y. Sakunai, O. Kajikawa, and H. Saito, Identification of canine lymphocyte subpopulations by immunofluorescence assay, *Am. J. Vet. Res., 45*: 2354-2358 (1984).
37. E. Holler, H. Kolb, N. Badenberger, R. Eckstein, G. Hoffmann-Fezer, R. P. Linke, W. Mempel, H. Rodt, and S. Thierfelder, Serological identification and separation of canine lymphocyte subpopulations, *Exp. Hematol., 12*: 774-781 (1984).

38. P. A. Trail and T. J. Yang, Characterization of canine T-lymphocyte subpopulations: The detection of Tμ and Tγ lymphocytes with homologous and heterologous immunoglobulins and the requirements for Fc receptor expression, *Cell. Immun., 74*: 182-191 (1982).
39. J. C. Wulff, G. E. Sale, H. J. Deeg, and R. Storb, Nonspecific acid esterase activity as a marker for canine T lymphocytes, *Exp. Hematol., 9*: 865-870 (1981).
40. R. Dalchau and J. W. Fabre, Identification and unusual tissue distribution of the canine and human homologues of Thy-1 (Θ), *J. Exp. Med., 149*: 576-590 (1979).
41. J. L. McKenzie and J. R. Fabre, Studies with a monoclonal antibody on the distribution of Thy-1 in the lymphoid and extracellular connective tissues of the dog, *Transplantation, 31*: 275-282 (1981).
42. D. R. Krawiec and C. C. Muscoplat, Development and characterization of a hybridoma-derived antibody (Aby 1A1) with specificity to canine thymocytes and peripheral T lymphocytes, *Am. J. Vet. Res., 45*: 491-498 (1984).
43. W. C. Ladiges, N. Durkopp, C. Urban, J. C. Wulff, and R. Storb, Monoclonal antibodies to canine cell surface antigens: A comparison of screening assays, *Hybridoma, 3*: 387-390 (1984).
44. M. Carreno, V. Esqueriazi, L. Fuller, M. Milgram, R. Alejandro, V. Pardo, and J. Miller, A monoclonal antibody affecting canine T cell reactions, *Fed. Proc., 45*: (1986).
45. J. A. Hansen, P. J. Martin, P. G. Beatty, E. A. Clark, and J. A. Ledbetter, Human T lymphocyte cell surface molecules defined by the workshop monoclonal antibodies ("T cell protocol"), in *Leucocyte Typing: Human Leucocyte Markers Detected by Monoclonal Antibodies* (A. Bernard, L. Boumsell, J. Dausset, C. Milstein, S. F. Schlossman, eds.), Springer-Verlag, New York, 1984, 195-212.
46. J. C. Wulff, H.-J. Deeg, and R. Storb, A monoclonal antibody (DT-2) recognizing canine T lymphocytes, *Transplantation, 33*: 616-620 (1982).
47. J. Szer, H. J. Deeg, P. Rieber, and R. Storb, Monoclonal antibody to human cytotoxic-suppressor T-lymphocytes cross-reacts with canine lymphocytes and inhibits cell-mediated lympholysis of canine cells, *Exp. Hematol., 13*: 641-646 (1985).
48. M. L. Schroeder, R. P. Warren, R. Storb, H. Goselink, S. Johnson, M. Brewer, Cell-mediated lympholysis in the dog, *Transplant. Proc., 7*: 411-413 (1975).
49. W. A. Buurman, A. J. J. M. Dremen, G. Groenewegen, R. J. M. M. Gres, C. J. van der Linden, and P. A. Vegt, Limiting dilution analysis of canine alloantigen-reactive T lymphocytes, *Transplantation, 35*: 363-367 (1983).
50. M. H. Breuning, B. S. Breun, M. Y. Engeloma, and P. Ivanyi, Activation of cytoxic T lymphocytes in HLA-A, -B and -C-identical responder-stimulator pairs, *Tissue Antigens, 24*: 81-89 (1984).
51. W. A. Buurman, C. J. van der Linden, A. J. J. M. Daemen, G. Groenewegen, R. F. C. Doveren, and G. Kootstra, Cell-mediated cytotoxicity toward class I and class II antigens on canine T and B lymphoblasts, *Tissue Antigens, 24*: 48-57 (1984).

52. C. Urban, J. C. Wulff, H. J. Deeg, R. F. Raff, N. Durkopp, and R. Storb, Analysis of alloreactive and cytotoxic canine lymphocytes and their precursors with murine monoclonal antibodies, *Transplantation, 35*: 469-473 (1983).
53. G. R. Betton, Natural cell-mediated cytotoxicity in the canine, in *The Canine as a Biomedical Research Model: Immunological, Hematological and Oncological Aspects* (M. Shufrime and F. O. Wilson, eds.) U.S. Department of Energy, Washington, D.C., 1980, pp. 99-126.
54. T. P. Loughran, H. J. Deeg, and R. Storb, Morphologic and phenotypic analysis of canine natural killer cells: Evidence for T-cell lineage, *Cell. Immunol., 95*: 207-217 (1985).
55. W. Newman, Selective blockade of human natural killer cells by a monoclonal antibody, *Proc. Natl. Acad. Sci. USA, 79*: 3858-3871 (1982).
56. K. Krumbacher, M. Happel, I. Doxiadis, and H. Grosse-Wilde, Enrichment of canine B-lymphocytes by Degalan bead columns, *Tissue Antigens, 25*: 111-114 (1985).
57. J. C. Wulff, M.-S. Tsoi, J. Aprile, H. J. Deeg, N. Durkopp, and R. Storb, Stimulation of canine lymphocyte subpopulations separated nonlytically by monoclonal anti-T and polyclonal anti-B cell antibodies, *Blut, 45*: 309-316 (1982).
58. C. A. Bowles, G. S. White, and D. Lucas, Rosette formation by canine peripheral blood lymphocytes, *J. Immunol., 114*: 399-402 (1975).
59. H. J. Deeg and R. Storb, Functional dichotomy of canine thoracic duct lymphocytes: Proliferation in mixed leukocyte culture and unresponsiveness to plant lectins, *J. Reticuloendothel. Soc. 29*: 395-405 (1981).
60. S. Maruyama, H. Kubagawa, and M. Cooper, Activation of human B cells and inhibition of their terminal differentiation by monoclonal antigen antibodies, *J. Immunol., 135*: 192-199 (1985).
61. E. Schmidt, H. J. Deeg, L. G. Lum, K. J. Kopecky, and R. Storb, Identification of immunoglobulin-secreting cells among canine peripheral blood mononuclear cells by the protein A hemolytic plaque assay, *Exp. Hematol., 11*: 193-201 (1983).
62. O. Prummer, A. Raghavachar, K. Siebert, T. M. Fliedner, In vitro induction of B cell differentiation in canine mononuclear blood cells: Bacterial lipopolysaccharide modulates the action of pokeweek mitogen, *J. Immunol. Meth., 75*: 193-199 (1984).
63. S. Krakowka and A. L. Wallace, In vitro properties of diffuse cytoplasmic esterase-positive canine mononuclear leukocytes, *Vet. Immunol. Immunopathol., 5*: 1-13 (1983).
64. E. M. Goodell, D. A. Blumenstock, and W. E. Bowers, Canine dendritic cells from peripheral blood and lymph nodes, *Vet. Immunol. Immunopath., 8*: 301-310 (1985).
65. J. A. Aprile and H. J. Deeg, UV irradiation of canine dendritic cells prevents mitogen induced cluster formation and lymphocyte proliferation, *Transplantation 42*: 653-660 (1986).

66. I. D. Bernstein, R. G. Andrews, S. F. Cohen, and B. E. McMaster, Normal and malignant human myelocytic and monocytic cells identified by monoclonal antibodies, *J. Immunol., 128*: 876-883 (1982).
67. R. G. Andrews, B. J. Torok-Storb, and I. D. Bernstein, Myeloid-associated differentiation antigens on stem cells and their progeny identified by monoclonal antibodies, *Blood, 62*: 124-132 (1983).
68. J. C. Wulff, S. C. Springmeyer, H. J. Deeg, and R. Storb, Canine bronchoalveolar cells: Antigen-presenting macrophages are Ia-positive, lymphocytes are of non-B lineage, *Blut, 47*: 263-270 (1983).
69. C. A. Holmberg, J. S. Manning, and B. I. Obsrun, Canine malignant lymphomas: A comparison of morphologic and immunologic parameters, *J. Natl. Cancer Inst., 56*: 125-129 (1976).
70. O. Onions, B- and T-cell markers on canine lymphosarcoma cells, *J. Natl. Cancer Inst., 59*: 1001-1006 (1977).
71. S. K. Dutta, M. W. Novilla, M. K. Baumgardner, and A. Ingling, Lymphocyte responsiveness to mitogens and quantitation of T and B lymphocytes in canine malignant lymphoma, *Am. J. Vet. Res., 39*: 455-458 (1978).
72. F. R. Appelbaum, G. E. Sale, R. Storb, K. Charrier, H. J. Deeg, T. Graham, and J. C. Wulff, Phenotyping of canine lymphoma with monoclonal antibodies directed at cell surface antigens: Classification, morphology, clinical presentation, and response to chemotherapy, *Hematol. Oncol., 2*: 151-168 (1984).
73. J. M. Pesando, P. Hoffman, and T. Conrad, Malignant human B cells express two populations of p24 surface antigens, *J. Immunol., 135*: 2709-2714 (1986).

10
Surface Antigens of Rabbit Lymphoid and Other Leukocytic Cells

J. MICHAEL WILKINSON
Royal College of Surgeons of England, London, England

I. INTRODUCTION

The rabbit has a long history as an experimental animal in biomedical research. This is in part due to its size, being small enough for economical breeding and handling but large enough to provide useful quantities of tissue and frequent blood samples. It has also proved to be an excellent model for a number of human disease conditions (1,2). Early work on tissue transplantation and histocompatibility was carried out in the rabbit (3-5), and it continues to be a useful model in this area (6-8). Probably the best model for rheumatoid arthritis is that of Dumonde and Glynn (9), which closely resembles human rheumatoid arthritis. The use of this antigen-induced model has been reviewed recently by Hunneyball (10) and has been shown to be dependent on the cellular immune response to the antigen. Atherosclerosis has been studied in either cholesterol-fed rabbits or in the Watanabe heritable hyperlipidemic (WHHL) rabbit (11), a model for human familial hypercholesterolemia (12). The role of macrophages in the development of atherosclerotic lesions has been emphasized by a number of groups (13-15). Other diseases that are studied using the rabbit as an experimental animal include syphilis (16,17), lung disease (18), diabetes (19), leprosy (20), and myasthenia gravis (21). In addition rabbits have been used as the host species for studying the pathogenosis of a number of viral diseases, including adult T-cell leukemia (22), malignant catarrhal fever (23), herpesvirus infection (24,25), and acquired immunodeficiency syndrome (AIDS) (26), where infection by the malignant rabbit fibroma virus has been proposed as a model for this disease (27,28).

All these disease states, and others, involve a perturbation of the immune system, and thus a detailed understanding of this system is of importance in gaining an insight into the pathogenesis of the disease concerned. Much of the early work on the humoral response to antigens and on the structure of immunoglobulins was carried out in the rabbit, and it was in this system that the phenomenon of allotypy was first described (29). The discovery of the unique allotype system associated with the variable region of the heavy chain has led to important insights into immunogenetics (30), and recent studies on the genes coding for these regions suggest that there are important differences between their organization and those of the analogous human and mouse proteins (31,32). In contrast to these studies, understanding of the rabbit cellular immune system has lagged behind that of man and mouse, and although there is clearly a general similarity, there may be important differences.

Rabbit lymphoid cells can be divided into the general categories of T and B cells (33,34). B cells are distinguished by antisera to surface immunoglobulin, by their mitogenic response to antiimmunoglobulin antisera (35) and by their adhereance to nylon wool (36). T cells have been characterized by a variety of heteroantisera to thymocytes (36-41) and can also form rosettes with papain-treated rabbit erythrocytes (42). T cells are also distinguished by their ability to respond to the mitogens Con A and PHA (39). Purified preparations of T and B cells have been isolated by specific killing of one or other subpopulation with a specific antiserum and complement (36-38,43) or by rosetting using antibody-coated erythrocytes (44,45). Other methods for the purification of T cells have involved depletion of B cells with nylon wool (36), by panning with antiimmunoglobulin antibody (46), or by absorption onto antibody-coated beads (47).

Using such methods the percentage of T and B cells in various lymphoid organs and peripheral blood have been determined (34,41,44,48), and subsets of T cells have been recognized (33,34,36,38,49). Fradelizi et al. (37) have defined a rabbit thymus lymphocyte antigen (RTLA), which characterizes thymocytes and peripheral T cells, while Chou et al. (40) have defined a rabbit bursal-equivalent antigen (RABELA), which characterizes B cells. These antigens are operationally defined, and no data have been obtained on the cell-surface molecules with which they are associated. The only rabbit lymphoid cell-surface molecule to be characterized using polyclonal antisera is a 12-Kd glycoprotein isolated from a thymocyte membrane preparation by Navran and Archer (50), which is able to inhibit the cytotoxicity of a goat anti-rabbit T-cell serum.

In addition to the interactions of T and B cells in the induction of the immune response, increasing attention has been given to the role of accessory cells. While the macrophage is of major importance in this respect, nonphagocytic cells may be of equal importance. These cells are the Langerhans cells of skin, veiled cells of afferent lymph, and interdigitating cells of lymph nodes (51). In studying the role of these cells in antigen presentation, the rabbit has proved to be of particular value in the investigation of veiled cells owing to the difficulty of obtaining them from smaller animals (52-54).

There are a number of difficulties in studying the cellular immune system of the rabbit as compared with that of the mouse. One of these is the difficulty of developing and maintaining inbred and congenic lines. Although inbred rabbit lines are available (55), rabbits are difficult to inbreed (56), and most investigators have preferred the use of outbred stocks. A second problem is the lack of transformed leukocyte cell lines, particularly those of defined function whose surface phenotype can be studied easily. A few cell lines are now available, and these are detailed in the following section.

II. RABBIT LEUKOCYTE CELL LINES

Attempts to transform rabbit lymphoid cells have not met with any great success. Cell lines which have been described in the literature are listed in Table 1.

A. TRSC-1

These cells were transformed with simian virus 40 (SV40) from the spleen cells of a hyperimmune rabbit producing antibody of restricted heterogeneity to Type III pneumococcal vaccine (57). Although this cell produces antibody specific for the original immunogen (58), this is intracellular and no surface or secreted immunoglobulin could be detected (59). Attempts to use this cell as a fusion partner with normal rabbit spleen cells in order to produce further antibody-producing cell lines were unsuccessful (59). No Fc or C3b receptors were detected, and it probably represents an early pre-B cell (59).

Table 1 Rabbit Transformed Cell Lines

Cell line	Transforming agent	Cell type	Ref.
TRSC-1	SV40	Immature pre-B cell	57-59
RL-5	Herpesvirus ateles	T cell	60
MF/120	Sheep-associated malignant catarrhal fever	NK cell	64
Ra-1	HTLV I	T cell	22
SV/6083	SV40	Macrophage	73
LPV/6056	Lymphotrophic papovavirus	Macrophage	73
HSV/6375	Herpesvirus sylvilagus	Macrophage	73

B. RL-5

This line (also known by the designations RLA, MD3, and EE-52) was transformed by herpesvirus ateles (60) by inoculation of the virus into the popliteal lymph node of a rabbit of the inbred B/J strain. The RL-5 cell line does not express surface immunoglobulin but does express a class I antigen of restricted heterogeneity (61). Glycoprotein preparations from this cell line have been used to raise monoclonal antibodies (62), as will be discussed below. These antibodies unequivocally demonstrate it to be a T-cell line. The functional subset to which it belongs is not known, but it has recently been shown to possess rearranged T-cell receptor α-chain gene transcripts (63).

C. MF/120

This cell line was isolated from the mesenteric lymph node of a rabbit infected with sheep-associated malignant catarrhal fever (64). Morphologically these cells resemble large granular lymphocytes. They have no surface immunoglobulin but react with antithymocyte serum (ATS). They show cytotoxicity towards kidney cells and cell lines from both rabbits and other species and are thought to be natural killer (NK) cells. They are able to transfer the infection to other rabbits by inoculation of whole cells (64). Other similar cell lines have since been derived and maintained in suspension culture. One of these, MF/746, gives surface immunofluorescence with the anti-T-cell antibodies L11/135 and W4/86 (see below) but not with 2C4, which recognizes class II antigens (65).

D. Ra-1

This and a number of other cell lines were transformed by co-culturing rabbit peripheral blood lymphocytes with a human T-cell line transformed with human T-cell leukemia virus (HTLV I) or by infecting rabbits with HTLV I by inoculation with either transformed human or rabbit T cells (22,66,67). Although the transformation of these cells is relatively easy, they not only express viral antigens on the cell surface but also carry infectious virus particles. They do not express surface immunoglobulin or receptors for IgG Fc, sheep erythrocytes, or complement (22). They give a positive reaction, by immunofluorescence, with the antibodies L11/135 and 2C4 (68,69) and are thus T cells which express class II antigens. In this they are like their counterparts derived from human peripheral lymphocytes (70-72).

E. SV/6083, LPV/6056, and HSV/6375

These cell lines have been derived recently by viral transformation of normal rabbit spleen cells by Kulaga et al. (73). They were transformed by SV40, lymphotropic papovavirus, and herpesvirus sylvilagus, respectively, and each line expresses appropriate viral genes. None of the cells contain rearranged immunoglobulin genes or express the T-cell antigen recognized by the L11/135 antibody and are thus unlikely to be of lymphoid origin. All three have been characterized as macrophagelike on the basis of cytochemical staining and the functional tests that they are phagocytic and are able to mediate antibody-dependent cell-mediated cytotoxicity. All three cell lines express message for class II genes, but only SV/6083 and LPV/6056 appear to express the gene product on the cell surface, as judged by reactivity with the 2C4 antibody. The authors suggest that these cell lines may be useful for the investigation of the expression of class II genes and also of antigen presentation in the rabbit.

In addition to these cell lines, a number of T-cell clones have been established which are IL-2 dependent. Cytotoxic T-cell lines have been obtained by growth from mesenteric lymph node cells that had been stimulated in mixed lymphocyte culture with mouse spleen cells (74). A minority of cell lines derived in this way showed cytotoxic activity for the mouse target cells, and this could be inhibited with ATS. Jackson et al. (75) have derived a helper T-cell clone from a rabbit hyperimmunized with group C streptococcal vaccine. This clone is surface Ig-negative and L11/135-positive and was shown to have helper activity in the induction of antibody specific for the immunizing antigen. The establishment of these and other such clones will be of great use in defining subsets of rabbit lymphoid cells and understanding their interactions.

III. MONOCLONAL ANTIBODIES RECOGNIZING LEUKOCYTE MARKERS

Our present understanding of the interactions and mechanisms underlying the cellular immune response in both man and mouse has come about, to a large extent, by the use of alloantisera and, more recently, monoclonal antibodies which can be used to recognize differentiation antigens defining functional subsets of lymphoid cells and which can be used to inhibit cellular interactions. With the development of monoclonal antibody production methods the way is now open to pursue this type of analysis in the rabbit. A number of monoclonal antibodies to rabbit leukocyte determinants have been prepared and characterized, and these are summarized in Table 2. Other antibodies which are less well characterized are summarized in Table 3. A variety of approaches has been used for characterization, with flow cytometry as the main method of defining the subsets of cells recognized. Other antibodies have been studied using inhibition of functional assays and complement-mediated cytotoxicity, and in many cases molecular data on the antigens recognized have been obtained. For convenience of discussion these antibodies have been divided into four groups, those which recognize T cells, those which recognize both T and B cells, those which recognize MHC antigens, and those which recognize other leukocytes. These groupings are shown in Table 4.

Table 2 Monoclonal Antibodies to Rabbit Leukocytes

Antibody	Subclass	Immunogen	Antigen	Target cells	Refs.
L11/135	G1	RL-5 glycoproteins	120 Kd gp	Th, T, PMN, MO	62, 76
L12/27	G1	RL-5 glycoproteins	NI	Th, T, B	62, 76
L12/201	G1	RL-5 glycoproteins	NI	Th, T, B	62, 76
L13/64	G2a	RL-5 glycoproteins	90/115 Kd gp	Th, T, B	62, 76
W4/28	G2a	RL-5 glycoproteins	90 Kd gp	Th, T, B	62, 76
W4/86	G1	RL-5 glycoproteins	90 Kd gp	Th, T, B	62, 76
L13/112	G1	RL-5 glycoproteins	42 Kd gp	—	98
9AE10	M	Spleen/MLN cells	25 Kd	Th, T	79
8AC8	G1	Spleen/MLN cells	ND	Th, T	81
2C4	G2a	Spleen cells	28/31/35 Kd	B, MO, VC	108
ART-A	G1	Thymocytes	95/105 Kd	T, B	95
ART-F	G1	Thymocytes	95 Kd	T, B	95
1.24	G1	Thymocytes	200 Kd	T, B, M	89
4.B9	M	Thymocytes/LN-T cells	ND	T, (B)	89

10.B3	G2a	Thymocytes/LN-T cells	ND	T, (B)	89
12.C7	G1	Thymocytes/LN-T cells	ND	T	89
10.C5	G2a	Thymocytes/LN-T cells	ND	T, B, M	89
3AE8	G1	Splenic B cells	NI	MO	116
ACM-1	G1	Thymocytes/Spleenic T cells	20 Kd	T, PMN	80
198	G1	Adherent blood leukocytes	165/95 Kd	M, MO, PMN	117
anti-61	G2b	Synthetic peptide	42 Kd	RL-5	102
RT1	G3	Splenic T cells	ND	Th, T, (B), PMN	91, 92
RT2	G2b	Splenic T cells	ND	Th, T, PMN	91, 92
RB1	M	Splenic B cells	ND	T, B, PMN	91, 92
RB2	M	Splenic B cells	ND	B	91, 92
RB3	M	Appendix B cells	ND	B	91, 92
RB4	M	Appendix B cells	ND	B	91, 92
RM1	G2b	Peritoneal exudate cells	ND	MO	91
RM2	M	Peritoneal exudate cells	ND	MO	91

Abbreviations: Th, thymocytes; PMN, polymorphonuclear leukocytes; M, monocytes; MO, macrophages; VC, veiled cells; MLN, mesenteric lymph node; NI, not identified; ND, not determined.

Table 3 Incompletely Characterized Antibodies

Antibody	Specificity	Refs.
3F5	Class II	109
1AF10	Class II	109
20.H1	Class II	111
4B1	Class I (K/D like)	101
5E2	Class I (T1/T6 like)	128
1B11	Class II	101
3A7	25-Kd protein kinase on B cells, MO, platelets	101
3F3	MO-specific	101
SRM-1	MO, erythrocytes	14

Table 4 Summary of Specificites of mAbs

T cell-specific	T and B cells	Class I	Class II	Others
L11/135	L12/27	L13/112	2C4	3AE8
9AE10	L12/201	anti-61	3F5	SRM-1
ACM-1	1.24	4B1	1AF10	RM1
4.B9	10.C5	5E2	1B11	RM2
10.B3	W4/28		20.H1	198
RT1	W4/86			3F3
RT2	L13/64			3A7
12.C7	ART-A			
8AC8	ART-F			
	RB1			
	RB2			
	RB3			
	RB4			

References for these mAbs are given in Tables 2 and 3 and in the text.

A. T-Cell-Specific Antibodies

Several of the antibodies described recognize essentially all thymocytes and circulating T cells and can thus be used as T-cell markers.

1. L11/135 (62,76)

This antibody recognizes a 120-Kd glycoprotein on thymocytes and T cells. This is the immunodominant antigen of the RL-5 cell line (62). After tunicamycin treatment the antigen was reduced in size to approximately 117 Kd and its antigenicity was found to be preserved even after heat treatment. It is thus a remarkably heat-stable protein whose antigenic structure is not modified by N-glycosylation. The antibody has proved effective in separating B and T cells by a panning technique (76). This technique has been used in the preparation of T-cell clones (75) and in a study of the pathogenicity of the bovine herpesvirus Movar 33/63 (24). L11/135 has also been used for the enumeration of T cells in studies of herpesvirus sylvilagus infection (25) and the immunopathology of experimental allergic encephalomyelitis (77). The study of Kramp et al. (25) demonstrates that the L11/135 antigen is shared by cottontail rabbit T cells. Although L11/135 can distinguish readily between B and T lymphocytes, the antigen has also been shown to be present on macrophages and neutrophils (78).

2. 9AE10 (79) and ACM-1 (80)

These antibodies have a similar tissue distribution to L11/135, in that they recognize all thymocytes and T cells and both have been shown to recognize the same antigen, which is a protein of 20-25 Kd. It has been suggested that this may be the rabbit equivalent of the mouse Thy-1 antigen (79), and this is supported by the reaction of 9AE10 with rabbit brain by membrane immunofluorescence. However, Chen et al. (80) have failed to absorb out 9AE10 activity with brain tissue and have cast doubt on this identification. McNicholas et al. (81) have carried out a functional analysis of the cells recognized by 9AE10 and have shown that they have the activities classically shown by T cells. While both antibodies recognize the same antigen, 9AE10, being an IgM, is better suited to techniques based on complement-mediated cytotoxicity, while ACM -1 is of greater use for fluorescence methods. Both antibodies react with the majority of peritoneal neutrophils but not macrophages (80).

9AE10 has been used to purify B cells from lymph nodes and spleen by complement-mediated lysis of T cells (82) in an investigation of mitogen-induced phosphorylation of lymphocyte cytosolic proteins and by antibody-mediated rosetting, using the technique of Wilson et al. (44), in an investigation of B-cell activation by antiimmunoglobulin antibodies (83). Wormmeester et al. (84) have also used it for the purification of both B and T cells by rosetting using an avidin-biotin system. 9AE10 has further been used to enumerate T cells by immunofluorescence after density gradient separation of B and T cells (85), after treatment of rabbits with dexamethasone (86), and in cerebrospinal fluid in a study of the effect of cyclosporin treatment of cryptococcal infections (87). Sobel et al. (77) used 9AE10 in their investigations and found that in large mononuclear cells of peripheral blood, a significantly higher percentage of cells stained with L11/135 than with 9AE10. ACM-1 has been used by Walstra et al. (88) to characterize T cells after purification from peripheral blood. Their work emphasizes the importance of a standardized method of separation in order to obtain reproducible T/B cell ratios.

3. 4.B9 and 10.B3 (89)

These antibodies have similar but not identical specificites. They recognize subpopulations of thymocytes, 25% in the case of 4.B9 and 80% in the case of 10.B3. They both recognize the majority of peripheral T cells and possibly 5-10% of B cells. 4.B9 has been used to identify T cells in a variety of lymphoid tissues in a study of T-cell activation (90). Further use is reported by Williams et al. (129).

4. RT1 and RT2 (91)

Two antibodies have recently been described by Ponsard et al. (91) which are reactive with antigens described as RT1 and RT2. The distribution of these antigens has been studied by complement-mediated cytotoxicity. The antibodies recognize essentially all thymocytes and T cells, but the antigen distribution is wider than that of RTLA (91). In particular, RT1 is found on the majority of peritoneal neutrophils while RT2 is present on a subpopulation (92). The antibodies have been used in an investigation of cells involved in the regulation of mitogen stimulation of spleenic T cells (93).

5. 12.C7 (89) and 8AC8 (94)

Two other antibodies have been shown to react with subsets of T cells. 12.C7 reacts with 60% of thymocytes and between 10-30% of T cells in lymph node, spleen, and peripheral blood but not with B cells or monocytes. It has been suggested that 12.C7 may recognize the cytotoxic/suppressor subset but no data are available to substantiate this (80). 8AC8 reacts with 40-80% of thymocytes and 50-96% of spleen or lymph node T cells (94). The 8AC8-positive cells were highly responsive to mitogen or antigen stimulation and to stimulation in a mixed lymphocyte reaction, and these cells may be the inducer/helper subpopulation, although again further data are required to answer this question.

B. Antibodies Reactive with T and B Cells

A number of antibodies recognize thymocytes, B cells, and T cells in such a way that a variety of subsets of these cells can be recognized. These are described briefly in this section.

Some new antibodies of this type have been reported by Loar et al. (130).

1. L12/27, L12/201 (62,76), 1.24, and 10.C5 (89)

L12/27 and L12/201 (76) both show differential staining of subsets of thymocytes and also stain all T and B cells and null cells, although the staining intensities of different subpopulations may differ. They clearly recognize different antigens but the nature of these antigens could not be determined by immunoprecipitation (62). L12/201 stains T cells more brightly than B cells, and this pattern of reactivity is shared by the antibodies 1.24 and 10.C5, which probably recognize the same molecule which may be the leukocyte-common antigen (89). These latter two antibodies also recognize monocytes. Sobel et al. (77) report the use of L12/201, and Williams et al. (129) of 1.24, for tissue staining.

2. W4/28, W4/86, L13/64 (62,76), ART-A, and ART-F (95)

These antibodies recognize similar subsets of glycoproteins of about 90 Kd. The antibodies W4/28, W4/86, and L13/64 are able to discriminate between different subsets of thymocytes and, while staining all T cells, only react with about half the population of splenic B cells, these being large cells which are strongly positive for μ chain (76). Apart from these similarities it is clear that they recognize different antigens as the three 90-Kd glycoproteins have been shown to be different by sequential immunoprecipitation (62). The L13/64 antibody immunoprecipitates a minor polypeptide of 115 Kd in addition to that of 90 Kd; this disappeared after tunicamycin treatment and a major component of 82 Kd was obtained (62). The relationship of the bands at 115 Kd and 90 Kd is not clear. Two other antibodies, ART-A and ART-F (95), show some similarity to L13/64. They both recognize most, if not all, thymocytes and T cells in the spleen and lymph nodes but only about 50% of B cells in these organs. ART-A immunoprecipitates two proteins of 95 Kd and 105 Kd but ART-F only one of 95 Kd. ART-F inhibits the binding of ART-A to RL-5 cells (95) and thus the two antibodies clearly recognize the same antigen; whether this is the same as that recognized by L13/64 can only be resolved by direct comparison.

3. RB1, RB2, RB3, and RB4

Four antibodies directed against antigens found on B cells have been described by Ponsard et al. (91). These antigens have been given the designations RB1, RB2, RB3, and RB4. The antibody to RB1 reacts with a majority of thymocytes and splenic T and B cells and also with a minority of neutrophils. It is thus similar in its specificity to some of the above antibodies. The antibodies to RB2, RB3, and RB4 all react with about 75% of B cells and with only small numbers of T cells. It is not clear what the significance of the B-cell staining is.

C. Antibodies to MHC Antigens

1. Class I Molecules

In the rabbit the existance of at least one class I locus, RLA-A, has been demonstrated serologically and has been shown to control allograft rejection (4,96,97).

Studies on class I gene expression have been carried out using the RL-5 cell line at both the protein and c-DNA levels (61,98-100) and have suggested that the rabbit expresses a more limited number of class I antigens than man or mouse. Surprisingly, in view of the high level of class I antigen expression on T cells, few monoclonal antibodies have been described which recognize them.

The antibodies L12/36 and L13/112 only recognize class I heavy chain when not associated with β_2-microglobulin and do not immunoprecipitate such chains from normal rabbit spleen cells (98). Two antibodies, 4B1 and 5E2, have recently been prepared (101). 4B1 recognizes K- or D-like class I molecules on all rabbit lymphocytes, but most strongly on T cells, while 5E2 recognizes a T1-like class I molecule (128).

A different approach has been used by Le Guern et al. (102), who have used synthetic peptides, based on the c-DNA and genomic sequences for the class I antigen expressed by the RL-5 cell line, as immunogen. Using a peptide corresponding to positions 61-73 of the N-domain, predicted to be a hydrophilic region of the protein, a number of antibodies reacting with the peptide were obtained. Of these, only one, designated anti-61, reacted with RL-5 cells but not with human cells that express class I. The specificity was confirmed by transfection of the rabbit class I gene into HeLa cells, which then also reacted with the antibody. This antibody, together with L13/112, has been used by Marchitto et al. (103) in an investigation of the association of class I MHC molecules with the surface of *Treponema pallidum* isolated from infected rabbits.

2. Class II Molecules

The class II locus, RLA-D, has been defined by the mixed lymphocyte reaction (104) and shown to code for alloantigens similar to class II antigens in other species (105). Studies of the class II gene family of the rabbit using c-DNA probes suggest that there are at least five α-chain and ten β-chain genes. These are homologous with the human DP, DQ, and DR subregion genes (106,107).

Three antibodies, 2C4, 3F5, and 1AF10, reacting with class II molecules, have been described (108,109). They all immunoprecipitate proteins with subunits of 28 Kd, 31 Kd, and 35 Kd, and limited sequence analysis suggests that they recognize either α or β chains of the DQ type (110). Preliminary data are available on two further antibodies to class II molecules, 1B11 and 20.H1. 1B11 recognizes what is probably a DP- or DR-like antigen (101), but no biochemical characterization has been carried out for 20.H1 (111). 2C4, 3F5, and 20.H1 are able to inhibit the mixed leukocyte reaction while 1AF10 is not (109,111).

2C4 has proved of particular use in investigating Ia expression on accessory cells. Donnelly and Prendergast (112) have studied Ia induction on macrophages in the eye in antigen-induced uveitis. Studies of antigen presentation by dendritic cells and macrophages have been carried out by Kapsenberg et al. (113) and by chondrocytes by Tiku et al. (114). 2C4 has also been shown to react strongly with veiled cells (115). Sobel et al. (77) have also used 2C4 in studies of Ia expression in tissues in allergic encephalomyelitis.

D. Antibodies Recognizing Other Leukocytes

Several antibodies have been described which react with leukocyte antigens other than those referred to above.

1. Macrophage-Specific Antibodies

A number of antibodies have been raised by immunization of mice with peritoneal exudate cells.

3AE8, described by Chen et al. (116), is reactive only with oil-induced peritoneal exudate macrophages; it does not react with T or B cells, neutrophils, or resident peritoneal or alveolar macrophages. It also cross-reacts with similar cells in both mouse and rat. The antigen recognized appears to be a membrane protein but attempts to identify this were unsuccessful.

SRM-1, prepared by Watanabe et al. (14) using thioglycolate-induced peritoneal exudate cells, reacts with monocyte/macrophage cells and also erythrocytes in peritoneal exudate, spleen, and peripheral blood as determined by flow cytometry and cytochemistry. The antibody was used for immunocytochemical staining of tissue macrophages in paraffin-embedded sections in an investigation of the role of macrophages in atherosclerosis. No further characterization in terms of subclass or antigenic specificity is available.

RM1 and RM2, raised against oil-induced peritoneal cells (91), show differential activity against cells from different organs. RM1, but not RM2, reacts with 30-40% of bone marrow cells, whereas RM2, but not RM1, recognizes 30-60% of peritoneal exudate cells. However, after attachment to a plastic surface, 48% of the adherent peritoneal exudate cells were found to have become positive for RM1, and it would seem that the RM1 antigen is characteristic of adherent cells.

3F3 is also largely macrophage-specific but reacts with some B cells in the appendix and with the TRSC-1 cell line (101).

2. Mab.198 (117)

This was induced by immunization of mice with rabbit adherent blood leukocytes. It reacts with granulocytes, monocytes, and tissue macrophages. The antigen recognized is a membrane protein with two noncovalently linked polypeptides of 165 Kd and 95 Kd. Mab.198 inhibits complement, but not Fc, receptor-mediated granulocyte functions. It is probable, therefore, that it recognizes the complement type 3 receptor (CR3).

3. 3A7 (101)

3A7 reacts with a 25 Kd protein which appears to be a protein kinase and is found on B cells, macrophages, platelets, and the TRSC-1 cell line (101).

E. Homologies with Antigens of Other Species

With the exception of the class I and II molecules referred to previously (Section III.C), it has not proved possible to identify, with any degree of certainty, the antigens recognized by the antibodies described above as being homologous with those described in any other species. For this purpose data on molecular characterization, including amino acid sequence data, tissue distribution, and correlation of expression with cellular function are all required. In no case is this the situation and thus identifications are, at best, tentative.

The antigen recognized by 9AE10 and ACM-1 has been identified as the rabbit homologue of the well-studied Thy-1 antigen (118), but there are some doubts about this identification and these have been noted above (80). On the basis of molecular size and its expression on all T cells, the L11/135 antigen may be the rabbit equivalent of the human T12 antigen (119), which also has an apparent molecular weight of 120 Kd. More problematic is the nature of the 90-Kd antigens which are identified by W4/28, W4/86, L13/64, ART-A, and ART-F. It is possible that one of these may be the equivalent of the heavily glycosylated 95-Kd glycoprotein identified on rat thymocytes with the antibody W3/13 (120), but the molecular data available is not sufficient to draw any firm conclusions. 1.24 recognizes a 200-Kd protein which may well be a leukocyte-common antigen (127). The 198 antibody recognizes a two-chain protein of 165 Kd and 95 Kd, and this may be similar to the LFA-1 and Mac-1 antigens (121).

As noted in Section III A5, functional studies suggest that 8AC8 recognizes the helper/inducer subset of T cells (94) and may therefore recognize an antigen homologous to the human T4 or the mouse L3T4 antigens (119,121). 12.C7, on the other hand, may recognize the cytotoxic/suppressor T-cell subset (89) and may recognize an antigen homologous to the human T8 or the mouse Ly 2/3 (119,121). As no molecular data have been obtained for these two antigens, these identifications must remain tentative.

IV. CONCLUSIONS

This review has attempted to gather together all the available data on monoclonal antibodies which recognize rabbit leukocyte antigens. In terms of defining differentiation antigens and molecules of functional importance, progress has so far been somewhat disappointing. Jackson et al. (76) have defined four subsets of thymocytes and two each of T and B cells by careful analysis of their reactivity with a panel of antibodies, but it was not possible to correlate any of these with a known function or stage of differentiation. Four subpopulations of thymocytes have also been demonstrated by Roholl et al. (122), and a tentative pathway of differentiation has been proposed, but it is not clear how these subpopulations correlate with those recognized by the monoclonal antibodies. Likewise, two subpopulations of B cells have been recognized by Watkins et al. (123) which seem to correlate with those demonstrated by Jackson et al. (76). Of these, the small cells which express low amounts of surface Ig are nonresponsive with B-cell mitogens, while the large cells, with a high expression of surface Ig, are responsive and are also those that are positive for the antibodies W4/28, W4/86, and L13/64.

Two antibodies which may recognize helper/inducer and cytotoxic/suppressor cells, respectively, have been described but there are no antibodies available which recognize the rabbit equivalent of T3 or the T-cell receptor molecule. Recent reports of the cloning of m-RNA from the α-chain (63) and genes for the β chain (124,125) of the rabbit T-cell receptor should allow the preparation of antibodies which recognize this structure by the use of synthetic peptides as antigens in an approach similar to that used by Le Guern et al. for the preparation of antibodies to class I antigens.

Despite the limited number of antibodies available, an increasing number of studies have been reported where monoclonal antibodies have been used to characterize rabbit leukocytes, and these investigations have been documented in Section III. These studies, together with those referred to in the introduction, give an indication of the wide variety of uses of the rabbit as an experimental model as evidenced by a recent workshop on rabbit immunogenetics and immunobiology (126). Further comparative work is required to define the antigens recognized by those antibodies which are already available, and other antibodies are required which will help towards a better understanding of the immune system of the rabbit.

ACKNOWLEDGMENTS

I wish to express my thanks to numerous colleagues who have provided me with information and data prior to publication. I am also grateful to the Wellcome Trust for financial support.

REFERENCES

1. R. R. Fox, Taxonomy and genetics, in *The Biology of the Laboratory Rabbit* (S. H. Weisbroth, R. E. Flatt, and A. L. Kraus, eds.), Academic Press, New York, 1974, pp. 1-22.
2. R. R. Fox, The rabbit as a research subject, *The Physiologist, 27*: 393-402 (1984).
3. P. B. Medawar, The behaviour and fate of skin autografts and skin homografts in rabbits, *J. Anat., 78*: 176-199 (1944).
4. R. G. Tissot, and C. Cohen, Histocompatibility in the rabbit. Identification of the major locus, *Tissue Antigens, 2*: 267-279 (1972).
5. C. Cohen, and R. G. Tissot, Specialized research applications: II Serological genetics, in *The Biology of the Laboratory Rabbit* (S. H. Weisbroth, R. E. Flatt, and A. L. Kraus, eds.), Academic Press, New York, 1974, pp. 167-177.

6. A. Gratwhol, I. Forster, and B. Speck, Histoincompatible skin and marrow grafts in rabbits on cyclosporin A, *Transplantation, 33*: 361-364 (1982).
7. L. T. Adler, J. E. Rehg, C. Cohen, and M. M. Le Beau, Graft-versus-host reactions and abrogation of allotype suppression following histoincompatible lymphoid cell transfers in rabbits, *Transplantation, 37*: 606-611 (1984).
8. E. Claasen, L. T. Adler, K. Saito, T. Yoshio, and F. L. Adler, Functional and histological studies of adoptive immunity in neonatally transplanted rabbits, *Immunology, 60*: 37-44 (1987).
9. D. C. Dumonde, and L. E. Glynn, The production of arthritis in rabbits by an immunological reaction to fibrin, *Br. J. Exp. Pathol., 43*: 373-383 (1962).
10. I. M. Hunneyball, Use of experimental arthritis in the rabbit for development of antiarthritic drugs, *Adv. Inflammation Res., 7*: 249-262 (1984).
11. Y. Watanabe, Serial inbreeding of rabbits with hereditary hyperlipidemia (WHHL-rabbit), *Atherosclerosis, 36*: 261-268 (1975).
12. L. M. Buja, T. Kita, J. L. Goldstein Y. Watanabe, and M. S. Brown, Cellular pathology of progressive atherosclerosis in the WHHL rabbit. An animal model or familial hypercholesterolemia, *Arteriosclerosis, 3*: 87-101 (1983).
13. M. E. Rosenfeld, A. Faggiotto, and R. Ross, The role of mononuclear phagocytes in primate and rabbit models of atherosclerosis, *Proc. 4th Leiden Conference on Mononuclear Phagocytes,* The Hague, Martinus Nijhoff, 1985, pp. 795-802.
14. T. Watanabe, M. Hirata, Y. Yoshikawa, Y. Nagafuchi, H. Toyoshima, and T. Watanabe, Role of macrophages in atherosclerosis. Sequential observations of cholesterol-induced rabbit aortic lesion by the immunoperoxidase technique using monoclonal antimacrophage antibody *Lab. Invest., 53*: 80-90 (1985).
15. T. Tsukada, M. Rosenfeld, R. Ross, and A. M. Gown, Immunocytochemical analysis of cellular components in atherosclerotic lesions. Use of monoclonal antibodies with the Watanabe and fat-fed rabbit, *Arteriosclerosis, 6*: 601-613 (1986).
16. K. Wicher, V. Wicher, S. M. Nakeeb, and S. Dubiski, Studies of rabbit testes infected with *Treponema pallidum.* I. Immunopathology, *Br. J. Vener. Dis., 59*: 349-358 (1983).
17. V. Wicher, and K. Wicher, Studies of rabbit testes infected with *Treponema pallidum.* III. Immunosuppressive activity of infiltrating mononuclear cells, *Br. J. Vener. Dis., 60*: 1-7 (1984).
18. B. Thompson, and Q. N. Myrcik, Characterisation and maturation of alveolar macrophages procured from BCG-induced pulmonary granulomas, *Exp. Lung Res., 9*: 237-253 (1985).
19. S. I. Roth, and H. H. Conaway, Spontaneous diabetes mellitus in the New Zealand white rabbit, *Am. J. Path., 109*: 359-363 (1982).
20. R. N. Mshana, D. P. Humber, M. Harboe, and A. Belehu, Nerve damage following intraneural injection of *Mycobacterium leprae* into rabbits presensitized to mycobacteria, *Clin. Exp. Immunol., 52*: 441-448 (1983).
21. G. Levi, R. Tarrab-Hazdai, and V. I. Teichberg, Prevention and therapy with electrolectin of experimental autoimmune myasthenia gravis in rabbits, *Eur. J. Immunol., 13*: 500-507 (1983).

22. I. Miyoshi, S. Yoshimoto, H. Taguchi, I. Kubonishi, M. Fujishita, Y. Ohtsuki, Y. Shiraishi, and T. Akagi, Transformation of rabbit lymphocytes with T-cell leukemia virus, *Gann, 74*: 1-4 (1983).
23. H. Bielefeld Ohmann, and L. A. Babiuk, Viral infections in domestic animals as models for studies of viral immunology and pathogenesis, *J. Gen. Virol., 66*: 1-25 (1986).
24. F. A. Osorio, D. L. Rock, and D. E. Reed, Studies on the pathogenesis of a bovine cytomegalo-like virus in an experimental host, *J. Gen. Virol., 66*: 1941-1951 (1985).
25. W. J. Kramp, P. Medveczky, C. Mulder, H. C. Hinze, and J. L. Sullivan, Herpesvirus sylvilagus infects both B and T lymphocytes *in vivo, J. Virol., 56*: 60-65 (1985).
26. J. M. Richards, J. M. Bedford, and S. S. Witkin, Rectal insemination modifies immune responses in rabbits, *Science, 224*: 390-392 (1984).
27. D. S. Strayer, E. Skaletsky, and J. L. Leibowitz, *In vitro* growth of two related leporipoxviruses in lymphoid cells, *Virology, 145*: 330-334 (1985).
28. D. S. Strayer, S. Sell, and J. L. Leibowitz, Malignant rabbit fibroma syndrome. A possible model for aquired immunodeficiency syndrome (AIDS), *Am. J. Path., 120*: 170-171 (1985).
29. J. Oudin, Allotypy of rabbit serum proteins. I. Immunochemical analysis leading to the individualization of seven main allotypes, *J. Exp. Med., 112*: 125-142 (1960).
30. T. J. Kindt, Rabbit immunoglobulin allotypes: Structure, immunology and genetics, *Adv. Immunol., 21*: 35-86 (1975).
31. K. E. Bernstein, C. B. Alexander, and R. G. Mage, Germline V_H genes in an a3 rabbit not typical of any one V_{Ha} allotype, *J. Immunol., 134*: 3480-3488 (1985).
32. J. L. Gallarda, K. S. Gleason, and K. L. Knight, Organisation of rabbit immunoglobulin genes. I. Structure and multiplicity of germ-line VH genes, *J. Immunol., 135*: 4222-4227 (1985).
33. C. Bona, B. Cinader, and S. Dubiski, Cellular immunology of the rabbit, *Ann. Immunol. (Paris), 128C*: 571-598 (1977).
34. S. Sell, The rabbit immune system: Characterisation of cell surface markers and functional properties of rabbit lymphocytes, *Mol. Immunol., 16*: 1045-1058 (1979).
35. S. Sell, E. Skaletsky, R. Holdbrook, D. S. Linthicum, and C. Raffel, Alternative hypotheses of lymphocyte surface immunoglobulin expression: B lymphocyte activation and B lymphocyte differentiation, *Immunol. Rev., 52*: 141-179 (1980).
36. D. Redelman, C. B. Scott, H. W. Sheppard, and S. Sell, *In vitro* studies of the rabbit immune system: II. Functional characterisation of rabbit T and B populations separated by adherence to nylon wool or lysis with anti-thymocyte serum and complement, *Cell. Immunol., 24*: 11-23 (1979).
37. D. P. Fradelizi, C. T. Chou, B. Cinader, and S. Dubiski, A membrane antigen of rabbit thymus cells, *Cell. Immunol., 7*: 484-501 (1973).

38. M. W. Fanger, A. C. Reese, M. D. Schoenberg, A. B. Stavitsky, and A. L. Reese, Evidence for T lymphocyte subpopulations in the rabbit, *J. Immunol., 112*: 1971-1980 (1974).
39. H. W. Shepperd, D. Redelman, and S. Sell, *In vitro* studies of the rabbit immune system: IV. Differential mitogen responses of isolated T and B cells, *Cell. Immunol., 24*: 34-44 (1976).
40. C. T. Chou, B. Cinader, and S. Dubiski, A membrane antigen of rabbit bursal equivalent cells, *Cell. Immunol., 28*: 334-340 (1977).
41. B. J. E. G. Bast, D. Catty, R. Manten-Slingerland, J. T. G. Jansen, D. H. Veldhuis, P. Roholl, and R. E. Ballieux, Surface Ig on rabbit lymphocytes. Rabbit B and T cells are distinct populations, *Eur. J. Immunol., 9*: 997-1003 (1979).
42. J.-M. Cavaillon, B. Cinader, C.-T. Chou, and S. Dubiski, Purification of rabbit B spleen cells by removal of adherent and of T cells, *J. Immunol. Methods, 26*: 1-10 (1979).
43. P. N. Shek, C.-T. Chou, S. Dubiski, and B. Cinader, Mitogen stimulation of rabbit spleen cells before and after complement-mediated cell kill with an antiserum directed against the thymus antigen RTLA, *Int. Arch. Allergy, 46*: 753-767 (1974).
44. B. S. Wilson, M. Teodorescu, and S. Dray, Enumeration and isolation of rabbit T and B lymphocytes by using antibody-coated erythrocytes, *J. Immunol., 116*: 1306-1312 (1976).
45. J. M. Cavaillon, C. Bona, P.-A. Cazenave, and B. Cinader, Purification of rabbit T-derived (Ig^-) lymphocytes, *J. Immunol. Methods, 14*: 355-359 (1977).
46. M. G. Mage, L. L. McHugh, and T. L. Rothstein, Mouse lymphocytes with and without surface immunoglobulin: Preparative scale separation in polystyrene tissue culture dishes coated with specifically purified anti-immunoglobulin, *J. Immunol. Methods, 15*: 47-56 (1977).
47. A. R. Rivas-Alcala, C.-T. Chou, B. Cinader, S. Dubiski, and M. F. Filosa, Regulatory influences on the response of rabbit T cells to concanavalin A and phytohaemagglutinin, *Scand. J. Immunol., 9*: 315-324 (1979).
48. T. N. S. Udupa, C.-T. Chou. J.-M. Cavaillon, B. Cinader, and S. Dubiski, The effect of temperature-dependent autorosettes on B/T cell ratios of purified rabbit peripheral blood lymphocytes, *J. Immunol. Methods, 33*: 201-212 (1980).
49. P. De Baetselier, M. Vaeck, W. De Smet, and Y. Ron, Antigen-induced proliferation assay for rabbit T lymphocytes. I. Characteristics of the response, *Immunology, 41*: 997-1003 (1980).
50. J. E. Navran, and S. J. Archer, Isolation and characterisation of a rabbit T lymphocyte specific antigen, *J. Immunol., 120*: 1429-1435 (1978).
51. B. M. Balfour, H. A. Drexhage, E. W. A. Kamperdijk, and E. C. M. Hoefsmit, Antigen presenting cells, including Langerhans cells, veiled cells and interdigitating cells, *Ciba. Found. Symp., 84*: 281-301 (1981).
52. B. Balfour, J. A. O'Brien, M. Perera, J. Clarke, T. Sumerska, and S. C. Knight, The effect of veiled cells on lymphocyte function, *Adv. Exp. Med. Biol., 149*: 447-454 (1982).

53. S. C. Knight, B. M. Balfour, J. O'Brien, L. Buttifant, T. Sumerska, and J. Clarke, Role of veiled cells in lymphocyte activation, *Eur. J. Immunol., 12*: 1057-1060 (1982).
54. S. C. Knight, B. Balfour, J. O'Brien, and L. Buttifant, Sensitivity of veiled (dendritic) cells to cyclosporine, *Transplantation, 41*: 96-100 (1986).
55. M. F. W. Festing, *Inbred Strains in Biomedical Research,* Macmillan, London, 1979.
56. C. K. Chai, Effect of inbreeding in rabbits: Skeletal variations and malformations, *J. Hered., 61*: 2-8 (1970).
57. J. J. Collins, P. H. Black, A. D. Strosberg, E. Haber, and K. J. Bloch, Transformation by simian virus 40 of spleen cells from a hyperimmune rabbit: Evidence for synthesis of immunoglobulin by the transformed cells, *Proc. Natl. Acad. Sci. USA, 71*: 260-262 (1974).
58. A. D. Strosberg, J. J. Collins, P. H. Black, S. Malamud, S. Wilbert, K. J. Bloch, and E. Haber, Transformation by simian virus 40 of spleen cells from a hyperimmune rabbit: Demonstration of production of specific antibody to the immunising antigen, *Proc. Natl. Acad. Sci. USA, 71*: 263-264 (1974).
59. E. Petit-Koskas, A. B. Schreiber, C. Favre, R. Chemler, B. Vray, V. Zurawski, G. Buttin, P. A. Cazenave, and A. D. Strosberg, Switched allotype expression in an immunoglobulin non-secreting rabbit lymphocyte cell line fused with gangliocytes, *Eur. J. Immunol., 11*: 388-392 (1981).
60. M. D. Daniel, R. D. Hunt, B. Fleckenstein, N. W. King, and J. K. Ingalls, The oncogenicity of herpesvirus ateles in rabbits, *Proceedings of the 3rd International Symposium on Oncogenesis and Herpesviruses,* Cambridge, Massachusetts, 1977.
61. E. S. Kimball, J. E. Coligan, and T. J. Kindt, Structural characterisation of antigens encoded by rabbit RLA-11 histocompatibility genes, *Immunogenetics, 8*: 201-211 (1979).
62. J. M. Wilkinson, D. L. Wetterskog, J. A. Sogn, and T. J. Kindt, Cell surface glycoproteins of rabbit lymphocytes: Characterisation with monoclonal antibodies, *Mol. Immunol., 21*: 95-103 (1984).
63. P. N. Marche, and T. J. Kindt, Two distinct T cell receptor α-chain transcripts in a rabbit T cell line: Implications for allelic exclusion in T cells, *Proc. Natl. Acad. Sci. USA, 83*: 2190-2194 (1986).
64. H. W. Reid, D. Buxton, I. Pow, J. Finlayson, and E. L. Berrie, A cytotoxic T-lymphocyte line propagated from a rabbit infected with sheep associated malignant catarrhal fever, *Res. Vet. Sci., 34*: 109-113 (1983).
65. H. W. Reid, personal communication.
66. I. Miyoshi, S. Yoshimoto, I. Kubonishi, M. Fujishita, Y. Ohtsuki, M. Yamashita, K. Yamato, S. Hirose, H. Taguchi, K. Niiya, and M. Kobayashi, Infectious transmission of human T cell leukemia virus to rabbits, *Int. J. Cancer, 35*: 81-85 (1985).
67. T. Akagi, I. Takeda, T. Oka, Y. Ohtsuki, S. Yano, and I. Miyoshi, Experimental infection of rabbits with human T cell leukemia virus type I, *Jpn. J. Cancer, 76*: 86-94 (1985).

68. Y. Uemura, S. Kotani, S. Yoghimoto, M. Fujishita, S. Yano, Y. Ohtsuki, and I. Miyoshi, Oral transmission of human T-cell leukemia virus type I in the rabbit, *Jpn. J. Cancer Res., 77*: 970-973 (1986).
69. I. Miyoshi, personal communication.
70. I. Miyoshi, I. Kubonishi, M. Sumida, S. Hiraki, T. Tsubota, I. Kimura, K. Miyamoto, and J. Sato, A novel T cell line derived from adult T cell leukemia, *Gann, 71*: 155-156 (1980).
71. I. Miyoshi, I. Kubonishi, S. Yoshimoto, and Y. Shiraishi, A T cell line derived from normal human cord leukocytes by co-culturing with human leukemic T cells, *Gann, 72*: 978-981 (1981).
72. I. Miyoshi, S. Yoshimoto, I. Kubonishi, H. Taguchi, Y. Shirashi, Y. Ohtsuki, and T. Akagi, Transformation of normal human cord lymphocytes by cocultivation with a lethally irradiated human T cell line carrying type C virus particles, *Gann, 72*: 997-998 (1981).
73. H. Kulaga, T. J. Kindt, and J. A. Sogn, Phagocytic rabbit cell lines expressing Class II MHC gene products: Establishment of cell lines by viral transformation, *J. Leukocyte Biol., 40*: 169-181 (1986).
74. D. Redelman, and E. Bussett, In vitro studies of the rabbit immune system: IX. Extended culture of rabbit cytotoxic cells and the generation of TCGF-dependant T lymphocyte lines, *J. Immunol. Methods, 56*: 371-379 (1983).
75. S. Jackson, T. M. Folks, D. L. Wetterskog, and T. J. Kindt, A rabbit helper T cell clone reactive against group-specific streptococcal carbohydrate, *J. Immunol., 133*: 1555-1557 (1983).
76. S. Jackson, T. M. Chused, J. M. Wilkinson, W. M. Leiserson, and T. J. Kindt, Differentiation antigens identify subpopulations of rabbit T and B lymphocytes, *J. Exp. Med., 157*: 34-46 (1983).
77. R. A. Sobel, R. C. van der Veen, and M. B. Lees, The immunopathology of chronic experimental allergic encephalomyelitis induced in rabbits with bovine proteolipid protein, *J. Immunol., 136*: 157-163 (1986).
78. D. W. Metzger, personal communication.
79. J. M. McNicholas, M. Raffeld, M. R. Loken, H. Reiter, and K. L. Knight, Monoclonal antibodies to rabbit lymphoid cells: Preparation and characterisation of a T cell-specific antibody, *Mol. Immunol., 18*: 815-822 (1981).
80. Z. Chen, D. W. Metzger, and F. L. Adler, Characterisation of a monoclonal antibody reactive with rabbit T lymphocytes and neutrophils, *Cell Immunol., 85*: 297-308 (1984).
81. J. M. McNicholas, J. R. Watkins, A. D. Johnson, and K. L. Knight, The use of a monoclonal anti-T cell antibody in defining functions of rabbit T lymphocytes, *Immunology, 43*: 635-641 (1981).
82. J. R. Dasch, and A. B. Stavitsky, Mitogen-induced phosphorylation of cytosolic proteins in rabbit T and B lymphocytes, *Mol. Immunol., 22*: 379-389 (1985).
83. H. Spieker-Polet, K. Hagen, and M. Teodorescu, The role of intercellular contacts in the activation of B lymphocytes by anti-immunoglobulin antibodies, *J. Immunol., 134*: 2827-2834 (1985).

84. J. Wormmeester, F. Stiekema, and K. De Groot, A simple method for immunoselective cell separation with the avidin-biotin system, *J. Immunol. Methods, 67*: 389-394 (1984).
85. C. Pontzer, and R. H. Keller, Rabbit peripheral blood T cell separation, *Fed. Proc., 67*: 934 (1983).
86. P. J. M. Roholl, and J. Wormmeester, Different T cell antigens and receptors for peanut agglutinin and *helix pomatia* agglutinin on steroid sensitive and resistant lymphocytes in the rabbit using immunofluorescence, *Immunobiol., 164*: 325-332 (1983).
87. J. R. Perfect, and D. T. Durack, Effects of cyclosporine in experimental cryptococcal meningitis, *Infect. Immun., 50*: 22-26 (1985).
88. K. Walstra, A. Gratwhol, I. Riederer, and B. Speck, B/T cell ratio of rabbit peripheral blood lymphocytes. Influence of separation technique on results, *J. Immunol. Methods, 79*: 143-147 (1985).
89. W. De Smet, M. Vaeck, E. Smet, L. Brys, and R. Hamers, Rabbit leukocyte surface antigens defined by monoclonal antibodies, *Eur. J. Immunol., 13*: 919-928 (1983).
90. M. Vaeck, W. De Smet, R. Hamers, and P. De Baetselier, Effects of anti-Ig reagents on T cell functions. I. Activation of rabbit T cells by anti-allotype antibodies, *Eur. J. Immunol., 12*: 953-960 (1982).
91. D. C. Ponsard, B. Cinader, C.-T. Chou, and S. Dubiski, Characterization of rabbit cells by monoclonal and polyclonal antibodies, *Immunology, 59*: 115-122 (1986).
92. Y.-Y. Liu, C.-T. Chou, B. Cinader, and S. Dubiski, T cell antigens and MHC determinants on rabbit granulocytes, *Immunol. Lett., 7*: 181-186 (1984).
93. D. C. Ponsard, C.-T. Chou, B. Cinader, and S. Dubiski, The rabbit immune system: Cells regulating the proliferative response of purified T cells to conconavalin A and phytohaemaglutinin, *Immunol. Lett., 13*: 63-69 (1986).
94. J. R. Watkins, J. M. McNicholas, M. R. Loken, and K. L. Knight, Characterisation of functionally distinct subpopulations of rabbit T lymphocytes, *Immunology, 53*: 659-667 (1984).
95. P. Guillet, P. Marche, J. Hoebeke, and A. D. Strosberg, Physicochemical studies on the antigen-antibody complexes of two monoclonal antibodies against rabbit thymocytes, *Mol. Immunol., 20*: 1059-1068 (1983).
96. C. Cohen, and R. G. Tissot, The effect of the RL-A locus and the MLC locus on graft survival in the rabbit, *Transplantation, 18*: 150-154 (1974).
97. C. K. Chai, Genetic studies of histocompatibility in rabbits: Identification of major and minor genes, *Immunogenetics, 1*: 126-132 (1974).
98. J. M. Wilkinson, M. L. Tykocinski, J. E. Coligan, E. S. Kimball, and T. J. Kindt, Rabbit MHC antigens: Occurrence of non-beta-2-microglobulin-associated Class I molecules, *Mol. Immunol., 19*: 1441-1451 (1982).
99. M. L. Tykocinski, P. N. Marche, E. E. Max, and T. J. Kindt, Rabbit Class I MHC genes: cDNA clones define full-length transcripts of an expressed gene and a putative pseudo gene, *J. Immunol., 133*: 2261-2269 (1984).

100. P. N. Marche, M. L. Tykocinski, E. E. Max, and T. J. Kindt, Structure of a functional rabbit Class I MHC gene: Similarity to human Class I genes, *Immunogenetics, 21*: 71-82 (1985).
101. W. J. Mandy, personal communication.
102. A.Le Guern, D. Wetterskog, P. N. Marche, and T. J. Kindt, A monoclonal antibody directed against a synthetic peptide reacts with a cell surface rabbit Class I MHC molecule, *Mol. Immunol., 24*: 455-461 (1987).
103. K. S. Marchitto, T. J. Kindt, and M. V. Norgard, Monoclonal antibodies directed against major histocompatibility complex antigens bind to the surface of *Treponema-pallidum* isolated from infected rabbits or humans, *Cell. Immunol., 101*: 633-642 (1986).
104. D. W. Lancki, R. G. Tissot, and C. Cohen, Histocompatibility in the rabbit. Genetic control of rabbit mixed leukocyte culture reactivity. *Transplantation, 27*: 79-86 (1979).
105. K. L. Knight, A. L. Leary, and R. G. Tissot, Identification of two Ia-like alloantigens on rabbit B lymphocytes, *Immunogenetics, 10*: 443-453 (1980).
106. C. Le Guern, P. N. Marche, and T. J. Kindt, Molecular evidence for five distinct MHC Class II α genes in the rabbit, *Immunogenetics, 22*: 141-148 (1985).
107. N. Sittisombut, and K. L. Knight, Rabbit major histocompatibility complex. I. Isolation and characterisation of three subregions of Class II genes, *J. Immunol., 136*: 1871-1875 (1986).
108. S. A. Lobel, and K. L. Knight, The role of rabbit Ia molecules in immune functions as determined with the use of an anti-Ia monoclonal antibody, *Immunology, 51*: 35-43 (1984).
109. R. S. Becker, A. Johnson, and K. L. Knight, Characterization of rabbit Ia molecules with allo- and monoclonal anti-Ia antibodies, *Fed. Proc., 44*: 555 (1985).
110. K. L. Knight, personal communication.
111. W. De Smet, E. Smet, L. Brys, and R. Hamers, A monoclonal antibody inhibiting the mixed leukocyte reaction in rabbit, *Abstracts 6th International Congress of Immunology, Toronto,* 1986, p. 68.
112. J. J. Donnelly, and R. A. Prendergast, Local production of Ia-inducing activity in experimental immunogenic uveitis, *Cell. Immunol., 86*: 557-561 (1984).
113. M. L. Kapsenberg, F. Stiekma, and W. Leene, Differential requirements for rabbit dendritic cells and macrophages in T lymphocyte proliferation induced by various mitogens, *Immunology, 55*: 301-310 (1985).
114. M. L. Tiku, S. Liu, C. W. Weaver, M. Teodorescu, and J. L. Skosey, Class II histocompatibility antigen-mediated immunologic function of normal articular chondrocytes, *J. Immunol., 135*: 2923-2928 (1985).
115. B. M. Balfour, and J. M. Wilkinson, unpublished observations.
116. Z. Chen, S.-E. Yen, and W. S. Walker, 3AE8: Monoclonal antibody defining inflammatory macrophages in three species, *Hybridoma, 3*: 141-149 (1984).

117. E. G. Smet, W. De Smet, L. Brys, and P. C. De Baetselier, Mab.198: a monoclonal antibody recognising the complement type 3 receptor (CR3) in the rabbit, *Immunology, 59*: 419-425 (1986).
118. D. G. Campbell, J. Gagnon, K. B. M. Reid, and A. F. Williams, Rat brain Thy-1 glycoprotein. The amino acid sequence, disulphide bonds and an unusual hydrophobic region, *Biochem. J., 195*: 15-30 (1981).
119. E. L. Reinherz, S. C. Meuer, and S. F. Schlossman, The human T cell receptor: Analysis with cytotoxic T cell clones, *Immunol. Rev., 74*: 83-110 (1983).
120. W. R. A. Brown, A. N. Barclay, C. A. Sunderland, and A. F. Williams, Identification of a glycophorin-like molecule at the surface of rat thymocytes, *Nature (Lond.), 289*: 456-460 (1981).
121. I. D. Walker, P. M. Hogarth, B. J. Murray, K. E. Lovering, B. J. Classon, G. W. Chambers, and I. F. C. McKenzie, Ly antigens associated with T cell recognition, *Immunol. Rev., 82*: 47-77 (1984).
122. P. J. M. Roholl, W. Leene, and J. W. M. Visser, T cell differentiation in the rabbit. I. Cytofluorometric analysis of a T cell antigen on lymphocytes from normal and dexamethasone treated animals, *Thymus, 5*: 153-165 (1983).
123. J. R. Watkins, M. R. Loken, and K. L. Knight, Two B cell subpopulations identified by flow cytometry, *Immunology, 56*: 315-320 (1985).
124. A. L. Angiolillo, E. Lamoyi, K. E. Bernstein, and R. G. Mage, Identification of genes for the constant region of rabbit T cell receptor β-chains, *Proc. Natl. Acad. Sci. USA, 82*: 4498-4502 (1985).
125. E. Lamoyi, A. L. Angiolillo, and R. G. Mage, An evolutionarily conserved rabbit T cell receptor β-chain variable region, *Immunogenetics, 23*: 266-270 (1986).
126. L. T. Adler, F. L. Adler, W. J. Mandy, L. S. Rodkey, and D. W. Metzger, Second international workshop on immunogenetics and immunology of the rabbit, *Cell. Immunol., 84*: 458-460 (1984).
127. R. Dalchau, J. Kirkley, and J. W. Fabre, Monoclonal antibody to a human leukocyte-specific membrane glycoprotein probably homologous to the leukocyte-common (L-C) antigen of the rat, *Eur. J. Immunol., 10*: 737-744 (1980).
128. C.-Y. Wang, C.-H. Chen, and W. J. Mandy, Identification of a rabbit class I-like thymocyte-specific antigen, *J. Immunol., 138*: 3352-3359 (1987).
129. K. A. Williams, T. S. Mann, M. Lewis, and D. J. Coster, The role of resident accessory cells in corneal allograft rejection in the rabbit, *Transplantation, 42*: 667-671 (1986).
130. L. D. Loar, D. Dennison, and S. Sell, Production and characterization of monoclonal antibodies to rabbit lymphocyte subpopulations I. Tissue immunofluorescence and flow cytometric analysis, *J. Immunol., 137*: 2784-2790 (1986).

11

Surface Antigens of Avian Blood Cells

J. RICHARD L. PINK
Central Research Units, F. Hoffmann-La Roche & Co. Ltd., Basel, Switzerland

DOUGLAS G. GILMOUR*
New York University School of Medicine, New York, New York

I. INTRODUCTION

Although there are important differences between avian and mammalian immune systems—for example, in the structure of lymphoid organs (1), the organization of immunoglobulin (Ig) genes (2), and the way in which B lymphocytes develop (3)—the functional similarities between the two types of immune system are striking. Chicken T cells with helper (4), suppressor (5), and cytotoxic (6) activities have been described, and their functions (at least for helper and cytotoxic cells) are major histocompatibility complex (MHC)-restricted (7,8). Chicken IL-1-like (9) and IL-2-like (10-12) lymphokines have been characterized. The avian immunoglobulin (Ig) classes [IgM, IgA, IgD, and an IgG-like class, which has also been referred to as IgY (13-15)] are functionally comparable to their mammalian counterparts, although as yet only in the case of μ heavy and λ light chains has a structural homology been established (16-18). Chicken MHC class I and class II antigens are structurally (19-22) and functionally (7,8,23,24) similar to their mammalian homologues, and chicken T-cell-surface proteins which resemble the mammalian T3 and T-cell receptor proteins have recently been identified (25).

Several other surface proteins present on avian blood cells have recently been characterized with polyclonal or monoclonal antibodies, but much less information is available concerning possible homology of these to mammalian cell-surface markers. In this review, we discuss antigens present on avian hemopoietic cells,

---

**Present address*: London, England.

with emphasis on those that have been biochemically characterized using monoclonal antibodies (mAbs) (Table 1). However, we do not cover work on Ig allotypes, and we deal only briefly with alloantigens (Table 2) and blood group antigens (except for MHC antigens) (Section III.A), since these topics have been reviewed recently (14,66-68).

II. MHC ANTIGENS

The chicken MHC, which was originally described as a blood group system (69, 70), determines three classes of alloantigen (71,72): B-F and B-L, which correspond to the mammalian MHC class I and II antigens, respectively, and B-G, which has no known mammalian counterpart (71) and has been referred to as an MHC class IV antigen (23). The B-G antigens, found only on erythrocytes (71) and their precursors (73), were discriminated from B-F and B-L using chickens recombinant for the B blood group system (74). B-G antigens can be distinguished from B-F and B-L by their different tissue distribution, different chemical structure, and lack of association with histocompatibility reactions (23,71,74,75), immune responsiveness (76), or disease resistance (77,78). No confirmed recombinants between B-F and B-L have been reported, and thus the position of B-L within the MHC has not been assigned with certainty. B-L antigens were discriminated from B-F on the basis of chemical structure and tissue distribution, by analogy with mammalian class I and II antigens (see below). The above work with alloantibodies was reviewed in detail by Gilmour (79).

A. B-G

The B-G antigens are genetically polymorphic proteins of molecular weight (MW) about 45,000 (a second protein with MW 30,000 precipitated by anti-B-G sera is probably a proteolytic breakdown product) (35,71,80). Although they are cell-surface proteins, there is so far no evidence that they are glycosylated. B-G antigens are not associated with β_2-microglobulin, but form polymers in the absence of reducing agents (80). They can be detected on embryonic erythrocytes from at least day 10 of incubation on (80; Simonsen, unpublished).

mAbs to B-G antigens were first made using CBA rather than BALB/c mice (33,34). It was relatively easy to produce mAbs which were specific for allodeterminants on these highly polymorphic antigens, which contrasts with the difficulty of making monospecific mAbs against mammalian MHC antigens (81). Thus when B^2/B^2 erythrocytes were used as immunogen, 13% of positive clones were monospecific for the donor haplotype in hemagglutination tests against a panel of six homozygous B haplotypes. mAbs showing similar monospecificity were later made against the other five haplotypes (33).

The B-G specificity of the above mAbs is based on tissue distribution and on genetic mapping. The anti-B2 mAb reacted in a rosette-forming cell assay with

Table 1 Surface Antigens of Avian Blood Cells Reacting with Monoclonal Antibodies

Cell lineage[a]	Name of antigen[b]	Apparent molecular weight ($\times 10^{-3}$)	Remarks	Refs.
Hem. (+ other)	B-F	40-45	MHC class I	26-28
Hem. (+ endothel.)	MB-1		Quail cells only	29, 154
Eryth. (+ other)	EE-1, CFA	45-48	Embryonic erythrocyte antigen	30-32
Eryth.	B-G	45	MHC class IV	30, 33-35
T	(see Table 3)	65	Mainly cortical thymocytes	36-40
T	CT-3	17, 19, 20	Homologous to T3	25
T	CATLA	48-50	Activated T cells	41
T	several mAbs		Peripheral T cells (see text)	42-46
B	Bu-1	70	Genetically polymorphic	39, 47-50
B	Ig	several		44, 51-54
B + mono.	B-L	30-35	MHC class II	55-57
Myelo. (immature)	(51-2, etc.)	170 + 190		58,59
Myelo. + lympho.	(L-17)	190 − 220	Homologous to T-200/B-220	39, 155
	(50-3-C)			59
	(17-B-2)	30		59
Myelo. + T + erythro.	(2-15, 22-3, etc.)			59
Myelo. + T	(49-44-A-1-C)			59
Myelo. + B (+ other)	(L-43)	23		39

[a]Hem., hemopoietic; endothel., endothelial; eryth., erythroid; T, B, thymus or bursa-derived lymphoid; mono, monocytic; myelo, myeloid.
[b]Bracketed names are those of relevant mAbs.

Table 2 Surface Antigens of Chicken Lymphocytes Reacting with Alloantisera (excluding MHC, Ig, and Bu-1 antigens; see Table 1)

		Tissue distribution (% + *ve* cells)				
Antigen	Expressing cell type	Thymus	Bursa	Spleen	PBL[a]	Refs.
Th-1	T cells	64	0-2	45	18	60, 61
Ly-4	T cells	25	0-2	53	75	61, 62
CA1-T, B, E	T cells, B cells, erythrocytes	100	<2	100	100	63
TA	T cells	80	<2	45	75	64
AT-1.1	T cells	50-70	<2	<2	<2	65
BA	B cells	<2	95	10	10	64

[a]PBL, peripheral blood lymphocytes.
Source: Ref. 67.

erythroid but not lymphoid precursor cells, inhibited erythroid but not granulocyte-macrophage colony formation, and did not inhibit the graft-versus-host competence of adult lymphocytes (73). It also stained only erythrocytes and no other peripheral blood cells in indirect immunofluorescence (Gilmour and Fredericksen, unpublished). In hemagglutination tests with cells from B blood group recombinant chickens (72,82), the mAb-detected specificities mapped to B-G. For example, anti-B15 reacted with B^{21r3} (BF-21, G15) (72) but not with B^{15r1} (BF-15, G21) erythrocytes; anti-B21 reacted conversely (Longenecker and Gilmour, unpublished). Some mAbs with narrowly polymorphic specificity have been reported: anti-B-G (21 + 23) (Coudert, personal communication, 1984) and anti-B-G (6 + 13) (80).

Other anti-B-G mAbs reacting with determinants found on erythrocytes of all haplotypes tested were shown to be B-G specific by direct and competitive radiobinding assays (30). They were used to immunoprecipitate B-G antigens from erythrocytes of 14 haplotypes for analysis by high resolution two-dimensional electrophoresis. Each B-G antigen had a characteristic highly reproducible pattern of polypeptides (35). Confirmation of allelic identities was made in several cases by analysis of immunoprecipitates made with specific alloantisera or a monospecific mAb. The patterns varied from single arrays to groups of up to 4-5 arrays of multiple polypeptides differing in relative mobility and isoelectric point. Most patterns included a major polypeptide of 48 Kd focusing near pH 6.9, which presumably corresponds with the 42-45-Kd or 47-Kd molecules reported elsewhere (71,80). Patterns characteristic of particular B-G alleles were also detectable in heterozygotes and in recombinants. The latter results confirmed mapping to B-G of the determinants detected by these mAbs (30). Some indirect evidence was presented that the patterns might be encoded by multiple gene sequences within B-G (35).

When preparing anti-B-G mAbs, Longenecker and Mosmann (83) noted the very widespread occurrence of "natural" (preimmune) antibodies to chicken erythrocytes. Such antibodies were detected by indirect hemagglutination tests in several species [mice, rats, humans, alligators, chickens (33,83,84)]. Most (but not all) of the antibodies react with MHC antigens rather than with species-specific determinants, because they are rendered operationally monospecific for B haplotypes by appropriate absorptions (83,84). The presence of these preformed antibodies is presumably responsible for the preferential strong early plaque-forming cell response of mice to the donor chicken MHC haplotype, and for the relative ease of producing mAbs which are sharply MHC-monospecific at appropriate dilutions. As noted above, such mAbs are B-G-specific. Most "natural" antierythrocyte antibodies in chickens were shown to be specific for B-G by immunofluorescence, but one out of 15 mAbs tested was specific for B-F (84).

In chickens, the existence of preimmune alloantibodies may be a factor in the powerful immunogenicity of B-G antigens, and in their low tolerogenicity.

It is a common observation that B blood group antigens (B-G + B-F) are highly immunogenic. B-G are probably more important in this respect, because in studies with B-recombinant chickens, antibody responses to B-F required the copresence of a B-G difference on the same erythrocyte, whereas B-G responses were independent of B-F differences (85). Such a difference could be readily explained by the presence of preimmune antibodies to B-G rather than B-F.

The low tolerogenicity of erythrocyte-specific antigens, presumably B-G, as compared with widespread tissue antigens, presumably B-F, was demonstrated by early observations that tolerance to skin grafts induced at hatching frequently coexists with absence of tolerance to erythrocytes (86)—the phenomenon of "split tolerance." This contrasted with the state of tolerance to both skin and erythrocytes, with long-continued erythrocyte chimaerism, which could be induced by embryonic parabiosis (87,88). More recent analysis (89) suggests that the susceptibility of embryos to B-G tolerance induction drops markedly just after day 15 of embryogenesis, at the time when maternal antibodies begin to be transferred from the yolk sac to the embryonic circulation (90). Erythrocytes among the cells used for tolerance induction would then be eliminated by the natural anti-B-G maternal antibodies, and split tolerance to B-F but not B-G would result.

The physiological function of B-G antigens is unknown. Any proposed function should account for the very widespread occurrence of natural antibodies to these antigens. Longenecker and Mosmann (83) suggest three possible explanations for this phenomenon: that chicken Ig germ-line V genes code for anti-B-G antibodies [unlikely, given the small number of such genes (2)] ; that bacteria or viruses either can carry histocompatibility antigens from one host to another, or themselves can cross-react with these antigens (unlikely, as the natural antibodies were also present in germ-free rats); or that the antibodies are autoimmune in origin, and directed against altered (for example, denatured) self histocompatibility antigens. We prefer this last explanation (91); it is possible, for example, that mammals make antibodies against their own class I antigens if these dissociate from β_2-microglobulin, and that these antibodies cross-react with B-G, which may itself represent a class I antigen unable to associate with β_2-microglobulin.

B. B-F

B-F antigens, immunoprecipitated from lysates of leukocytes (19) or erythrocytes (92,93) with B blood group alloantisera, consist of a specific polypeptide of MW 40-45,000 noncovalently bound to a smaller protein (MW 12,500), avian β_2-microglobulin. This evidence for their correspondence with mammalian MHC class I antigens was confirmed by the finding of considerable homology between the partial amino terminal amino acid sequences of chicken leukocyte B-F and mammalian H-2, HLA, and GPLA sequences (20,21). There is also close (45%) homology between the amino terminal sequences of avian and mammalian (murine) β_2-microglobulin (94). The functional evidence for assignment of B-F to class I relates to a (B-F + B-L) chromosomal region, which was originally discriminated from B-G in recombinant chickens. This region, and not B-G, was associated with acute skin graft rejection and with graft-versus-host and mixed leukocyte reactions (23,71,74,75). It may encode more than one B-F antigen (26).

No monospecific mAbs against B-F allo-antigens have been made, although these antigens have much the same high degree of polymorphism as B-G (72,95, 96). Included among mAbs with partial polymorphic specificity are an anti-F (19 + 15) (26), an anti-F (19 + 15 + 13) (28), and another reacting with F4, 12, 13, and 21, but not with F14, 15, and 19 (27). A further group of monoclonals reacted strongly with 14 out of 17 haplotypes but weakly, if at all, with F4, 6, and 13, and were thus directed toward a widely shared but perhaps not strictly monomorphic determinant (26).

Some of these mAbs were used to confirm the immunochemical results, and to demonstrate B-F antigens on all cells in blood by indirect immunofluorescence (IIF) (26,27). Erythrocytes stained only weakly (27). In further IIF staining, B-F was shown on cultured macrophages and Concanavalin A-induced T-cell blasts, as well as on bursal and thymic lymphoid cells. In the central lymphoid organs, cortical (less mature) cells were only weakly stained (27,28). B-F was present on thymic mesenchyme but could not be demonstrated in brain and liver except on a few isolated liver cells, perhaps Kupffer cells (27). In earlier hemagglutinin-absorption studies with alloantibodies, B antigens (presumably B-F) were detected on cells in spleen and bone marrow (97) and in liver but not in brain or muscle (98).

B-F antigens are first detectable by hemagglutination on erythrocytes soon after hatching (80), but can be detected on chick embryo fibroblasts (CEF) by mixed agglutination of erythrocytes and CEF, using either B blood group alloantisera or anti-CEF alloantisera (99). Although CEF were potent immunogens for specific polymorphic antigens (presumably B-F) shared with erythrocytes (99), it has been difficult to demonstrate B-F on CEF by IIF; it was necessary to use a very powerful mAb, with an IIF titre of 1:50,000 against erythrocytes and lymphocytes, to demonstrate B-F on CEF by conventional IIF (Gilmour, unpublished). The expression of B-F on CEF is clearly very weak. In this work, using either alloantibody or mAb, there was a marked diminution of B-F antigen expression, often to negativity, following infection and transformation by Rous sarcoma virus (Gilmour, 1985, unpublished). This effect was transformation-specific because the related nontransforming virus RAV-1 had no effect. These observations have been confirmed with monoclonal antibody using the fluorescence-activated cell sorter and a cellular ELISA test (Gogusev et al., 1986, unpublished).

C. B-L

B-L antigens are similar to mammalian class II antigens in their structure and tissue distribution (100). Several mAbs to B-L, all detecting monomorphic determinants, have been made (55-58). Anti-B-L alloantisera or mAbs precipitate three types of polypeptide, corresponding to the α, β, and invariant chains of mouse or human class II antigens, from lysates of biosynthetically labeled lymphocytes (101,102). When immunoprecipitates from several haplotypes were studied by two-dimensional gel electrophoresis, a single nonpolymorphic α chain of AMW 34,000 was observed, whereas two polymorphic β chains (AMW 30-35,000) could be distinguished on the basis of differences in size as well as antigenicity (103) and isoelectric point (102). All the proteins carried N-linked carbohydrates, which were of the high-mannose type on the invariant chain, but of complex type on α and β polypeptides (102). A DNA sequence of two exons corresponding to the β chain β_2 and transmembrane domains was obtained by Auffray et al. (22), who used a human DQβ probe to detect cross-hybridizing sequences in a chicken genomic DNA library. The B-L sequences were about equally homologous at the amino acid level (55%) to DQ, DR, DP, I-A, and I-E mammalian class II β chains (22).

B-L antigens are present on B cells and monocytes in blood, and B cells, macrophages, and dendritic cells in bursa, spleen, and thymus (55-57,71,104, 105). The percentages of macrophages (adherent leukocytes) staining with anti-B-L sera were reported to be different in different tissues, being highest in spleen (c. 75%) and lowest in thymus (10%) (105), whereas thymic dendritic cells were all strongly B-L-positive. B-L antigens are first detected in the bursa of day-12 embryos, and later (day 17) appear in spleen (104). B-L-positive macrophages and dendritic cells were found early (day 13) in the thymus. Both these cell types derive from circulating precursors which enter the primary lymphoid organs along with lymphoid precursor cells (56). B-L antigens have also been demonstrated on endothelial cells in bursal capillary blood vessels (57), and may be expressed or inducible on other endothelial cell types, as is the case in mammals (106).

III. ERYTHROCYTE ANTIGENS

A. Blood Groups

The erythrocytes carry a series of blood group antigens determined by the erythrocyte alloantigen (Ea) loci, of which there are 13 (66,107). Only 12 independent (unlinked) loci exist, because Ea-A and Ea-E are closely linked with a recombination frequency of about 0.5 centimorgans (108). The Ea-B locus contains the B-G and B-F components of the MHC. The Ea antigens are detected on erythrocytes by hemagglutination with alloantisera, and the A, B, and C antigens have also been detected on blood lymphocytes by lymphoagglutination (109) and by immunoadherence (110). The B-F antigens of Ea-B are responsible for strong histocompatibility reactions, and the Ea-C antigens are associated with weak variable histocompatibility responses (111). Two of the Ea loci are associated with viruses. The Ea-R locus codes for an antigen R^1 allelic to absence of antigen determined by a silent allele Ea-r. R^1 is closely associated with dominant susceptibility (Tv-B^{S1}) to subgroup B leukosis-sarcoma (L-S) viruses (112). Despite this finding, there has been no success in attempts to detect cell membrane receptors for L-S virus by immune sera against erythrocytes. The Ea-K locus has been shown (113) to be identical with the previously described *Vaccinia* hemagglutinogen (Vh) locus, which was detected by agglutination of chicken erythrocytes by extracts of *Vaccinia* and other viruses (114,115). A series of multiple alleles at Ea-K gave genotypes which were quantitatively associated with *Vaccinia* hemagglutination titre, with, for example $K^1K^1 > K^2K^2 > K^3K^3 >$ kk (113). The latter recessive genotype showed absence of agglutinability by *Vaccinia* virus extracts and thus corresponded with the genotype vhvh.

B. Embryonic Antigens

Erythrocytes from embryonic chicks or from young birds (less than about 4 months old) carry antigenic determinants which are absent from adult erythrocytes (116,117). This antigenicity is associated with a glycoprotein, or family of closely related glycoproteins, of MW 48,000 (118,119), called either embryonic antigen, or chicken fetal antigen (CFA). Antisera against embryonic erythrocytes recognize several different determinants on this glycoprotein, as can be shown by sequential absorbtion of the sera with erythrocytes from different avian species (120). Also, immature erythrocytes (i.e., erythrocyte precursors in adult bone marrow, especially in birds which have been made anemic by phenylhydrazine treatment) carry some but not all of the antigenic determinants associated with the embryonic glycoprotein (117,121).

Monoclonal antibodies to the embryonic protein have been prepared (30,31) and used for immunochemical and histological studies of the antigen. Although it is not detectable on adult erythrocytes, it is present at low levels on normal adult leukocytes (30,122-124) and in varying amounts on a wide variety of other tissues, including gut epithelium, kidney tubules, hepatocytes, connective tissue in many organs, muscle endomysium, neural ectoderm, and retina (32). The antigen precipitated from retinal cells and muscle tissue was similar in size to the erythrocyte antigen, but had a slightly more basic mean isoelectric point when analyzed by two-dimensional gel electrophoresis (32). In addition, embryonic antigen is present on normal chick fibroblasts as well as on a variety of virus-transformed fibroblast and hemopoietic cell lines (123-129).

The antigenic complexity, wide tissue distribution, and variation in isoelectric point of the embryonic glycoprotein suggest that its antigenicity might be associated with carbohydrate residues, and there is some direct biochemical evidence for this idea (119). In this respect the embryonic determinants could resemble the I/i human erythrocyte antigens, which are carried on polylactosamine chains attached (on red cells) mainly to the band 3 glycoprotein, but which are also found on other (e.g., lymphoid) cells (130-132). However, the mobility in gel electrophoresis of the embryonic antigen differs from the mobilities of the band 3 protein and of antigens present on immature rodent erythrocytes (132), so that close homology between the avian and mammalian glycoproteins is unlikely.

Less well characterized than the embryonic antigen are an "immature" erythrocyte antigen (AMW 140,000) present on red cell precursors from anemic birds, but not on normal adult or embryonic circulating erythrocytes (133); and several "adult" antigens which are preferentially expressed on erythrocytes from adult birds. Three proteins of AMWs 102,000, 85,000, and 40,000 have been identified as carrying "adult antigen" specificities (118). The 40,000 AMW component may be the B-G antigen, as two mAbs which bound preferentially to adult cells (although still reacting weakly with erythrocytes from newly hatched chicks) were B-G-specific (30).

In young chicks three types of erythrocyte can be found: (a) cells carrying embryonic antigen only (in birds up to 60 days old); (b) cells expressing both embryonic and adult antigens (from hatch up to about 4 months of age); and (c) cells carrying adult antigens only (from 10 days of age on) (119,134). Distinct stem cells give rise to the adult and embryonic antigen-bearing populations (stem cells for the double-positive erythrocytes could not be distinguished from stem cells for the embryonic antigen positive population) (135). As previously mentioned, precursors of adult erythrocytes express at least some embryonic antigen specificities; however, colony-forming precursors (CFU-E) for adult and embryonic erythrocytes can be distinguished using sera against the adult or embryonic antigen complexes (135). These antigen systems have recently been reviewed by Dietert (136).

IV. LYMPHOCYTE ANTIGENS

Antigens specific for thymic, bursal, T, or B cells have been detected by xenoantisera, alloantisera (Table 2), or mAbs. Although many authors have used xenoantisera for the study of lymphocyte tissue distribution or function, only in a few cases have the relevant antigens been biochemically characterized, and this section will concentrate mainly on antigens detected by mAbs (Table 1).

A. T-Cell Antigens

Several authors have described mAbs whose main reactivity is against cortical thymocytes. It is likely that these antibodies react with similar or related antigens. The antibody α-TD-1 described by Peault et al. (36,37) reacted with about 80% of chicken or quail thymocytes, but with only 1-2% of peripheral (splenic) lymphocytes, and not at all with blood cells. The staining of thymocytes was confined to cortical cells; the staining was strong throughout the cortex, with the exception of a layer of subcapsular cells which stained less strongly. Four other mAbs with similar, but not identical, activity to α-TD-1 have been studied—CF-1 and CT-1a (38), X.14 (39), and J10A4 (40). The tissue distributions of the antigens detected by these mAbs are given in Table 3. All four antibodies precipitated a glycoprotein with a major component of MW 63-65,000, and minor components of higher MW [103,000 (38) or 125,000 and 180,000 (39)] from thymocytes. No material was precipitated from thymocytes by α-TD-1, but this may be due to (for example) low affinity of the α-TD-1 antibody, and does not exclude that the same molecules are detected by all four mAbs. The ontogenetic development of the antigens detected by CT-1, α-TD-1, and J10A4 was similar, the percentage of positive cells in the thymus increasing from about 10% to over 70% between days 8 and 10 in the quail (36) or 12 and 14 in the chicken (38).

The fact that these antibodies detect similar, but apparently not identical, determinants suggests that they might react with a glycoprotein which undergoes modification during differentiation from cortical thymocytes to peripheral T cells. Other glycoproteins whose glycosylation state and antigenicity are altered during differentiation include the T-200 and (probably) the Thy-1 antigens in mice (137), and the embryonic antigen in chicks (see Section III.B). However, other reasons for the differences in reactivity of the anti-chick cortical thymocyte mAbs discussed above—for example, differences in the strains of chickens examined—are not excluded.

Other monoclonal antibodies reacting with chicken T cells have been described more recently. The CT-3 mAb reacts with about 30% of thymocytes and essentially all peripheral T cells and recognizes a complex of 3 polypeptides (MWs 20,000, 19,000, and 17,000) homologous to the mammalian T3 antigen complex (25). The two larger chains are N-glycosylated. Under less dissociating conditions, two additional polypeptides (MWs 49,000 and 38,000) homologous to mammalian T-cell receptor α and β chains are co-precipitated by the mAb. The antibody was mitogenic for adult chick splenic T cells and reacted (in a fluorescence assay) with about 5% of thymocytes, but no spleen cells, from 12-day embryos (25). The Inn-CH-16 mAb reacts with a chicken activated T-lymphocyte-specific antigen (CATLA), which is present on the great majority of Concanavalin A-activated T cells, but not on nonactivated T cells or on B cells (41). Whether CATLA is related to an IL-2 receptor is unclear, as its reported MW (49,000) is different from that of mammalian IL-2 receptors (55,000) (138). The Inn-CH-T1 mAb reacts with 70% of thymocytes and 65% of peripheral blood lymphocytes (i.e., all or most peripheral T cells), but not with bursa cells (42). Several other mAbs reacting with still undefined subsets of peripheral T cells, as well as

Table 3 Tissue Distribution of Antigens Detected by Four Monoclonal Antibodies Reacting with Avian Cortical Thymocytes

	Reactivity (% positive cells) with					
Antibody	Chick total thymocytes	Chick medullary thymocytes[a]	Chick spleen lymphocytes	Chick bursa cells	Quail total thymocytes	Refs.
α-TD-1	75-80	–	<1	<1	80	36, 37
CT-1	91	+	3	<0.05	Cortex +[a]	38
CT-1a	91	N.D.[b]	3	<0.05	0	38
X.14	65-85	–	1-2	1	N.D.	39
J10A4	80	Some cells +	20	<1	N.D.	40

[a]As determined by immunofluorescence on tissue sections.
[b]N.D., not determined.

with some thymocytes, are available (42-45); one of these reacts with a genetically polymorphic determinant (45).

Xenoantisera have been used to precipitate several different molecules from chicken T cells. Antigens of Mw about 65,000 and 45,000, present on the majority of thymocytes and a minority (5-15%) of peripheral lymphocytes, have been described (37,139); the former might be related to the antigens detected by the mAbs listed in Table 3. The latter was not associated with β_2-microglobulin and showed no evidence of genetic polymorphism; whether it is related to a human T-cell antigen (T-10) of similar size and tissue distribution (140) is unclear. Other xenoantigens precipitated from chicken thymocytes by sera raised in turkeys or rabbits had MWs of about 170-180,000, 135,000, 100,000, and 75,000 (141) (in nonreducing conditions). Two mAbs used by the same authors precipitated (from thymocytes) molecules of MWs 185,000 and 135,000, which may be related to the xenoantigens.

Although attempts to use xenoantisera to define functional T-cell subsets in the chicken have been partially successful (141), two mAbs which react with antigens perhaps homologous to the mammalian CD4 (L3T4) and CD8 (Lyt-2) antigens could be more useful (142). Also, a molecule biochemically similar to Thy-1 has been isolated from chicken brain (143), but is not detectable on lymphocytes; and an avian transferrin receptor has been detected by a specific mAb on virus-transformed macrophages (58,144).

B. B-Cell Antigens

Although several groups have described mAbs reacting with chicken B cells, it seems likely that, so far, all of these have been directed either against Ig molecules (Table 1) or against the Bu-1 alloantigen originally described by Gilmour et al. (60). The best characterized of the anti-Bu-1 mAbs is L-22 (39,47,48), which reacts with the Bu-1a allelic gene product. Other anti-Bu-1a (49,50) and an anti-Bu-1b (50) mAb are available.

The Bu-1 antigen is a protein of MW 70,000 found on all bursal and peripheral B cells (39,60), but is also present on a subpopulation of adherent cells in bursa and thymic medulla, and on large, vacuole-containing macrophage-like cells in the liver (48). It is not detectable on blood monocytes or on plasma cells in Harder's gland. It is first observed during development in 9-day embryos, on lymphoid (and possibly myeloid) precursor cells entering the bursa; and can be induced in vitro on 16-day embryo bone marrow cells (thought to be B-cell precursors) (145). These facts, together with the observations that very few Bu-1-positive cells populate the embryonic thymus, suggests that at least some lymphoid precursor cells are already precommitted to the B or T lineages before they enter the bursa or thymus (48). Nothing is known of Bu-1 function, but *Bu-1* genotype is correlated with the levels of B-L expression on bursal cells of different chicken strains (146). Other B-cell antigens are described in Ref. 44.

C. *ev* Loci

The chromosomal DNA of most chickens contains sequences homologous with portions of the gene sequences of the avian leukosis-sarcoma viruses. These are transmitted in the germ line and probably arose from past events of integration. Studies of their antigenic expression in cultured chick embryo fibroblasts have led to the discovery of at least 21 distinct endogenous retrovirus (*ev*) loci in the chicken genome (147,148).

Endogenous viral envelope antigen was first detected on plasma cells by immunofluorescence techniques (149) and was later found to be determined by the *ev 6* locus (150). This *ev 6* antigen was found in much smaller quantities on bursal lymphocytes (151) and on thymocytes (152) by more sensitive radioimmunochemical techniques. The quantitative expression was greater on lymphoblasts produced by in vitro mitogenic stimulation of B or T lymphocytes (152). It was later shown that the increased expression in lymphoblasts was a property shared by the antigenic products of several *ev* loci, and may thus have been related merely to the increased rate of synthesis of most cellular proteins. In contrast, the high expression of envelope antigen in plasma cells was associated with only one (*ev 6*) of the loci studied (153). The much increased expression of *ev 6* antigen is thus a specific concomitant of the differentiation of B cells to plasma cells.

V. MYELOID LINEAGE ANTIGENS

In this section are briefly summarized studies on mAbs which react with cells of the myeloid (granulocyte/macrophage) lineage in chicken blood or bone marrow. (Anti-MHC antibodies are excluded—see Section II.) Many patterns of reactivity with erythroid and T or B lymphoid cells, as well as myeloid cells, are shown by these mAbs. Often, information about reactions with normal cell types (e.g., thrombocytes) is lacking, so our discussion of these mAbs is brief and intended to encourage further work in this field rather than to be exhaustive.

Several mAbs reacting with immature myeloid cell lines (obtained by transformation with avian myeloblastosis virus), but not with lymphoid or erythroid cells, have been described by Kornfeld et al. (59); three of these precipitated antigens with MWs between 100,000 and 190,000 from the cell lines. All reacted with 4-5% of normal chicken bone marrow cells (58,59).

A mAb reacting with all blood cell lineages except mature erythrocytes was described by Peault et al. (29). This antibody, MB-1, was prepared by immunization with quail μ chains and reacted not only with these but with quail endothelial as well as hemopoietic cells. The extensive cross-reaction might be due to activity towards carbohydrate. No reaction with chicken cells was observed, making this antibody, and others with similar species specificity (e.g., 25), useful for studies on quail-chick chimeras. The antigen has been futher characterized (154).

L-17, a mAb detecting an antigen probably homologous to the mammalian L-CA/T-200/B-220 antigen family (reviewed in Ref. 137), reacts with all myeloid and lymphoid cells in blood and lymphoid organs, but not with erythrocytes or thrombocytes (39). Like the mammalian antigen the chicken protein had MW about 180,000 on thymus cells, and 190,000 + 210,000 on B (bursal) lymphocytes. Other mAbs with similar specificity exist (44,155). MAb 50-3-C reacted with cell lines of myeloid and lymphoid origin, as well with normal thymus and bursa cells; 50-3-C also reacted with erythroblasts (59). 17-B-2 precipitated a 30,000 MW protein, clearly not homologous to L-CA, whereas the molecule detected by 50-3-C was not characterized and could be the L-17-binding antigen (59).

Other mAbs have been described as reacting with myeloid, erythroid, and T lymphoid cells; myeloid and T lymphoid cells; or myeloid and B lymphoid cells (Table 1). The latter antibody (L-43) also reacted with fibroblasts and epithelial cells (Pink, unpublished) and precipitated a molecule of MW 23,000 from B lymphocytes. In view of the fact that polyclonal rabbit antisera which react specifically with macrophages (105) or thrombocytes (156) are not difficult to prepare, one can hope that mAbs specific for these cell types as well as for different granulocyte lineages could soon become available.

VI. SUMMARY

Three points stand out when the list of avian blood cell antigens detected by mAbs is considered. Not unexpectedly, some antigens dominate the responses of mice to particular types of chicken cell: B-G on erythrocytes, Bu-1 on bursa cells, the TD-1 family of antigens on thymocytes (the same is not necessarily true of myeloid cells, against which several types of mAb have been produced following immunization with either normal cells or virus-transformed cell lines). More surprising is the observation that antibodies to genetically polymorphic determinants (e.g., on B-G, B-F, and Bu-1) can dominate the response; these antibodies can be extremely useful and underline the necessity of working with well-characterized chicken lines when raising mAbs. Finally, of all the mAb-detected antigens described here, only a few—the MHC class I and II antigens, CT-3, Ig molecules, L-CA/T-200 antigens and perhaps CD4, CD8 and T cell receptor molecules (157)—show clear homology to mammalian cell-surface antigens. However, given the functional similarity of avian and mammalian immune systems, it seems likely that additional homologous antigens will soon be described and will enable avian immunologists to combine knowledge gained from experiments on mammals with all the advantages inherent to avian systems.

REFERENCES

1. L. N. Payne and P. C. Powell, The lymphoid system, in *Physiology and Biochemistry of the Domestic Fowl, Vol. 5* (B. M. Freeman, ed.), Academic Press, London, 1984, p. 277.

2. J.-C. Weill, M. Leibowitch, and C.-A. Reynaud, Questioning the role of the embryonic bursa in the molecular differentiation of B lymphocytes, *Current Topics in Microbiol. and Immunol., 135*: 111 (1987).
3. J. R. L. Pink, O. Lassila, and O. Vainio, B lymphocytes and their self-renewal, in *Avian Immunology: Basis and Practice* (A. Toivanen and P. Toivanen, eds.), CRC Press, Boca Raton, Florida, 1987, Vol. I, p. 65.
4. G. J. Thorbecke, M. A. Palladino, and S. P. Lerman, Lymphoid cell cooperation in immune responses of the chicken—a review, *Cont. Topics in Immunobiol., 9*: 91 (1980).
5. M. D. Grebenau, S. P. Lerman, M. A. Palladino, and G. J. Thorbecke, Suppression of adoptive antibody responses by addition of spleen cells from agammaglobulinemic chickens "immunised" with histocompatible bursa cells, *Nature, 260*: 46 (1976).
6. K. Fahey and J. J. York, Cytotoxic activity of avian lymphoid cells in *Avian Immunology: Basis and Practice* (A. Toivanen and P. Toivanen, eds.), CRC Press, Boca Raton, Florida, 1987, Vol. I, p. 179.
7. O. Vainio, C. Koch, and A. Toivanen, B-L antigens (Class II) of the chicken major histocompatibility complex control T-B cell interaction, *Immunogenetics, 19*: 131 (1984).
8. D. L. MacCubbin and L. Schierman, MHC-restricted cytotoxic response of chicken T cells: Expression, augmentation and clonal characterization, *J. Immunol., 136*: 12 (1986).
9. Y. Hayari, K. Schauenstein, and A. Globerson, Avian lymphokines. II: Interleukin-1 activity in supernatants of stimulated adherent splenocytes of chickens, *Dev. Comp. Immunol., 6*: 541 (1982)
10. K. Schauenstein, A. Globerson, and G. Wick, Avian lymphokines: I. Thymic cell growth factor in supernatants of mitogen-stimulated chicken spleen cells, *Dev. Comp. Immunol., 6*: 533 (1982).
11. M. Schnetzler, A. Oommen, J. S. Novak, and R. M. Franklin, Characterisation of chicken T cell growth factor, *Eur. J. Immunol., 13*: 560 (1983).
12. O. Vainio, M. J. H. Ratcliffe, and T. Leanderson, Chicken T-cell growth factor: Use in the generation of a long-term cultured T-cell line and biochemical characterisation, *Scand. J. Immunol., 23*: 135 (1986).
13. A. A. Benedict and K. Yamaga, Immunoglobulins and antibody production in avian species, in *Comparative Immunology* (J. J. Marchalonis, ed.), Blackwell Scientific Publications, Oxford, 1976, p. 335.
14. A. A. Benedict and J. M. Berestecky, Special features of avian immunoglobulins, in *Avian Immunology: Basis and Practice* (A. Toivanen and P. Toivanen, eds.), CRC Press, Boca Raton, Florida, 1987, Vol. I, p. 113.
15. C.-L. H. Chen, J. E. Lehmeyer, and M. D. Cooper, Evidence for an IgD homologue on chicken lymphocytes, *J. Immunol., 129*: 2580 (1982).
16. J. A. Grant, B. Sanders, and L. Hood, Partial amino acid sequences of chicken and turkey immunoglobulin light chains. Homology with mammalian λ chains, *Biochemistry, 10*: 3123 (1971).
17. C.-A. Reynaud, A. Dahan, and J.-C. Weill, Complete sequence of a chicken light chain immunoglobulin derived from the nucleotide sequence of its mRNA, *Proc. Natl. Acad. Sci. USA, 80*: 4099 (1983).

18. A. Dahan, C.-A. Reynaud, and J.-C. Weill, Nucleotide sequence of the constant region of a chicken μ heavy chain immunoglobulin, *Nucl. Acids Res., 11*: 5381 (1983).
19. A. Ziegler and J. R. L. Pink, Chemical properties of two antigens controlled by the major histocompatibility complex of the chicken, *J. Biol. Chem., 251*: 5391 (1976).
20. E. S. Vitetta, J. W. Uhr, J. Klein, F. Pazderka, E. J. Moticka, R. F. Ruth, and J. D. Capra, Homology of (murine) H-2 and (human) HLA with a chicken histocompatibility antigen, *Nature, Lond., 270*: 535 (1977).
21. H. Huser, A. Ziegler, R. Knecht, and J. R. L. Pink, Partial aminoterminal amino acid sequences of chicken major histocompatibility antigens, *Immunogenetics, 6*: 301 (1978).
22. C. Auffray, G. Behar, A. Billault, Y. Bourlet, and F. Guillemot, Structure and expression of chicken Class II (B-L) antigen β chain genes, results presented at *Avian Immunology Workshop,* Inssbruck, 1985.
23. M. Crone and M. Simonsen, Avian major histocompatibility complex, in *Avian Immunology: Basis and Practice* (A. Toivanen and P. Toivanen, eds.), CRC Press, Boca Raton, Florida, 1987, Vol. II, p. 25.
24. K. Halan, R. Boyd, and G. Wick, Chicken major histocompatibility complex and disease, *Scand. J. Immunol., 14*: 607 (1981).
25. C.-L. H. Chen, L. L. Ager, G. L. Gartland, and M. D. Cooper, Identification of a T3/T cell receptor complex in chickens, *J. Exp. Med., 164*: 375 (1986).
26. M. Crone, M. Simonsen, K. Skojdt, K. Linnet, and L. Olsson, Mouse monoclonal antibodies to class I and class II antigens of chicken MHC. Evidence for at least two class I products of the *B* complex, *Immunogenetics, 21*: 181 (1985).
27. J. R. L. Pink, M. W. Kieran, A.-M. Rijnbeek, and B. M. Longenecker, A monoclonal antibody against chicken MHC class I (B-F) antigens, *Immunogenetics, 21*: 293 (1985).
28. R. Sgonc, K. Hala, and G. Wick, Relationship between the expression of Class I antigen and reactivity of chicken thymocytes, *Immunogenetics* (in press).
29. B. M. Peault, J.-P. Thiery, and N. M. Le Douarin, Surface marker for hemopoietic and endothelial cell lineages in quail that is defined by a monoclonal antibody, *Proc. Natl. Acad. Sci. USA, 80*: 2976 (1983).
30. M. M. Miller, R. Goto, and S. D. Clark, Structural characterisation of developmentally expressed antigenic markers on chicken erythrocytes using monoclonal antibodies, *Dev. Biol., 94*: 409 (1982).
31. K. Kline, J. P. Allison, B. McIntyre, and B. G. Sanders, Immunochemical characterisation of differentiation and age-related cell surface antigens expressed by chicken erythrocytes, *Cancer Res., 44*: 3576 (1984).
32. M. M. Miller and J. R. L. Pink, Chick embryonic erythrocyte antigen—tissues sharing expression, *Exp. Cell Res., 167*: 295 (1986).
33. B. M. Longenecker, T. R. Mosmann, and C. Shiozawa, A strong preferential response of mice to polymorphic antigenic determinants of the chicken MHC, analyzed with mouse hybridoma (monoclonal) antibodies, *Immunogenetics, 9*: 137 (1979).

34. B. M. Longenecker and T. R. Mosmann, Nomenclature for chicken MHC (B) antigens defined by monoclonal antibodies, *Immunogenetics, 13*: 25 (1981).
35. M. M. Miller, R. Goto, and H. Abplanalp, Analysis of the B-G antigens of the chicken MHC by two-dimensional gel electrophoresis, *Immunogenetics, 20*: 373 (1984).
36. B. Peault, M. Coltey, and N. M. Le Douarin, Tissue distribution and ontogenetic emergence of differentiation antigens on avian T cells, *Eur. J. Immunol., 12*: 1047 (1982).
37. B. Peault, J. R. L. Pink, M. Coltey, B. Bruner, and N. M. Le Douarin, Surface markers of avian T lymphocytes as defined by a monoclonal antibody and antisera, in *Embryonic Development: Genetic Aspects* (M. M. Burger and R. Weber, eds.), A. R. Liss, New York, 1982, p. 435.
38. C. H. Chen, T. C. Chanh, and M. D. Cooper, Chicken thymocyte-specific antigen identified by monoclonal antibodies: Ontogeny tissue distribution and biochemical characterisation, *Eur. J. Immunol., 14*: 385 (1984).
39. J. R. L. Pink and A.-M. Rijnbeek, Monoclonal antibodies against chicken lymphocyte surface antigens, *Hybridoma, 2*: 287 (1983).
40. E. Houssaint, E. Diez, and F. V. Jotereau, Tissue distribution and ontogenic appearance of a chicken T lymphocyte differentiation marker, *Eur. J. Immunol., 15*: 385 (1985).
41. K. Hala, K. Schauenstein, N. Neu, G. Krömer, H. Wolf, G. Böck, and G. Wick, A monoclonal antibody reacting with a membrane determinant associated with T cell activation in the chicken, *Eur. J. Immunol., 16*: 1331 (1986).
42. K. Hala, N. Neu, R. L. Boyd, H. Wolf, G. Böck, and G. Wick, Monoclonal antibodies against B and T chicken peripheral blood lymphocytes, *Immunology, 165*: 269 (1983) (Abstr.).
43. O. Mazzelia, L. Cauchy, F. Coudert, and J. Richard, Chicken thymocyte-specific antigens identified by monoclonal antibodies, *Hybridoma, 5*: 319 (1986).
44. C. H. Chen and M. D. Cooper, Identification of cell surface molecules on chicken lymphocytes with monoclonal antibodies, in *Avian Immunology, Basis and Practice* (A. Toivanen and P. Toivanen, eds.), CRC Press, Boca Raton, Florida, 1987, Vol. I, p. 137.
45. O. Vainio, T. Veromaa, E. Eerola, and P. Toivanen, Characterization of 2 monoclonal antibodies reactive with subpopulations of chicken lymphocytes, in *Avian Immunology* (W. T. Weber and D. L. Ewert, eds.), A. R. Liss, New York, 1987, p. 87.
46. H. Wolf, K. Hala, R. L. Boyd, and G. Wick, MHC- and non-MHC-encoded surface antigens of chicken lymphoid cells and erythrocytes recognised by polyclonal xeno-, allo- and monoclonal antibodies, *Eur. J. Immunol., 15*: 305 (1984).
47. J. R. L. Pink, O. Vainio, and A.-M. Rijnbeek, Clones of B lymphocytes in individual follicles of the bursa of Fabricius, *Eur. J. Immunol., 15*: 83 (1985).
48. E. Houssaint, E. Diez, and J. R. L. Pink, Ontogeny and tissue distribution of the chicken Bu-1a antigen, *Immunology* (in press).
49. A. A. Benedict, T. Fredericksen, and D. G. Gilmour, unpublished results.

50. T. Veromaa, O. Vainio, E. Eerola, and P. Toivanen, unpublished results.
51. T. C. Chanh, C.-L. H. Chen, and M. D. Cooper, Mouse monoclonal antibodies to chicken V_H idiotypic determinants: Reactivity with B and T cells, *J. Immunol., 129*: 2541 (1982).
52. J. T. Wright, C. L. Chen, H. Kubagawa, and M. D. Cooper, in *Avian Immunology* (W. T. Weber and D. L. Ewert, eds.), A. R. Liss, New York, 1987, p. 81.
53. A. A. Benedict, unpublished results.
54. G. Koch, Monoclonal antibodies to biliary IgA of the chicken, results presented at the *Avian Immunology Workshop,* Innsbruck, 1986.
55. D. L. Ewert, M. S. Munchus, C. H. Chen, and M. D. Cooper, Analysis of structural properties and cellular distribution of avian Ia antigen by using monoclonal antibody to monomorphic determinants, *J. Immunol., 132*: 2524 (1984).
56. P. D. Oliver and N. M. Le Douarin, Avian thymic accessory cells, *J. Immunol., 132*: 1748 (1984).
57. F. P. Guillemot, P. D. Oliver, B. M. Peault, and N. M. Le Douarin, Cells expressing Ia antigens in the avian thymus, *J. Exp. Med., 160*: 1803 (1984).
58. J. A. Schmidt, J. Marshall, M. J. Hayman, G. Doderlein, and H. Beug, Monoclonal antibodies to novel erythroid differentiation antigens reveal specific effects of oncogenes on the leukemic cell phenotype, *Leukemia Research, 10*: 257 (1986).
59. S. Kornfeld, H. Beug, G. Doederlin, and T. Graf, Detection of avian hematopoietic cell surface antigens with monoclonal antibodies to myeloid cells, *Exp. Cell. Res., 143*: 383 (1983).
60. D. G. Gilmour, A. Brand, N. Donnelly, and H. A. Stone, Bu-1 and Th-1, two loci determining surface antigens of B or T lymphocytes in the chicken, *Immunogenetics, 3*: 549 (1976).
61. T. L. Fredericksen and D. G. Gilmour, Two independent T lymphocyte antigen loci in the chicken, Ly-4 and Th-1, *Immunogenetics, 14*: 535 (1981).
62. T. L. Fredericksen, B. M. Longenecker, F. Pazderka, D. G. Gilmour, and R. F. Ruth, A T-cell antigen system of chickens: Ly-4 and Marek's disease, *Immunogenetics, 5*: 535 (1977).
63. J. Galton and J. Ivanyi, Immunofluorescent detection of differentiation antigens (CA1) in the chicken, *Eur. J. Immunol., 7*: 241 (1977).
64. J. Galton and J. Ivanyi, Detection of bursa and thymus-specific alloantigens in the chicken, *Eur. J. Immunol., 7*: 457 (1977).
65. A. T. Waytes, L. D. Bacon, and N. R. Rose, AT-1.1: A thymus-specific alloantigen of chickens, *Immunogenetics, 20*: 359 (1984).
66. D. G. Gilmour, Blood groups, in *Physiology and Biochemistry of the Domestic Fowl, Vol. 5* (B. Freeman, ed.), Academic Press, New York, 1985.
67. L. Lehtonen, D. G. Gilmour, and P. Toivanen, Alloantigenic markers of chicken T and B lymphocytes, in *Avian Immunology: Basis and Practice* (A. Toivanen and P. Toivanen, eds.), CRC Press, Boca Raton, Florida, 1987, Vol. I, p. 127.
68. J. M. Foppoli, L. K. Ching, A. A. Benedict, J. Ivaryi, J. Derka, and E. K. Wakeland, *Immunogenetics, 8*: 385 (1979).
69. W. E. Briles, W. H. McGibbon, and M. R. Irwin, On multiple alleles effecting cellular antigens in the chicken, *Genetics, 35*: 633 (1950).

70. D. G. Gilmour, Segregation of genes determining red cell antigens at high levels of inbreeding in chickens, *Genetics, 44*: 14 (1959).
71. J. R. L. Pink, W. Droege, K. Hala, V. C. Miggiano, and A. Ziegler, A three-locus model for the chicken major histocompatibility complex, *Immunogenetics, 5*: 203 (1977).
72. W. E. Briles, N. Bumstead, D. L. Ewert, D. G. Gilmour, J. Gogusev, K. Hala, C. Koch, B. M. Longenecker, A. W. Nordskog, J. R. L. Pink, L. W. Schierman, M. Simonsen, A. Toivanen, P. Toivanen, O Vainio, and G. Wick, Nomenclature for chicken major histocompatibility (B) complex, *Immunogenetics, 15*: 441 (1982).
73. B. M. Longenecker and T. R. Mosmann, Restricted expression of an MHC alloantigen in cells of the erythroid series, *J. Supramol. Str., 13*: 395 (1981).
74. K. Hala, M. Vilhelmova, and J. Hartmanova, Probable crossing-over in the *B* blood group system of chickens, *Immunogenetics, 3*: 97 (1976).
75. M. Vilhelmova, V. C. Miggiano, J. R. L. Pink, K. Hala, and J. Hartmanova, Analysis of the alloimmune properties of a recombinant genotype in the major histocompatibility complex of the chicken, *Eur. J. Immunol., 7*: 674 (1977).
76. I. Y. Pevzner, C. L. Trowbridge, and A. W. Nordskog, Recombination between genes coding for immune response and the serologically determined antigens in the chicken *B* system, *Immunogenetics, 7*: 25 (1978).
77. J. Plachy and V. Albrecht, Genetic control of Rous sarcoma regression in inbred lines of chickens, *Fol. Biol., 27*: 363 (1981).
78. W. E. Briles, R. W. Briles, R. E. Taffs, and H. A. Stone, Resistance to a malignant lymphoma in chickens is mapped to subregion of major histocompatibility (*B*) complex, *Science, 219*: 977 (1983).
79. D. G. Gilmour, Blood groups, in *Physiology and Biochemistry of the Domestic Fowl, Vol. 5* (B. M. Freeman, ed.), Academic Press, London, 1984, p. 363.
80. J. Salomonsen, K. Skjodt, M. Crone, and M. Simonsen, The chicken erythrocyte-specific MHC antigen, *Immunogenetics, 25*: 373 (1987).
81. G. Möller (ed.), Hybrid myeloma monoclonal antibodies against MHC products, *Immunol. Revs., 47*: 1 (1979).
82. C. Koch, K. Skjodt, A. Toivanen, and P. Toivanen, New recombinants within the MHC (B-complex) of the chicken, *Tissue Antigens, 21*: 129 (1983).
83. B. M. Longenecker and T. R. Mosmann, "Natural" antibodies to chicken MHC antigens are present in mice, rats, humans, alligators and allogeneic chickens, *Immunogenetics, 11*: 293 (1980).
84. N. Neu, K. Hala, and G. Wick, "Natural" chicken antibodies to red blood cells are mainly directed against the B-G antigen and their occurrence is independent of spontaneous autoimmune thyroiditis, *Immunogenetics, 19*: 269 (1984).
85. K. Hala, J. Plachy, and J. Schulmannova, Role of the B-G region antigen in the humoral immune response to the B-F-region antigen of chicken MHC, *Immunogenetics, 14*: 393 (1981).
86. O. Stark, B. Frenzl, and V. Kren, Dissociation of two types of immunologic tolerance induced in newborn chicks, *Transpl. Bull., 28*: 92 (1961).

87. M. Hasek and T. Hraba, Immunological effects of experimental embryonal parabiosis, *Nature, Lond., 175*: 764 (1955).
88. R. E. Billingham, L. Brent, and P. B. Medawar, Quantitative studies on tissue transplantation immunity III. Actively acquired tolerance, *Phil. Trans. Roy. Soc. (Ser. B.), 239*: 359 (1956).
89. C. Havele, T. G. Wegmann, and B. M. Longenecker, Tolerance and autoimmunity to erythroid differentiation (B-G) major histocompatibility complex alloantigens of the chicken, *J. Exp. Med., 156*: 321 (1982).
90. A. Buxton, Antibody production in avian embryos and young chicks, *J. Gen. Microbiol., 10*: 398 (1954).
91. J. R. L. Pink, C. Koch, and A. Ziegler, Immuno-ornithological conversation, in *The Immune System, Vol. 1* (C. M. Steinberg and I. Lefkovits, eds.), Karger, Basel, 1981, p. 69.
92. R. T. Kubo, K. Yamaga, and H. A. Abplanalp, Isolation and partial characterisation of the major histocompatibility antigen in the chicken, in *Avian Immunology* (A. A. Benedict, ed.), Plenum Press, New York, 1977, p. 209.
93. A. Ziegler and J. R. L. Pink, Structural similarity of major histocompatibility antigens on leukocytes and erythrocytes, *Immunochem., 15*: 515 (1978).
94. K. Skjodt, K. G. Welinder, M. Crone, S. Verland, J. Salomonsen, and M. Simonsen, Isolation and characterization of chicken and turkey beta-2 microglobulin, *Mol. Immunol., 23*: 1301 (1986).
95. M. Simonsen, M. Crone, C. Koch, and K. Hala, The MHC haplotypes of the chicken, *Immunogenetics, 16*: 513 (1982).
96. M. Simonsen, K. Hala, and E. M. Nicolaisen, Linkage disequilibrium of MHC genes in the chicken I. The *B-F* and *B-G* loci, *Immunogenetics, 10*: 103 (1980).
97. V. Benda, and K. Hala, Relative distribution of B antigens in erythrocytes and some other chicken tissues, *Folia Biol., 18*: 301 (1972).
98. L. D. Waters, and J. Bennett, An attempt to demonstrate erythrocyte antigen in brain, liver, and muscle tissue in White Leghorns, *Poultry Sci., 50*: 975 (1971).
99. I. Hlozanek, and K. Hala, The detection of B red blood cell allele on chick embryo fibroblasts, *Folia Biol., 15*: 474 (1969).
100. D. L. Ewert, and M. D. Cooper, Ia-like alloantigens of the chicken, in *Ia Antigens and Their Analogs in Man and Other Animals* (C. S. David and S. Ferrone, eds.), CRC Press, Boca Raton, Florida, 1982, p. 1.
101. J. R. L. Pink, Lectin-binding products of the chicken major histocompatibility complex, *Folia Biol. (Prague), 25*: 333 (1979).
102. F. Guillemot, P. Turmel, D. Charron, N. le Dourrin, and C. Auffray, Structure, biosynthesis, and polymorphism of chicken MHC Class II (B-L) antigens and associated molecules, *J. Immunol., 137*: 1251 (1986).
103. M. Crone, J. Jensenius, and C. Koch, Evidence for two populations of B-L (Ia-like) molecules encoded by the chicken MHC, *Immunogenetics, 13*: 381 (1981).
104. D. L. Ewert, and M. D. Cooper, Ia-like alloantigens in the chicken: serologic characterisation and ontogeny of cellular expression, *Immunogenetics, 7*: 521 (1978).

105. R. Peck, K. K. Murthy, and O. Vainio, Expression of B-L (Ia-like) antigens on macrophages from chicken lymphoid organs, *J. Immunol., 129*: 4 (1982).
106. G. Wick, K. Hala, H. Wolf, R. L. Boyd, and K. Schauenstein, Distribution and functional analysis of B-L/Ia-positive cells in the chicken, *Mol. Immunol., 21*: 1259 (1984).
107. D. G. Gilmour, Blood groups, in *Physiology and Biochemistry of the Domestic Fowl, Vol. 2* (D. J. Bell and B. M. Freeman, eds.), Academic Press, London, 1971, p. 883.
108. W. E. Briles, New evidence for close linkage between the A and E blood group loci of the chicken, *Genetics, 60*: 164 (1968).
109. L. W. Schierman and A. W. Nordskog, Relationship of erythrocyte to leukocyte antigens in chickens, *Science, 137*: 620 (1962).
110. S. Y. Wong, F. Pazderka, B. M. Longenecker, G. R. J. Law, and R. F. Ruth, Immobilization of lymphocytes at surfaces by alloantibodies, *Immunol. Commun., 1*: 597 (1972).
111. L. W. Schierman and A. W. Nordskog, Evidence for a second blood group-histocompatibility system in chickens, *Transplantation, 3*: 44 (1965).
112. L. B. Crittenden, W. E. Briles, and H. A. Stone, Susceptibility to an avian leukosis-sarcoma virus: Close association with an erythrocyte isoantigen, *Science, 169*: 1324 (1970).
113. K. S. Brown, W. E. Briles, and E. R. Brown, Vaccinia virus hemagglutination receptor in chickens determined by K isoantigen locus, *Proc. Soc. Exp. Biol., NY, 142*: 16 (1973).
114. D. G. Gilmour, Blood groups in chickens, *Brit. Poultry Sci., 1*: 75 (1960)
115. D. G. Gilmour and A. C. Allison, Inheritance of susceptibility of chicken erythrocytes to haemagglutination by poxviruses and phospholipids, *Virology, 37*: 237 (1969).
116. B. G. Sanders, Developmental disappearance of a fowl red blood cell antigen, *J. Exp. Zool., 167*: 165 (1968).
117. J.-P. Blanchet, The chick erythrocyte membrane antigens: Characterisation and variation during embryonic and post-embryonic development, *Dev. Biol., 48*: 411 (1976).
118. V. Krsmanovic, J. P. Blanchet, T. B. Greenland, and M. Aupoix, Immunochemical properties of embryonic and adult specific antigens of chicken erythrocytes, *Exp. Cell Res., 120*: 409 (1979).
119. K. Kline, J. P. Allison, and B. G. Sanders, Chemical and immunological characterisation of developmentally expressed chicken erythroid surface membrane antigens, *Dev. Biol., 91*: 389 (1982).
120. R. R. Dietert and B. G. Sanders, Serological dissection of a chicken onco-developmental antigen, *Dev. Comp. Immunol., 2*: 181 (1978).
121. C. H. Nelson, N. H. Patel, and B. G. Sanders, Chicken fetal antigen expression on the definitive erythroid maturation series in the bone marrow of the adult chicken, *J. Exp. Zool., 212*: 101 (1980).
122. R. R. Dietert, H. A. Lewin, M. A. Qureshi, and L. B. Kass, Chicken fetal antigen. Association with lymphoid development and differentiation, *J. Exp. Zool., 220*: 65 (1982).

123. P. C. Powell, K. J. Hartley, B. M. Mustill, and M. Rennie, The occurrence of chicken fetal antigen after infection with Marek disease virus in three strains of chicken, *Oncodev. Biol. Med., 4*: 261 (1983).
124. K. K. Murthy, R. R. Dietert, and B. W. Calnek, Demonstration of a chicken fetal antigen (CFA) on normal splenic lymphocytes, Marek's disease lymphoblastoid cell lines and other neoplasms, *Int. J. Cancer, 24*: 349 (1979).
125. O. Perisic, J. M. Biquard, J.-P. Blanchet, T. B. Greenland, and V. Krsmanovic, Normal or retrovirus-infected cultured chicken embryo cells express the 48000 D age-related antigen characteristic of embryonic chicken erythrocytes, *Differentiation, 18*: 175 (1981).
126. B. G. Sanders, J. P. Allison, and K. Kline, Monoclonal antibody to chicken fetal antigens on normal erythroid cells and hematopoietic-lymphoid tumor cell lines, *Cancer Res., 42*: 4532 (1982).
127. V. Krsmanovic, J.-P. Blanchet, I. Park, and I. Raynaud, Expression of differentiation and age-related antigens on chicken erythroleukemia cells transformed by avian erythroblastosis virus (AEV), *Exp. Cell. Res., 147*: 351 (1983).
128. C. H. Nelson, J.-P. Allison, K. Kline, and B. G. Sanders, Chicken fetal and adult antigen expression on erythroleukemia cells before and after induced differentiation, *Cancer Res., 42*: 4625 (1982).
129. B. G. Sanders and K. Kline, Fetal tumor membrane-associated antigens: Genetic and immunological implications, *Trans. Am. Mic. Soc., 94*: 470 (1975).
130. C. H. Nelson, K. Kline, J. R. Ellison, and B. G. Sanders, Hematopoietic differentiation cell surface antigen switching in the bone marrow of different aged chickens, *Differentiation, 26*: 36 (1984).
131. R. Childs and T. Feizi, Differences in carbohydrate moieties of high molecular weight glycoproteins of human lymphocytes of T and B origins revealed by monoclonal autoantibodies with anti-I and anti-i specificities, *Biochem. Biophys. Res. Comm., 102*: 1158 (1981).
132. M. Fukuda, M. N. Fukuda, and S. Hakomori, Developmental change and genetic defect in the carbohydrate structure of Band 3 glycoprotein of human erythrocyte membrane, *J. Biol. Chem., 254*: 3700 (1979).
133. V. Krsmanovic, O. Perisic, J.-P. Blanchet, S. Y. Lee, and T. Greenland, Identification of two types of immature antigenic molecules on chicken red cells, *Exp. Cell. Res., 140*: 433 (1982).
134. J.-P. Blanchet, J. Samarut, and V. Nigon, Chick erythrocyte membrane antigens. Their expression in irradiated chicks grafted with haematopoietic tissues from different origins, *Exp. Cell. Res., 102*: 9 (1976).
135. J. Samarut, J.-P. Blanchet, and V. Nigon, Antigenic characterisation of chick erythrocytes and erythropoietic precursors: Identification of several definitive populations during embryogenesis, *Dev. Biol., 72*: 155 (1979).
136. R. R. Dietert, Oncodevelopmental antigens in avian species, in *Avian Immunology: Basis and Practice* (A Toivanen and P. Toivanen, eds.), CRC Press, Boca Raton, Florida, 1987, Vol. II, p. 71.

137. J. R. L. Pink, Changes in T-lymphocyte glycoprotein structures associated with differentiation, *Comtemp. Topics Mol. Immunol., 9*: 89 (1983).
138. W. J. Leonard, J. M. Depper, G. R. Grabtree, S. Rudikoff, J. Pumphrey, R. J. Robb, M. Krönke, P. B. Svetlik, N. J. Peffer, T. A. Waldmann, and W. C. Greene, Molecular cloning and expression of cDNAs for the human interleukin-2 receptor, *Nature, 311*: 626 (1985).
139. J. R. L. Pink, B. Fedecka-Bruner, M. Coltey, B. M. Peault, and N. M. Le Douarin, Biochemical characterisation of avian T lymphocyte-specific antigens, *Eur. J. Immunol., 11*: 517 (1981).
140. C. Terhost, A. van Agthoven, K. Leclair, P. Snow, E. Reinherz, and S. Schlossman, Biochemical studies of the human thymocyte cell surface antigens T6, T9 and T10, *Cell, 23*: 771 (1981).
141. K. N. Traill, G. Böck, R. L. Boyd, K. Ratheiser, and G. Wick, Ontogeny of surface markers on functionally distinct T cell subsets in the chicken, *Eur. J. Immunol., 14*: 61 (1984).
142. M. Chan, C. L. Chen, L. L. Ager, and M. D. Cooper, Identification of the avian CD4 and CD8 homologues, *Fed. Proc., 46*: 49 (1987).
142. K. Hala, personal communication, 1986.
143. J. A. P. Rostas, T. A. Shevenan, C. M. Sinclair, and P. L. Jeffrey, The purification and characterisation of a Thy-1-like glycoprotein from chicken brain, *Biochem. J., 213*: 143 (1983).
144. H. Beug, A. von Kirchbach, G. Döderlein, J.-F. Conscience, and T. Graf, Chicken hematopoietic cells transformed by seven strains of defective avian leukemia viruses display three distinct phenotypes of differentiation, *Cell, 18*: 375 (1979).
145. A. Brand, J. Galton, and D. G. Gilmour, Committed precursors of B and T lymphocytes in chick embryo bursa of Fabricius, thymus and bone marrow, *Eur. J. Immunol., 13*: 449 (1983).
146. T. L. Fredericksen and D. G. Gilmour, Influence of genotypes at a non-MHC B lymphocyte alloantigen locus (Bu-1) on expression of Ia (B-L) antigen on chicken bursal lymphocytes, *J. Immunol., 134*: 754 (1985).
147. U. G. Rovigatti and S. M. Astrin, Avian endogenous viral genes, *Current Topics in Microbiol. and Immunol., 103*: 1 (1983).
148. E. H. Humphries, M. L. Danhof, and I. Hlozanek, Characterization of endogenous viral loci in five lines of White Leghorn chickens, *Virology, 135*: 125 (1984).
149. M. S. Halpern, W. S. Mason, D. L. Ewert, D. T. Deery, and J. M. England, Expression of endogenous retroviral envelope antigen in Ig(+) B cells of immunized $15I_5 \times 7_1$ chickens, *J. Immunol., 126*: 1198 (1981).
150. M. S. Halpern, D. L. Ewert, L. J. Flores, K. Y. Lin, and J. M. England, Endogenous retroviral envelope antigen in plasma cells, *J. Immunol., 127*: 698 (1981).
151. D. L. Ewert, and M. S. Halpern, B cell expression of endogenous retroviral envelope antigen: Biochemical and immunofluorescence characterization, *J. Immunol., 129*: 1724 (1982).
152. D. L. Ewert, O. Vainio, and M. S. Halpern, Increased endogenous retroviral gene expression is a consequence of lymphocyte activation, *J. Immunol., 131*: 3036 (1983).

153. D. L. Ewert, J. H. Chalmers, R. A. McBride, and M. S. Halpern, Individual *ev* loci determine characteristic patterns of endogenous retroviral envelope antigen expression during lymphocyte maturation, *Virology, 133*: 128 (1984).

154. M. Labastie, T. J. Poole, B. M. Péault, and N. M. Le Douarin, MB7, a quail leukocyte endothelium antigen: Partial characterization of the cell surface and secreted forms in cultured endothelial cells, *Proc. Natl. Acad. Sci. USA, 83*: 9016 (1986).

155. E. Houssaint, S. Tobin, J. Cihak, and U. Lösch, A chicken leukocyte-common antigen: Biochemical characterization and ontogenetic study, *Eur. J. Immunol., 17*: 287 (1987).

156. K. N. Traill, G. Böck, R. Boyd, and G. Wick, Chicken thrombocytes. Isolation, serological and functional characterisation using the flourescence-activated cell sorter, *Dev. Comp. Immunol., 7*: 111 (1983).

157. E. L. Reinherz, T-cell receptors: Who needs more? *Nature, 325*: 660 (1987).

12

Biochemistry, Tissue Distribution, and Ontogeny of Surface Molecules Detected on *Xenopus* Hemopoietic Cells

MARTIN F. FLAJNIK, ELLEN HSU,* JAMES F. KAUFMAN, and LOUIS DU PASQUIER
Basel Institute for Immunology, Basel, Switzerland

I. INTRODUCTION

Among the models used to study the phylogenetic and ontogenetic aspects of the immune system, the anuran amphibian *Xenopus* (the clawed toad or South African frog) occupies a privileged position. Representative of the first terrestrial vertebrates that appeared about 350 million years ago, it is an important landmark from the phylogenetic viewpoint (1). Moreover, its embryonic and larval development, like those of other anurans, have been exploited for a long time by developmental biologists and immunologists for ontogenetic studies. Because of these interesting aspects, the *Xenopus* immune system has been fairly well analyzed.

Most elements of the immune system described in mammals also exist in *Xenopus*. The lymphoid system, although simpler than that of mammals, is organized in a similar way. The thymus, spleen and gut-associated lymphoid tissues function approximately in the same manner as in mammals, and the collaboration between T cells and B cells is similar in both mammals and amphibians (2). Responses of the *Xenopus* T and B cells to various mitogens and factor production seem to follow the same rules as in mammals (3-9). A major histocompatibility complex (MHC) encodes polymorphic class I, II, III, and IV molecules which (at least for the class I and II antigens) show strong structural homologies with their mammalian counterparts (10-16). As in mammals, the MHC of *Xenopus* controls acute

**Present affiliation*: Columbia University College of Physicians and Surgeons, New York, New York.

graft rejection, the mixed leukocyte reaction (MLR), the restriction of collaboration between T and B cells, the genesis of cell-mediated lympholysis (CML), the graft-versus-host reaction (gvh), and thymic education (10,17-20).

Xenopus immunoglobulins consist of only three heavy chain isotypes and an as yet unknown number of light chain classes. Two of the heavy chain isotypes are present in serum in polymeric form like IgM, and the third, IgY, has analogies but so far no proven structural homologies with mammalian IgG (21-26).

These similarities are certainly numerous enough to justify the use of *Xenopus* as a model for the study of the immune system. In fact, since the immune system is simpler, (fewer cells, fewer Ig isotypes, lower antibody diversity, etc.), it is possible to examine certain immune responses with greater ease than in mammals.

The most attractive aspect of *Xenopus* immunology is the opportunity to study the ontogeny of the immune response (27). The embryos and tadpoles are free of maternal influences and are accessible from the earliest stages of development. Although they are exposed to many of the same antigenic challenges as the adult, *Xenopus* tadpoles express a different antibody repertoire than the adults as judged by the affinity and isoelectric points of anti-hapten antibodies (28-35). MHC expression also changes during ontogeny; tadpoles do not express the adult form of the class I molecules, but do express the same class II antigens as the adult (76). At metamorphosis there are profound changes in the immune system with a new influx of hemopoietic cells, a change in the antibody repertoire and the establishment of tolerance to newly arising adult-specific antigens (36-38).

In addition to these ontogenetic aspects, *Xenopus* offers the possibility, because of polyploidization relationships between the various species, to study the role of gene duplication on certain elements of the immune system (39).

With so much to study there is an obvious need for defined strains and immunological reagents. A few partially inbred (i.e., homozygous at the MHC) strains and clones of interspecies hybrid animals have been developed (40-45). These helped to define some of the above-mentioned characteristics of the *Xenopus* immune system (Table 1). With respect to reagents which will constitute the main subject of this chapter, antisera and monoclonal antibodies have been raised with varying success depending on the antigens studied. It has been easy to raise anti-Ig reagents and difficult to obtain reagents against antigens defining cell subpopulations and MHC molecules. In our attempts to raise these reagents we have produced antibodies directed against structures with no known immunological functions, but, as described later, some have been useful in other ways.

This chapter will first detail the production and the analysis of the reagents. Their use in elucidating various aspects of the regulation of expression of the MHC antigen and Ig determinants, as well as the differentiation of B cells, will then be

Table 1 Strains and Clones of MHC-Defined *Xenopus*

Strain	MHC haplotypes	Species
LG6	*a/c*	
LG7	*a/c*	
LG15	*a/c*	*X. laevis–X.*
LG17	*a/c*	*gilli* hybrids
LG46	*a/c*	(isogenic clones)
LG5	*b/c*	(13,17,41)
LG14	*a/d*	
LG3	*b/d*	
		X. laevis–X.
LM3	*w/y*	*muelleri* hybrids
LM22	*w/z*	(isogenic clones)
LM34	*w/z*	(45)
F	*f* (40)	
G	*g* (40)	
J	*j* (44)	*X. laevis*
A8	*r* (43)	
K	*k* (19)	

described. In a later section, technical parameters for the production of new and better reagents will be considered. This is a valid point, since the molecular biology studies in lower vertebrates will call for more specific reagents, either to be used to screen expression libraries, or to determine the expression product of an as yet uncharacterized gene.

II. REAGENTS

A. Anti-MHC

The first anti-*Xenopus* MHC reagents produced were alloantisera raised against cells coming from MHC-typed individuals (10). These sera were used to immunoprecipitate class I and class II molecules from the cell surface of *Xenopus* hemopoietic cells (see Figs. 1 and 2). Cross-reactive xenoantisera were used to characterize class II molecules (14,15). Finally, with the use of these presently defined reagents, partial purification became possible, enabling the production of better antibodies against the MHC components.

1. MHC Structure

Class I molecules consist of a polymorphic heavy chain of 40-45 kilodaltons (Kd) depending on the haplotype which encodes them (13). They bear one asparagine-linked glycan and are associated noncovalently with a nonglycosylated molecule of 13 Kd, presumably β_2-microglobulin (β_2-m; Fig. 1). These molecules can be immunoprecipitated with specific alloantisera or with xenoantisera that have been raised against *Xenopus* cells.

Class I molecules are expressed by cells in all tissues of the organism as determined by immunofluorescence on frozen sections. They are expressed in the highest amounts in hemopoietic tissue and skin (76). At this time, we have no evidence that multiple polymorphic class I molecules are expressed. We have also failed to find Qa or T1-like class I molecules either on the surface of hemopoietic cells or secreted in the serum.

The α and β chains (30-33 Kd) of *Xenopus* class II molecules are noncovalently associated transmembrane glycoproteins (14). The α chains bear three N-linked glycans (2 complex, 1 high mannose). The β chains bear two N-linked glycans (1 complex, 1 high mannose) and, like mammalian β chains, have an increased gel mobility under nonreducing conditions. Both chains are polymorphic as judged by isoelectric focusing (IEF) of class II molecules encoded by different haplotypes (15). It is not yet known how many class II loci are present. From N-terminal sequencing data, it appears that there are at least 2 α chains and 5 β chains encoded by the *f* haplotype (Fig. 2).

Class II molecules are produced by macrophages and B cells, and preliminary evidence indicates they are also made by thymocytes and peripheral T cells. They are not expressed by erythrocytes or elicited peritoneal macrophages (14).

2. Alloantisera

Alloantisera are raised by skin grafting histoincompatible frogs of known MHC type (determined by MLR), allowing the skin grafts to be rejected (16-20 days) and then immunizing with hemopoietic cells (10,31). The frogs are boosted after one month and test-bled after another month. Most of the alloantibody at this point, as tested by ELISA, is of the IgY class. The sera can now be tested by hemagglutination, hemolysis, or immunoprecipitation with cells or cell lysates from the immunizing strain (10,13,31). For reasons we do not understand, the skin graft rejection is essential in order to produce a "strong" alloantiserum.

In general, these sera have to be absorbed on splenocytes from siblings. This is possible only when MHC-typed families already exist. These antisera are very heterogenous in their ability to recognize class I, class II, or class IV molecules as well as in the number of public determinants recognized. Alloantisera made in the LM3 strain against *X. laevis* MHC haplotypes often show extensive cross-reactions. It is difficult to produce antisera against MHC molecules encoded by

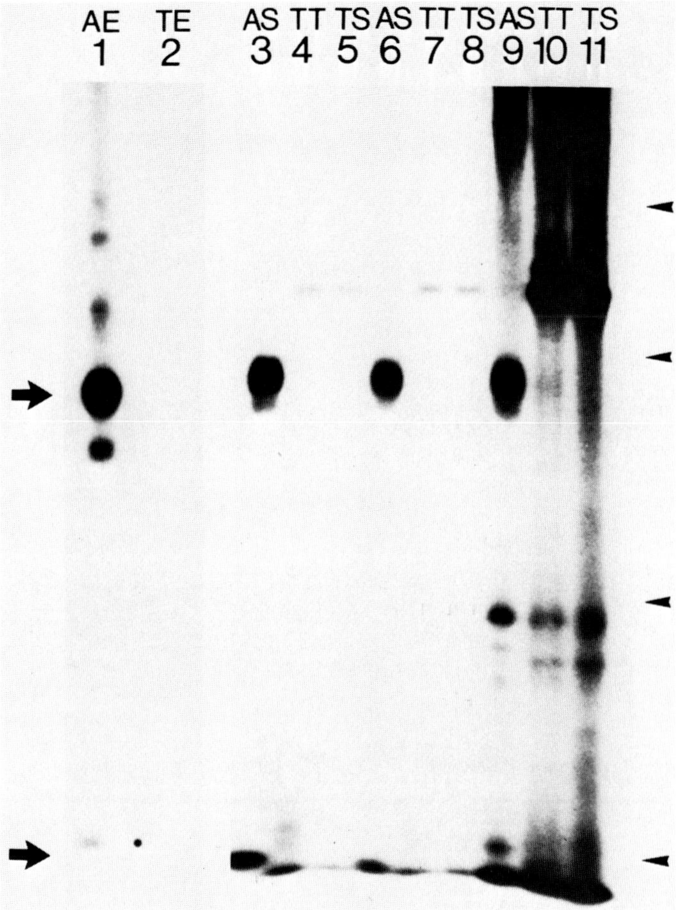

Figure 1 Immunoprecipitation of class I molecules from lysates of iodinated cell-surface proteins from LG3 tadpoles and adults. Mobilities of standards are indicated on the right from top to bottom: BSA, 68 Kd; ovalbumin, 45 Kd; carbonic anhydrase, 30 Kd; lysosyme, 14 Kd. The large arrows on the left point out the class I heavy chain (42 Kd) and β_2-m bands (13 Kd). The β_2-m runs with the dye front in lanes 6 and 9. Lysates were incubated with alloantisera (lanes 1-8) or mouse xenoantisera (lanes 9-11). AE = adult erythrocytes, TE = tadpole erythrocytes, TT = tadpole thymocytes, TS = tadpole spleen, AS = adult spleen. Note that although many background bands are immunoprecipitated from tadpole lysates with xenoantisera, no class I molecules are precipitated. The bands in the 68-Kd region in lane 1 are candidates for MHC-linked erythrocyte antigens.

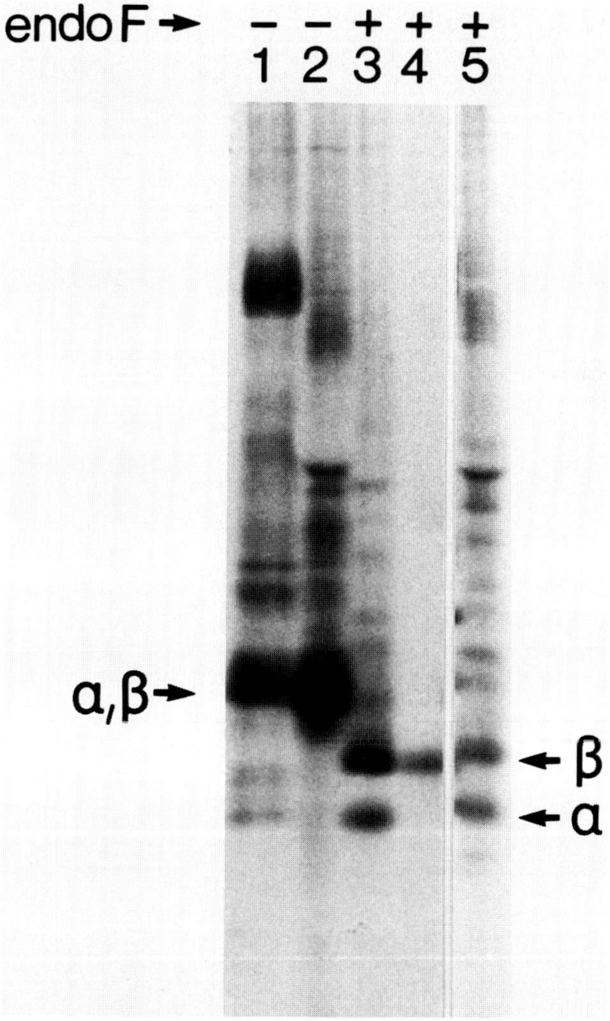

Figure 2 Immunoprecipitations of class II molecules from cell lysates of biosynthetically labeled (^{35}S-methionine) proteins from F strain tadpoles (lane 5) and adults (lanes 1-4). Class II molecules were precipitated with an A.TH anti-*Xenopus* serum (lane 1) or a rabbit serum directed against human class II molecules (lanes 2-5, Ref. 14). This antiserum recognizes only the β chain under denaturing conditions (lane 4). After removal of asparagine-linked carbohydrates, both tadpole and adult α and β chains have the same approximate mobilities (lanes 3,5) and are identical in IEF (76).

the *j* haplotype except when they are produced by animals of the G strain. In this case, sera usually react against molecules of all the MHC classes. Reciprocally, good anti-MHC alloantisera can be raised in the J strain against the *g* haplotype. Antisera with anti-class I and anti-class IV activity can be produced between all members of the LG family (Table 1). It is easiest to prepare reagents reacting with class I molecules encoded by the *c* or *d* haplotype. Immunoprecipitations of typical class I and class IV molecules are displayed in Figure 1.

A biochemically unidentified molecule is detected by immunofluorescence on the thymic epithelium of tadpoles with an LG6 anti-LG3 alloantiserum (76). The molecule appears to be MHC-linked since it is found on the thymus epithelium of members of the LG family that have the *b* or *d* haplotype. It is expressed in high amounts by the medulla and is found at the time of the first outpocketing of the thymus from the embryonic pharyngeal (endodermal) epithelium. It is not the polymorphic adult class I molecule, since absorption of this antiserum on LG3 erythrocytes does not abolish the fluorescence on the thymus epithelium. What effect, if any, this molecule has on the immune system is not known.

3. Xenoantisera Raised in Mice

Mouse anti-*Xenopus* hemopoietic cell sera have been obtained after immunizing intraperitoneally with 2×10^7 leukocytes and boosting 1 to 2 months later the same way. The mice are bled 5 to 7 days after the last injection. It has been a matter of luck as to whether anti-class I antisera are obtained in this manner. We screen these sera by immunoprecipitation. Of course, many other molecules are also immunoprecipitated, as shown in Figure 1. Some of these mouse anti-*Xenopus* antisera recognize allelic polymorphisms of *Xenopus* by immunoprecipitating class I molecules encoded by some haplotypes better than from others. None of the xenoantisera we have raised immunoprecipitate class I molecules from tadpole lysates. We have not yet systematically determined which class I molecules share the most common antigenic determinants that are recognized by xeno- or alloantisera.

In contrast to the haphazard method of procuring anti-class I xenoantisera, anti-class II sera are not difficult to obtain. Shinohara et al. (46,47) have shown that by immunizing mice of the A.TH (I-E class II negative) strain with cells from the A.TL (I-E class II positive) strain, alloantisera with broad species reactivities can be obtained. They demonstrated that these alloantisera react, as assayed by cytotoxicity, with fish and frog leukocytes. Reciprocally, when A.TH mice were injected with fish or frog cells, antisera were obtained which reacted with leukocytes from I-E positive mouse strains. They were never able to immunoprecipitate class II molecules from radioactively labeled molecules in frog or fish lysates. We have repeated their immunization protocols and have found that 6 out of 7 A.TH mice immunized with frog leukocytes have anti-frog class

II activity in their sera (Fig. 2). We have not yet tested these antisera on I-E positive mouse strains but, unfortunately, they do not immuniprecipitate class II molecules from trout or lamprey hemopoietic cell lysates.

4. Cross-Reactive Xenoantisera

Several rabbit anti-human MHC xenoantisera have been useful in the biochemical analysis of *Xenopus* MHC antigens. One particular antiserum, a rabbit anti-human DR serum (anti-p29boost), was used to identify and characterize *Xenopus* class II molecules (Fig. 2; Ref. 14). Class II molecules immunoprecipitated with this antiserum are essentially identical with those immunoprecipitated with alloantisera and the A.TH anti-frog xenoantisera.

A large number of rabbit antisera produced against purified human and chicken MHC molecules have been tested by immunoprecipitation from labeled spleen and blood lysates from a variety of lower vertebrates. Depending on the species tested, various molecules are recognized and in each case must be rigorously examined for their relationship to MHC molecules. As was found with *Xenopus*, the antisera against class I α chain and class II β chain seem to be the most cross-reactive. However, these cross-reactions are not due to a few special determinants conserved throughout evolution. Rather, very small subpopulations of immunogen-specific antibodies cross-react with MHC-like molecules of a given species, and these cross-reacting subpopulations are different for different species. Indeed, extremely strong rabbit sera can cross-react as alloantisera within a particular species. These data, as well as the criteria for identification of MHC molecules in a lower vertebrate, have recently been discussed (48).

B. Species-Specific Reagents: Anti-*Xenopus gilli*

1. Xenoantisera Raised Between *Xenopus* Species

Antisera were raised against *X. gilli* antigens by repeatedly immunizing *X. laevis* with LG15 blood cells in order to examine the genetic linkage of these antigens with MHC or Ig loci (49). Two series of alloantibodies (acidic and basic), as determined by IEF, were detected by lysis of LG15 erythrocytes. Erythrocytes from offspring from *X. laevis-X. gilli* hybrids (either small eggs from LG15 fertilized with *X. laevis* sperm to allow segregation of *X. laevis* and *X. gilli* chromosomes or small eggs from triploid LLG fertilized with *X. laevis* sperm so that resulting offspring have supernumary *X. gilli* chromosomes) expressed either none, one, or both of these "antigens." The basic set of alloantibodies were never seen alone, but the acidic bands of lysis sometimes were. Two of these antisera (A38 and A39) have now been tested by immunoprecipitation on lysates from LG15 surface-labeled erythrocytes or metabolically labeled splenocytes (Fig. 3). Both these sera immunoprecipitate molecules of 80 and 170 Kd from cell-surface-labeled erythrocytes (Fig. 3). The A39 serum also precipitates class I molecules

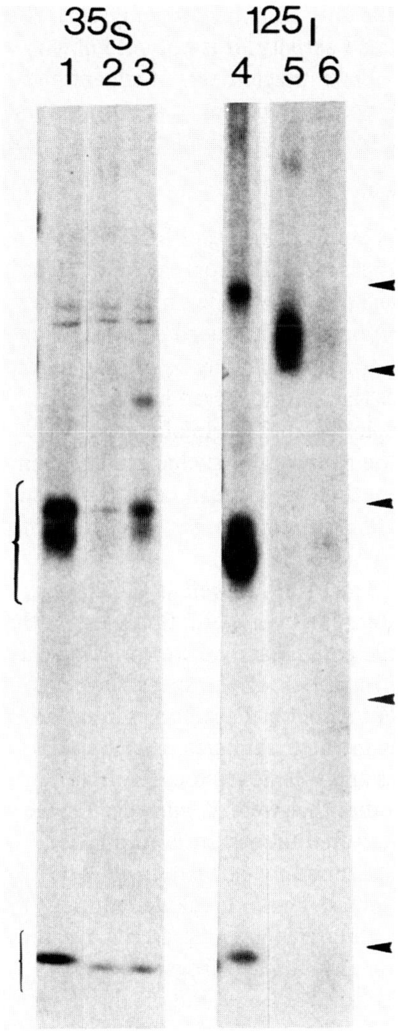

Figure 3 Immunoprecipitations from LG15 biosynthetically labeled leukocytes (lanes 1-3) or cell-surface-labeled erythrocytes (lanes 4-6) lysates with alloantisera (LG3 anti-LG15; lanes 1,4) or xenoantisera (*X. laevis* anti-LG15: A38, lanes 2,5; A39, lanes 3-6). Markers on the right are 92 Kd, 68 Kd, 45 Kd, 30 Kd, 14 Kd. Brackets on the left encompass the class I heavy chain molecules (40-45 Kd) and β_2-m (12-14 Kd) since the gels were run under reducing conditions MHC encoded erythrocyte antigens co-migrate with class I heavy chains (lane 4). The molecule at 90 Kd in lane 4 is an erythrocyte antigen not encoded by the MHC.

from LG15 lysates along with a 60-Kd molecule only from leukocyte lysates. The A38 serum also has a small amount of anti-class I activity. It is not yet known which of these antigens are recognized by the basic or acidic sets of alloantibodies. Combining immunoprecipitation and IEF with these types of antisera should allow us to genetically map the *Xenopus* MHC in the hyperdiploid species hybrids.

2. Monoclonal Anti-*X. gilli* Leukocyte Antigen

For over a century the amphibian embryo has been a useful tool for developmental biologists. Since we now have partially inbred MHC homozygous strains and isogenic clones of *Xenopus*, immunological questions concerning tolerance and hemopoietic cell development from embryonically produced chimeras can be addressed (50-53). There are several cell markers which may be used to determine the percentages of blood cells in animals that have received hemopoietic stem cell grafts as embryos. Frogs tolerate triploidy so that triploid and diploid grafts containing hemopoietic stem cells can be reciprocally exchanged between embryos (54,55). Cells from the blood, spleen, thymus, etc. can later be stained with any DNA dye (Feulgen propidium iodide, mithramycin, etc.) to determine the percentage of cells derived from the embryonic graft (56).

The previously described xenoantisera, A38 and A39, as well as alloantisera, can be used in MHC-disparate chimeras to determine by immunofluorescence the percentage of cells derived from the embryonic graft. Since we were making embryonic chimeras between *X. laevis* (J strain) and one of the species hybrids (LG15), we attempted to produce anti-*X. gilli* monoclonal antibodies in order to be able to detect LG15 hemopoietic cells in these chimeras. CAF*1* strain mice were immunized with LG15 thymocytes and splenic leukocytes. In order to increase the possibility of procuring antibodies that were *X. gilli*-specific, we coated the immunizing cells with a heat-inactivated mouse antiserum raised against *X. laevis* blood cells. We hoped to block immunogenic sites shared between *X. laevis* and *X. gilli* cell-surface molecules. The monoclonal antibody RC5 from this fusion as tested by ELISA on glutaraldehyde fixed cells, reacted only with leukocytes from LG15 but not from any *X. laevis* frogs. All leukocytes from thymus and spleen are stained with this antibody, but erythrocytes are negative (see Figs. 11 and 12). The monoclonal antibody also recognizes a determinant on LG15 tadpole leukocytes. RC5 has been used to determine the extent of chimerism of thymocytes and splenic leukocytes in adult chimeras made between J and LG15 embryos (50).

C. Anti-Adult-specific Reagents

1. Monoclonal Antibody g2C11

This antibody was obtained by immunizing mice with hemopoietic cells of the G strain. The monoclonal antibody stains exclusively a determinant on adult

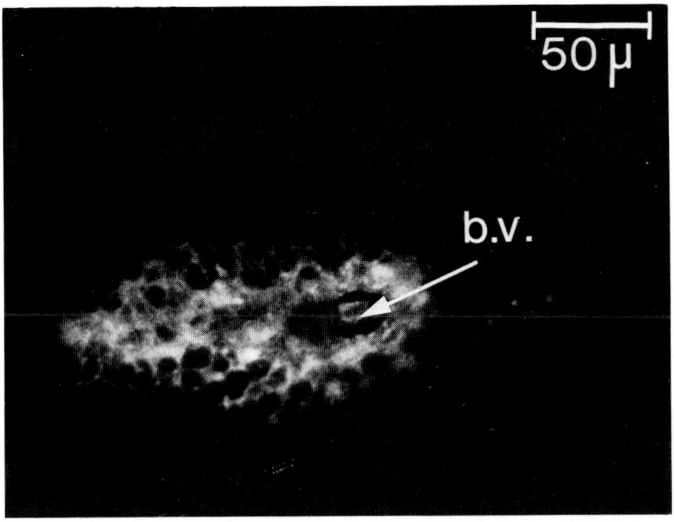

Figure 4 Frozen section of spleen stained with the monoclonal antibody G2C11. Procedures are detailed in Ref. 20; b.v. = blood vessel.

tissue and immunoprecipitates a 15-Kd molecule from spleen cell lysates. The location of the determinant is most peculiar; it shows a gradient of intensity of immunofluorescence on sections, with high intensity near the blood vessel, and almost or completely negative when far from the blood vessel (Fig. 4). The molecule seems to diffuse freely in all the tissue (kidney, liver, spleen) where it has been localized. It is not present in the brain.

2. Anti-Adult β Globulin Xenoantiserum

When rabbits are immunized with *Xenopus* red cells they invariably produce a large amount of antibody against a serum protein migrating in the β globulin fraction and belonging to the lipoportein fraction, as evidenced by Sudan staining of the immunoelectrophoretic gel. This factor, present in the serum and on the surface of red cells and leukocytes, exists only in adults. It normally appears during the last week of metamorphosis. Immunization with total serum does not yield antibodies to this molecule; it may be necessary that it is presented on the cell surface to be antigenic. Tadpoles blocked in their development with chemicals that inhibit thyroid function produce the molecules after 4 months of blockage.

3. Monoclonal Antibody F1F6

This antibody was obtained after immunizing mice with erythrocytes from the F strain. In the radioimmunoassay used for its detection, it was found to bind better

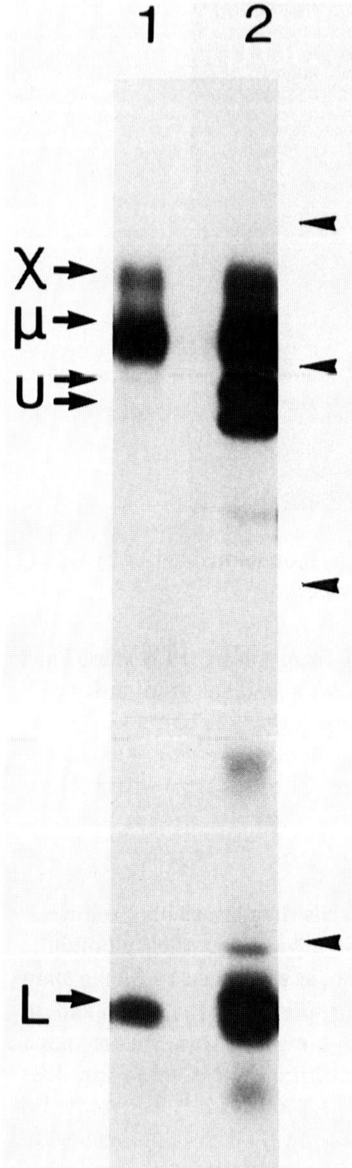

Figure 5 Iodinated *Xenopus* serum immunoglobulins immunoprecipitated with monoclonal antibodies (both directed against light chains). Markers noted on the right from top to bottom (92 Kd, 68 Kd, 45 Kd, 30 Kd). Very little ν chain is associated with the light chains recognized by the monoclonal antibody in lane 1.

to F erythrocytes than to strain G, but it nevertheless binds to erythrocytes from all strains. It immunoprecipitates a 13-Kd molecule from erythrocyte and leukocyte lysates (see Fig. 13) and recognizes a determinant on both tadpole and adult erythrocytes. F1F6 is often used as a control in ontogenetic and immunofluorescence studies.

D. Anti-Immunoglobulin

1. Ig Structure

Xenopus laevis has three classes of immunoglobulins: IgM, IgX, and the IgG analog IgY (Figs. 5, 7). A series of monoclonal antibodies have been raised against *Xenopus* Ig. There are reagents directed against IgM and IgY heavy chains, V_H (which recognizes the heavy chains of all three isotypes), and light chains (22, 26). The biochemical properties of the Ig heavy chains are presented in Table 2. The three isotypes are present in the sera of tadpoles and adults. IgY is markedly depressed in sera from thymectomized animals (36). The recently discovered third Ig class, IgX, is found in the serum in widely varying amounts depending on the animals examined, and is a polymer like the "conventional" IgM (pentamers or hexamers; Ref. 26). It is not yet known whether IgM and IgX are made by the same cells by a switching mechanism, are receptors on different populations of B cells, or are co-expressed by the same cell as are mammalian IgM and IgD.

Anti-light chain monoclonal antibodies distinguish several populations of nonglycosylated light chains. Three light chain bands, with mobilities of 25-30 Kd, can be detected by SDS-PAGE, and these yield three types of distinct peptide maps after digestion with enzyme (22). It is not yet known how any of these peptides or the light chains themselves are related. The J chain migrates faster than the light chains on SDS-PAGE under reducing conditions and bears asparagine-linked glycans. It appears as a fast-moving band on alkaline-urea gels, has a peptide map very different from Ig light chains, and is associated with IgM.

Table 2 Biochemical Properties of *Xenopus* Immunoglobulins

Ig class	Heavy chain MW	Heavy chain MW deglycosylated	Structure
IgM	73 Kd (μ)	60-62 Kd	pentamer/hexamer
IgX	80 Kd (χ)	64 Kd	pentamer/hexamer
IgY	66 Kd, 69 Kd (ν)	66 Kd	monomer

2. Anti-Immunoglobulin Xenoantisera

The serum from various species of *Xenopus* can be passed over protein A columns to yield very pure Ig preparations that can be injected into rabbits or mice. Mouse antisera usually react with the Ig of all species of *Xenopus*. They can be made specific for one species by absorption on Sepharose 4B derivatized with the Ig from other species.

Such reagents were prepared against *X. gilli* (36 chromosomes) and *X. ruwenzoriensis* (108 chromosomes) IgM to study Ig expression in interspecies polyploid hybrids (57). These antisera were used since we failed to raise *X. gilli*- or *X. ruwenzoriensis*-specific monoclonal antibodies. Only *X. laevis*-specific monoclonal antibodies were obtained.

In order to avoid annoying cross-reactions, the source of many past misinterpretations, certain laboratories raise their anti-Ig antisera against deglycosylated Ig (58).

3. An Anti-*X. laevis*-specific IgM Monoclonal Antibody, 14G1

The lymphocytes of a mouse immunized with Ig from *X. laevis* were fused with the myeloma Sp2/0 and hybridomas were screened for specific anti-*X. laevis* Ig by radioimmunoassay on *X. laevis* Ig and various *Xenopus* species Ig in parallel. One hybridoma, producing an IgG_1 anti *X. laevis* IgM, was obtained. Of all the species tested, 14G1 reacts with the IgM of *X. laevis* and perhaps slightly with *X. tropicalis* (22).

4. Anti-Ig Heavy Chain Isotype Monoclonals

The first anti-*Xenopus* IgM monoclonal (6.16) antibody was obtained by Bleicher and Cohen (3). Since then, many anti-IgM and IgY heavy chain monoclonal antibodies have been produced (22,26). Anti-V_H specific antibodies have also been obtained, but await further characterization (22). There have been no reported antibodies directed against allotypic determinants.

When tested on serum from *Rana* and *Bufo* species, none of the anti-IgM monoclonal antibodies reacted, while one anti-IgY and some anti-V_H did. We were able to confirm some reports by Steiner's group (59) that in *Rana catesbiana, R. pipiens,* and *Bufo marinus* the light chain is not disulfide bonded to the IgY heavy chain, and that while *X. laevis* and *B. marinus* both have two IgY heavy chains differing only in carbohydrate, in *R. catesbiana* the two IgY heavy chains have very different peptide maps. In *X. laevis* all the heavy and light chains are covalently bonded.

E. Anti-T-Cell Antibodies

In spite of numerous attempts to produce a monoclonal antibody with reactivity against *Xenopus* T cells, only one has been described (60). Nagata hyperimmunized mice with *Xenopus* thymocytes of the J strain (see Table 1). One monoclonal antibody (XT-1) stains 90-95% of thymocytes from all strains of frogs but peripheral T cells (approximately 30% of splenic leukocytes) from only the J strain. Cells that stain with this antibody are present in the thymus by 7 days after fertilization, and are found in the spleen, liver, and kidney by 20 days after fertilization (61). Adult percentages of cells staining with this monoclonal antibody are reached at midlarval stages. early thymectomy abrogates the appearance of cells bearing the determinant recognized by XT-1.

When XT-1 positive splenocytes are obtained by protein-A Sepharose chromatography after binding the antibody to the cells, there is an enrichment for cells that proliferate in response to T-cell mitogens and allogeneic cells in MHC (77). Depletion of cells bearing this marker does not completely abrogate the responses to T-cell mitogens and allogeneic cells. Thus, XT-1 probably is not a pan-T reagent but instead recognizes a determinant on a molecule expressed by a subset of T cells.

The molecule to which XT-1 binds has not been identified and likewise it is not known whether the MHC is somehow involved in its retention on peripheral T cells from only the J strain of *Xenopus.* Family studies should now be carried out to determine whether the MHC controls its expression. Because this reagent reacts only with splenocytes from the J strain, it is not the everyday type of anti-T-cell reagent that is needed in our field. It should prove useful, however, in studying the development of the T-cell system in tadpoles and adults.

III. ANTIGENIC EXPRESSION

The reagents described in the previous section have been used to study the *Xenopus* immune system.

A. Ontogenetic Aspects

1. MHC Expression

IEF analysis has demonstrated that the same class II molecules are expressed by tadpoles and adult hemopoietic cells (Fig. 2; Flajnik et al., submitted). In contrast, the adult class I molecules are not expressed by tadpoles (Fig. 1; Ref. 31; Flajnik et al., submitted). They appear on all tissues at the metamorphic climax. We are now trying to determine whether the absence of class I antigens has any effect on the tadpole's immune system. For example, are class I restricted T cells present in tadpoles? Since none of the different antisera tested immunoprecipitate class I molecules from tadpole lysates, we feel that they do not express any class I antigens.

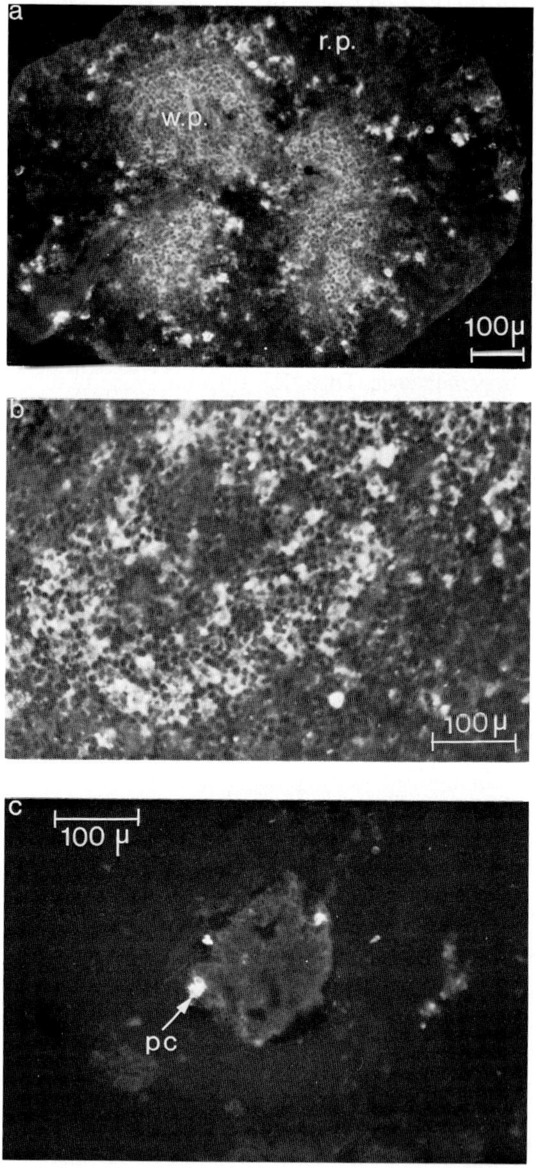

Figure 6 Staining of various frozen tissue sections with anti-Ig monoclonal antibodies. a, Tadpole spleen with 10A9 anti-IgM (22); r.p. = red pulp; w.p. = white pulp. b, Adult spleen with 10A9, section corresponds to one B-cell-rich white pulp area. c, Tadpole thymus with 10A9; pc = plasma cell. d, Adult thymus with

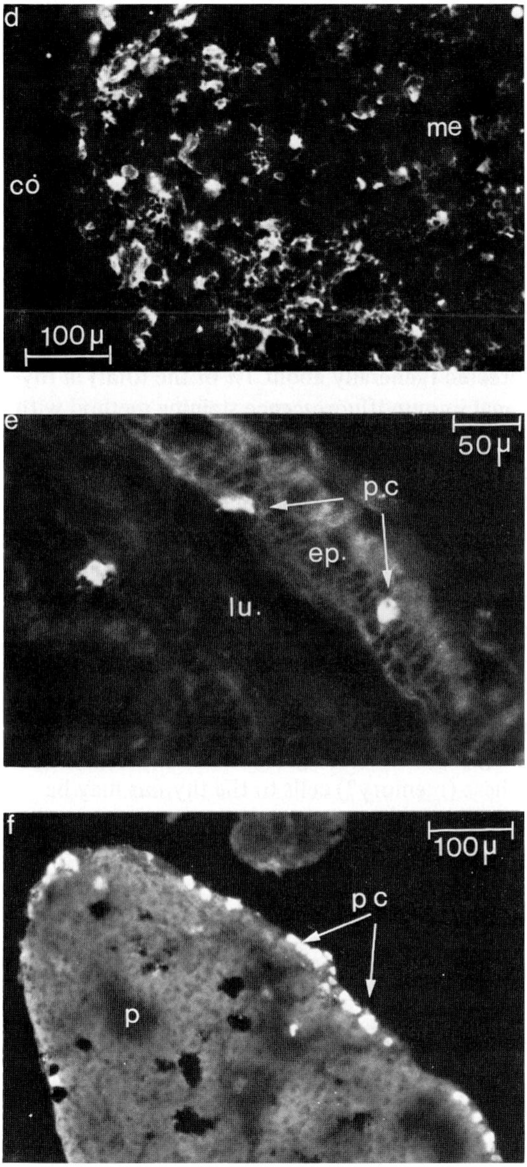

10A9 (anti-IgM) and 11D5 (anti-IgY). The medulla (me) is rich in plasma cells. Cortex (co) does not contain many. e, Posterior region of the adult intestine stained with 10A9; pc = plasma cells. f, Adult liver with 10A9. The peripheral hematopoietic layer is rich in plasma cells (pc) but not the parenchyme (p).

2. Ig Expression

Pre-B cells with cytoplasmic Ig can first be detected in the liver at stage 46 (5 days postfertilization; Ref. 63) and in the spleen from its earliest differentiation (62). IgM is found in tadpole peritoneal fluid at stage 49 (12 days of development) when cells bearing surface IgM are first detected by immunofluorescence (34,62). IgY is first detected in peritoneal fluid at stage 51 (17 days postfertilization; Ref. 34). As in mammals, the liver and spleen of tadpoles and adults contain many B cells (Figs. 6a and b). The B cells are accumulated in the splenic white pulp in both tadpoles and adults. The intestine also contains accumulations of B cells that predominantly produce IgM and IgX (Fig. 6e; Ref. 26). IgM (and IgX) is the secretory Ig of reptiles and amphibians (64).

Although B cells cannot be detected (generally about 1% of the total) in thymocyte suspensions by conventional immunofluorescence staining method with anti-Ig monoclonal antibodies (see Fig. 12, Refs. 2,57), it has been demonstrated by *in situ* protein-A plaques and *in vitro* Ig synthesis experiments that the thymus definitely contains B cells (65). Many plasma cells can be detected in the thymus by section staining in tadpoles and adults (Figs. 6c and d). They are probably not detected by conventional live-cell immunofluorescent staining procedures, because these Ig-secreting cells no longer have surface Ig. It is clear from biosynthetic-labeling studies that B cells in the thymus preferentially make IgY, whereas those in the spleen, intestinal mucosae, and liver produce all three isotypes (Fig. 7). It has been suggested that the preferential expression of IgY by thymic B cells may be either due to their intrinsic properties in the thymus or, alternatively, a result of the homing patterns of antigen-driven B cells (65). If the latter is true, the homing of these (memory?) cells to the thymus may be part of a regulatory mechanism acting on these cells. The thymus contains T cells that appear to have increased "suppressor" activity, whereas splenic T cells are better "helpers" (65).

B. Genetic Regulation

1. Allelic Exclusion

Using the various reagents mentioned in the previous section (anti-*X. laevis* μ, anti-*X. gilli ruwenzoriensis* reagents), the expression of surface IgM was studied by immunofluorescence in various *Xenopus* species hybrids having increasing number of chromosomes: (*X. laevis-X. gilli*) hybrids 36 chromosomes; (*X. vestitus-X. laevis*) hybrids, 54 chromosomes; (*X. laevis-X. ruwenzoriensis*) hybrids, 72 chromosomes; (*X. laevis-X. gilli-X. vertitus*) hybrids, 72 chromosomes. Whether the hybrids were diploid or polyploid, a lymphocyte produced only one Ig at a time, i.e., there was evidence for allelic exclusion (58). This suggested that the selection presumed to make a lymphocyte synthesize only one antibody

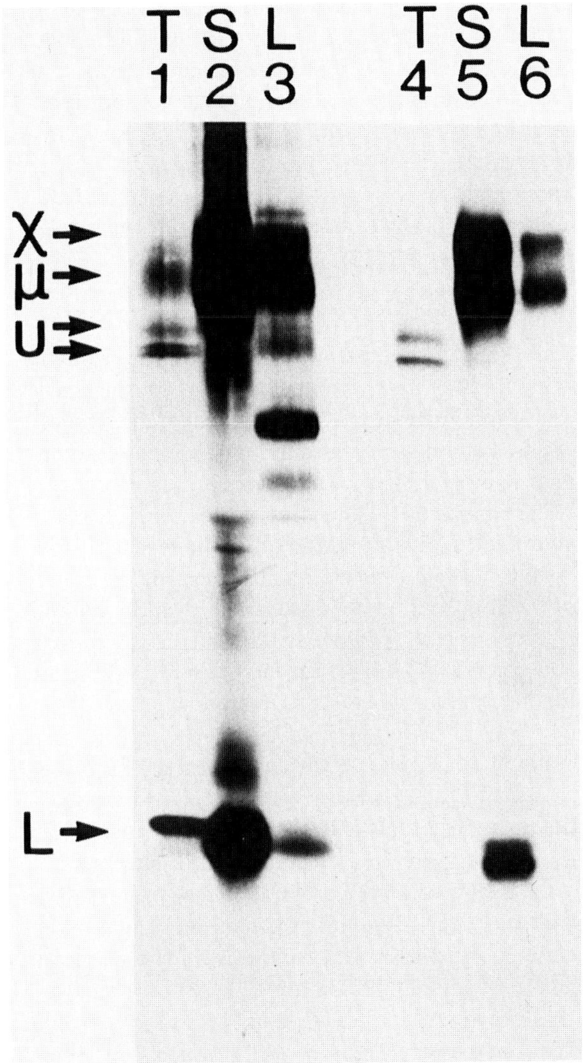

Figure 7 Immunoprecipitation of biosynthetically labeled secreted immunoglobulins from thymus (lanes 1,4), spleen (lanes 2,5), and liver (lanes 3,6) cultures. Igs were immunoprecipitated either with a rabbit anti-*Xenopus* Ig (Ref. 22, lanes 1-3) or with an anti-light chain monoclonal antibody (lanes 4-6, same as used in Fig. 5, lanes 4-6). Note the increase in the relative expression of IgY in the thymus culture (lanes 1,3) and the preferential association of the "upper" light chain with ν heavy chain (lane 1, Ref. 22).

is high and that allelic exclusion existed in the ancestors of amphibians which appeared 300 million years ago. The apparent lack of cells producing multiple Ig in polyploid hybrids having more than one pair of functional Ig genes suggests that if a stochastic model for allelic exclusion is correct, the frequency of multiple successful rearrangements has to be very low, resulting in a huge waste of lymphocyte precursors. Given the particularity of the frog development, in which the development of a well-functioning immune system with a reasonable antibody diversity occurs within 3 weeks, it has been argued that the stochastic model cannot be the correct one in *Xenopus* (58).

2. Speculation on Isotypes in Polyploid *Xenopus*

Xenopus laevis (36 chromosomes) appears to have undergone an entire genome duplication. It will be interesting to determine whether the genes for the heavy chains of the two IgM isotypes, μ and χ, are genetically linked as are the genes encoding the different isotypes in mammals, or are found on different chromosomes. There are two clusters of hemoglobin genes in *X. laevis*, each encoding all of the larval and adult α and β chains (66). There also may be two Ig gene clusters in *Xenopus*, one containing the μ gene and the other the χ gene. If the duplication event occurred by autopolyploidization, then afterwards the μ and χ genes could have diverged. If the duplication event occurred by allopolyploidization through a cross between two ancestral *Xenopus*, each having 18 chromosomes, then the divergence of the genes will have preceded the polyploidization event. If the gene encoding the heavy chain of IgY is found in one cluster and not the other, this will strongly favor the allopolyploidization mechanism. It will be exciting to determine whether *X. tropicalis* (20 chromosomes) has both the μ and χ genes.

One might also consider the possibility that IgM and IgX are two ancient distinct isotypes and that the influence of polyploidy manifests itself elsewhere. For instance, it may occur at the light chain level, or within a real single isotype form recognized by monoclonal antibodies. Immunoprecipitation of IgM from the supernatant of culture done in the presence of tunicamycin show several heavy chains ranging between 61,700 and 60,000 daltons (22). These could represent the production of a duplicated locus, since *X. laevis* with its 36 chromosomes already represent a polyploid species of *Xenopus* with respect to the more primitive and simpler *X. tropicalis.*

C. Functional Studies with B Cells

1. Mitogen Studies

With their anti-IgM monoclonal antibody (6.16), Bleicher and Cohen (3) performed panning studies which demonstrated that B-cell-depleted populations of spleen cells were enriched in their ability to proliferate after stimulation with

T-cell mitogens such as PHA or Con A. Responses to alloantigens in MLC were also enriched. Proliferation in response to a B-cell mitogen, LPS, was unchanged or only slightly depressed in B-cell-depleted populations. They further showed that the proliferation in response to LPS was not B-cell-specific and that extensively purified LPS was unable to induce any proliferation (67). Thus, it appeared that contaminating molecules in LPS preparations were the actual "mitogens" that stimulated *Xenopus* splenocytes to proliferate. Hsu and Leanderson (manuscript submitted) have now shown that at the dosages used in mouse and human studies, LPS does not stimulate much proliferation but does induce maturation in B cells as evidenced by protein-A plaques. LPS induces secretion of IgM and IgX, followed by small amounts of IgY after 7 days of culture (26).

Schwager and Hadji-Azimi have shown that both pokeweed mitogen and the Ig fraction of rabbit anti-*Xenopus* IgM are potent stimulators of B-cell proliferation and differentiation (23,24). B-cell responses to pokeweed mitogen are dependent on T-cell involvement, and both IgM and IgX are secreted in culture supernatants. Stimulation with anti-IgM appears to be T-cell independent, but only IgM is secreted.

The effects of phorbol myristate acetate (PMA) on B cells has been examined (25). Although it is a powerful mitogen causing 80% of resting splenic leukocytes to enter S phase, stimulation to Ig secretion is highly variable. B cells lose surface Ig, and blasts with cytoplasmic Ig are observed, but usually few protein-A plaque-forming cells are found.

Monoclonal anti-Ig coupled to Sepharose sometimes stimulate ^{3}H-thymidine uptake, but Ig secretion is completely suppressed (unpublished results). Of those that have been tried, 10A9 anti-IgM and 1E9 anti-light chain have been successful, while 14B4 anti-V_H and 13B2 anti-light chain were negative.

2. Ig Re-expression After Capping

We have recently tested the efficacy of panning and the kinetics of re-expression of IgM after capping using Bleicher's anti-IgM antibody (6.16). Splenic leukocytes were purified by Ficoll (2), washed in L-15 medium containing 5% FCS (L-15/FCS), resuspended to between 3 and 6 × 10^6 cells per ml and put onto 6.16-coated plastic dishes. Panning was carried out essentially as described by Bleicher and Cohen (3). For adult cells, and tadpole splenocytes pooled from 50 to 100 individuals, 6-well Costar plates were used and 2 ml of cells were put into each well. They were kept at 4°C for 90 minutes and nonadherent cells were collected by washing 4 times with 5 ml of L-15/FCS. The adherent cells were placed at 27°C with 5% CO_2 for 7 hours and were then retrieved by vigorous pipetting. The cells were washed, counted, and put into culture at 10^6 cells per ml in 24-well Costar plates. They were kept at 27°C and analyzed at different time intervals.

Unseparated leukocytes, nonadherent cells, and adherent cells at 10, 36, 64, 96, and 168 hours after panning were tested for IgM staining with 6.16 (Figs. 8, 9).

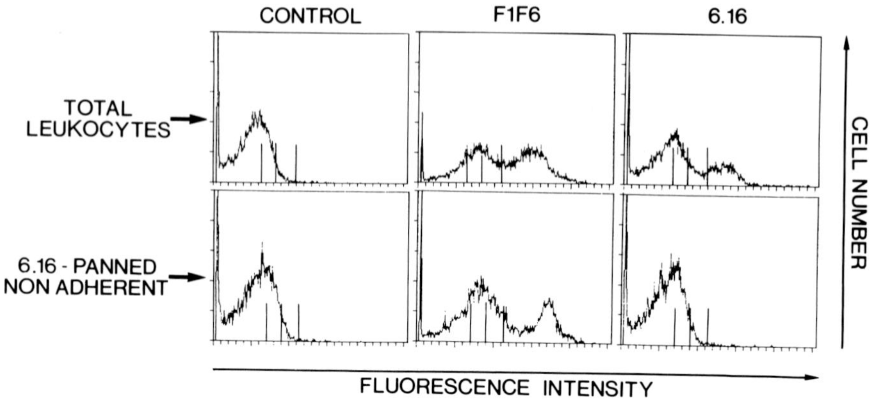

Figure 8 FACS analyzer profiles of control or nonadherent to anti-IgM coated plates splenic leukocytes stained with 6.16 (αIgM) or F1F6 (anti-13 Kd).

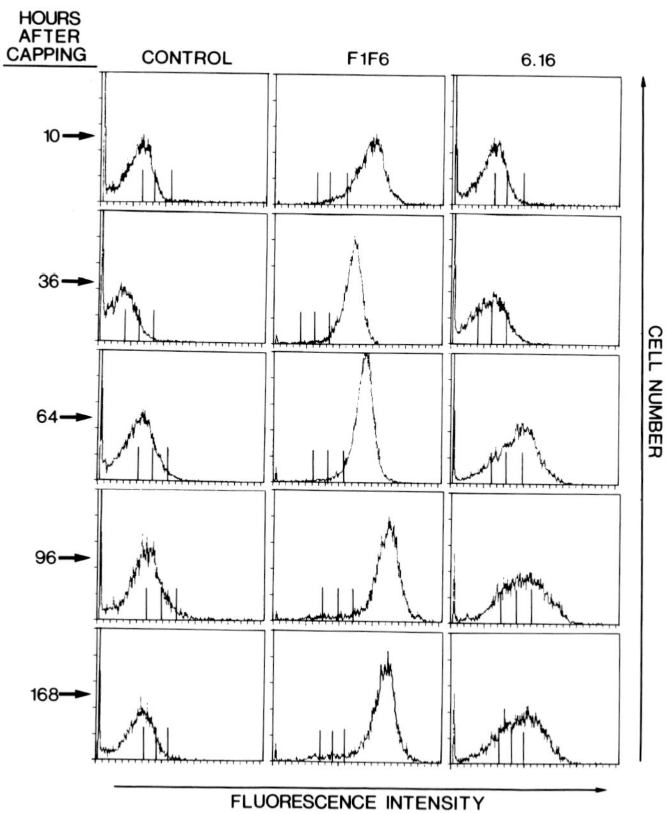

Figure 9 FACS analyzer profiles of anti-IgM adherent cells allowed to cap their IgM receptors and re-express after various time periods in culture. Stained as in Figure 8.

As a control, the monoclonal antibody F1F6, described in Section II, was used. Cells were resuspended to 5×10^6 per ml in APBS (113 mM NaC1, 9.3 mM Na_2HOP_4, 1.4 mM KH_2PO4, 0.67 mM $CaC1_2$, 0.37 mM $MgC1_2$) containing 0.1% BSA and 0.05% NaN_3 (A/B/A), and 0.1 ml of cells was incubated with 0.1 ml of monoclonal supernatants in 96-well round-bottom microtiter plates for 1 hour at 4°C. They were washed 3 times with A/B/A and incubated with goat anti-mouse Ig coupled to fluorescein (Nordic) for another hour at 4°C. The cells were washed twice and resuspended in 1 ml of A/B/A containing 0.02 mg/ml propidium iodide (which stains the nuclei of dead cells so that they are gated out of the analysis) and analyzed on a FACS analyzer.

Generally 15-30% of the splenic leukocytes are stained with anti-IgM monoclonal antibodies such as 6.16 (Fig. 8). The monoclonal antibody F1F6 stains all cells but shows a bimodel distribution. When B cells are removed by panning on 6.16-coated dishes, all 6.16 positive cells are absent in this nonadherent population and most of the cells in the bright F1F6 positive peak are also gone. There is no membrane re-expression of IgM after 10 hours of culture, but it gradually increases in expression until 96 hours after capping when it becomes maximal (Fig. 9). The 168-hour profile is virtually identical. All of the cells re-express IgM molecules since the staining is not bimodal as one expects from negative and positive cell populations; anti-Ig light chain monoclonal antibodies do show a bimodal staining distribution. In contrast to its staining on unseparated leukocytes, F1F6 stains all the adherent cells with equal intensity, falling in the brightly staining peak of the unseparated cells (Fig. 9). Taken together, the data strongly suggest that the 6.16 adherent cells are B cells and that IgM and the molecule recognized by F1F6 do not co-cap.

When the same experiment was attempted with tadpole B cells, approximately 30% failed to re-express their receptors. We believe that the cells which do not re-express IgM after capping may be immature B cells. After receiving a negative signal from the anti-IgM, these immature cells are effectively deleted as has been described for B cells from other organisms (68). We feel that, like adult B cells, all of the tadpole splenocytes which stick to the 6.16-coated wells bear surface IgM since: (a) no cells stick to plates coated with nonspecific monoclonal antibodies of the same isotype, and (b) there is less than 0.3% macrophage contamination as determined by nonspecific esterase staining of 6.16-adherent tadpole cells. (For adherence of macrophages, it is essential to allow cells to adhere at physiological temperatures for approximately 2 hours. Ninety minutes at 4°C is not sufficient.) It will be interesting to determine the nature of the tadpole cells that fail to re-express IgM after capping. Perhaps the B-cell differentiation events are carried out in the spleen and liver of the tadpole and switch to the bone marrow in adults. The same experiments should now be carried out with cells from adult bone marrow.

The percentage of B cells (Ig positive cells) in tadpole spleens is generally higher than that of adults, ranging from 30-50% (Fig. 10, Ref. 58). The deter-

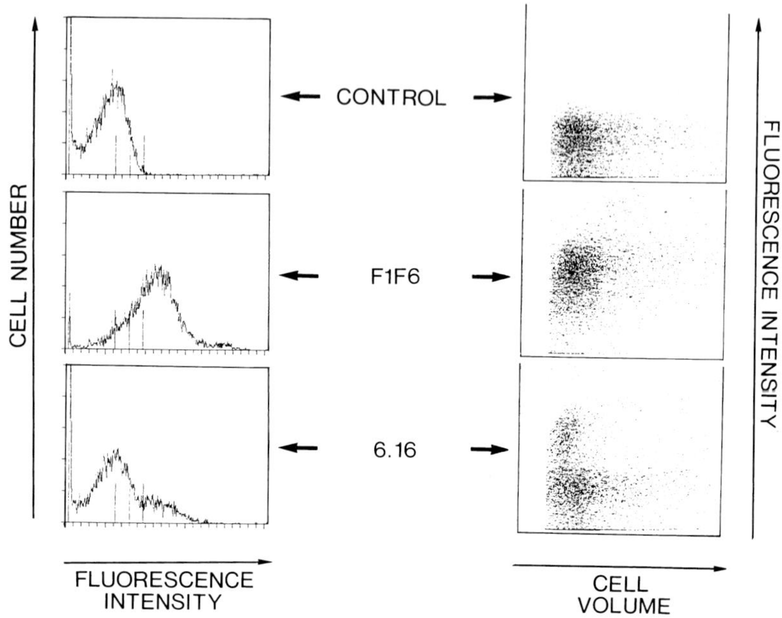

Figure 10 FACS analyzer profiles of tadpole splenic leukocytes stained with 6.16 or F1F6.

minant (molecule recognized by F1F6 does not show an increased level of expression in tadpole B cells as it does in adults.

The FACS analyzer measures the Coulter volume of cells instead of light scatter. Volume-versus-fluorescence dot plots of total splenocytes (including erythrocytes) stained with 6.16 and F1F6 are shown in Figure 11. Depending on the animal examined, B cells usually appear in the lowest cell volume of the leukocyte peak. In both cases (splenocytes from a *X. laevis* J animal or from LG15), 6.16 stains the small leukocytes while F1F6 stains the small cells and erythrocytes brightly. The second leukocyte population, which includes T cells, stains less well with F1F6 and not at all with 6.16. Tadpole splenocytes do not show a bimodal volume distribution (Fig. 10). Nevertheless, the small cells stain with 6.16, but F1F6 appears to show no preference in its staining of tadpole cells.

IV. TECHNICAL ASPECTS

A. Methods of Immunoprecipitation (69)

We, like many others, have had problems determining which molecules are immunoprecipitated by certain monoclonal antibodies. There are three immuno-

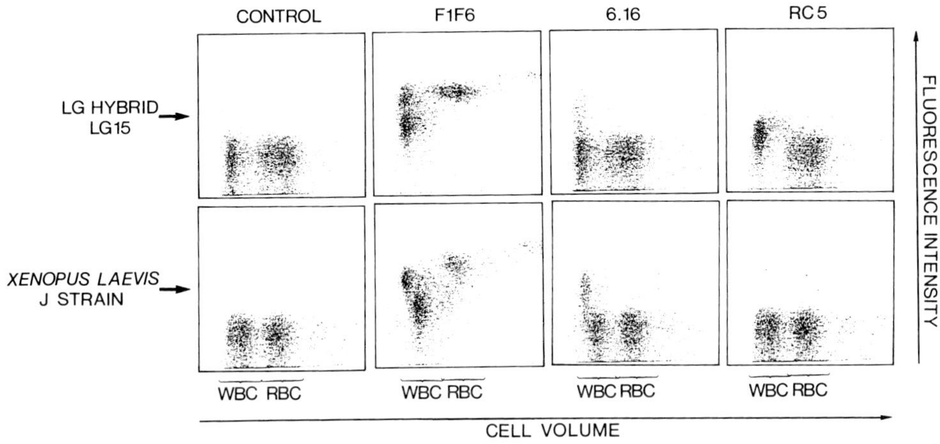

Figure 11 Cell volume versus log fluorescence intensity analysis of adult LG15 or JJ spleen cells (leukocyte and erythrocyte) stained with 6.16, F1F6, or RC5.

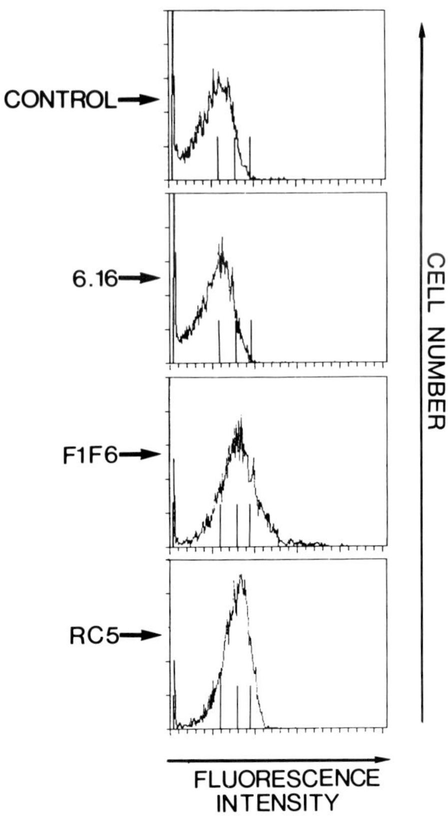

Figure 12 FACS analyzer profiles of LG15 adult thymocytes stained with 6.16, F1F6, or RC5.

precipitation techniques that we employ, SPIT (Solid Phase Immunoisolation Technique), protein-A, and "prebinding." Some monoclonal antibodies that stain cells recognize other molecules on the cell surface besides proteins (e.g., nucleic acids, glycolipids), and these, obviously, will never be observed on a protein gel. Chromatography methods which detect these other classes of molecules must then be adopted.

1. Spit Method

We find it useful to screen our fusions by immunofluorescence on the FACS analyzer. It is an unbiased method and allows us to choose monoclonal antibodies which recognize subpopulations of splenocytes at the outset. After the screening on cells or tissues, we then test by immunoprecipitation using the SPIT method (70). This consists of coating 96-well polyvinylchloride microtiter plates with an affinity purified anti-mouse Ig reagent (e.g., Kirkegaard and Perry). Wells are coated with 0.1 ml of 0.1 mg/ml of the reagent overnight at 4°C. The anti-mouse Ig solution can be collected and reused once or twice more. After washing the wells with APBS/2% BSA/0.1% NaN_3 several times, 0.2 ml of monoclonal supernatant is added and the plate is kept at room temperature for 2-3 hours. The supernatants are aspirated and 0.2 ml more of the same antibody is added in order to saturate the anti-Ig reagent. After 2 more hours at room temperature, the plates are washed twice and 0.1 ml of a radioactive lysate from cells that have been biosynthetically or cell-surface radiolabeled (lysis buffer: 20 mM Tris-C1 pH8, 1 mM $MgC1_2$, 150 mM NaC1, 2% NP40, 0.1 mM phenylmethylsulfonylfluoride freshly added) is added and left overnight at 4°C. The next day, the plate is washed with cold lysis buffer and the immune complexes are collected by pipetting LSB (Laemmli sample buffer: 50 mM Tris-C1 pH 6.8, 2% SDS, 10% glycerol, 0.1% bromophenol blue, ± 5% 2-mercaptoethanol) into each well. The fluid is then put in Eppendorf tubes, boiled, and loaded onto gels.

2. Protein-A

The second method, protein-A Sepharose immunoprecipitation, was described by Kessler (71). Radioactive lysates are first "precleared" to remove any molecules that bind to Sepharose or protein-A. Antibodies (monoclonals, xenoantisera, or alloantisera) are mixed with the precleared lysates and are left overnight on ice in Eppendorf tubes. If the monoclonal antibodies are of the IgM class, the next day one must add an anti-IgM reagent produced in an animal (goat or rabbit) whose IgG classes bind well to protein A (72). When alloantisera are used, we add a monoclonal antibody which binds frog IgG since frog Ig does not bind well to protein-A. Protein-A beads (50% v/v stored at 4°C in NET-NO: 150 mM NaCl, 5 mM EDTA, 0.5% NP40, 50 mM Tris-C1 pH8, 0.05% NaN_3, 1 mg/ml ovalbumin) are added to the precipitate and they are rotated for one hour at 4°C. The beads are washed three times in NET-NON (NET-NO with 0.5 M more NaC1) with 20-minute rotations. They are washed twice more in NET-N (NET-NO without ovalbumin). During the first NET-N wash, the beads are transferred to fresh Eppendorf tubes since radioactive material from the lysate may stick nonspecifically to the sides of the first tube, which increases background. The complexes are released from the beads with LSB. The beads are vortexed, boiled, and the sample is loaded onto SDS gels (73).

When immunoprecipitating with monoclonal antibodies, we generally use the SPIT method since it is fast, both IgM and IgG monoclonal antibodies work well, and low affinity antibodies which do not immunoprecipitate by the protein-A method may work by SPIT. The disadvantage of SPIT is that backgrounds are often worse since lysates are not "precleared" as they are with the protein-A method. Because there is usually a high amount of protein (10-20% FCS) in monoclonal supernatants, no blocking step between the goat anti-mouse and monoclonal antibody steps are necessary. By altering the coating and blocking steps, one can also use complex antisera in the SPIT assay.

3. Prebind

Some monoclonal antibodies do not immunoprecipitate by the SPIT or protein-A methods, possibly because they do not bind to their antigens in detergent lysates. In these cases, we attempt "prebind" experiments (74). Leukocytes are biosynthetically labeled long enough to allow most of the radiolabeled proteins to reach the cell surface (in *Xenopus* we label for 21-25 hours). The monoclonal antibody is added to the cells and incubated for one hour on ice in medium containing 0.1% NaN_3. The cells are washed and then lysed in lysis buffer. The complexes are then collected by either SPIT or protein-A as described above. To be sure to only immunoprecipitate the biosynthetically labeled cell-surface molecules, one must add excess (6-fold) cold lysate at the time of lysis. This ensures that antibodies that come off of their antigens during lysis will not bind internally labeled proteins.

RC5 has been one of these troublesome antibodies that never immunoprecipitated molecules from LG15 radiolabeled molecules in detergent lysates. When the prebind method was employed, a molecule of approximately 200 Kd was immunoprecipitated from LG15 but not J spleen lysates. This molecule may be the *Xenopus gilli* homolog of the common leukocyte antigen (75).

B. Strategies for Monoclonal Antibody Production

1. General Findings

We have performed many fusions using cells as the immunogen and have obtained few useful reagents. Many monoclonal antibodies that we have produced are directed against molecules on or in cells but very few that are directed against MHC antigens or subpopulations of hemopoietic cells. We have produced many (like

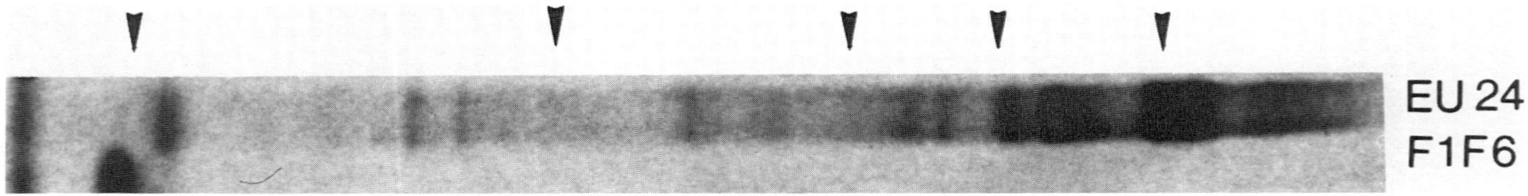

Figure 13 Immunoprecipitations of erythrocyte iodinated cell-surface proteins by SPIT with Eu24 and F1F6. Markers: 92 Kd, 68 Kd, 45 Kd, 30 Kd, 14 Kd.

F1F6) which are useful as controls in some experiments. Monoclonal antibodies against nuclear, cycloplasmic, and membrane molecules have been obtained which may be useful someday, but not for our purposes now. When immunizing with cells, we often produce monoclonals against carbohydrate or protein determinants shared between many different molecules on the cell surface. They immunoprecipitate a "ladder" of proteins from radiolabeled cells (Fig. 13). These type of antibodies often show ubiquitous staining patterns on frozen sections (Fig. 14). Immunizations with *Xenopus* cells using mice often lead to production of these types of monoclonal antibodies, possibly because of the phylogenetic distance between these two species. It has not been difficult for investigators, as evidenced by this book, to raise interesting anti-cell monoclonal antibodies when cells from other mammalian species have been used as the immunogen.

One finding that can be very misleading is the fact that the serum of the mouse, the spleen of which is used for fusion, may contain some antibodies against the desired determinant (e.g., MHC), as detected by a sensitive radioimmunoprecipitation assay, but yet the fusion will yield no monoclonal antibodies against this determinant. This result is likely due to the fact that many of the antibodies

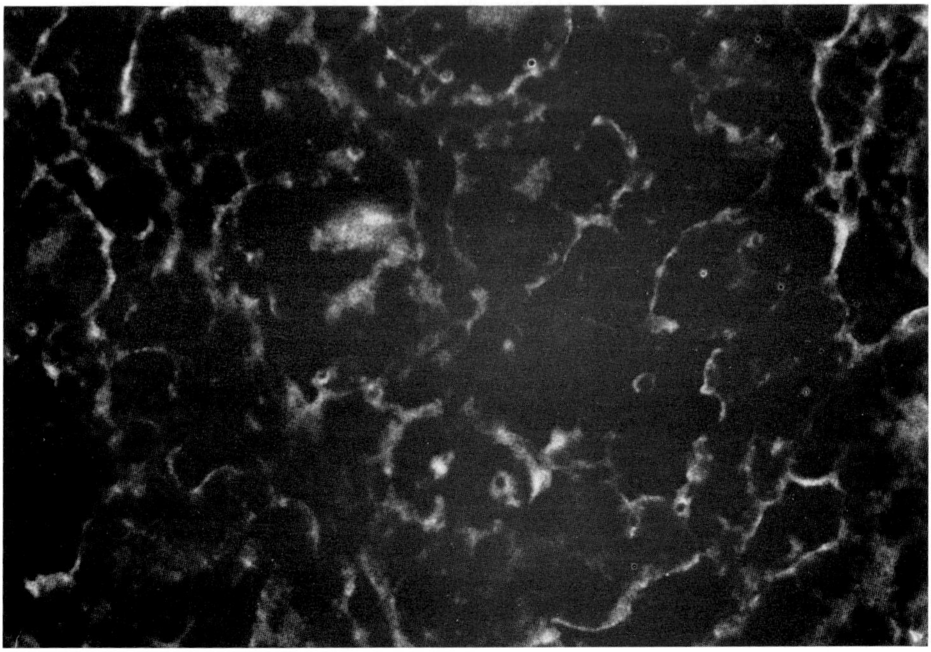

Figure 14 Frozen sections of adult liver stained with Eu24.

present in the serum fail to precipitate anything labeled from the lysate of the cells. It is difficult to estimate which faction of the total antibodies the specific anti-MHC antibodies represent. It can be probably very low since screening up to 400 hybridomas per fusion from such mice yielded no anti-MHC hybridomas.

2. Strategies

Immunization with purified Ig has never failed although some anti-carbohydrate antibodies have also been obtained from these fusions. We find it important, whenever possible, to avoid immunizations with cells only. To produce anti-MHC monoclonals, we have stopped cell immunization protocols and are now painstakingly purifying the molecules before immunizing. Twenty-one fusions were necessary before Nagata could produce one anti-T-cell reagent (61). For anti-T-cell subset antibodies, it may be useful to try cross-priming with purified mammalian molecules such as Thy-1, CD4, or CD8 after injections with *Xenopus* thymocytes. The hybrids resulting from such a fusion could be tested on *Xenopus* cells.

It is important to maintain a concrete goal when producing monoclonal antibodies against *Xenopus* antigens. Performing fusions after immunizing with cells to see what will "fall out" is simply a waste of time. It is important to spend the time to determine the best ways to increase the probability of producing useful reagents. Purifying the immunogen or narrowing the number of immunogens by injection of immune complexes or membranes is important.

Our major goals at this time are to produce monoclonals against MHC molecules, T-cell subsets, and the IgX molecule. Since the adult class I molecule is absent in tadpoles, it is important to obtain an anti-class I or β_2-m reagent to determine whether there are tadpole-specific class I molecules and also whether other types of class I antigens (Qa or T1-like) are present in adult or tadpole *Xenopus*. Anti-T-cell subset antibodies, besides being useful tools for immunological studies, are important reagents to analyze whether there are shifts in the T-cell populations during ontogeny. Since the IgX (third isotype) is IgM-like in several respects, it will be interesting to determine its cell distribution and continue with biochemical studies.

V. CONCLUSIONS

This chapter may be disappointing in that we do not yet know anything about "differentiation antigens" as described in mammals which define different ontogenetic steps of hemopoietic lineages. However, we hope the description of the ontogeny and tissue distribution of several of the well-known MHC and Ig proteins of *Xenopus*, as well as molecules recognized by several other monoclonals and antisera, will entice those who work in comparative immunology to produce reagents to answer questions raised in this chapter.

ACKNOWLEDGMENTS

We thank Masayuki Miyasaka for help with cell staining and Carolyn Harley for typing the manuscript. The Basel Institute for Immunology was founded and is supported by Hoffmann-La Roche.

REFERENCES

1. H. R. Kobel, *Monitore Zool. Ital., 8*: 119 (1981).
2. B. Blomberg, C. C. A. Bernard, and L. Du Pasquier, *Eur. J. Immunol., 10*: 869 (1980).
3. P. A. Bleicher and N. Cohen, *J. Immunol., 127*: 1549 (1981).
4. N. Green (Donnelly) and N. Cohen, *Cell. Immunol., 48*: 59 (1979).
5. S. Tochinai, *Immunology, 31*: 125 (1976).
6. M. R. H. Collie, R. J. Turner, and M. J. Manning, *Eur. J. Immunol., 5*: 426 (1975).
7. L. Du Pasquier and J. D. Horton, *Immunogenetics, 3*: 105 (1976).
8. J. D. Horton, J. J. Rimmer, and T. L. Horton, *Dev. Comp. Immunol., 1*: 119 (1977).
9. D. Watkins and N. Cohen, *Dev. Comp. Immunol., 9*: 819 (1985).
10. L. Du Pasquier, X. Chardonnens, and V. C. Miggiano, *Immunogenetics, 1*: 482 (1975).
11. M. F. Flajnik, J. F. Kaufman, and L. Du Pasquier, *Dev. Comp. Immunol., 9*: 771 (1985).
12. M. F. Flajnik, J. F. Kaufman, E. Hsu, and L. Du Pasquier, *Dev. Comp. Immunol., Suppl. 3*: 9 (1984).
13. M. F. Flajnik, J. F. Kaufman, P. Reigert, and L. Du Pasquier, *Immunogenetics, 20*: 433 (1984).
14. J. F. Kaufman, M. F. Flajnik, L. Du Pasquier, and P. Reigert, *J. Immunol., 134*: 3248 (1985).
15. J. F. Kaufman, M. F. Flajnik, and L. Du Pasquier, *J. Immunol., 134*: 3258 (1985).
16. T. Nakamura, A. Sekizawa, T. Fujii, and C. Katagiri, *Immunogenetics, 23*: 181 (1986).
17. C. C. A. Bernard, G. Bordmann, B. Blomberg, and L. Du Pasquier, *Immunogenetics, 9*: 443 (1979).
18. C. C. A. Bernard, G. Bordmann, B. Blomberg, and L. Du Pasquier, *Eur. J. Immunol., 11*: 151 (1981).
19. T. Nakamura, *Transplantation, 40*: 393 (1985).
20. M. F. Flajnik, L. Du Pasquier, and N. Cohen, *Eur. J. Immunol., 15*: 540 (1985).
21. I. Hadji-Azimi and J. Schwager, *Dev. Comp. Immunol., 6*: 703 (1982).
22. E. Hsu and L. Du Pasquier, *Mol. Immunol., 21*: 257 (1984).
23. J. Schwager and I. Hadji-Azimi, *Differentiation, 27*: 182 (1984).
24. J. Schwager and I. Hadji-Azimi, *Differentiation, 30*: 29 (1985).
25. E. Hsu, T. Lenderson, and R. M. Franklin, *Ann. Inst. Pasteur/Immunol., 136D*: 105 (1985).

13

Differentiation Antigens of Swine Lymphoid Tissues

JOAN K. LUNNEY
Agricultural Research Service, U.S. Department of Agriculture, Beltsville, Maryland

MARK D. PESCOVITZ*
National Cancer Institute, National Institutes of Health, Bethesda, Maryland

I. INTRODUCTION

In this review we plan to summarize what is currently known about monoclonal antibody (mAb)-defined differentiation antigens of swine lymphoid tissues. Because of the abundance of data, we will emphasize antigen expression on isolated lymphoid cells and will include, where available, data on tissue expression of cell subset-specific antigens.

For ease of discussion we have divided swine lymphoid differentiation antigens into three categories: (a) antigens associated with the swine major histocompatibility complex (MHC), designated the swine leukocyte antigen (SLA) complex; (b) antigens expressed on a broad range of peripheral blood mononuclear cell (PBMC) subsets, such as the leukocyte function antigen-1 (LFA-1); and (c) antigens expressed on discrete cellular subsets such as T or B cells. In discussing these differentiation antigens we will use nomenclature that was recently introduced for the human differentiation antigens (1,2).

We would like to emphasize at the outset that this review is being written at a time when several laboratories have new panels of mAb, which they are just in the process of characterizing. It is clear that in the next few years there will be many more mAb available with which to delineate more fully swine lymphoid differentiation antigens.

**Present affiliation*: University of Minnesota, Minneapolis, Minnesota.

II. SWINE MAJOR HISTOCOMPATIBILITY COMPLEX ANTIGENS (SLA ANTIGENS)

A. Background

Swine MHC antigens, or SLA antigens, have been defined by alloantisera testing, by cellular typing, and by immunochemical methods using families of outbred swine (3-5) or SLA inbred miniature swine (6,7). The class I MHC antigens are divided into two categories, the traditional class I transplantation antigens and the class I-like differentiation antigens. The class I transplantation antigens are characterized by their expression on all PBMC, by the molecular weight (MW) of their immunoprecipitated antigens (polymorphic heavy chain of approximately 45,000 dalton, encoded by the MHC complex, associated noncovalently with the nonpolymorphic β_2-microglobulin light chain of 12,000 dalton) and by their ability to cause rapid allograft rejection (8). These antigens were named, following the human nomenclature, the SLA-A,B,C antigens (9). The class I-like differentiation antigens have been described in other species, e.g., T1a and Qa antigens in mice; these antigens map close to the MHC complex, are expressed only on subsets of lymphoid cells, and have molecular weights that are similar or slightly smaller than the traditional class I antigens (10). The existence of such class I-like differentiation antigens in swine has not yet been reported, although there is at least one mAb that may react with a T1a-like antigen of swine (Pescovitz et al., manuscript in preparation).

Recently the class I heavy chain genes from the *dd* SLA haplotype have been cloned, and some have been shown to be expressed in transfected mouse L cells (11,12). There are seven class I genes, designated PD1, PD14, PD6, PD15, PD7, PD8, and PD4, in the pig. Interestingly, this appears to be the lowest number for any species yet analyzed, since mice have up to 36 class I genes and humans about 20 (R. Ehrlich and D. Singer, manuscript in preparation). As the sequence of each of these individual genes becomes available and their cellular expression characterized, it should be easier to define their locus reactivity and to identify the swine equivalent of the mouse Qa and T1a class I-like genes.

The class MHC II antigens, also known as the Ia (immune response associated) antigens, are characterized by their higher level of expression on B cells and macrophages and by the MW of their cell surface antigens (α chain of approximately 35,000 dalton and β chain of approximately 28,000 dalton) (8). Class II SLA antigens were originally defined by mixed lymphocyte reactivity. Identification of recombinant swine enabled researchers to develop class II-specific serologic reagents (4,13,14). The class II loci are encoded by the SLA-D region and, in accordance with accepted human nomenclature, will be designated SLA-DR,DQ, DP (2). Data presented below indicate that there are at least two sets of expressed SLA class II antigens which, because their exact genetic mapping is unknown, will be provisionally termed SLA-DRw and SLA-DQw. Southern blots of restriction fragments from genomic DNA from SLA inbred miniature swine using cDNA probes indicate that the pig has genomic DNA encoding α and β chains homologous to all three SLA class II loci, thus suggesting the existence of SLA-DPw antigens as well (D. H. Sachs et al., unpublished data). Further studies will be necessary to determine how many class II locus products are expressed in the pig.

Because of the importance of the MHC complex in tissue transplantation and other immunologic research, D. H. Sachs and his colleagues developed the SLA inbred miniature swine (6,7). The entire herd of animals was derived from an original set of two miniature swine. Three independent SLA haplotypes (sets of SLA class I and class II-linked genes), designated SLA^a, SLA^c, and SLA^d, have been characterized in these swine. Homozygous animals are designated $SLA^{a/a}$ or, for convenience, *aa*. Two independent SLA recombinant haplotypes, SLA^f and SLA^g, have been detected; each expresses the $SLA\text{-}A^cB^cDR^dDQ^d$ gene products (14). No difference has yet been found between these two recombinant haplotypes.

SLA histocompatibility typing with swine alloantisera has defined unique private specificities of individual alleles of several SLA locus products, as well as shared public determinats of the same proteins (4). Since all mAb to swine differentiation antigens have been produced in rodents, they tend to recognize species-specific, i.e., more public, determinants of each antigen. In some cases mAb recognizing polymorphic determinants of differentiation antigens have been produced. Based on published data on rodent mAb to human MHC, or HLA, antigens, it is likely that most mAb to polymorphic SLA antigenic determinants will react with epitopes shared between different SLA specificities, and only rarely would an mAb be found that reacts with a unique (private) SLA antigenic determinant, or specificity (4,15). Moreover, since panels of cells bearing known SLA specificities are only available in France (4), the range of SLA specificities recognized by these mAb has not yet been tested. Cells from the SLA inbred miniature swine express just three independent SLA haplotypes and represent therefore only a small panel of SLA specificities. They have, however, been used successfully to map mAb-defined polymorphic determinants to either the SLA class I or class II gene products. The availability of SLA recombinant animals has greatly aided this research.

In this review, we will use the term alloantigenic determinant to mean an antigenic epitope that has been shown to be polymorphic in swine of different SLA haplotypes. A polymorphic determinant is one that varies within the species but whose mapping is unknown, and a monomorphic determinant is an epitope of an antigen which does not vary within the species.

B. mAb Reactive with Class I SLA Antigens

mAb reactive with class I SLA antigens are listed in Table 1. The top half of the table lists mAb that react with polymorphic determinants of SLA class I antigens, as defined by their differential reactivity on cells from SLA inbred miniature

Table 1 mAb Reactive with SLA Class I Antigens

		Characterization of specificity									
		Alloantigen reactivity[a]					SLA transfected cells[b]				
mAb	Ig class	*dd*	*cc*	*gg*	*aa*	outbred	PD1	PD14	Biochemistry[c] Antigen MW (X 10^3)	Defined in species[d]	Refs.
A. *Polymorphic Reactivity*											
74-11-10	IgG2b, k	+	±	±	+	P	+	+	45,12	swine	16
2.2.13		+	+	NT	+	P	–	–	45,12	swine	e
2.12.3	IgM	+	–	NT	–	P	–	+	45,12	swine	e
2.28.1	IgM	+	+	NT	+	P	+	–		swine	e
2.32.1	IgG	+	–	–	–	P	–	+		swine	e
H21A	IgM	–	–	–	–	P	NT			bovine	17
CA48P-A	IgM	+	+	+	±	P	NT			mouse	17
CA4C-A	IgM	+	±	±	±	P	NT			mouse	17
H11A	IgG2a	+	+	+	+	P	NT			bovine	17
H58A	IgG2a	+	+	+	+	P	NT		45,12		17
H17A	IgG2	–	–	–	–	P	NT			bovine	17
H22A	IgG2a	NT	NT	NT	NT	P	NT				17
3A6		±	+	+	+	NT	NT		45,12	human	18

B. *Monomorphic Reactivity*

PT85	IgG2a, k	+	+	+	+	+	+	+	45,12		17
2.4.11	IgG1	+	+	NT	+	+	+	+	45,12	swine	e
2.13.3	IgG1	+	+	NT	+	NT	NT		45	swine	e
2.27.3	IgG	+	+	NT	+	+	+	+	45,12	swine	e
FMD2	IgG2b	NT	NT	NT	NT	+	NT		44,12	swine	19
IIB2	IgG2a	NT	NT	NT	NT	+	NT		44,12	bovine	f
7-34-1	IgG2a	+	+	+	+	+	–	–	45,12	swine	20
3B3		+	+	+	+	NT	NT			human	18
9455SA		+	+	+	+	NT	NT		45,12	human	g
D4.37HL252		+	+	+	+	NT	NT			rat	21

[a]mAb reactivity was assessed by mAb-mediated cytotoxicity assay, by cell ELISA assay, or by FMF analysis on PBL from SLA inbred miniature swine or from outbred swine. Reactivity with outbred swine is designated as polymorphic (P) or monomorphic (+).
[b]L cells that have been shown to express the PD1 or PD14 class I SLA gene products were assayed as described above for mAb binding (12).
[c]Radiolabeled extracts of swine cells were immune precipitated with the mAb noted, facilitated with protein A bearing *S. aureus* bacteria with or without anti-mouse immunoglobulin. The eluted antigens were analyzed on SDS-polyacrylamide gel electrophoresis and molecular weight determined in relation to known standards.
[d]Some mAb were originally shown to react with class I MHC antigens of other species and then shown to cross-react with pig cell-surface antigens, implying reactivity with SLA class I antigens.
[e]Ivanoska et al., unpublished data.
[f]Letesson et al., personal communication.
[g]Commercially available.

swine of *dd, cc, gg,* and *aa* haplotypes and from outbred swine. The bottom half of the table lists mAb that react with monomorphic determinants of class I antigens. In some cases these mAb were tested on mouse fibroblast, or L cell, lines that had been transfected with, and shown to express, either the PD1 or PD14 SLA class I gene products.

From the data presented in Table 1 it is clear that mAb can be divided into several groups. Some, e.g., 74-11-10, react with polymorphic determinants of SLA class I antigens but also recognize the gene products of at least two separate class I genes, PD1 and PD14, as determined by reactivity with transfected L cells (12,16). Sequential gel precipitation analysis using this mAb and alloantibodies that have been selected to react with only one locus product confirm this multilocus reactivity. There are other mAb, e.g., 2.12.3 and 2.32.1, that have just recently been derived (Ivanoska et al., unpublished data), that react with polymorphic determinants of class I antigens and recognize the PD14 but not the PD1 gene product. Since only two of the seven class I SLA genes have been identified as surface antigens on transfected L cells (12), it is unknown if these two mAb react with the product(s) of other class I genes. This determination will have to await the successful expression of each complete SLA class I gene in appropriate tissue culture cells. Since some of these genes might code for SLA class I-like differentiation antigens, cells other than fibroblasts may be required for successful gene expression. If either or both of these mAb recognize a unique determinant of the PD14 gene product, then they would represent the first mAb reactive with a private SLA specificity. Studies using panels of SLA typed cells must be performed to establish this point.

The mAbs that react with monomorphic determinants of SLA class I genes can also be divided into several groups (Table 1). There are those such as PT85 that react with all cells of every pig tested and with the two SLA transfected L cells. These mAb probably recognize a monomorphic determinant of all classical SLA class I genes. Other mAb, like 2.28.1, react with cells from every pig tested yet only react with PD1 transfected L cells, indicating it may be recognizing a monomorphic determinant of a single gene locus (Ivanoska et al., unpublished data). If it is shown that this mAb is unreactive with the products of the other SLA class I genes, then it could be very useful for determining the locus reactivity of other antibodies, by using binding inhibition, lysostrip analysis, and/or immunochemical methods. Thus, even though a test antibody might not bind to *dd* PBMC (and therefore not to L cells that were transfected with *dd* SLA class I genes), one could still verify that the antibody bound to the same locus product on other SLA haplotype cells using this locus-specific, monomorphic mAb. A third type of mAb recognizing monomorphic determinants of SLA class I genes is exemplified by mAb 7-34-1. This mAb reacts with cells of all pigs and precipitates a class I type molecule, yet is unreactive with SLA transfected L cells (12). This might be an mAb to swine β_2-microglobulin, the light chain of the SLA class I antigen, which would not be produced by the mouse L cells, or, equally likely, it could be reactive with a monomorphic determinant of another SLA class I gene that has not yet been expressed on transfected cells.

Hybridomas secreting mAb specific for SLA class I antigens have most frequently been produced with cells from mice that were immunized against swine antigens or against antigens of a variety of livestock species (Table 1) and not from mouse anti-mouse alloimmunizations. Early data looking at mouse alloantisera specific for class I MHC antigens showed that cross-reactive antibodies, recognizing class I MHC antigens of other species, occurred only infrequently and only in certain sera during a given immunization protocol (22). Our own screen of mAb reactive with class I MHC antigens of other species for anti-swine cross-reactivity confirmed these results. Of 15 mouse anti-mouse, 8 mouse anti-rat, and 2 rat anti-mouse class I MHC mAb only one mAb cross-reactive with pig cells was found (23; Lunney, unpublished data). Davis and his colleagues specifically tried to produce mAb that had interspecies cross-reactivity by immunizing mice with cells from one species and then boosting with cells from one to three other species prior to fusion (17). In his published report 7 of the 15 anti-class I mAbs reactive with cow, sheep, goat, and/or horse antigens cross-reacted on pig cells (which were rarely used in his immunization protocols). When murine anti-HLA-A,B mAb were screened, French workers found no cross-reactions and we found three weakly cross-reactive mAbs out of a total of 8 tested (23,24). These results contrast sharply with antisera reactive with class II MHC antigens, where, as will be discussed below, alloantisera and mAbs show significant interspecies cross-reactivity.

In summary, a growing panel of mAb reactive with class I SLA antigens have been developed. Most mAb were produced by immunization against swine antigens and appear to react with monomorphic determinants, or broadly polymorphic determinants, of one or more SLA class I gene products. However, a few mAb have been identified that exhibit more restricted reactivity and may be recognizing unique, private SLA class I specificities.

C. mAb Reactive with Class II SLA Antigens

mAb reactive with swine class II MHC antigens are listed in Table 2. When class II SLA-specific mAb were analyzed for polymorphic reactivity, almost none exhibited differential reactions on cells from SLA inbred swine. The only mAbs that appeared to recognize polymorphic determinants were 9B, 227 and Genox 3.53. Each of these mAbs appears to have a low affinity interaction with swine class II antigens, as indicated by their significantly decreased titers against swine cells and by their inability to precipitate class II glycoproteins from extracts of cells that bound the mAb and, therefore, they are not very useful for most analyses (23; Lunney et al., unpublished data).

Since swine class II antigens are just now being cloned, L-cell transfectants expressing sets of gene products are not yet available for identifying locus specificity.

Table 2 mAb Reactive with SLA Class II Antigens

		Characterization of specificity							
		Alloantigen recognition[a]							
mAb	Ig class	*dd*	*cc*	*gg*	*aa*	outbred	Biochemistry[b]	Reactivity Other species[c]	Refs.
SLA-DRw									
MSA3	IgG2b, k	+	+	+	+	+	35,28		25
ISCR3	IgG2b, k	+	+	+	+	+	35,28	I-E	26
40B	IgG2a, k	+	+	+	+	+	35,28	I-E-III	27,28
9B	IgG2a, k	+	–	+	+	NT[d]	–	I-E-III	27,28
40E	IgG2a, k	+	+	+	+	NT	35,28	I-E-III	27,28
39D	IgG2a, k	+	+	+	+	NT	35,28	I-E-III	27,28
40K	IgG2a, k	+	+	+	+	NT	35,28	I-E-III	27,28
39G	IgG2a, k	+	+	+	+	NT	35,28	I-E-III	27,28
40D	IgG2a, k	+	+	+	+	+	35,28	I-E-III	27,28
7A	IgG2a, k	+	+	+	+	+	35,28	I-E-II	27,28
74C	IgG3, k	+	+	+	+	+	35,28	I-E-II	28,29
DC2.06	IgG1	+	+	+	+	+	35,28	HLA-DR	30,31

SLA-DQw									
TH16B	IgG2a, k	+	+	+	+	+	34,27	bovine	17,32
H42A	IgG2a, k	+	+	+	+	+	34,27		17,32
TH21A	IgG2a, k	+	+	+	+	+	34,27	bovine	17,32
TH22	IgG2a, k	+	+	+	+	+	34,27	bovine	17,32
RH1A	IgG2a, k	+	+	+	+	+	34,27		17,32
SLA class II									
227	IgG1, k	–	–	NT	+	NT	–	HLA-D	33,23
Genox 3.53		+	–	NT	+	NT	–	HLA-D	34,23
H4	IgG3	NT	NT	NT	NT	+	NT	HLA-D	17
TH4B	IgM	+	+	NT	+	+	NT	bovine	17
TH14B		NT	NT	NT	NT	+	NT	bovine	17
TH81B		NT	NT	NT	NT	+	NT	bovine	17

[a]Analyses performed as described in legend 1 of Table 1.
[b]Analyses performed as described in legend 3, Table 1, except all gels run under nonreducing conditions. A dash denotes no immunoprecipitation with a given mAb though other mAb were positive on the same gel.
[c]Reactivity of some mAb was first characterized on the genes or species shown and then were used to analyze swine class II antigens.
[d]NT = not tested.

However, unlike SLA class I proteins for which no MW or significant isoelectric point differences are evident, the swine class II gene products have both minor MW, and major isoelectric point, differences (28, Fig. 1). In addition, the molecular weight differences of class II, or Ia antigens, are enhanced under nonreducing conditions. All of the anti-mouse I-E mAb that cross-react with swine Ia antigens

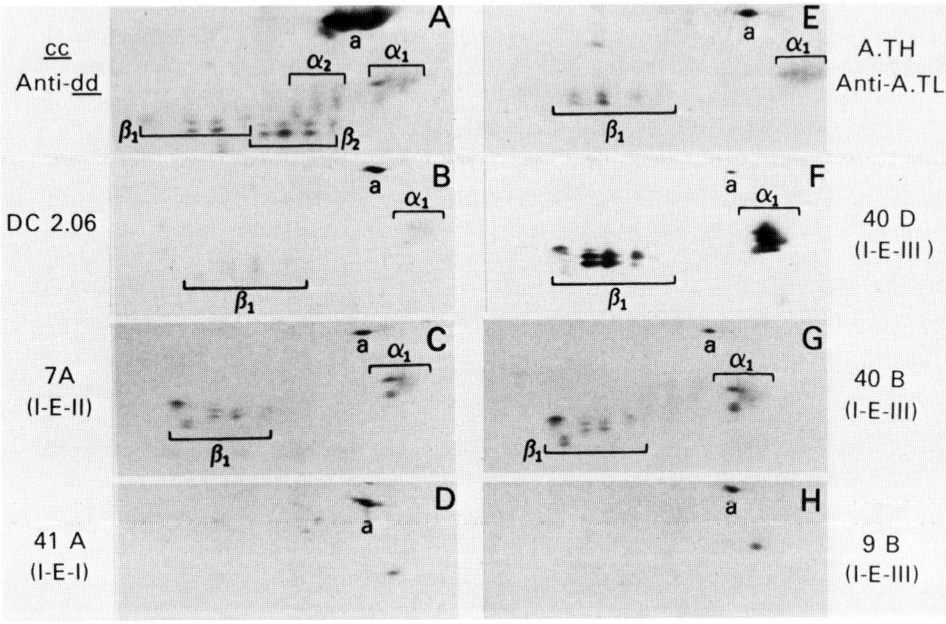

Figure 1 Two-dimensional gel electrophoresis of extracts of SLA^{dd} cells precipitated by mouse anti-Ia monoclonal antibodies. SLA^{dd} cells were labeled with ^{35}S-methionine overnight, extracted with a Nonidet P40 buffer, and aliquots immunoprecipitated with the alloantisera or mAb noted in the figure followed by *S. aureus* Cowan bacteria. The bound material was eluted and run in two-dimensional gel electrophoresis, isoelectric focusing followed by SDS-PAGE. The small spot noted as "a" is actin. The large smears over "a" are the heavy chains of the SLA class I antigens that are very similar both in isoelectric point and molecular weight. The light chain, β_2-microglobulin, has been cut off these autoradiograms. The class II antigens, SLA-DRw, are represented by the alpha chain α_1 and the beta chain β_1, while the SLA-DQw antigens are the α_2 and β_2 subsets. Spots representing the SLA-DPw antigens could be in either of these sets of spots in A or might not be precipitated by the swine alloantiserum. B, C, E, F, G, and H show different mAb that cross-react with SLA-DRw antigens. D shows a non-cross-reactive mAb. No anti-SLA-DQw mAb were tested in this set of experiments. (Reprinted from *J. Immunol., 130*: 2790 (1983).)

precipitated the higher molecular weight set of class II antigens (Fig. 1C, F, G). Because of the homology of HLA-DR antigens with I-E antigens, the anti I-E reactive swine Ia antigens will be provisionally designated SLA-DRw. The other dominant, lower molecular weight set of swine class II antigens will be designated the SLA-DQw antigens in analogy to HLA-DQ antigens. The SLA-DR and SLA-DQ subsets of swine class II antigens have been demonstrated to be independent sets of antigens by sequential immunoprecipitation analysis using mAb 40D and TH16 (32). SLA-DPw proteins may also be included in the Ia antigens precipitated in these gels, but antibodies that react with this subset of swine Ia antigens have not yet been identified nor has it been confirmed that the putative SLA-DP genes are transcribed into surface proteins. Future DNA and cell transfection experiments will help define the true genetic complexity of the SLA-D region, including the numbers of expressed α and β genes for each locus.

In the human, the major mixed lymphocyte reaction (MLR) stimulatory loci are the HLA-DR and HLA-DQ loci; the HLA-DP locus is defined by secondary MLR reactivity (35). Inhibition of alloantigen-stimulated blastogenesis in swine revealed that the anti-SLA-DQw mAb were able to inhibit the MLR response 10 to 100 times more effectively than anti-SLA-DRw mAb (32). This may indicate that the SLA-DQw locus is the more stimulatory locus in a swine MLR in analogy with the I-A locus product which generates the stronger MLR response in mice. Studies with other mAb must be performed to confirm these observations.

Interspecies cross-reactivity of antibodies to MHC antigens were first described for rodent class II antigens by Sachs et al. and mapped to the mouse I-A subregion (36). Extension of these studies to other species revealed that mouse alloantisera exhibited strong cross-reactions with human and pig antigens but in this case it was the anti-I-E antibodies that were the most reactive (37-40). Shinohara and colleagues further demonstrated that these anti-Ia cross-reactions extended down the evolutionary scale as far as frogs and fishes (41,42). Analysis of interspecies cross-reactions were probed further after Pierres and his associates developed panels of mAb reactive with mouse I-A and I-E locus products and characterized them all for alloreactivity and for Ia epitopes recognized (27,29). Using these mAb we were able to show that none of Pierres' 8 anti-I-A mAb, or of our 7 anti-I-A mAb, cross-reacted strongly on pig Ia antigens (28); likewise two rat anti-mouse class II mAb failed to cross-react (23). Only anti-I-E mAb exhibited interspecies Ia cross-reactions, and only those mAb reactive with epitopes II and III were positive on swine class II antigens (28). It is interesting to note that epitopes II and III contain all the polymorphic epitopes of the I-E antigens. In summary, the SLA-DRw antigens are recognized by mAb reactive with epitopes II and III of the mouse I-E antigen.

Another pattern emerged when mAb reactive with bovine class II antigens were analyzed on pig cells; 7 of 9 mAb exhibited cross-reactions with swine class II antigens (17). Immunoprecipitation analyses revealed that all of these mAb reacted with the lower MW SLA-DQw antigens (32). Thus, anti-mouse I-E mAb cross-react with SLA-DRw antigen, while anti-bovine Ia mAb react with the SLA-DQw antigens. This may indicate that there are unique evolutionary relationships between molecules coded by the different SLA-D region loci. Studies with mAb reactive with different locus products, including the HLA-DP antigens, and with Ia antigens of other species should help to unravel these evolutionary interactions.

In summary, antigens encoded by at least two separate SLA-D region loci have been identified and characterized using several different mAb reactive mainly with monomorphic determinants of each locus product. The positive mAb were generally produced in immunizations against other species and later identified as cross-reactive with swine Ia antigens. MAb that recognize unique, polymorphic determinants of swine Ia antigens await future fusions using purified antigens, such as have been performed by Barber and his colleagues (personal communication), or new SLA-D gene transfectants as immunogens, or the generation of a swine myeloma fusion partner and then the production of swine anti-swine mAb.

III. DIFFERENTIATION ANTIGENS EXPRESSED ON BROAD LYMPHOID CELL POPULATIONS

A. Introduction

Other than the MHC antigens there are many conceivable antigens which are species-, but not cell type-, specific. In a xenogeneic immunization, mAb against these would be produced; in fact in both of our hybridoma fusions many such mAb were isolated (16). The function and analogous mAb for other species of most of these mAb is unknown. However, some mAb that react with all lymphocytes in the pig have known human or murine analogs. One of these, anti-LFA-1, actually cross-reacts among the species. The well-characterized mAb reactive with broad lymphoid cell populations are discussed below and summarized in Tables 3 and 4.

B. Leukocyte Function Antigen I (LFA-1) mAb

In both humans and mice, antibodies to LFA-1, or CD18, block proliferative response of lymphocytes, cytotoxic activity of T lymphocytes and natural killer cell reactivity (43,44). It is from this effect on lymphocyte function that their name was derived. The human and murine LFA-1 proteins are composed of a 95,000 MW β chain and a 175,000 MW α chain (43,44). The β chain is shared with the Mac-1 protein in association with a 165,000 MW α chain, and with a protein of unknown function in association with a 150,000 MW α chain (45,46). A panel of five different CD18 mAb, three reacting with the human common β chain (44,47), one reacting with the Mac-1 α chain, and one reacting with the human LFA-1 α chain, were screened for reactivity on porcine lymphocytes. Only the three mAb, MHM23, H5B9, and H52, that reacted with the β chain subunit reacted also with pig lymphocytes (J. Hildreth and M. Pescovitz, manuscript in preparation). Immunoprecipitation of solubilized, radiolabeled swine PBMC with the three β chain reactive mAb yielded a β chain of 95,000 MW, identical to the human beta chain MW, and a heavy chain of 175,000 MW, consistent with LFA-1. MHM23 also precipitated a third chain of 150,000 MW, which is identical in MW to the human P150, although by two-dimensional gel electrophoresis it is more acidic in the pig than in the human. Neither of the three β chain-specific antibodies precipitated a 165,000 MW Mac-1 α chain, even when a radiolabeled macrophage preparation was analyzed (J. Hildreth and M. Pescovitz, manuscript in preparation). The reason for this is unknown but could indicate that either a separate Mac-1 α chain does not exist in the pig or that the pig Mac-1 α chain is associated with a non-cross-reactive β chain.

Flow microfluorometric (FMF) analysis of PBMC disclosed that all cells were reactive with the LFA-1 antibody in a bimodal distribution with a minor bright peak containing 20-30% of the cells and a major dull peak containing the remainder. Dual parameter FMF analysis indicated that all of the macrophages, as defined by staining with mAb 74-22-15, were contained within the bright population. All of the CD1 (mAb 76-7-4)-reactive B cells were contained in the dull population, and the $CD4^+$ and $CD8^+$ T cells were divided between the bright and dull populations (J. Hildreth et al., manuscript in preparation). This bimodel distribution and expression of CD18 on macrophages, on B cells, and on T cells is similar to that seen on human cells (44).

Detailed functional analysis of the role of the LFA-1 antigen was performed by the addition of the anti-LFA-1 β chain antibodies to various in vitro cellular assays. These mAb partially inhibited suboptimal mitogen-induced responses, and completely inhibited the allogeneic MLR at an early stage. CTL activity was nearly completely inhibited by the LFA-1 antibodies at the effector stage and, as seen with human CTL, this inhibition was additive to that produced by a CD8 antibody (48). Finally, NK-mediated killing was completely eliminated by the presence of the anti-LFA-1 subunit antibody. All of these in vitro effects have been reported previously for both human and mouse LFA-1 antibodies. Due to the lack of availability of porcine CD18 α subunit-specific mAb, it is uncertain if LFA-1 is actually involved in these interactions or if p150, or the elusive porcine Mac-1, is actually the critical protein. The development of porcine LFA-1 α subunit-specific antibodies, which will allow the resolution of this dilemma, is currently in progress (J. Hildreth, personal communication).

C. Common Leukocyte Antigen mAb

There is one mAb, 74-9-3, that reacts with the porcine common leukocyte antigen (16). This resulted from a fusion between cells from a BALB/c mouse immunized with porcine thymocytes and the SP2/0 myeloma. Immunoprecipitation with this antibody from extracts of whole PBMC produces a pattern of three polypeptides identical to that reported for the human and rodent common leukocyte antigens with molecular weights of 180,000, 195,000, and 210,000. FMF analysis with this mAb yields a single uniform and brightly staining population of cells. No functional studies have been done with this mAb.

D. Other Pan-Lymphocyte-Reactive mAb

Several other mAb have been generated from fusions involving cells from BALB/c mice immunized with porcine cells (16; W.R. Lie et al., and B. Barber et al., personal communications). These mAb reacted with the entire population of porcine lymphocytes. Other than the demonstration of their lack of reaction with class I MHC antigens and of their FMF distribution on all cells, no additional information is available.

IV. DIFFERENTIATION ANTIGENS EXPRESSED ON SPECIFIC LYMPHOID CELL POPULATIONS

A. Introduction

Historically, distinct lymphoid cell populations were identified by physical properties, such as adherence to glass or nylon wool, or by their ability to rosette with red cells or complement-coated cells, or by their phagocytic activity (49, 50). Some xenoantisera reactive with specific cell subsets were generated; however, these required extensive absorptions to be useful and displayed significant batch to batch variability (51,52). The development of monoclonal antibody technology provided an alternative method for examining the presence of specific cell-surface antigens. The development of such mAb in other species, as described in other chapters in this book, allowed the identification of specific cell subtypes within the already identified broader categories of B cells, T cells, and macrophages, and allowed the elucidation of functional interactions between cells. More recently mAb to certain cell types such as T cells have been used clinically to alter immune responses to tumors or to engrafted organs (53,54).

The great utility of mAb in other species has stimulated attempts to generate mAb against porcine cellular subsets. This was of particular importance in the case of cell subset-specific mAb because, as opposed to class II MHC and LFA-1 mAb, available mAb for other species did not cross-react with porcine tissues (16). A large panel of cell population-specific mAb has been generated by investigators from around the world and is summarized in Tables 3 and 4, and described below. The best-defined mAb functionally are those that react with swine T cells. In many cases a direct analogy can be made with mAb to human antigens based on biochemistry of the antigen, on the function of cells reactive with the mAb, and

Table 3 mAb Reactive with Swine Lymphoid Cells

mAb	Ig class	Specificity	Refs.
MSA4	IgG2a	CD2, pan-T cell	25
Mac 80	IgG2a	CD2, pan-T cell	a
Mac 83	IgM	CD2, pan-T cell	a
74-12-4	IgG2b, k	CD4, helper T cells	16,55
76-2-11	IgG2a, k	CD8, cytotoxic T cells	16,55
122/28	IgG2a, k	CD8, cytotoxic T cells	56
295/33	IgG2a, k	CD8, cytotoxic T cells	56
76-7-4	IgG2a, k	CD1, B cell subset, thymocytes, Langerhans cells	16
8/1	IgG2b	resting T cells, thymocytes	b
PT81	IgG2b	50% T cell, some null cells	17
MSA2	rat IgG	T-cell subsets	25
76-6-7	IgM, k	pan-T cell and macrophage	16
74-22-15	IgG1, k	macrophages, granulocytes	16
74-22-15A	IgG2b, k	macrophages, granulocytes	16
C4, F2, A2		macrophages, granulocytes	c
76-5-28	IgM, k	macrophages and T subsets	16
MSA1	rat IgG	myeloid cells (RBC, monocytes, etc.)	25
1A11, 1D10, 2D7	IgG1, k	B cells (pig Ig M)	57
2EZ, 3B11, 5C9	IgG1, k	B cells (pig Ig M)	57
28.4.1, PIg47B	IgG1, k	B cells (pig Ig M)	58,17
28.6.1, PIg45A	IgG2b	B cells (pig Ig M)	58,17
H5B9, H52, MHM23	IgG1, k	LFA-1 beta chain	d
74-9-3	IgM, k	common leukocyte antigen	16
PNK-I		NK cells	59
PNK-E		NK cells	59
A_3G12	IgG1	platelets	e

[a]R. Binns et al., personal communication.
[b]U. Koszinowski et al., personal communication.
[c]J. Sanchez-Viscaino et al., personal communication.
[d]J. Hildreth and M. Pescovitz, manuscript in preparation.
[e]J.-J. Letesson et al., personal communication.

Table 4 Summary of mAb Reactive with Specific PBMC Cell Subsets

mAb	Cells recognized			Summary
	T	B	macrophage	
MSA4	+++	+/−	+/−	CD2, pan-T cell
Mac80	+++	+/−	NT	CD2, pan-T cell
Mac83	+++	+/−	NT	CD2, pan-T cell
74-12-4	++	−	−	CD4, class II T_h or T_c
76-2-11	++	−	−	CD8, class I T_c or T_h
122/28	++	−	−	CD8, class I T_c or T_h
295/33	++	−	−	CD8, class I T_c or T_h
mAb to IgM	−	++	−	B cell, anti-IgM
76-7-4	−	++	−	CD1, peripheral B cell, thymocytes
74-22-15	−	−	+++	macrophage, granulocyte
MSA1	−	−	++	myeloid cells
H5B9	++	+	+++	LFA-1
H52	++	+	+++	LFA-1
MHM23	++	+	+++	LFA-1
76-6-7	++	+/−	+++	macrophage and T cells
76-5-28	+	−	+++	macrophage, T-cell subset

on the distribution of cells that bear the antigen. A recent nomenclature meeting divided the anti-human T-cell mAb into several clusters and gave each group a cluster of differentiation (CD) number (1). For those anti-swine mAb that closely parallel the human examples, the same CD number was applied. For example, the three anti-swine T-cell mAb that react with cytotoxic T cells (CTL) are classified as CD8, the same group to which the anti-human CTL mAb belong. There are two major T-cell proteins which have yet to have mAb to their porcine analog identified, those being the CD3, or T3, protein and the T-cell receptor. The generation of mAb to these antigens will be an important task for future research.

B. T-cell-specific mAb

1. CD2-specific mAb

The CD2 antigen is the sheep red blood cell receptor expressed on all mature swine T cells (25). mAb to this protein block the ability of T cells to rosette. Recent functional analyses suggest that the CD2 antigen may be involved in thymic T-cell development (60). Hammerberg and Schurig reported the first anti-porcine CD2-specific mAb, MSA4 (25). Binns has produced two additional

CD2-specific antibodies, Mac 80 and Mac 83, as determined by the ability of the antibodies to block sheep red blood cell rosetting (personal communication). The three mAb react with spatially related, and possibly the same, epitope(s) since both Mac 80 and Mac 83 inhibit the binding of MSA4 to PBMC as assessed by FMF analysis (M. Pescovitz, unpublished data). The antibody MSA4 was generated with cells from a (BALB/c X C3H/He)F_1 mouse immunized with porcine thymocytes fused to the SP2/0 fusion partner. The MW of the MSA4 protein is 50,000 dalton in the reduced state when immunoprecipitation is performed with radiolabeled PBMC (M. Pescovitz et al., manuscript in preparation).

Single parameter FMF analysis of PBMC with the three CD2 mAb showed a dominant positive peak of approximately 40-60% of the cells, a negative peak, and a dull shoulder between the two which contains approximately 15% of cells. Dual parameter FMF analysis was performed with MSA4 and various other porcine specific mAb. It was found that all of the $CD4^+$ and $CD8^+$ cells were contained within the MSA4 bright population, however, the former two antibodies combined stained only about 90% of the bright population. The remaining 10% were $MSA4^+$ but $CD8^-$ and $CD4^-$ (M. Pescovitz et al., manuscript in preparation). The MSA4 dull population was found to be stained with the CD1 antibody (specific in PBMC for B cells) and also to a slight degree by the macrophage-specific antibody 74-22-15. Therefore, the dull population was composed of both B cells and macrophages. In fact, when a nylon wool-adherent, B-cell population was examined with MSA4, it was noted that B cells did stain weakly with this antibody (M. Pescovitz, unpublished data). The staining of B cells with CD2 type antibody has been reported for activated B cells in humans (61). There is no report of human macrophage staining with the CD2 antibody. The level of expression of the CD2 marker on B cells and macrophages is 1/8 to 1/16 that of T cells. This difference can explain the specificity of sheep red blood cell rosetting for porcine T cells (62). FMF analysis of thymocytes showed that only 1% of thymocytes failed to express the CD2 marker. The role of these cells, of whether they are prethymocytes or some contaminating population, is uncertain. As expected from the pan-T-cell reactivity of the MSA4, the antibody plus complement will eliminate the cells that respond to mitogen and to allogeneic lymphocytes in a proliferative response (25; M. Pescovitz et al., manuscript in preparation). In addition CTL effectors are completely eliminated with MSA4 plus complement, as reported in humans for such antibodies. MSA4 weakly blocks CTL activity when the antibody is present at the effector stage. Finally, the MSA4 antibody plus complement will completely eliminate the cells responsible for NK-mediated killing of the erythroleukemia cell line, K562, thereby classifying porcine NK cells as T-cell-like (M. Pescovitz et al., manuscript in preparation).

2. CD4-specific mAb

The CD4, or T4, protein is found on class II-specific T cells, both helper and cytotoxic cells (63). There is only one report of such an antibody for swine (55), mAb 74-12-4, also known as PT4, resulted from a fusion between cells from a BALB/c mouse immunized with pig thymocytes and the SP2/0 myeloma line. Immunoprecipitation performed from radiolabeled whole PBL using this 74-12-4 mAb generated a single band at 50,000 MW under reducing conditions (16). This MW is nearly identical to that reported for the antigen defined by CD4 mAb, OKT4 or Leu 3 mAb in humans (64), and by the L3T4 or GK1.5 mAb in mice (65). This similarity in MW distribution was supportive of the designation of this as the CD4 molecule.

The 74-12-4 mAb was initially characterized as being present on nylon wool-nonadherent cells (T cells) and absent from the nylon wool-adherent fraction (B cells) and from the glass-adherent fraction (macrophages) as determined by single parameter FMF analyses (16). Among the peripheral blood population approximately 20-40% of resting PBMC and approximately 30-70% of nylon wool non-adherent cells are reactive with the 74-12-4 mAb. The FMF profile of either whole PBL or nylon wool nonadherent T cells shows a single positive peak and a single negative peak which is in contrast with the profile from 76-2-11 mentioned below. Subsequent analysis using dual parameter FMF, counterstaining with mAb 74-22-15 (macrophage specific), with MSA4 (CD2, pan-T-cell marker), with 76-7-4 (subset of peripheral B cells), or with antibodies to pig immunoglobulin (B cells) confirmed the isolated distribution of the 74-12-4 marker to T-cell populations in the peripheral blood (M. Pescovitz, unpublished data). Such analysis with the anti SLA class II mAb 40D showed that about one third of resting CD4$^+$ cells expressed class II MHC antigens (66).

Thymocytes were also examined for the presence of 74-12-4 marker by both FMF analysis and in situ immunohistochemistry (M. Pescovitz, manuscript in preparation). Approximately 60% of thymocytes were positive in a single peak with the 74-12-4 antibody. Dual parameter FMF analysis showed that all these cells also expressed the MSA4, or CD2, marker and the majority were also dual expressors for the CD8 marker, a finding quite similar to that reported for both murine and human tissues. When frozen sections of thymus were stained with the 74-12-4 marker, it was seen that nearly all cortical thymocytes were positive for the 74-12-4 marker, whereas only 20-30% of medullary thymocytes expressed this marker. Within porcine duodenum, the 74-12-4$^+$ cells are enriched in the lamina propria and are rare among the intraepithelial lymphocytes (H. Salmon et al., unpublished data).

In both humans and mice the CD4$^+$ cells are involved primarily in proliferative responses to soluble antigens and to surface MHC antigens and in providing help for antibody production. In addition in these species there is a strong correlation between CD4$^+$ cytotoxic cells and target specificity for class II MHC antigens. A similar correlation is seen with the porcine CD4$^+$ cells. If PBL were treated with 74-12-4 antibody and complement prior to stimulation with either lysozyme, Con A, PHA, or a second-party allogeneic stimulator cell, a marked to complete reduction in the proliferative response was seen (55). More importantly, this inhibition was also produced by adding the antibody without complement into the proliferative culture. The antibody had to be present however, at a early time point in the proliferative response to have an effect. This indicated, as seen in other species, that the CD4 protein is involved in some early proliferative function. Unpublished reports (I. Casal, L. Enjuanes, and E. Vinuela, personal communication) demonstrated that, in vitro, the antibody response to African swine fever virus was also blocked by the CD4 antibody.

The effect of the CD4 antibody on porcine class II-specific CTL has not been addressed due to the difficulty in generating class II-specific CTL in this species. However, when typical class I-specific CTL were treated with CD4 antibody no effect on their lytic activity was seen (55). This indicates that at least the class I specific CTL are not $CD4^+$. In addition NK-mediated killing as performed using the assay of Koren et al. (67) was not decreased by treatment of effector cells with 74-12-4 and complement, indicating that porcine NK cells did not bear the CD4 antigen.

3. CD8-specific mAb

There are two reports of porcine anti-CD8-specific mAb in the literature, one referring to an anti-PT8 mAb, 76-2-11 (55), and the second referring to two anti-S-L2 mAb, 295/33 and 122/28 (56). All of these mAb were generated with cells from BALB/c mice immunized with porcine thymocytes and then fused to the SP2/0 myeloma cells. The MW of the CD8 protein in the pig is 35,000 in the reduced state and 70,000 in the nonreduced state (16,56). This MW distribution is identical to that reported for the protein precipitated by the human T8 and Leu2 mAb (68).

FMF analysis with the CD8 antibody discloses that 24-38% of PBL and 40-60% of nylon wool-nonadherent T cells stained positive with the antibodies (16,56). The profile, however, differs from the CD4 antibody in that 3 peaks are identified: a bright population, a duller population that expresses approximately 1/4 the amount of antigen, and a negative population. More detailed dual parameter FMF analysis indicated that all 76-2-11 positive cells were contained in the $CD2^+$ (T cell) population (M. Pescovitz et al., manuscript in preparation). In addition the $CD8^+$ cells did not express the macrophage marker or two B-cell markers, surface Ig or CD1 antigen. Of greater interest, though, are the results obtained with dual parameter analysis using anti-class II MHC mAb and the CD4 antibody. All $CD8^+$ cells expressed the class II marker, SLA-DRw, detected by mAb 40D (66). This distribution of Ia on porcine T cells was noted earlier (69) and differs from humans and mice for both of which resting T cells fail to express Ia antigens (70). All canine and guinea pig T cells express Ia antigens, although there is no T subset specificity (71,72). This also contrasts with the dual parameter analyses reported above for the CD4 antibody where only about 1/3 of the $CD4^+$ cells expressed the Ia antigens (66). When CD4 was used for dual parameter analysis with CD8 it was noted that the dull population of $CD8^+$ cells also express the CD4 antigen (55). This dual positive population makes up approximately 15-20% of total peripheral T cells. Although a minor population, these dual expressor cells must include the Ia^+CD4^+ cells mentioned above. A similar dual expressor population has been noted in certain disease states of humans and in patients receiving immunosuppression but not in normal controls (73).

In contrast to the two positive peaks noted among the PBMC, only a single positive and a single negative peak were noted when thymocytes were stained with 76-2-11 (M. Pescovitz et al., manuscript in preparation). This constituted approximately 50-60% of the thymocyte population. Dual parameter FMF analysis indicated that all of these $CD8^+$ thymocytes were also positive with the CD2 (T-cell) mAb. In addition, when the $CD8^+$ cells were stained with the CD4 mAb the majority of the thymic population was seen to be dual expressors of CD4 and CD8, which contrasts to the peripheral blood where only a minority are dual expressors for these mAb. Therefore, among the thymic population CD4 and CD8 mAb divide the thymocytes into four populations: double negatives, double positives, and positive for either the CD4 or CD8 mAb alone (M. Pescovitz et al., manuscript in preparation).

Immunohistochemistry was also performed using the CD8 antibody which disclosed that all of the cortical thymocytes expressed the CD8 antigen, whereas only approximately 10-20% of medullary thymocytes expressed the CD8 protein (M. Pescovitz et al., manuscript in preparation). This indicates that the cortical thymocytes are the dual expressors of CD8 and CD4 and is consistent with the current hypothesis for thymic differentiation in mice and humans that suggests that as cells migrate from the cortex to the medulla they acquire a more mature phenotype and express only the CD4 or CD8 antigen (74). Swine intraepithelial gut lymphocytes are predominantly $CD8^+$ (H. Salmon et al., personal communication).

Functional analysis was also performed using the CD8 mAb with and without complement to block certain in vitro functions. Proliferative responses to the soluble antigens lysozyme or (T,G)-A-L, to the T-cell mitogens, PHA, or Con A, to the B-cell mitogens, LPS, pokeweed mitogen or *Staphylococcus aureus*, or to second-party allogeneic stimulators were unaffected by pretreatment of responder cells with antibody plus complement or by having the antibodies present during the proliferative response (55,56). This is in contrast to that reported above for the CD4-specific antibody but is consistent with the results reported for other species in which the $CD8^+$ cells had only a minimal function in proliferative responses. In contrast to these findings, both precursor and effector CTL cells were highly sensitive to PT8 and complement treatment (55,56). In addition the presence of the 76-2-11 CD8 mAb without complement blocked CTL-mediated lysis (55). These results indicate that porcine classic CTL are $CD8^+$ and that CD8 antigen is involved in CTL-mediated killing, perhaps as hypothesized for the human studies, as an adherence molecule.

Porcine NK cells, as generated by the method by Koren et al. (67), are also sensitive to the effects of CD8 plus complement-mediated killing, indicating that porcine NK cells express the CD8 antigen (M. Pescovitz et al., manuscript in preparation). However, in contrast to the results with CTL, this NK-mediated killing is not inhibitable by the presence of the CD8 antibody at the effector stage of the assay.

The function ot the dual expressing $CD4^+/CD8^+$ dull cells seen in the peripheral blood is uncertain, however, some data indicates that these cells are not CTL. This data derives from the fact that killing with CD8 mAb and complement at the beginning of the CTL assay will eliminate killing, and eliminate the CD8 bright population as detected by FMF analysis at the end of the 7-day culture, even though a large population of CD8 dull cells remained (55). In humans, data suggested that the CD8 dull population has a suppressor function although the role of the CD8 mAb on suppressor-cell activity in the pig has not yet been examined.

4. CD1-specific mAb

In humans, the CD1, or T6, antigen is a class I-like differentiation antigen. It has similar biochemical properties to class I-like MHC antigens, in that mAb to CD1 precipitate a 45000 MW heavy chain and a 12000 MW light chain (75). Unlike class I MHC antigens, the CD1 antigen has a restricted tissue distribution, it is localized to the cortical thymocytes and is thought to be similar to the murine T1a antigen (76). The in vivo role of this antigen is, as yet, unknown. There is one report in the literature of a CD1-specific mAb for swine, 76-7-4, that resulted from the fusion of splenocytes from a BALB/c mouse immunized with porcine thymocytes to the SP2/0 myeloma line (16). Immunoprecipitation from radioiodine-labeled whole PBL yielded a class I-like protein with a 40,000 MW heavy chain and a 12,000 MW light chain (16). The heavy chain in this instance is somewhat lighter than that seen with antigens precipitated by anti-SLA class I-specific mAb, e.g., 74-11-10, while the MW of the light chain is identical to that of β_2-microglobulin. This relative MW is similar to that reported for the human T6 antigen (75).

FMF analysis on whole PBMC yielded a percentage of positive cells that was similar to that seen when staining with anti-surface immunoglobulin (16). In addition, the positive cells were restricted to the nylon wool-adherent cell populations, the B cells. This B-cell specificity was reconfirmed by two dimensional FMF analysis in that none of the CD4 or CD8 positive cells were stained with the CD1-specific antibody (M. Pescovitz, manuscript in preparation). In addition, macrophages, as detected by 74-22-15 mAb, also were not stained with the CD1 antibody. However, when staining with the CD1 antibody was compared to that resulting from an antibody to surface immunoglobulin it was found that all of the CD1 positive cells were surface Ig^+, which confirms the results on purified populations. Not all surface Ig^+ cells, though, were positive with the CD1-specific antibody; only 1/2 to 2/3 of the B cells were stained with the CD1 antibody. The functional difference, if any, between the $CD1^+$ and $CD1^-$ B cells is unknown.

FMF analysis of a single cell suspension of thymocytes showed approximately 60% of thymocytes stained with the CD1-specific antibody (16). This thymic reactivity explained the initially apparent paradox in the generation of a B-cell-specific antibody following an immunization with thymocytes, a B-cell-deficient population of cells. Dual parameter FMF analysis showed that, in general, both $CD4^+$ and $CD8^+$ cells were distributed in both the $CD1^+$ and $CD1^-$ populations (M. Pescovitz et al., manuscript in preparation). An interesting finding, however, was the relative reciprocity of CD1 antigen expression compared with classic class I MHC antigens, in that the brightest cells for the class I-specific antigen were negative for CD1 antigen and vice versa, which has also been noted for the H-2D and T1a antigens (76).

Immunohistochemistry was also performed on thymus and skin using the CD1-specific antibody (M. Pescovitz et al., manuscript in preparation). When thymus was stained, it was apparent that the majority of the $CD1^+$ cells were in the cortex, in fact 90-100% of cortical cells were $CD1^+$. Contrary to this, only 5-10% of the medullary cells expressed the CD1 antigen. Therefore the CD1 protein is a marker for cortical versus medullary thymocytes. The apparent reciprocity with the class I-specific antibody seen on FMF analysis was further confirmed in the immunohistochemistry, in that the class I-specific antibody stained only the medullary cells and not the cortical cells. The thymic distribution of the porcine CD1 antigen is identical to that reported for the human mAb (77) and also for the murine ThB antibody (78), although the latter precipitated a different molecular weight protein. Further confirmation of the CD1-like specificity of the 76-7-4 antibody was seen when porcine epidermal sheets were stained with 76-7-4 in immunofluorescence. Here, dendritic-like cells (i.e., porcine Langerhans cells) stained very brightly with 76-7-4 (M. Pescovitz et al., manuscript in preparation). This presence of the CD1 antigen on Langerhans cells was also clearly seen in human tissues (79).

No functional analysis of the cells bearing the CD1 marker in the thymus or among the peripheral B cells were performed. Further analysis of the B-cell population, such as distribution of specific Ig classes or functional activity in vitro, e.g., antibody generation, would be a fruitful area for future investigations.

5. Other T-cell-reactive mAb

mAb 8/1. Koszinowski has recently developed another T-cell-reactive mAb 8/1 (personal communication). The MW of the antigen has not been determined. This antibody stains 5-50% of bone marrow cells, 100% of thymocytes, and nearly all peripheral T cells. Immunoperoxidase staining of lymph nodes and spleen showed that $8/1^+$ cells were found in the T-cell-specific areas. The 8/1 antigen is apparently not present on activated cells. CTL precursors and T helper precursors are eliminated by treatment with 8/1 and complement; CTL effectors and activated T helpers are not eliminated by this treatment. Further characterization of this antibody is underway.

mAb PT81. Kelly et al. have characterized the mAb, PT81, which resulted from (B10.A(3R) × BALB/c) F_1 mice immunized with porcine thymocytes (80). This mAb reacts with 25% of splenic mononuclear cells, 66% of thymocytes, and 38% of porcine PBMC. In the presence of complement it lysed 37% of PBMC and 47% of T cell purified by sheep erythrocyte rosetting. It also binds 10-15% of null cells. Removal of $PT81^+$ cells, by treatment with mAb and complement, significantly (by 80%) reduces the proliferative response of PBL to PHA, Con A, PWM, and soybean agglutinin.

mAb MSA2. Hammerberg and Schurig developed MSA2 from a Sprague Dawley rat immunized with pig PBMC (25). MSA2 reacts with 45% of PBMC, 75% of sheep erythrocyte rosette positive T cells, 11% of rosette negative cells, 60% of thymocytes, 56% of splenocytes, 12% of bone marrow cells, and 8% of glass-adherent cells. It does not react with neutrophils or red blood cells. Depletion of PBMC with MSA2 and complement results in a 50-80% reduction in the proliferative response to the mitogens Con A, PHA, and PWM.

mAb 76-6-7. mAb 76-6-7 resulted from a fusion between splenocytes from a BALB/c mouse immunized with porcine thymocytes and the SP2/0 myeloma (16). On FMF analysis the mAb stains all glass-adherent cells very strongly and all T cells less well. It is apparently negative on B cells. It also stains all thymocytes, 65% of lymph node cells, 37% of bone marrow cells, 56% of splenocytes, and 78% of granulocytes. Treatment of a population of PBL with this mAb and complement eliminates the cells needed for allogeneic mixed lymphocyte responses. The antigen appears to be highly immunogenic, since several other mAb (PT91 and PT37) of similar FMF appearance were generated by Davis et al. (17; M. Pescovitz et al., unpublished observation). There is no known analog in other species.

C. Macrophage-specific mAb

1. 74-22-15 mAb

This antibody resulted from a fusion between cells from a BALB/c mouse immunized against porcine thymocytes and the SP2/0 myeloma (16). Recently, using the methodology reported by Radbruch et al. (81), an Ig heavy chain class switch mutant of the 74-22-15 IgG1 hybridoma was selected and shown to bear the IgG2b heavy chain (M. Pescovitz et al., unpublished data). This mAb has the same staining characteristics as the parent line, is easier to purify on protein A Sepharose, and, of greater importance, is now cytotoxic in the presence of complement. The molecular weight of the precipitated protein is 215,000.

FMF analysis of whole PBMC with 74-22-15 showed that approximately 10-15% of cells are stained as a single, very intense peak with the 74-22-15 antibody (16). This population is confined to the glass adherent population in that approximately 90% of the glass-adherent cells are positive for the 74-22-15 antibody, and the nylon wool-nonadherent, T-cell-enriched population does not stain with this antibody. These findings have been reconfirmed by dual parameter FMF analysis in that the CD4, CD8, and CD1 antigens are not expressed on cells which also bear the 74-22-15 antigen (M. Pescovitz, unpublished data). As mentioned above, the MSA4 dull cells are made up partially of 74-22-15 positive cells. Approximately 1/2 of the 74-22-15 positive PBMC also express class II MHC antigens (F. Popitz et al., unpublished data). This distribution of Ia on macrophage-like cells has also been noted in humans and mice where only a portion of resting macrophages expressed class II MHC antigen (82,83). FMF analysis of a single cell suspension of thymus showed that very few if any of these cells express 74-22-15 antigen, therefore the generation of this antibody was fortuitous in that an antibody was generated against a minor contaminant cell population. The antibody also stains 100% of granulocytes. The function of the 74-22-15 positive cells in in vitro reactions is still under investigation. Preliminary data however indicates that the 74-22-15$^+$ cells do not have NK activity.

Sanchez-Vizcaino and his colleagues (personal communication) have produced several mAb, C4, AZ, and F2, that appear to have similar reactivity to 74-22-15. Immunocytochemical studies show that all four mAb stain macrophages in the cortex and medulla of the thymus. All stain the red pulp, including the ellipsoids in the spleen, densely, as well as the interfollicular areas and the germinal centers of secondary follicles of lymph nodes.

2. 76-5-28 mAb

This antibody resulted from fusion of cells from a BALB/c mouse that was immunized with porcine thymocytes to the SP2/0 myeloma cells (16). The MW of the protein is 25,000. Single parameter FMF analysis on purified populations suggests that 76-5-28 antigen is restricted to a macrophage- or glass-adherent population; in addition it binds to 39% of granulocytes (16). This distribution is also apparently confirmed with dual parameter FMF analysis (M. Pescovitz and J. Lunney, unpublished data). However, preliminary functional experiments suggest that the 76-5-28 antigen also is present on T cells in that treatment with 76-5-28 antibody and complement of responder populations eliminates the ability of that population to respond to a mitogenic stimulus (F. Popitz et al., unpublished data). In addition, treatment with 76-5-28 and complement decreases the number of 74-12-4 positive cells that remain. The explanation for the apparent discrepancy between the FMF analysis and the functional analysis is unknown but may result from efficient killing by this IgM mAb of a very weakly staining population of cells.

3. MSA1 mAb

MSA1 resulted from the fusion of Sprague Dawley splenocytes that were immunized with porcine PBMC and the SP2/0 myeloma (25). This mAb reacts with 26% of PBMC, 22% of $SRBC^+$ PBMC, 30% of $SRBC^-$ PBMC, 8% of thymocytes, 22% of splenocytes, 86% of bone marrow cells, and 99% of adherent cells. It also reacted with 97% of granulocytes and red blood cells. Treatment of PBL with MSA1 and complement reduced by 70-90% the proliferation caused by the mitogens Con A, PHA, and PWM.

D. B-cell-reactive mAb

1. IgM-reactive mAb

mAb reactive with porcine immunoglobulin M (IgM) have been produced in several laboratories as part of their efforts to produce panels of mAb reactive with all porcine immunoglobulin isotypes (57,58). After establishing that their mAb reacted with IgM purified from serum, these researchers proceeded to test many of their anti-IgM mAb for reactivity with B cells in PBMC and in tissue sections and demonstrated that they exhibited the expected B-cell subset specificity. The top section of Table 5 lists these anti-swine IgM hybridomas.

2. CD1-specific mAb

In discussing T-cell-specific mAb an unusual pattern of reactivity for the CD1 mAb, 76-7-4, was described. This mAb reacted with 60% of porcine thymocytes and with porcine Langerhans cells, like its human equivalent (16). However, unlike the CD1 mAb reactive with human cells, 76-7-4 binds to a significant proportion (~50%) of mature B cells in PBMC using two-dimensional FMF analysis. The relevance of this $76\text{-}7\text{-}4^+$ IgM^+ B-cell subset is as yet unknown.

3. mAb Reactive with Other Immunoglobulin Isotypes

Even though many immunoglobulin (Ig) isotypes are found in the greatest abundance in the serum or secretions, they most likely will also be found on low amounts in specific B-cell populations. Moreover, no listing of mAb reactive with swine lymphoid differentiation antigens would be complete without a short discussion of mAb reactive with Ig isotypes.

Table 5 lists the mAb that have been well characterized for their reactivity with swine Ig isotypes. Most of these mAb have been tested for epitope reactivity by competition assays (although not between laboratories yet). This data indicates that each Ig isotype has at least two, and possibly four, separate epitopes recognized by the murine mAb. In their studies, van Zaane and Hulst (58) have potentially identified, by differential mAb reactivity, two subsets of swine IgG

Table 5 mAb Reactive with Swine Immunoglobulins

Binding specificity				
Pig isotype	Epitope[a]	Hybridoma	Mouse Ig isotype	Refs.
IgM	a	1A11	IgG1	57
	a	1D10	IgG1	57
	a	2D7	IgG1	57
	a	2E2	IgG1	57
	a	3B11	IgG1	57
	b	5C9	IgG1	57
	A	28.4.1	IgG1	58
	B	28.6.1	IgG2b	58
	x[c]	PIg45A	IgG2b	17
	x[c]	PIg47B	IgG1	17
IgG	a	1B4	IgG1	b
	a	1F9	IgM	b
	a	1H11	IgM	b
	a	3G12	IgM	b
	a	4A7	IgM	b
	b	3H2	IgG1	b
	c	3H7	IgG1	b
	A	23.3.1b	IgG1	58
	A	34.32.1	IgG1	58
	B	34.36.1	IgG1	58
	C	23.5.1b	IgG1	58
	C	23.7.1b	IgG1	58
	C	23.9.1b	IgG1	58
	C	34.14.1a	IgG2b	58
	C	34.31.1	IgG1	58
IgG1	A	23.49.2	IgG1	58
	A	34.5.1.a	IgG1	58
	A	34.6.1.a	IgG1	58
	A	34.8.1.a	IgG1	58
	A	34.11.1a	IgG1	58
	A	34.16.1a	IgG1	58
	A	34.18.2a	IgG1	58
	A	34.20.2	IgG1	58
	B	34.9.2a	IgG2a	58
	B	34.10.1	IgG1	58
	B	34.19.2a	IgG2a	58
	C	23.2.3b	IgG1	58

(Table 5 *continues*)

Table 5 (*continued*)

Binding specificity				
Pig isotype	Epitope[a]	Hybridoma	Mouse Ig isotype	Refs.
	C	23.29.1	IgG1	58
	C	23.34.3	IgG1	58
IgG1 (pH 5.0)	D	34.17.2a	IgG1	58
IgG2	A[d]	23.1.1b	IgG2a	58
	A[d]	23.43.3b	IgG2b	58
	B	34.1.1a	IgG1	58
	B	34.2.1a	IgG1	58
	B	34.3.1a	IgG1	58
	C	34.4.1a	IgG1	58
IgA	a	3H5	IgG1	b
	x[c]	1F11	IgG1	b
	x	3B8	IgG1	b
	x	3D11	IgG1	b
	x	5E2	IgG1	b
	x	6D11	IgG1	b
	A	27.8.1	IgG1	58
	B	27.9.1	IgG1	58
	x	27.10.1	IgG1	58
Light chain	L1[e]	3C10	IgG1	b
	L1[e]	4H6	IgG1	b
	L2[e]	3D8	IgG1	b
	L	27.1.1	IgG2b	58
	L	27.2.1	IgG1	58
	L	27.3.1	IgG1	58
	L	27.7.1	IgG1	58
	L	28.2.1	IgG2b	58
	L	28.5.1	IgG1	58
	L	34.15.1a	IgA	58
	L	PIg31B	IgG1	17

[a]Epitope bound was determined in separate laboratories, for each set of mAb, by inhibition analyses. It is not yet known if/what the relationship is between the epitopes defined to date.
[b]P. Paul, W. Mengeling, and R. van Deusen, manuscript in preparation.
[c]X = no epitope assignment has yet been determined.
[d]Both of these mAb react with an allotypic determinant of swine IgG2.
[e]Light chain reactivity has not yet been divided into epitopes recognized, although Paul et al. has determined that two separate light chains are recognized by their mAb.

as well as potential allotypic determinants of swine IgG2. Paul and his collaborators (manuscript in preparation) have demonstrated two separate swine Ig light chains that are probably analogous to the κ and λ light chains found in other species, although their exact identification has not yet been established.

This panel of mAb reactive with swine Ig isotypes should be very useful for B-cell differentiation studies in this species, as well as for the analysis of Ig isotypes produced in a wide range of porcine immune responses.

E. Natural Killer (NK) Cell-specific mAb

Kim has reported the development of two mAb, PNK-I and PNK-E, reactive with porcine NK cells (59). These resulted from a fusion of BALB/c splenocytes immunized against porcine large granular lymphocytes with the myeloma cell line P3.X63.Ag8.653, and screening the hybridomas for effect on NK-mediated killing. PNK-I and complement kills 14% of PBMC and blocks NK killing in the absence of complement. PNK-E also kills 15% of PBMC in the presence of complement, but, as opposed to PNK-I, it enhances NK-mediated killing in the absence of complement. Neither mAb has an effect on antibody-dependent cell-mediated cytotoxicity. The molecular weights of the antigens and possible analogs in other species are unknown.

F. Platelet-specific mAb

Letesson and Coppe (personal communication) have developed an antibody A_3G12 that reacts specifically with porcine platelets as determined by immunogold staining and transmission electron microscopy. The molecular weight of the antigen and any functional role are unknown.

V. IMPORTANCE OF THESE mAb TO SWINE DIFFERENTIATION ANTIGENS FOR FUTURE RESEARCH IN SWINE IMMUNOLOGY

The understanding of swine immunology has expanded significantly. As described in detail above, mAb to most important SLA antigens as well as mAb to many cell-subset-specific antigens are now well characterized and available for future research studies. No other veterinary species has such a well-characterized panel of mAb to such a wide range of lymphoid differentiation antigens. Clearly, several crucial mAb specificities are still missing, such as an anti-T-cell receptor or anti-SLA-DP locus antigen, and will require more research effort. However, with the current panel of mAb many important immunological studies can be approached using modern mAb tools.

Analysis of this large panel of mAb already suggests some questions for future research. Many mAb react with more than one cell type. This may reflect some common differentiation pathway such as might be demonstrated by the reactivity of mAb with both macrophages and granulocytes, or with B cells and thymocytes. Many of the mAb-defined antigens must have some important function, since they have been conserved among widely different species as indicated by the similarities in function, in biochemical size, etc.; some to the extent that mAb cross-react among the species (e.g., LFA-1). Further work including perhaps the generation of additional mAb and comparison of results with mAb in other species should aid in defining more clearly these important common function and delineating them from species specific determinants and/or functions.

Transplantation surgeons have demonstrated the usefulness of swine as a model for transplantation of a wide range of tissues and organs, including the liver, kidney, heart, and bone marrow (84). The close physiological similarity of pigs to humans, along with the availability of the large panels of mAb to similar lymphoid differentiation antigens for these two species, should greatly aid in the development of mAb treatment protocols for humans based on developmental research in swine.

Analyses of swine immune responses to infectious diseases or to new subunit antigen vaccines will be greatly enhanced by the availability of this full panel of mAb reagents. In addition, the successful production of transgenic swine expressing bovine growth hormones (85), and of transgenic mice expressing SLA genes (86), suggests future possibilities of producing more healthy, disease-resistant swine by genetic engineering.

VI. AVAILABILITY OF HYBRIDOMA CELL LINES

All hybridoma cell lines generated in the authors' laboratories have been made available to The American Type Culture Collection so that they are easily accessible by all scientists. The authors recommend that all of the hybridoma cell lines producing anti-swine cell mAb be made available to such collections.

VII. SUMMARY

Over the past several years a number of laboratories have been involved in the production of mAb against porcine lymphocyte antigens. This chapter reviews both published and unpublished work dealing with these mAb. The mAb available for analysis were divided into 3 groups: (a) MHC-reactive mAb, (b) mAb reactive with all mononuclear cells but non-anti-MHC; and (c) subpopulation-specific mAb.

The anti-MHC mAb were divided into those which react with class I and class II SLA antigens. The anti-class I SLA mAb were further divided into those reactive with monomorphic and polymorphic determinants based on differential reactivity with cells from SLA inbred miniature swine and with murine fibroblasts transfected with isolated SLA class I genes. The class II SLA-reactive mAb were divided in SLA-DRw- and SLA-DQw-specific mAb and were distinguished by antigen MW on SDS-polyacrylamide gel electrophoresis.

The broadly reactive, non-anti-MHC mAb include mAb specific for the swine analog of the common leukocyte antigen and of the leukocyte function-associated (LFA-1) antigen. The LFA-1 mAb reacts with all PBMC and profoundly inhibits in vitro T-cell blastogenesis, and CTL and NK cell lytic reactivity.

The subpopulation-specific mAb include antibodies which recognize members of each major mononuclear cell subset: T cells, B cells, macrophages, and natural killer cells. The largest amount of data exists for the T-cell-specific mAb. Analogs exist for the CD2 antigen (pan-T cell, anti-sheep red blood cell receptor, T11), CD4 (T helper cell, MHC class II-specific, T4), and CD8 (cytotoxic/suppressor cell, MHC class I-specific, T8). The designation of each analog was based on biochemistry of the antigen, distribution of positive cells in the blood and in lymphoid organs, and function of the cells reactive with the mAb. For B cells, mAb reactive with swine IgM (as well as with many other Ig isotypes) are available as well as a CD1-reactive mAb that in swine also recognizes a subset of peripheral blood B cells. For macrophages, mAb reactive with monocytes and granulocytes are available as well as one that recognizes all myeloid cells. Finally for natural killer cells, two mAb have been produced. Many of the antibodies are available through the American Type Tissue Collection. Current and potential uses for the mAb are addressed.

ACKNOWLEDGMENTS

We would like to thank our colleagues from around the world who provided us with their data, some before publication, to be included in this chapter. The authors would like to thank Ms. Patty Hobbs for her expert typing of the manuscript and Drs. Ralph Quinones, Hyun Lillehoj, H. Ray Gamble, and David H. Sachs for their critical review of the chapter. Finally, the authors would like to acknowledge Dr. David H. Sachs, in whose laboratory much of this work was performed, for his support and guidance of their research and for his foresight in recognizing 15 years ago the important role of swine in current immunologic and transplantation research.

REFERENCES

1. A. Bernard, L. Boumsell, and C. Hill, in *Leukocyte Typing: Human Leukocyte Differentiation Antigens Detected by Monoclonal Antibodies* (A. Bernard, L. Boumsell, J. Dausset, C. Milstein, and S. F. Schlossman, eds.), Springer-Verlag, New York, 1984, p. 9.
2. W. F. Bodmer, E. Albert, J. G. Bodmer, J. Dausset, F. Kissmeyer-Nielsen, W. Mayr, R. Payne, J. J. van Rood, Z. Trnka, and R. L. Walford, *Immunogenetics, 20*: 593 (1984).

3. M. Vaiman, C. Renard, P. Lafage, J. Ameteau, and P. Nizza, *Transplant., 10*: 155 (1970).
4. M. Vaiman, P. Chardon, and C. Renard, *Immunogen., 9*: 353 (1979).
5. D. Viza, J. R. Sugar, and R. M. Binns, *Nature, 227*: 949 (1970).
6. D. H. Sachs, G. Leight, J. Cone, S. Schwarz, L. Stuart, and S. Rosenberg, *Transplant., 22*: 559 (1976).
7. J. K. Lunney, M. D. Pescovitz, and D. H. Sachs, in *Swine in Biomedical Research* (M. E. Tumbleson, ed), Plenum, New York, 1986, pp. 1821-1836.
8. D. H. Sachs, in *Fundamental Immunology* (W. E. Paul, ed.), Raven Press, New York, 1984, p. 303.
9. D. White and J. Lunney, *Transplant Proc., 11*: 1170 (1979).
10. L. Hood, M. Steinmetz, and B. Malissen, *Ann. Rev. Immunol., 1*: 529 (1983).
11. D. S. Singer, R. D. Camerini-Otero, M. L. Satz, B. Osborne, D. Sachs, and S. Rudikoff, *Proc. Natl. Acad. Sci. USA, 79*: 1403 (1982).
12. M. L. Satz, L.-C. Wang, D. S. Singer, and S. Rudikoff, *J. Immunol., 135*: 2167 (1985).
13. J. R. Thistlethwaite, Jr., L. R. Pennington, J. K. Lunney, and D. H. Sachs, *Transplant., 35*: 394 (1983).
14. L. R. Pennington, J. K. Lunney, and D. H. Sachs, *Transplant., 31*: 66 (1981).
15. R. Fauchet, J. G. Bodmer, L. J. Kennedy, M. C. Mazzilli, C. Müller, C. Raffaux, and P. Richiardi, in *Histocompatibility Testing* (E. D. Albert, M. P. Baur, and W. R. Mayr, eds.), Springer-Verlag, New York, 1984, p. 211.
16. M. D. Pescovitz, J. K. Lunney, and D. H. Sachs, *J. Immunol., 133*: 368 (1984).
17. W. C. Davis, L. E. Perryman, and T. C. McGuire, in *Hybridoma Technology in Agricultural and Veterinary Research* (N. J. Stern and H. R. Gamble, eds.), Rowman and Allanheld, Totowa, New Jersey, 1984, p. 121.
18. B. F. Haynes, M. E. Hemler, D. L. Mann, G. S. Eisenbarth, J. Shelhamer, H. S. Mostowski, C. A. Thomas, J. L. Strominger, and A. S. Fauci, *J. Immunol., 126*: 1409 (1981).
19. J.-J. Letesson et al., *Vet. Immunol. Immunopathol.,* in press.
20. W.-R. Lie, M. F. Rothschild, and C. M. Warner, *Fed. Proc., 45*: 987 (1986).
21. D. Smilek, H. C. Boyd, D. B. Wilson, C. M. Zmijewski, F. W. Fitch, and T. J. McKearn, *J. Exp. Med., 151*: 1139 (1980).
22. E. Ivaskova, P. Ivanyi, M. Mickova, and P. Demant, *Tissue Antigens, 6*: 286 (1975).
23. J. K. Lunney, B. A. Osborne, J.-J. Metzger, G. L. Gilliland, S. Rudikoff, and D. H. Sachs, *Fed. Proc., 40*: 1053 (1981).
24. J.-L. Teillaurd, D. Crevat, P. Chardon, J. Kalil, C. Goujet-Zalc, G. Mahouy, M. Vaiman, M. Fellous, and D. Pious, *Immunogenetics, 15*: 377 (1982).
25. C. Hammerberg and G. Schurig, *Vet. Immunol. Immunopath., 11*: 107 (1986).
26. M. Watanabe, T. Suzuki, M. Taniguchi, and N. Shinohara, *Transplant., 36*: 712 (1983).
27. M. Pierres, F. M. Kourilsky, J.-P. Rebouah, M. Dossetto, and D. Caillol, *Eur. J. Immunol., 10*: 950 (1980).

28. J. K. Lunney, B. A. Osborne, S. O. Sharrow, C. Devaux, M. Pierres, and D. H. Sachs, *J. Immunol., 130*: 2786 (1983).
29. M. Pierres, P. Mercier, M. Madsen, C. Mawas, and T. Kristensen, *Tissue Antigens, 19*: 289 (1982).
30. D. J. Charron and H. O. McDevitt, *Proc. Natl. Acad. Sci. USA, 76*: 6567 (1979).
31. B. A. Osborne, J. K. Lunney, L. Pennington, D. H. Sachs, and S. Rudikoff, *J. Immunol., 131*: 2939 (1983).
32. J. K. Lunney, W. C. Davis, and M. D. Pescovitz, *Fed. Proc., 44*: 554 (1985).
33. L. A. Lampson and R. Levy, *J. Immunol., 125*: 293 (1980).
34. F. M. Brodsky, P. Parham, C. J. Barnstable, M. J. Crumpton, and W. F. Bodmer, *Immunol. Rev., 47*: 3 (1979).
35. G. M, T. Schreuder, I. Doxiadis, J. Parlovlict, and H. Grosse-Wilde, in *Histocompatibility Testing* (E. D. Albert, M. P. Baur, and W. R. Mayr, eds.), Springer-Verlag, New York, 1984, p. 243.
36. D. H. Sachs, G. W. Humphrey, and J. K. Lunney, *J. Exp. Med., 146*: 381 (1977).
37. J. K. Lunney and D. H. Sachs, *J. Immunol., 122*: 623 (1979).
38. J. K. Lunney, D. L. Mann, and D. H. Sachs, *Scand. J. Immunol., 10*: 403 (1979).
39. T. L. Delovitch and J. A. Falk, *Immunogenetics, 8*: 405 (1979).
40. P. Ivanyi, E. Gyodi, G. Gyorffy, H. Pavljokova, E. Ivaskova, and G. Petranyl, *Scand. J. Immunol., 6*: 431 (1977).
41. N. Shinohara, D. H. Sachs, N. Nonaka, and H. Yamamato, *Nature, 292*: 362 (1981).
42. N. Shinohara and D. H. Sachs, in *Ia Antigens, Vol. I, Mice* (S. Ferrone and C. S. David, eds.), CRC Press, Boca Raton, Florida, 1982, p. 219.
43. D. Davignon, E. Martz, T. Reynolds, K. Kürzinger, and T. A. Springer, *J. Immunol., 127*: 590 (1981).
44. J. E. K. Hildreth, F. M. Gotch, P. D. K. Hildreth, and A. J. McMichael, *Eur. J. Immunol., 13*: 202 (1983).
45. A. Fisher, A. Durandy, G. Sterkers, and C. Griscelli, *J. Immunol., 136*: 3198 (1986).
46. K. Kürzinger, M. K. Ho, and T. A. Springer, *Nature, 296*: 668 (1982).
47. J. E. K. Hildreth and J. T. August, *J. Immunol., 134*: 3272 (1985).
48. T. A. Springer, D. Davignon, M.-K. Ho, K. Kürzinger, F. Martz, and F. Sanchez-Madrid, *Immunol. Reviews, 68*: 171 (1982).
49. P. M. Outteridge, R. M. Binns, and S. T. Licence, *Int. Archs. Allergy Appl. Immun., 67*: 18 (1982).
50. H. Salmon, *Int. Archs. Allergy Appl. Immun., 60*: 262 (1979).
51. H. Salmon, *Ann. Immunol. (Paris), 129C*: 571 (1978).
52. H. Johnson, Jr., J. K. Lunney, D. H. Sachs, and M. W. Flye, *Transpl., 29*: 477 (1980).
53. H. Schreiber, *Adv. in Cancer Res., 41*: 291 (1984).
54. A. B. Cosimi, R. B. Colvin, G. J. Jaffers, J. V. Giorgi, F. L. Delmonico, T. C. Fuller, and P. S. Russell, *Transpl. Proc., 16*: 1459 (1984).

55. M. D. Pescovitz, J. K. Lunney, and D. H. Sachs, *J. Immunol., 134*: 37 (1985).
56. S. Jonjic and U. Koszinowski, *J. Immunol., 133*: 647 (1984).
57. P. S. Paul, R. A. van Deusen, and W. L. Mengeling, *Vet. Immunol. Immunopath., 8*: 311 (1985).
58. D. van Zaane and M. M. Hulst, submitted for publication.
59. Y. B. Kim, M. Czajkowski, and G. A. Munson, in *Natural Killer Activity and Its Regulation* (T. Hoshino, H. S. Koren, and A. Uchida, eds.), Excerpta Medica, 1980, p. 250.
60. D. A. Fox, R. E. Hussey, K. A. Fitzgerald, A. Bensussan, J. F. Daley, S. F. Schlossman, and E. L. Reinherz, *J. Immunol., 134*: 330 (1985).
61. K. H. G. Mills, C. P. Wormon, and J. C. Cawley, *Eur. J. Immunol., 13*: 379 (1983).
62. R. M. Binns, *Vet. Immunol. and Immunopath., 3*: 95 (1982).
63. S. C. Meuer, S. F. Schlossman, and F. L. Reinherz, *Proc. Nat. Acad. Sci. USA, 79*: 4395 (1982).
64. P. E. Rao, M. A. Talle, P. C. Kung, and G. Goldstein, *Cell Immunol., 80*: 310 (1983).
65. D. P. Dialynas, Z. S. Quan, K. A. Wall, A. Pierres, J. Quintans, M. Loken, M. Pierres, and F. W. Fitch, *J. Immunol., 131*: 2445 (1983).
66. M. D. Pescovitz, F. Popitz, D. H. Sachs, and J. K. Lunney, in *Advances in Gene Technology: Molecular Biology of the Immune System* (J. W. Streilein et al., eds.), ICSU Press, New York, 1985, p. 271.
67. H. S. Koren, D. B. Amos, and Y. B. Kim, *Proc. Nat. Acad. Sci. USA, 175*: 5127 (1978).
68. J. A. Ledbetter, R. L. Evans, M. Lipinski, C. Cunningham-Rundles, R. A. Good, and L. A. Herzenberg, *J. Exp. Med., 153*: 310 (1981).
69. J. R. Thistlethwaite, Jr., L. R. Pennington, J. K. Lunney, and D. H. Sachs, *Transplant., 35*: 394 (1983).
70. H.-S. Ko, S. M. Fu, R. J. Winchester, D. T. Y. Yu, and H. G. Kunkel, *J. Exp. Med., 150*: 246 (1979).
71. H. J. Deeg, J. C. Wulff, S. DeRose, G. E. Sale, M. Brown, M. A. Brown, S. C. Springmeyer, P. J. Maitin, and R. Storb, *Immunogenetics, 16*: 445 (1982).
72. R. Burger, I. Scher, S. O. Sharrow, and E. M. Shevach, *Immunol., 51*: 93 (1984).
73. S. Berrih, C. Gaud, M. A. Bach, H. Le Brigand, J. P. Binet, and J. F. Bach, *Clin. Exp. Immunol., 45*: 1 (1981).
74. R. Scollay and K. Shortman, *Thymus, 5*: 245 (1983).
75. Y. Bushkin, M. J. Chorney, E. Diamante, S. M. Fu, and C. Y. Wong, *Mol. Immunol., 21*: 821 (1984).
76. E. A. Boyse, *Cell, 38*: 1 (1984).
77. E. R. Reinherz, P. C. Kung, G. Goldstein, R. H. Levey, and S. F. Schlossman, *Proc. Nat. Acad. Sci. USA, 77*: 1588 (1980).
78. R. D. Stout, M. Yutoku, A. Grossberg, D. Pressman, and L. A. Herzenberg, *J. Immunol., 115*: 508 (1975).

79. K. A. Haines, T. J. Flotte, T. A. Springer, I. Gigli, and G. J. Thorbecke, *Proc. Natl. Acad. Sci. USA, 80*: 3448 (1983).
80. K. W. Kelley, W. C. Davis, H. Salmon, J.-M. Aynaud, and M. Oliver, *Fed. Proc., 43*: 1681 (1984).
81. A. Radbruch, B. Liesegang, and K. Rajewsky, *Proc. Natl. Acad. Sci. USA, 77*: 2909 (1980).
82. H. V. Raff, L. J. Picker, and J. D. Stobo, *J. Exp. Med., 152*: 581 (1980).
83. C. Cowing, S. H. Pincus, D. H. Sachs, and H. B. Dickler, *J. Immunol., 121*: 1680 (1978).
84. M. D. Pescovitz and D. H. Sachs, in *Human Class II Histocompatibility Antigens: Theoretical and Practical Aspects-Clinical Relevance* (S. Ferrone, B. Solheim, and E. Moller, eds.), (1985).
85. R. E. Hammer, V. G. Pursel, C. E. Rexroad, R. J. Wall, D. G. Bolt, K. M. Ebert, R. D. Palmiter, and R. L. Brinster, *Nature, 315*: 680 (1985).
86. W. I. Frels, J. A. Bluestone, R. J. Hodes, M. R. Capecchi, and D. S. Singer, *Science, 228*: 577 (1985).

14

Differentiation Antigens and Functional Characteristics of Bovine Leukocytes

CYNTHIA L. BALDWIN, W. IVAN MORRISON, and JAN NAESSENS
International Laboratory for Research on Animal Diseases, Nairobi, Kenya

I. INTRODUCTION

Studies of immune responses in animals other than those regarded as "laboratory animals" have previously suffered from a lack of reagents with which to identify leukocyte cell populations. With the advent of monoclonal antibody (mAb) technology a plethora of reagents has been developed in recent years which identify leukocyte differentiation antigens in many species, including domestic animals (see other reviews included in this volume). It is now clear that the general organization of the immune system is basically similar among mammals. For instance, the human T-lymphocyte differentiation antigens, CD4 and CD8, have analogues among mice, rats, cattle, swine, and sheep (1-8). The availability of such reagents makes it feasible to study in more detail immunological mechanisms and their role in controlling infectious diseases in domestic animals.

Reagents are available for use in cattle which identify differentiation antigens of T lymphocytes and subpopulations of T lymphocytes (1,2,9-11), which identify monocytes and tissue macrophages (12,13), and which react with antigens common among various leukocyte lineages, such as those shared by monocytes and granulocytes or by monocytes and T lymphocytes (10,12). Bovine B cells can be identified by the expression of surface immunoglobulin (sIg) of various isotypes (14,15). In addition, monoclonal antibodies to monomorphic or polymorphic determinants on class I and class II major histocompatibility complex (MHC) antigens can be used to evaluate the level of maturation or activation of cells of different lineages (9,12,16-19).

A functional role has not been determined for all of the antigens described for bovine leukocytes. However, the biochemical characteristics of some of the antigens, along with tissue distribution and functional properties of the cells that

Table 1 Brief Summary of Differentiation Antigens of Bovine Leukocyte Populations

Section and subject	Antigen recognized	Identifying antibodies	Leukocyte populations expressed on	Refs.
II. T cells	BoT4	IL-A11, IL-A12	Class II restricted T cells	1,17
	BoT8	IL-A17	Class I restricted T cells	2,17
	BoT3	IL-A27, IL-A28, BLT-1	Mature T cells	20 11
	BoT2	IL-A26 B26A CH128A, CH61A	Majority T cells	20 9 21
	–	J6, J5	T-cell blasts	10
	–	P13	Some T-cell blasts	22
	–	BT3/8.12	Some T cells, monocytes, granulocytes	10,23
	–	J3	Some mature T cells, monocytes	
	–	P5	T cells, monocytes	12
III. B cells	IgG	*IL-A2*	B cells	–
	IgM	B5/4.1.4	B cells	14,15
	IgD?	B4/27	B cells	14
IV. Monocytes and granulocytes	–	IL-A25	Alveolar macrophages	13
	–	IL-A23	Monocytes, macrophages, fibroblasts	13
	–	P8, IL-A22, IL-A24	Monocytes, granulocytes	12 13
V. MHC	Class I MHC	P12, P3, W6/32	All cells	12 22 16
	B_2-mgl[a]		B1.1G6	All cells
	Class II MHC	R1, H4, TH21A J11 a-HLA-DR,[b] B2 Val 7C7	Some monocytes, macrophages, B cells, T-cell blasts	12 9 18 19

[a]B_2-mgl = beta$_2$-microglobulin.
[b]a-HLA-DR = commercial mAb against HLA-DR (DAKOPATTS, Copenhagen, Denmark).

express them, indicate that they are analagous to antigens defined in other species. Moreover, some reagents that identify differentiation antigens of human leukocytes cross-react with similar molecules of cattle leukocytes (see Section V). These will be included in this review. Such similarities allow a functional role to be postulated for some of the antigens.

Bovine differentiation antigens and associated functions, where known, will be dealt with as indicated in Table 1. In the case of T-cell differentiation antigens, our nomenclature is based on that applied to human differentiation antigens, which are grouped into clusters of differentiation (CD) (24). Bovine antigens have been allocated the same number as the CD number of the analogous human molecule, but using the prefix 'Bo' for bovine, as has been done for the bovine leukocyte antigens (BoLA) coded for by the MHC, and "T" for T-cell antigen. Thus "BoT4" is a molecule on bovine T lymphocytes equivalent to a CD4 molecule.

II. T LYMPHOCYTES

A. Introduction

T-cell differentiation antigens have provided useful tools for studying cellular interactions as well as mechanisms of activation of lymphoid cells. Many of the T-cell differentiation antigens of cattle have analogues in humans. The bovine T-cell antigens have largely been classified in this section according to their analogy with those of humans (see Table 2).

Mature T cells in humans can be distinguished as a group from other lymphocytes, monocytes, or granulocytes by expression of the T11 (CD2) antigen, which is the receptor for sheep red blood cells (RBC) as detected by rosetting techniques (E rosette) (25,26), by T3 (CD3), the nonvariant polypeptide chain which is noncovalently associated with the T-cell receptor (27,28), or by T1 (CD5) (27-29), the human analogue of Ly1 in the mouse (30). T11 appears to be on all peripheral T cells and on the majority of thymocytes. In contrast, T3 and T1 are mature T-cell markers: they are expressed by all peripheral T cells but are found on only 10% of thymocytes, all of which are found in the thymic medulla. In cattle, mAb are available which react with the bovine analogue of human T11 (BoT2) and possibly also T3 (BoT3), as described in Section II.B.

T cells of humans may be subdivided into two major subsets, namely those restricted by interaction with class I MHC antigens and those restricted by class II MHC antigens (31-34). The two subsets of T cells express CD8 or CD4 antigens, respectively, or their analogues in other species (1-8). Within the CD4$^+$ and CD8$^+$ subsets, T cells may have varying functions. CD4$^+$ cells can act as helper cells to both B cells and other T cells as well as having cytotoxic and suppressor activities (35,36). CD8$^+$ T cells include both cytotoxic and suppressor cells (32, 33). Recently human T cells have been divided into two other distinct, nonoverlapping categories. CD11 is expressed by suppressor T cells, whereas mAb 9.3

Table 2 T-Cell Differentiation Antigens

Antigen	Antigen biochemistry	Reacting mAb	Isotype of mAb	Tissue localization	Function	Human analogue	Refs.
$BoT2_1$	55 Kd	CH128A	IgG1	All peripheral T cells	E-rosette receptor,	CD2	21
		IL-A26	IgM	(50% PBM), cortical	alternative pathway	(T11)	20
		B26A	IgM	and medullary thymocytes	of T-cell activation		9
		CH61A	IgG1				21
BoT3	22 Kd	BLT-1	IgM	All peripheral T cells	Nonvariant component	CD3	11
		IL-A27 (?)	IgG1	(50% PBM), medullary	of T-cell receptor	(T3)	20
		IL-A28 (?)	IgM	thymocytes			20
BoT4	52, 54 Kd	IL-A11	IgG2a	70% thymocytes (cortical	Class II MHC restricted	CD4	1,17
		IL-A12	IgG2a	and medullary), 30% of PBM,	T cells	(T4)	1,17
				50% of peripheral T cells			
				($BoT8^-$ T cells)			

BoT8	32, 34 Kd	IL-A17	IgG1	70% thymocytes (cortical and medullary), 20% of PBM, 40% peripheral T cells ($BoT4^-$ T cells)	Class I MHC restricted	CD8 (T8)	2,17
'Blast'	100 Kd, gp[a]	J5	IgG2b	Transient on all activated T cells	Probably function in cell multiplication, growth factor receptor?	nk[b]	10
	100 Kd, gp	J6	IgG1				10
'Blast'	160 Kd	P13	IgM	Some T-cell blasts, cytokeratin	Possibly cell multiplication?	nk	22
"Shared"	150, 158 Kd	BT3/8.12	IgG2a	Some T cells, monocytes, granulocytes	Unknown	nk	10,23
		J3	IgG1	Some mature T cells, monocytes	Unknown	nk	10
		P5	IgM	Most or all T cells, monocytes	Unknown	nk	12

[a]gp = glycoprotein.
[b]nk = not known.

recognizes the remaining T cells, including helper cells, cytolytic cells, and cytolytic precursors. Antibodies against CD11 also react with monocytes and granulocytes. Both categories (those expressing CD11 or reacting with mAb 9.3) include $CD4^+$ and $CD8^+$ T cells (37). The bovine analogues of CD4 and CD8, BoT4 and BoT8, respectively, and the functional properties of lymphocytes that express these differentiation antigens are discussed in Section II.C.

Antigens specifically associated with cell activation are also found on various lymphoid populations. Some have been identified as being receptors for growth factors, such as interleukin 2 (IL-2) (38,39) or transferrin (40). MAb P13, J5, and J6 identify T-cell blast antigens of cattle (10,22) and are described in Section II.D. Although their analogues in other species are not known, some similarities are evident.

In addition to the specific T-cell markers of cattle, three other cell markers, BT3/8.12 (23), J3 (10), and P5 (12), are discussed in Section II.E. These react with T cells as well as monocytes but not with normal B cells. BT3/8.12 and P5 react with granulocytes as well.

B. Pan-T-lymphocyte Markers: BoT2 and BoT3

Immunologists working with bovine lymphocytes have struggled for years with the difficulty of reliably identifying T cells. There are many published methods for identification of bovine T lymphocytes by rosetting with sheep RBC, which have given varying degrees of success (41-44). The most successful method includes treatment of the RBC with 2-aminoethylisothiouronium (AET) prior to reacting with the lymphocytes, centrifugation of the cells to facilitate rosette formation, and caution in handling the rosetted cells. Using this method, it is possible to identify 50-63% of bovine peripheral blood mononuclear cells (PBM) as expressing the E-rosette receptor (44; Baldwin, unpublished results).

The lectins peanut agglutinin and *Helix pomatia* agglutinin have also been used as markers for bovine T lymphocytes, the latter requiring the use of neuraminidase-treated cells (45,46). However, it is now clear that such lectins also react with nonlymphocytic cells, including macrophages (47). Moreover, the dilution of lectin used in staining cells is critical in order to facilitate distinction between T and B lymphocytes, probably because of the relatively low avidity of the lectin-ligand interaction (47). On the other hand PNA reacts strongly with cortical thymocytes and thus is useful for distinguishing cortical and medullary thymocytes in cell suspensions.

Several monoclonal antibodies have been produced which react with the bovine differentiation antigen BoT2. The conclusion that this antigen is analogous to CD2 in humans is based on the ability of the antibodies to block E-rosette formation or inhibit immunofluorescence staining of PBM by other mAb which are able to block E-rosette formation Furthermore, two of the mAb precipitate a molecule of about 55 Kd, which is similar to the 50-Kd molecular mass of the human T11 molecule (21). BoT2 is not present on B cells, monocytes, or granulocytes. Usinger and Splitter (48) have reported that up to 10% of E-rosetting cells also have sIg, and Lewin et al. (9) have reported that 5% of PBM stain with both anti-sIg antibodies and B26A, a mAb which detects the E-rosette receptor (21). By analysis of dual fluorescence staining with an antibody to IgM (B5/4.1.4) and mAb IL-A26 (anti-BoT2) using the fluorescence-activated cell sorter (FACS), we have not found any lymphocytes which express sIg in addition to expressing BoT2 (20). Lymphocytes expressing BoT2 comprise 45-80% of PBM with a mean of about 62% (Fig. 1; Table 3; 9). FACS profiles of staining with mAb against BoT2 indicate that the antigens are expressed at a fairly high density on PBM

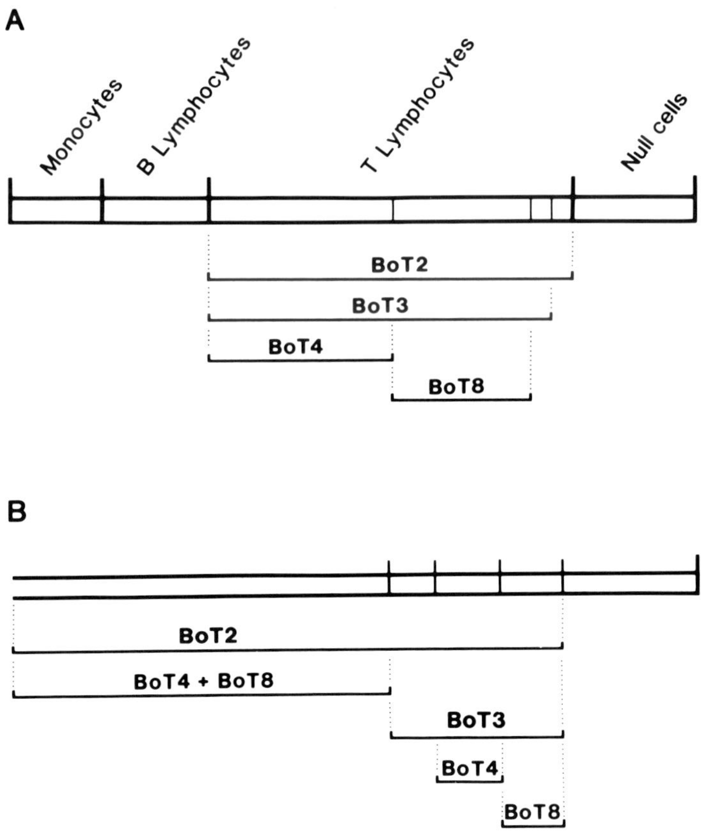

Figure 1 Schematic representation of relative proportion of mononuclear cells expressing the differentiation antigens BoT2, BoT3, BoT4, and BoT8 in (A) PBM and (B) thymus.

Table 3 Percentage of Bovine PBM Expressing the T-cell Differentiation Antigens BoT4, BoT8, BoT3, and BoT2[a]

Animal	BoT8	BoT4	BoT8 + BoT4	BoT2	BoT3	BoT3/BoT2 X 100%	(BoT4 + BoT8)/BoT3 X 100%
C-22	26.4	32.6	59.0	60.7	62.9	102%	94%
C-165	32.1	38.7	70.8	74.8	65.6	88%	108%
B-641	30.4	33.6	64.0	66.9	70.1	105%	91%
B-487	21.7	38.9	60.6	69.0	66.9	97%	91%
C-481	24.2	28.9	53.1	58.2	58.6	101%	91%
B-734	30.6	30.1	60.7	63.5	55.4	87%	110%
C-24	25.4	22.7	48.4	46.3	51.2	111%	95%
Mean ± SD	27.3 ± 3.8	32.2 ± 5.7	59.5 ± 7.2	62.8 ± 9.1	61.5 ± 6.8	98.7 ± 8.8	97.1 ± 8.3

[a]BoT8 was detected by mAb IL-A17, BoT4 by IL-A12, BoT2 by IL-A26, and BoT3 by IL-A28.

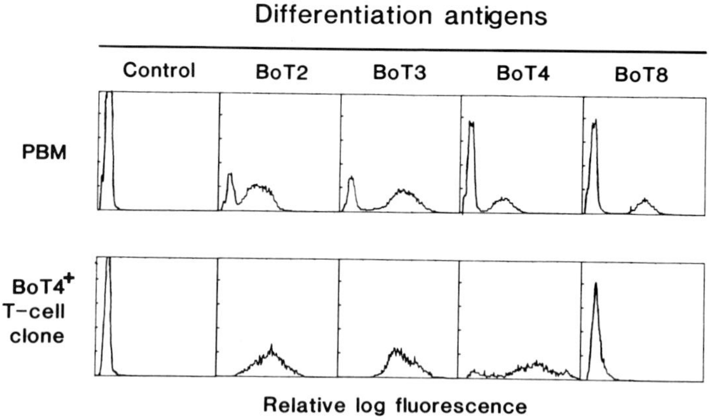

Figure 2 FACS profile of PBM (top row), and BoT4$^+$ T-cell clone (bottom row), stained with mAb reactive with T-cell differentiation antigens. The control was cells with no mAb. BoT2 was identified by mAb IL-A26, BoT3 by mAb IL-A28, BoT4 by mAb IL-A12, and BoT8 by mAb IL-A17. Intensity of fluorescence is presented as a log scale, identical for all mAb. The ordinate is relative cell numbers.

(Fig. 2). The BoT2$^+$ cells, together with those identified as monocytes either by nonspecific esterase staining (49) or by mAb (12,13), and those identified as B cells by expression of sIg (14,15), account for about 80-90% of total mononuclear cells in the peripheral blood in adult cattle. However, calves less than 1 year of age and some adults can have as much as 30% of PBM not identifiable by these markers (Baldwin et al., unpublished results). The function of these cells remains unknown, although work is currently in progress to define this, and a mAb, IL-A29, has been raised which reacts uniquely with a portion of these cells (unpublished).

In humans, mAb have been produced which react with three distinct epitopes on the T11 antigen (50). Epitope 1 ($T11_1$) is ascribed with rosetting of RBC, and mAb to this epitope block rosette formation. In cattle, mAb IL-A26, B26A, CH61A, and CH128A all block rosette formation of bovine lymphocytes by greater than 95% and are therefore attributed with recognizing $BoT2_1$ (20,21).

Monoclonal antibodies to the other T11 epitopes in humans do not block rosette formation, but they can be distinguished from one another by the fact that $T11_3$ is only expressed on activated lymphocytes; its expression is very rapid, within 2 hours, after stimulation (51). When mAb to $T11_2$ and $T11_3$ are combined they stimulate T-cell proliferation even in the absence of monocytes or IL-1 (51). Stimulation of T lymphocytes via the T11 molecule is believed to constitute a pathway of T-cell activation which is alternative to that mediated by the T-cell receptor complex. Reinherz suggests that this is important in intrathymic ontogeny, during which cells responding to self MHC antigens are rendered nonresponsive (51).

Co-staining inhibition studies of bovine PBM using a mAb to $BoT2_1$ and another mAb, CH61A, have shown that the two mAb react with the same cell population (21). Furthermore, CH61A also precipitates a molecule of 55 Kd (21) but it does not block E-rosette formation. On this basis, it is believed to recognize an epitope analogous to human $T11_2$ ($BoT2_2$).

Monoclonal antibodies to BoT2 have proven very useful as pan-T-cell markers, and are expressed on activated as well as resting T lymphocytes (Fig. 2). Cloned bovine T-cell populations specific for either alloantigens or autologous cells infected with the protozoan parasite *Theileria parva* express BoT2 at high density (Fig. 2); these include clones with helper or cytotoxic function. In the peripheral blood all of the T cells which express either of the subset markers BoT4 and BoT8 are within the BoT2$^+$ population (see Section II.C) (Fig. 1; Table 3). Staining of cryostat sections of thymus by the immunoperoxidase technique and FACS analysis of thymic suspensions indicate that the about 80% of thymocytes express BoT2 (9,20). This is in agreement with results of Renshaw who showed that the majority of fetal bovine thymocytes formed E rosettes (52).

There is evidence that mAb to $T11_1$ can uniformly block cytolytic activity of human alloreactive T-lymphocyte clones (53). We found that mAb IL-A26 in some instances blocked cytotoxicity of a bulk population of bovine alloreactive lymphocytes generated in vitro in a mixed leukocyte culture (MLC) by more than 50%, whereas in other instances it had no effect on cytotoxicity.

A mAb believed to react with the bovine analogue of T3 (BoT3) has been described by Rabinovsky and Yang (11). This antibody, BLT-1, reacts with 92% of nylon nonadherent lymphocytes and with all peripheral lymphocytes reactive with an anti-bovine thymocyte serum. At ILRAD, we have also developed two mAb (IL-A27 and IL-A28) of the IgG1 and IgM isotypes which are tentatively ascribed to recognition of BoT3, based on tissue distribution and functional characteristics (20, Fig. 2). They are pan-T-cell mAb when used with PBM and do not react with monocytes, granulocytes, or B lymphocytes. Using PBM from seven cattle we found a small but distinct population of PBM that expresses BoT2 but not BoT3, as well as a small population that expresses BoT3 but not BoT4 or BoT8 (Fig. 2, Table 3). The results indicate that the majority of, but not all, mature bovine T cells express BoT3, BoT2, and either BoT4 or BoT8.

In the thymus the picture is radically different. Only about 28% of thymocytes express BoT3, based on results by Rabinovsky and Yang (11) and Baldwin et al. (20), and the majority of these are within the thymic medulla based on tissue staining. This is in agreement with results of staining of human thymocytes and thymus sections with mAb against CD3 (27,29). This property is useful for rapidly distinguishing mAb reactive with BoT3 from those recognizing BoT2; not only does BoT2 stain a higher proportion of thymocytes (Fig. 1), but cells expressing BoT2 are found in both the cortex and the medulla (20). Rabinovsky and Yang (11) reported that thymic hormones could induce expression of BoT3 on bovine thymocytes, suggesting that it is a marker of mature T cells.

Results of immunoblotting experiments performed by Rabinovsky and Yang (11) indicate that a 22-Kd molecule is recognized by the mAb BLT-1. In man and mouse, T3 is composed of several glycoprotein subunits with molecular masses ranging from 20 to 27 Kd with one major component around 20 Kd (54, 55). The ability of a mAb to identify more than one subunit of a complex molecule is very much dependent on the epitope with which it reacts and the labeling and extraction method used to characterize the antigen. Characterization of BoT3 using mAb directed towards different epitopes may reveal that it also is composed of several subunits of varying molecular weights. It has not yet been possible to precipitate any molecules with mAb IL-A27 or IL-A28.

Preliminary studies with BLT-1 failed to show functional similarities with antibodies against human T3; the antibody was not mitogenic and did not block PHA-induced proliferation. Studies with IL-A27, however, indicate that antibodies against BoT3 can activate T cells to proliferate. When attached to Sepharose 4B beads as well as in solution, mAb IL-A27 is able to stimulate proliferation of PBM (20) in a manner similar to that observed with mAb to CD3 molecules in humans (56). In contrast, mAb IL-A12, which reacts with BoT4, has no stimulatory ability whether in soluble form or fixed to Sepharose 4B beads (20). Incubation of PBM with either mAb (IL-A27 or IL-A12) attached to Sepharose 4B beads has shown that rosetting of PBM around the beads occurs in an antigen-specific manner. For instance, soluble mAb IL-A27 blocks all rosetting of PBM with IL-A27-coated beads, but has no effect on rosetting with IL-A12-coated beads. We have found a difference in the magnitude of stimulation by IL-A27 among cattle which is not related to the ability of the PBM to produce T-cell growth factor (TCGF) in vitro (Baldwin, unpublished results). The relatively low response of PBM from some animals seems to correlate with the presence of monocytes, since monocyte-depleted PBM give a more consistent response among animals.

Monoclonal antibody IL-A27 gave low levels (33%) of blocking of cytotoxicity by uncloned populations of cytotoxic effectors. The capacity to inhibit cytotoxicity is not enhanced when the antibody is linked to Sepharose 4B beads. In the same assays where IL-A27 inhibited cytotoxicity, mAb IL-A28, an IgM antibody that also reacts with BoT3, enhanced killing. In some other assays, similar potentiation of cytotoxicity was observed with mAb IL-A27. The reason for this is unclear, but may relate to enhanced contact between effector and target cells through cross-linking by the mAb or by triggering cytolytic cells in a nonspecific manner as T3 does with human T cells (57). The discrepancies between the functional effects of mAb BLT-1, mAb IL-A27, and mAb to CD3 molecules in humans may result from differences in the isotypes of the antibodies as suggested previously (11), or because they recognize different epitopes on the molecule which are associated with different functions.

C. T-lymphocyte Subset Markers: BoT4 and BoT8

BoT4 is the bovine equivalent of CD4 in humans (1,17), whereas BoT8 defines the reciprocal T-cell subset in cattle, analogous to CD8 in humans (2,17). Although these are nonoverlapping populations in PBM, these antigens are shared by a large proportion of thymocytes (Figs. 1 and 3). Together the antibodies stain about 60% of PBM (Table 3) and about 75% of thymocytes. Most cattle have slightly more BoT4$^+$ cells in their PBM than BoT8$^+$, and calves generally have a lower proportion of both in their PBM than adult cattle (Table 4). In adult cattle, BoT4 and BoT8 together account for the majority of BoT2$^+$/BoT3$^+$ lymphocytes in PBM.

BoT4 is expressed on approximately 30% of bovine PBM (1, Table 3) with a range of 20-40%. BoT8 is found on about 18% of PBM (2), but ranges from 10 to 32% (2; Table 3). These are similar to the proportions of CD4$^+$ and CD8$^+$ cells in the peripheral blood of humans (58,59), SBU-T4$^+$ and SBU-T8$^+$ cells in sheep (4), and PT4$^+$ and PT8$^+$ cells in swine (6). In thymic cell suspensions, BoT4 and BoT8 are each expressed on about 70% of the cells and over 60% express both markers based on dual fluorescence staining (Fig. 3) and additive staining with mAb to BoT4 and BoT8. Thymocytes which express only BoT4 or BoT8 also express BoT3 (20, Fig. 1). This is similar to results in other species.

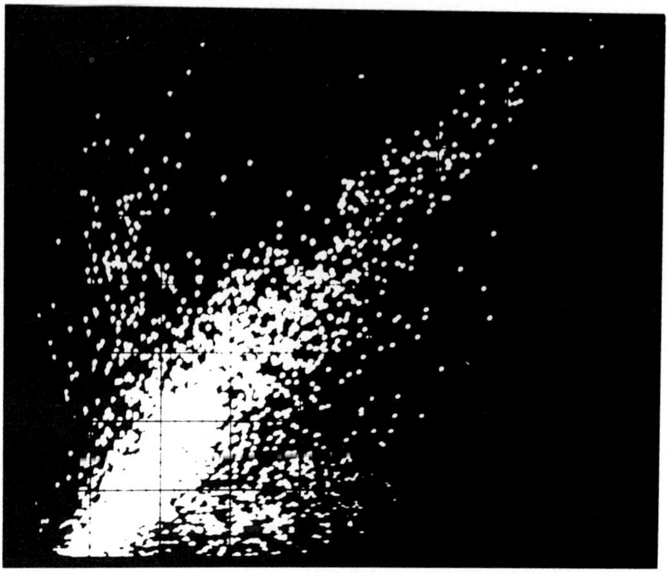

Figure 3 FACS analysis of dual fluorescence of a thymocyte suspension stained with mAb IL-A12 (BoT4) and mAb IL-A17 (BoT8). Thymocytes were prepared, and dual fluorescence staining conducted, essentially as described by Ellis et al. (2). The majority of thymocytes express both BoT4 and BoT8. Small populations (about 5%) express only one or other of the markers.

Table 4 Expression of T-cell and B-cell Differentiation Antigens by PBM from Calves and Adult Cattle

Group[a]	Differentiation antigen sIg	BoT4	BoT8	Total[b] %
Calves	27.5[c] ± 4.2	20.7 ± 4.9	13.1 ± 2.3	61.3%
Adults	35.2 ± 8.4	28.1 ± 11.6	27.7 ± 7.6	85.0%

[a]Calves were less than 1 year (n = 8); adults were over 2 years (n = 12).
[b]The sum of the percentage sIg$^+$, BoT4$^+$, and BoT8$^+$ cells is indicated.
[c]The mean ± SD are indicated. Percentage "+" cells were derived from FACS analysis of fluorescence staining. All staining was done at the same time. sIg was detected by heteroantiserum, BoT4 by mAb IL-A12, and BoT8 by mAb IL-A17.

$BoT4^+$ and $BoT8^+$ lymphocytes can be distinguished on the basis of functional activities as distinct subsets of cells. When PBM are sorted by the FACS into either $BoT4^+$ and $BoT4^-$ populations, or into $BoT8^+$ and $BoT8^-$ populations, marked differences in the capacities of the populations to respond to mitogens or alloantigens are observed. $BoT4^+$ and $BoT8^-$ populations proliferate very well to phytohemagglutinin (PHA), concanavalin A (Con A), or alloantigens without requiring exogenous growth factors, e.g., TCGF or monocytes. Bovine lymphocytes are able to proliferate to mitogens without monocytes if the culture medium contains 2-mercaptoethanol (60). The reciprocal populations, $BoT8^+$ or $BoT4^-$, however, do not proliferate, or proliferate to a much lesser degree than the $BoT4^+$ and $BoT8^-$ populations (Fig. 4). When TCGF is added to cultures of $BoT8^+$ cells, proliferation is enhanced, but often is still less than that seen with $BoT4^+$ or $BoT8^-$ cells (Fig. 4). The addition of monocytes to these cultures does not increase the response of $BoT8^+$ cells (2).

The results indicate that $BoT4^+$ PBM are able to generate the necessary growth factors for proliferation, whereas $BoT8^+$ PBM cannot. There is some indication,

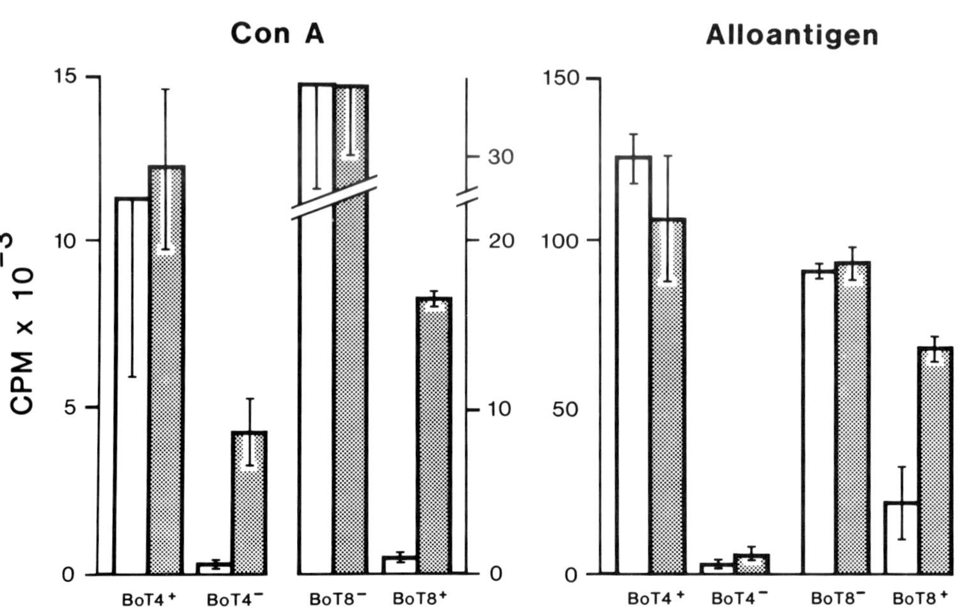

Figure 4 Proliferative responses of PBM sorted by the FACS into either $BoT4^+$ and $BoT4^-$ populations by mAb IL-A12, or into $BoT8^-$ and $BoT8^+$ populations by mAb IL-A17, as described elsewhere (1). Sorted populations were stimulated with either Con A or allogeneic PBM (alloantigen) without addition of exogenous TCGF (open bars) or in presence of TCGF (dotted bars). Proliferation was assessed by incorporation of [^{125}I] iododeoxyuridine and is reported as counts per minute (CPM).

Table 5 Production of Soluble Growth Factors by BoT4$^+$ Alloreactive T-cell Clones

	TCGF activity of supernatant from cells stimulated by[a]		
BoT4$^+$ clone	Medium	Con A	Allogeneic PBM
2.4	79[b]	9,104	1,381
4.8	401	4,510	4,809
4.3	389	1,792	446

[a]Stimulator cells were fixed with glutaraldehyde (1). 5×10^5 responder cells were stimulated with 2×10^6 stimulator cells or 2.5 μg Con A/ml, in 2 ml medium in 24-well culture dishes. Background responses are either medium controls or from clones stimulated with autologous stimulator cells. Supernatents were collected after 24 hr and filtered through a 0.45-μm filter.
[b]Supernatants were assayed for growth factor activity by culturing with a TCGF-dependent T-cell line. Proliferation was assessed by incorporation of [^{125}I]iododeoxyuridine after 48 hr of culture and is expressed as counts per minute of incorporated radioactivity. Supernatants were assayed in cultures at 50% v/v.

as well, that even in the presence of exogenous TCGF and/or monocytes, BoT8$^+$ cells often have a lower intrinsic capacity to proliferate. It may be that fewer cells within the population are able to respond, or that the cells respond slower initially (require more time to enter the first mitotic cycle), or that they divide fewer times during the assay period (have a longer cell cycle).

The isolation of alloreactive bovine T-cell clones (17) has made it possible to evaluate the functions of T cells within the BoT4$^+$ and BoT8$^+$ populations on an individual basis. Antigen-specific proliferation assays have indicated that BoT4$^+$ clones overall have a greater ability to proliferate than BoT8$^+$ clones without addition of exogenous TCGF (1), confirming results obtained with FACS-sorted PBM. Evaluation of supernatants of BoT4$^+$ clones have shown that they secrete soluble growth factors (Table 5) when stimulated with the appropriate alloantigen or Con A.

Studies with BoT8$^+$ clones which are cytolytic for autologous cells infected with the protozoan parasite *Theileria parva* have provided evidence that some BoT8$^+$ clones also produce the necessary growth factors required for proliferation (Table 6). Thus, they are able to proliferate when cultured with appropriate stimulator cells which have been gamma or UV-irradiated or fixed with glutaraldehyde. So, although BoT4$^+$ cells may have a greater tendency towards self-contained proliferative responses, BoT8$^+$ cells are not incapable of proliferating

Table 6 Proliferation of Cytolytic BoT8$^+$ Clones Reactive with Cells Infected with *T. parva* When Stimulated by Gamma or UV-irradiated, or Glutaraldehyde-fixed Stimulators Without Addition of Exogenous TCGF (Blocking by mAb IL-A12 and IL-A17[a])

		Treatment of stimulator cells and presence of mAb				
Clone	No stimulators	UV irradiated	Glutaraldehyde fixed	Gamma irradiated	Gamma irradiated/ mAb IL-A12	Gamma irradiated/ mAb IL-A17
14.1	670[b] ± 554	6,107 ± 970	559 ± 164	8,121 ± 364	6,207 ± 918	677 ± 84
14.58	340 ± 87	128,981 ± 8,944	44,951 ± 1,201	161,025 ± 16,907	223,507 ± 56,601	117,816 ± 2,837

[a]Responders were seeded at 10^5 cells/well and stimulated with 2×10^5 cells/well for 5 days. Stimulator cells were prepared and cultured essentially as described elsewhere (1).
[b]Proliferation was assessed by counts per minute of incorporated [^{125}I] iododeoxyuridine.

without addition of exogenous growth factors. Similar results have been found with Ly2$^+$ lymphocyte clones (61), the murine equivalent of CD8.

Using bulk populations of cytolytic effectors generated in mixed leukocyte cultures (MLC) of PBM from cattle sensitized to the appropriate alloantigens in vivo by skin grafting (62), it has been shown that the BoT8$^+$ population contains cytolytic cells (2). These results were obtained by sorting cells from a MLC into BoT8$^+$ and BoT8$^-$ populations with the FACS and subsequently testing them on target cells expressing high levels of class I MHC antigens. The ability of the BoT8$^+$ cells to kill was greater than that of the unsorted population. Similarly, when the effector population was depleted of BoT4$^+$ cells, no reduction in cytolytic activity was found when tested on targets expressing both class I and class II MHC antigens (1). Cytolytic cells may be present within the BoT4$^+$ population; however, the proportion of cells that are cytolytic effectors may be lower than in the BoT8$^+$ population. A further consideration is that class II antigen expression is generally not as high as class I expression on the target cells used.

Studies with alloreactive T-cell clones, however, have demonstrated that BoT4$^+$ cells may be cytolytic (17). Bulk MLC of bovine PBM may contain cells which suppress cytotoxic activity of BoT4$^+$ cells, as suggested by Vidovic et al. (63), to occur in MLC of murine lymphocytes. Mastro and Hurley have generated suppressor cells by stimulating lymph node cells with Con A or tumor-promoting phorbol esters. Both types of suppressor cells, which arise from different precursor populations as assessed by binding of peanut agglutinin, are able to inhibit MLC proliferation (Mastro and Hurley, personal communication). Their effect on cytolytic activity of either the BoT4$^+$ or BoT8$^+$ population has not yet been determined.

The hallmark of CD4 and CD8 lymphocytes and their analogues in mice is their restriction of recognition of foreign antigen in conjunction with class II or class I MHC antigens, respectively (31-34), although exceptions have been noted (64). In cattle, MHC antigens coded for by one class I BoLA locus (the A locus) have been defined by alloantisera and mAb (12,16,17,65). Studies with BoT8$^+$ cytotoxic T-cell clones specific for lymphoblasts infected with *T. parva* have clearly demonstrated that they are restricted by class I MHC molecules (66). Similarly, evidence has been obtained that alloantigen-specific BoT8$^+$ clones are specific for class I MHC antigens (17). Polymorphic reagents are not yet available to adequately define polymorphic determinants on bovine class II MHC molecules. However, using BoT4$^+$ alloantigen-specific T-cell clones, Teale and coworkers (17) have demonstrated that their restriction pattern does not correlate with expression of BoLA A-locus products. Additional evidence to support the contention that they are class II-restricted comes from the observation that the proportion of target cells killed in cytotoxicity assays by BoT4$^+$ clones correlates with the proportion of targets that express class II MHC antigens, as detected by mAb that react with monomorphic epitopes on class II molecules (see Section V). Some of these mAb, including one antibody directed against HLA-DR which cross-reacts with bovine class II molecules, are able to block cytolytic activity of BoT4$^+$ alloantigen-specific clones but not BoT8$^+$ clones (17). Conversely, antibodies to monomorphic epitopes on bovine class I MHC molecules can block cytotoxicity of some BoT8$^+$ clones but not BoT4$^+$ clones (17). The ability of the antibodies to block varies among clones, and may relate to their affinity as has been suggested for human and murine clones (67-69).

CD4 and CD8 molecules have been postulated to interact with nonpolymorphic portions of class II and class I MHC molecules, respectively, on the target cell (36,70). By analogy, BoT4 and BoT8 molecules may be required by some T cells to provide adequate interaction of the T-cell receptor with either MHC alloantigens or autologous MHC antigens in conjunction with foreign antigens. Blocking studies using mAb IL-A11, IL-A12, and IL-A17 have shown little or no effect of these mAb on the proliferative responses of PBM to stimulation by mitogens or allogeneic cells, or on generation of cytolytic effectors in MLC (1,2). However, variable levels of blocking of cytotoxicity (0-64%) by mAb IL-A17 have been observed when bulk cultures of alloreactive cytotoxic cells generated in MLC with PBM from cattle primed with alloantigens in vivo are incubated with IL-A17 in cytotoxicity assays (Fig. 5; 2). Blocking was found for both primary and secondary stimulated MLC in vitro although blocking decreased after the second stimulation from 64 to 35%. Similarly, *Theileria*-specific MHC-restricted cytotoxic T lymphocytes (CTL) generated in vivo in animals undergoing challenge with *T. parva* could be inhibited to variable degrees (10-60%) by incubation with mAb IL-A17 (Morrison, unpublished).

When tested on alloreactive T-cell clones, inhibition of proliferation or cytotoxicity of some but not all clones by mAb IL-A11/IL-A12 or IL-A17 has been

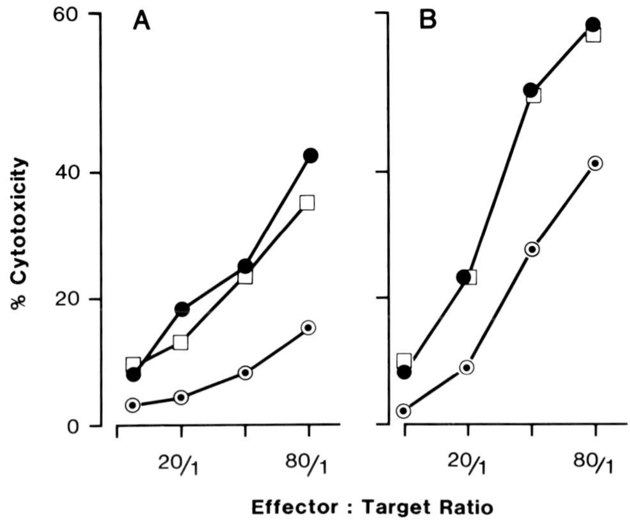

Figure 5 Inhibition of cytotoxicity by effector cells generated in vitro by stimulation in a MLC either one time (A), or two times (B). Effector PBM were from a cow which had been immunized in vivo by skin grafting (59). The ability of mAb IL-A17 (open circles), mAb W6/32 (squares), or no mAb (closed circles) to inhibit cytotoxicity was assessed. Cytotoxicity assays and blocking were carried out as described previously (1).

observed. MAb IL-A12 blocked the proliferation of three out of five $BoT4^+$ clones by 50% or more (1). Similar inhibition of the cytotoxic activity of some of these clones, by mAb directed against BoT4, has been detected (17). Variable levels of blocking of cytotoxicity by mAb IL-A17 has also been found among $BoT8^+$ clones (17; Table 6).

From these results, it is clear that at the clonal level these mAb are capable of inhibiting either proliferation or cytotoxicity to variable degrees. The failure to detect inhibition of proliferation of bulk MLC by mAb to BoT4 may be due to the presence of significant numbers of $BoT4^+$ cells which are not susceptible to blocking by the antibodies and to the participation of $BoT4^-$ T cells in these proliferative responses. Conversely, the finding that cytotoxicity of bulk populations was inhibited by IL-A17 indicates that a major proportion of the cytotoxic cells in these populations is susceptible to blocking.

Biochemical characterization of both BoT4 and BoT8 has demonstrated similarities of the physical characteristics of these molecules with analogues in other species, although differences are also observed. BoT4 has been precipitated as two polypeptide chains of 52 and 55 Kd, while only one chain of a similar molecular mass was precipitated in the case of human Leu-3 (55 Kd) (3), and murine L3T4 molecule (52 Kd) (71). Both polypeptide chains of BoT4 appear to be expressed

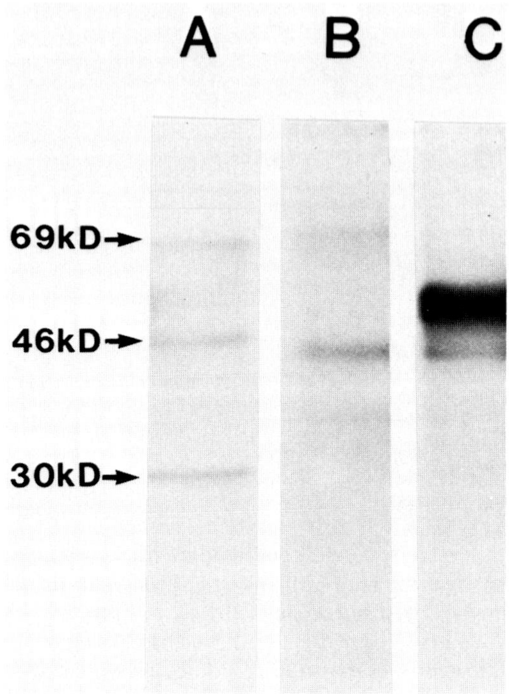

Figure 6 SDS-PAGE of molecules precipitated by mAb IL-A12 (BoT4) from a BoT4+ T-cell line or from a BoT4⁻ cell line which had been labeled by iodination of surface molecules as described elsewhere (63). Lane A, molecular weight markers; lane B, BoT4⁻ cell line; lane C, BoT4+ cell line.

in similar concentrations on the membranes (Fig. 6). It has been suggested that the two chains may occur as a result of posttranslational modifications (1). BoT8 also occurs as two chains on both thymocytes and mature T lymphocytes (2). The BoT8 doublet on bovine lymphocytes, which is composed of molecules of 34 and 35 Kd, is similar in molecular mass to the two chains of PT8 on swine T lymphocytes, 33-35 Kd, found by Jonjic and Koszinowski (72), although Pescovitz et al. only found one chain (73). It differs from analogues in other species which occur as doublets only on thymocytes, and as singular entities on mature T lymphocytes (3-5).

Overall, the similarities of BoT4 and BoT8, and of the T lymphocytes which express them, to the analogues in other species are striking, and the minor differences not unexpected. These reagents have provided tools to probe the involvement of the lymphocyte subsets in immune responses of cattle to pathogens. In cattle infected with *T. parva*, they have been used to characterize BoT8+ cytotoxic T-cell clones which are restricted by class I MHC molecules and specific for *T. parva* strain-specific antigens (60), as well as BoT4$^+$ clones which are also strain restricted and express helper activity (74).

D. T-lymphocyte Blast Antigens

Three mAb, J5, J6, and P13, react exclusively with bovine T-lymphocyte blasts (10,22). None of these mAb react with resting PBM. In addition, J5 and J6 have been tested with lymph node cells, thymocytes, bone marrow cells, neutrophils, fibroblasts, and bovine leukosis virus-infected B cells and found to be negative on all (10). J5 and J6 are believed to react with different epitopes of the same molecule. Although they demonstrate reciprocal inhibition of binding, and both precipitate molecules of 100 Kd, only the binding of J6 is sensitive to treatment of the target cells with trypsin, chymotrypsin, or proteinase K (10). Both J5 and J6 react with all sIg$^-$ lymphoblasts following stimulation of PBM with Con A or pokeweed mitogen. Expression of the molecule is maximal at 24 hr after stimulation with Con A, whereas B cells stimulated by pokeweed mitogen remain negative for both J5 and J6 throughout the culture period.

Continuously cultured T-cell lines show variation in the kinetics of expression of J5 and J6 (10). An alloreactive cell line expressed the J5/J6 molecule maximally at 3 days after stimulation and became negative by day 7. No cycling of expression was found with an antigen-independent/TCGF-dependent cell line continually cultured in the presence of TCGF. This suggests that a difference in cell cycle and activation may occur between these two cell lines. It may indicate that the TCGF-dependent line does not return to G_0, but is continually in a blast state. Continuous expression of the J5/J6 molecule has also been found on bovine lymphocytes transformed into continually proliferating cells by infection with *T. parva.* This observation promotes speculation that the molecule may be synthesized during the S phase in the cell cycle. If this speculation is correct, it appears that antigen-responsive T-cell lines enter an obligate prolonged G_0/G_1 after each antigenic stimulus as determined by periodic absence of expression of the J5 and J6 T-cell-restricted blast markers.

The blast antigens recognized by mAb J5 and J6 have some similarities with cell-surface molecules described in other species. The molecular weight of the J5/J6 precipitated molecule under reducing conditions (100 Kd) is the same as that for the transferrin receptor (40), but differs by the fact that it is not expressed on non-T cells of hematopoietic origin, and under nonreducing conditions the molecule does not form a dimer of 200 Kd (Naessens, unpublished). Neither J5 nor J6 are able to block proliferation of a TCGF-dependent T-cell line (10), indicating that neither molecule is involved in uptake of required nutrients or growth factors, or that the reactivity of the mAb with the particular epitope is inadequate to block either uptake of such factors or the response of the cell.

The T-cell blast antigen recognized by P13 differs from that of J5 and J6, as only a portion of blast cells express the P13 determinant following Con A or PHA stimulation (22). P13 is also expressed somewhat later than the J5/J6 molecule, i.e., day 4 to 5 after stimulation. However in MLC, 70% of the blast cells express P13 by day 7 (22). P13 precipitates a molecule of about 160 Kd from the surface of lymphoblasts; it also reacts with a cytokeratin-like molecule of approximately 55 Kd within bovine epithelial cells (Morrison, unpublished). The kinetics of expression and cellular distribution of the P13 molecule is similar to blast antigens on alloreactive T-cell blasts described in man and mouse (22). The function of these blast antigens is not known.

E. T-lymphocyte Markers Shared with Monocytes and Granulocytes

Before the advent of the more restricted T-lymphocyte differentiation antigens described above, these mAb were very useful for delineating T cells from B cells. MAb P5 (12) recognizes most, if not all, T cells in PBM; the number of positive cells in the PBM of 25 cattle was found to range from 44 to 83% (12). It has been demonstrated that most blast cells arising in cultures stimulated with Con A or with allogeneic cells are $P5^+$, indicating that the majority of the responsive cells are T cells. P5 also reacts with monocytes, the majority of which can be distinguished from T cells in PBM on the basis of their size using forward-angle light scattering analysis on the FACS.

Expression of the cell-surface molecule recognized by mAb P5 has a bimodal distribution on PBM, with the mean fluorescence of the "P5-high expressors" being 3-fold greater than that on the "P5-low expressors" (12). The proportion of P5-low and P5-high expressors varies among individual cattle. Monocytes are always high expressors of P5, whereas thymocytes, which also express P5, are all low expressors. Lymphocyte antigens with a bimodal distribution have been described in other species; thus, PT8 in swine (6) has low expression on some $PT4^+$ PBM, and Ly1 in mice has low expression on some $Ly2,3^+$ lymphocytes (75) and on a small subpopulation of B cells (76,77). Although no functional relevance can be assigned to expression of the antigen recognized by P5, it has been gainfully employed as a reagent for distinguishing T cells from B cells (12).

Monoclonal antibodies BT3/8.12 and J3 react with different epitopes on the same molecules (10). Although the epitope recognized by BT3/8.12 is expressed by some but not all T cells (15), by 15-20% of thymocytes, and by monocytes and granulocytes, the epitope defined by mAb J3 is only found on a proportion of mature T cells and monocytes (10). The epitope recognized by J3 is also susceptible to neuraminidase and β-N-acetylglucosaminidase treatment, whereas that recognized by BT3/8.12 is not. On lymphocytes, mAb BT3/8.12 is able to completely inhibit the binding of mAb J3, whereas mAb J3 can only partially inhibit binding of BT3/8.12 (10). This shows that the lymphocyte membrane contains sialylated ($J3^+$) as well as nonsialylated ($J3^-$) molecules. The expression, or lack

Table 7 Proportion of BoT4$^+$ PBM from Individual Cattle Which React with mAb BT3/8.12

Animal	Percentage of cells reacting with mAb or expressing antigen indicated			% BoT4$^+$ PBM reacting with mAb BT3/8.12
	BT3/8.12	BoT4	BT3/8.12 + BoT4	
C-234	57	27	71	48%
C-447	47	23	48	100%
C-165	54	27	55	100%
C-197	62	32	78	50%
C-196	57	31	78	32%
C-210	49	25	63	44%
Mean ± SD	54 ± 6	28 ± 3	66 ± 12	62 ± 30%

thereof, of BT3/8.12 reactivity does not change after normal PBM are activated. PBM sorted into BT3/8.12$^+$ and BT3/8.12$^-$ populations with the FACS, and subsequently stimulated with Con A and TCGF, retain their original phenotype (10).

There is no correlation between reactivity with BT3/8.12 and expression of BoT4 or BoT8 on T lymphocytes. MAb BT3/8.12 reacts with approximately 50% of PBM (10; Table 7), with a range of 47 to 62% in six cattle tested (Table 7). In two of these cattle, virtually all BoT4$^+$ PBM reacted with BT3/8.12, in three cattle about half of the BoT4$^+$ PBM reacted with BT3/8.12, and in one animal about one third of the BoT4$^+$ PBM reacted with BT3/8.12 (Table 7). In some experiments, staining of alloreactive T-cell clones, defined as BoT4$^+$ or BoT8$^+$, have indicated a greater tendency for mAb BT3/8.12 to react with BoT8$^+$ clones than with BoT4$^+$ clones (Newson and Teale, personal communication). However, it is clear that both BoT4$^+$ and BoT8$^+$, cytolytic and noncytolytic clones may or may not react with BT3/8.12. Thus, no correlation has been established for cell functions and expression of the molecule recognized by BT3/8.12.

The determinants recognized by BT3/8.12, J3, and P5 are expressed on transformed T and B cells: a bovine lymphoid tumor cell line which expresses sIg, BL20 (78), reacts with BT3/8.12 and P5; and both T and B cells infected with *T. parva* are positive for BT3/8.12, J3, and P5 determinants (10,22, Newson, personal communication). These studies suggest that expression of the "BT3/8.12 gene" occurs in B and T lymphocytes when cell growth is deregulated and lineage-specific differentiation and possibly function are lost (10) since negative T-cell clones acquire the BT3/8.12 molecule after transformation with *T. parva*.

The function of the antigens defined by mAb BT3/8.12, J3, and P5 remains elusive. Furthermore, the significance of why T cells and monocytes retain the exclusive capacity to sialylate the BT3/8.12 molecule, giving rise to the J3 epitope, is not known. Perhaps they are important molecules in cell communication or growth regulation in normal lymphocytes.

III. B LYMPHOCYTES

A. Introduction

For many years polyspecific heteroantisera against bovine immunoglobulins have proven useful for identifying bovine B cells by their expression of surface immunoglobulin (sIg) (79). Isotype-specific heteroantisera which react with IgM, IgG1, IgG2, or IgA have been produced in goats (80). Using such reagents it is possible to examine the relative proportion of sIg^+ cells in various lymphoid tissues, attribute immunological responses to B cells, and deplete B cells from cell populations (46,81) in order to examine immunological responses of other cell types, such as T cells. However, very little is known about the expression of the various Ig isotypes during ontogeny and activation of bovine B lymphocytes. In the case of activated B cells, the lectin peanut agglutinin has been found to react with germinal center B cells (47,82) and no doubt could be used, as in other species (83), for isolation of these cells for functional studies.

B cells also express complement and Fc receptors, which may be considered differentiation markers and can be identified by rosetting techniques. However, by simultaneously rosetting with erythrocyte-antibody-complement (EAC) complexes to detect complement receptors, and staining by immunofluorescence to detect sIg, it has been demonstrated that not all bovine B cells have complement receptors. Approximately 15-20% of sIg^+ PBM do not form EAC rosettes (79; Baldwin, unpublished results). Furthermore, monocytes also express complement receptors (79). The usefulness of Fc receptors as B-cell markers is limited by the fact that at least half of all B cells do not express Fc receptors (79,84), and some T cells and monocytes express Fc receptors (79). Monoclonal antibodies and isotype-specific heteroantisera (Table 8), therefore, not only provide more comprehensive tools with which to identify B cells than rosetting techniques, but the specific isotype of the sIg, as well as the isotype of cytoplasmic and secreted immunoglobulin of B cells, can be identified.

B. Monoclonal Antibodies to Surface Immunoglobins

At ILRAD, several mAb have been developed which react with various Ig isotypes (Table 8). Wells and Kar developed a mAb, IL-A2, which is specific for IgG (unpublished results). Using a radioimmune assay employing purified bovine Ig of different isotypes they showed that IL-A2 reacts with both IgG1 and IgG2 but

Table 8 Monoclonal Antibodies Which Identify Bovine Ig of Various Isotypes

Bovine antigen	Identifying mAb	Isotype of mAb	Refs.
IgG1,2	IL-A2	IgG	Wells and Kar, personal communication
IgM	B5/4.1.4	IgG1	14,15
IgD?	B4/27.23.4	IgG2a	15; Pinder, personal communication

Table 9 Tissue Distribution of B Cells Reacting with mAb B5/4.1.4 and B4/27.23.4 in Bovine Lymphoid Tissues[a]

	% Cells reactings with mAb in different compartments					
Identifying mAb	PBM[b]	Spleen	Lymph node	Tonsil	Thymus	Bone marrow
B4/27.23.4	26	12	40	59	2	4
B5/4.1.4	26	43	47	22	1	0

[a]Part of the data were derived from Pinder et al. (15).
[b]All of the data except that for PBM were obtained from one animal.

not IgM. It was subsequently demonstrated that mAb IL-A2 was able to precipitate bovine Ig from serum, and the isotype of the precipitated Ig was identified by immunoelectrophoresis as IgG. From approximately 15 animals tested, IL-A2 reacted with less than 5% of PBM (Black et al., personal communication).

Pinder and co-workers developed two mAb, B5/4.1.4 and B4/27.23.4, which react with bovine B cells (14,15). B5/4.1.4 is specific for bovine IgM (14), whereas there is evidence that B4/27.23.4 may detect bovine IgD (Pinder and Roelants, personal communication). B5/4.1.4 reacts with a slightly higher proportion of cells from the spleen and lymph node (Table 9), and sometimes PBM (15), but with fewer tonsillar cells than does B4/27.23.4. Furthermore, mAb B4/27.23.4 does not co-cap with B5/4.1.4 or with an anti-IgG Ab (Pinder and Roelants, personal communication). In tissue sections, both mAb give surface staining of small lymphocytes in spleen and lymph node follicles, but very few positive cells in the paracortical areas of lymph nodes or periarteriolar regions of the spleen. In addition, B5/4.1.4. gives cytoplasmic staining of small numbers of cells in the lymph nodes and spleen (15; Morrison and MacHugh, unpublished data). Only B5/4.1.4 precipitates serum Ig, and is specific for IgM (14). Taken together, these similarities and differences of reactivity of B5/4.1.4 and B4/27.23.4 are

Table 10 Percentage of PBM Reactive with mAb B5/4.1.4 and with Heteroantiserum Specific for Bovine IgM

Group	Animal	Reagents used for staining PBM: Heteroantiserum[a]	Reagents used for staining PBM: mAb B5/4.1.4
A.	C589	16	8
	B944	32	23
	C193	37	20
	C22	50	31
	Mean ± SD	38 ± 14	21 ± 10
B.	B654	10	9
	C167	11	12
	C234	12	8
	C580	13	10
	B641	13	12
	C320	16	12
	C18	18	18
	C196	20	19
	C25	22	17
	C165	22	24
	B487	31	29
	B166	33	33
	C19	33	29
	Mean ± SD	20 ± 8	18 ± 8

[a]Heteroantiserum, reactive with bovine IgM, was produced in a goat by immunizing with purified bovine IgM.

consistent with B4/27.23.4 reacting with IgD, but conclusive proof by immunoprecipitation is not yet available.

Using B5/4.1.4 in a dual fluorescence assay with the mAb to BoT3 or BoT2 (see Section II), we have shown that none of the PBM tested express both markers indicating that it is specific in its reactivity with bovine B cells (20). The numbers of sIg^+ cells detected in the PBM of cattle using mAb B5/4.1.4 or heteroantisera varies considerably between individual animals, ranging from 10 to 50% with heteroantisera and from 8 to 33% with mAb B5/4.1.4, in 17 cattle tested (Table 10). We have also found that adult cattle generally have more sIg^+ cells in PBM than do calves (Table 4).

Pinder et al. (14) reported that B5/4.1.4 detects some heterogeneity of serum IgM among cattle. The heterogeneity was in the intensity of binding, as detected both by indirect immunofluorescence staining and in radioimmunoassays. Nonetheless, all cattle tested had some reactivity. In about 25% of cattle tested, the percentage of $sIgM^+$ cells detected by B5/4.1.4 is significantly lower than the number of sIg^+ cells detected by heteroantisera (Black and Olobo, personal communication; Table 10, Group A). These findings suggest that B5/4.1.4 may react with a high frequency IgM allotype. Alternatively differences such as those reported for group A in Table 10 could be attributable to heterogeneity between different animals in the affinity of binding by mAb B5/4.1.4.

IV. MONOCYTES, MACROPHAGES, AND GRANULOCYTES

A. Introduction

Cells of the monocytic lineage comprise a heterogeneous population, both morphologically and functionally. They are found in a variety of tissues and play a role in controlling both the afferent (inductive) and efferent (effector) limbs of immune responses (reviewed by Van Furth, 85). In cattle, mononuclear-phagocytic cells are most accessible in the peripheral blood, lungs, and mammary gland. Populations of cells containing 70-90% monocytes can be obtained by adherence of PBM to plasma-coated gelatin surfaces; further enrichment of such populations for monocytes, to over 95% purity, can be achieved by sorting with the FACS using a monocyte-specific mAb (60). Pulmonary macrophages may be isolated by lung lavage (13), and mammary gland macrophages may be obtained in large quantities by infusion of sterile saline (86) or by inducing inflammatory responses with stimulants such as lipopolysaccharide (87). Characterization of these cells has relied on nuclear morphology, phagocytosis of latex particles, expression of receptors for complement and immunoglobulin Fc (79,88), nonspecific esterase activity (49), peroxidase activity, and acid phosphatase activity (86,88). Such characteristics are often not exclusively expressed by monocytic cells and therefore cannot be considered as lineage-specific markers.

A variety of mAb have been developed in humans and mice to define cells of the monocytic lineage (89-92), but none of these clearly define function of the cells or lineage specificity, though in some instances there is evidence that variation in function is correlated with differences in expression of cell-surface antigens (93-98). Several mAb have been produced to identify cells of the monocytic lineage in cattle (Table 11). Although with one exception the molecules recognized by these mAb have not been characterized biochemically, nor have functional roles been ascribed either to the molecules or to the cells expressing them, the mAb have the capacity to discriminate among cell populations within the monocytic/myeloid lineage of cattle and will no doubt prove useful in functional studies.

Table 11 Monoclonal Antibodies Reactive with Monocytes, Macrophages, and Granulocytes[a]

mAb	Isotype of mAb	Fusion immunization	Reacts with			
			Monocytes	Pulmonary macrophage	Mammary gland macrophage	Granulocytes
IL-A25	IgG1	pul. macro.[b]	–	++++	–	–
IL-A23	IgG1	pul. macro.	±	+++	+	–
P8	IgG2a	monocytes	+	nd[c]	nd	+
IL-A22, IL-A24	IgG1	pul. macro.	++	++	+	+

[a]All mAb described in this table are referenced from Ellis et al. (13) except for P8, from Lalor et al. (12).
[b]Pulmonary macrophages.
[c]nd = not done.

B. Monocyte/Macrophage Markers

Two mAb will be discussed in this section: IL-A23 and IL-A25, produced by Ellis and co-workers at ILRAD (13). Although the results described herein are for mononuclear cells of cattle, these mAb also react with similar specificity with sheep and goat cells. MAb IL-A25 was derived from a hybridoma established from a fusion with spleen cells from a mouse immunized with bovine pulmonary macrophages. It reacts with a molecule uniquely expressed by pulmonary macrophages, as neither monocytes from the peripheral blood nor mammary gland macrophages react with the mAb (Table 11). It appears to be truly a differentiation antigen of the monocyte/macrophage lineage, as it is not expressed by granulocytes, fibroblasts, transformed lymphoblastoid cells or blasting T cells (alloreactive T-cell clones) (13; see Tables 11 and 12).

A second mAb, IL-A23, also reacts with about 50% of pulmonary macrophages but differs from IL-A25 in that it reacts with about 50% of peripheral blood monocytes and 33% of mammary gland macrophages. MAb IL-A23 also reacts with fibroblasts thereby differing from the other mAb described in this section (13). The molecule recognized by mAb IL-A23 has a variable expression on monocytes among cattle, when compared with other mAb (IL-A22 and IL-A24, see below) which react with the maiority of blood monocytes. In some animals, it is

Table 12 Cellular Distribution of Differentiation Antigens Expressed on Monocytic Cells

	Percentage positive[a] cells on		Expression on[c]		
mAb	PBM	Monocyte-[b] depleted PBM	NBC 13	BL3	Fibroblasts
IL-A25	0%	0%	–	–	–
IL-A23	7%	0%	–	–	+
P8	11%	0%	nk[d]	nk	–
IL-A22	9%	0%	–	+	–
IL-A24	9%	0%	+	+	–

[a]Adapted from Ellis et al. (13), Lalor et al. (12), and Goddeeris et al. (60).
[b]The PBM used contained approximately 12% ANAE$^+$ cells. PBM depleted of monocytes had less than 1% ANAE$^+$ cells (60).
[c]NBC 13 is a non-T, non-B lymphoblastoid cell line from a BLV-infected cow; BL3 is a null cell from a BLV-negative cow (99). The fibroblasts were a cell line derived from bovine thymus.
[d]nk = not known.

expressed only at low levels on a small proportion of the monocytes, whereas in others it is present on most of the monocytes (13). Interestingly, mAb IL-A23 reacts strongly with the majority of monocytes from animals in the later stages of infection with *T. parva* (MacHugh and Morrison, unpublished data), suggesting that the mAb may recognize a molecule on monocytes associated with activation of the cells.

C. Monocyte/Granulocyte Markers

Three mAb have been generated which react with granulocytes as well as with monocytes: P8, IL-A22, and IL-A24 (Tables 11 and 12). P8 was derived from a fusion using spleen cells from a mouse immunized with a monocyte-enriched population of PBM (12). It reacts strongly with large PBM which have α-naphthyl acetate esterase activity. It does not react with resting, blasting, or transformed B or T lymphocytes (Table 11), making it a very useful marker for identifying monocytes in PBM populations. Its reactivity with pulmonary or mammary gland macrophages is not known. $P8^+$ cells from PBM have been shown to supply the necessary accessory function in responses of peripheral blood lymphocytes to Con A (60), and to be the stimulatory cell in allogeneic mixed leukocyte reactions (100).

Ellis and colleagues (13) have produced two additional mAb, IL-A22 and IL-A24, with similar specificities, which react with 40 and 31% of bone marrow cells, respectively. These mAb also react with mononuclear phagocytes of goats and sheep. Although both mAb usually react with greater than 90% of monocytes, they sometimes exhibit minor disparities in the proportion of monocytes with which they react in PBM of individual cattle, suggesting that they recognize different molecules or different epitopes on the same molecule. Their target antigen is on less than 25% of mammary gland macrophages, but about 50% of pulmonary macrophages. mAb IL-A24 also has been found to react with a lymphoblastoid cell line, NBC 13, derived from a cow infected with bovine leukemia virus (Ellis, personal communication), thus distinguishing the epitope it recognizes from that of mAb IL-A22 (Table 12). In addition, both mAb IL-A22 and IL-A24 react with BL3, another lymphoblastoid cell line from a nonbovine-leukosis virus-infected cow. mAb IL-A24 has been shown to precipitate two polypeptides of about 75 Kd and 110 Kd from blood monocytes (13). Purified immunoglobulin of IL-A24 blocks antigen-specific proliferation of T cells to keyhole limpet hemocyanin, presumably by blocking the ability of monocytes to act as accessory cells (13).

V. BoLA MOLECULES

A. Introduction

As stated earlier alloantisera have been used to define BoLA specificities encoded by one class I locus (101,102). There is also unconfirmed serological evidence for additional class I products (103) and for class II polymorphic specificities (104). A number of monoclonal antibodies have also been produced which recognize monomorphic or polymorphic determinants on bovine class I or class II molecules (9,12,16,17,19,66,105). Moreover, many antisera and mAb produced against human class I and class II products (HLA) cross-react with bovine MHC molecules (9,106-112). The significance of cross-reacting epitopes between HLA and BoLA is unclear.

There is some evidence obtained by Bensaid and co-workers (16), from studies using sequential immunoprecipitation with mAb and alloantisera against polymorphic epitopes, that more than two BoLA class I products are expressed on the surface of bovine cells. The class I molecules were composed of a heavy chain of 44-45 Kd associated with a β_2-microglobulin light chain which has a molecular mass of 12 Kd. Bensaid et al. (16) have used B1.1G6, a mAb which reacts with human β_2-microglobulin, either free or complexed with heavy chain, to demonstrate the presence of β_2-microglobulin bound to class I heavy chains in the membrane of bovine lymphocytes (111,112) (Table 13). mAb W6/32, which recognizes an epitope formed by association of HLA class I (A, B, and C) heavy chains with β_2-microglobulin (109,110) and displays a similar reactivity in cattle (16), precipitates all conventional BoLA class I molecules (16). In addition, a

Table 13 Identification of BoLA Class I and Class II Antigens by mAb

BoLA class	mAb	Isotype of mAb	Antigen biochemistry	Refs.
I	P3[a]	IgG2a	12, 44-45 Kd	16
I	P12	IgM	nk[b]	22
I	W6/32	IgG2a	12, 44, 45 Kd	16,106,108, 109,110
I	B1.1G6	IgG2a	12 Kd[c]	111,112
II	R1	IgM	26-29, 32-34 Kd	12,113
II	J11	IgG1	29, 31 Kd	see Fig. 7
II	H4	IgG3	27, 35 Kd	9,114
II	TH21A	IgG2b	nk	9
II	HLA-DR[d]	IgG2a	27, 31, 34 Kd	115
II	B2Va17C7[b]	IgG1	27, 32 Kd	19

[a]These mAb recognize polymorphic determinants.
[b]nk = not known.
[c]B1.1G6 reacts with β_2-microglobulin both in free form and in association with class I heavy chains.
[d]mAb to HLA-DR is 1.35.

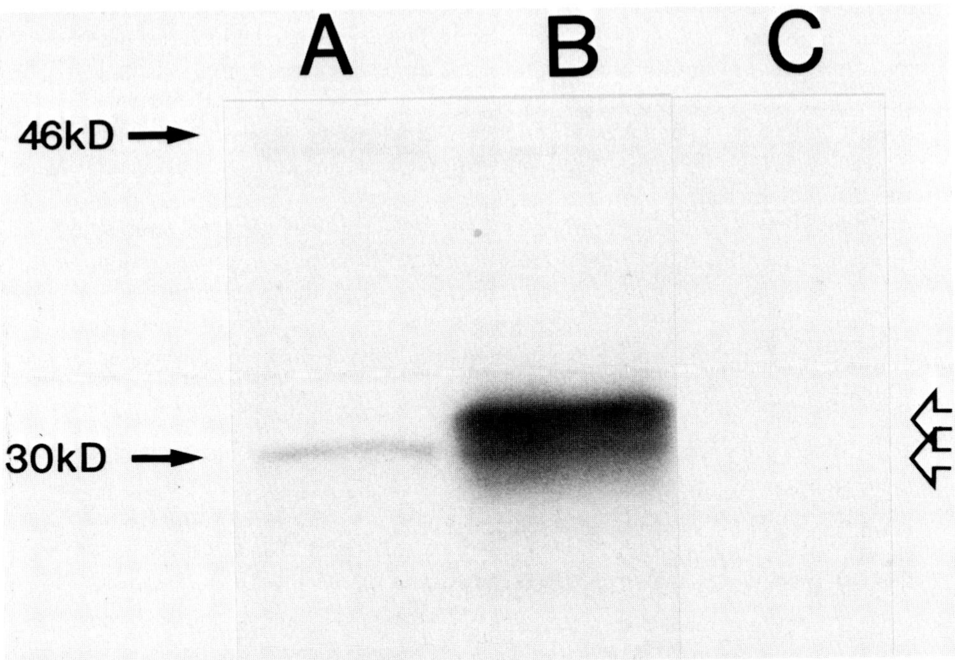

Figure 7 SDS-PAGE of molecules preipitated by mAb J11 (lane B) and an unrelated antibody (lane C), from the surface of Con A blasts labeled with ^{35}S-methionine as described elsewhere (10). Molecular weight markers are in lane A, indicated by arrows on the left. MAb J11 precipitated two bands of 31 and 28 Kd.

class I-like molecule similar to the human T6 (CD1) molecule has been characterized with a mAb TH97A (116); this molecule, which is composed of 44 Kd and 12 Kd polypeptides, is expressed on cortical thymocytes and on dendritic cells in peripheral lymphoid tissues.

MAb specific for human HLA-DR gene products and antisera against murine I-A or I-E gene products have been used by Levy et al. (18,115) to precipitate molecules of 27, 31, and 34 Kd, believed to represent the polypeptide chains of the bovine class II molecule (Table 13). MAb R1 (12,113) and mAb J11 (Fig. 7), which also recognize nonpolymorphic BoLA class II epitopes, precipitate molecules with molecular masses of 26-29 Kd and 32-34 Kd, believed to be analogous to the α chain and β chain, respectively, of class II molecules of other species. These studies illustrate the similarities of BoLA class II molecules with those of man and mouse, both in biochemical characteristics and in expression of common epitopes. Staining of cloned T cells with different mAb against class II antigens, some of which were produced by Davis at Washington State University, results in different patterns of staining, suggesting that the different mAb may see different class II products.

B. Class I

Monoclonal antibodies P12 and P3 (12), which recognize nonpolymorphic and polymorphic epitopes, respectively, on BoLA class I molecules, have been employed to examine the distribution of class I MHC molecules in lymphoid tissues of cattle (Table 14). Class I MHC distribution is contrasted with class II distribution in Table 14. In PBM and spleen, 100% of cells express class I molecules, whereas only 5-13% of thymocytes have detectable class I molecules. In sections of bovine thymus, expression of class I molecules is confined to mature lymphocytes in the medulla. Medullary epithelial cells also react strongly with these mAb, whereas there is only very weak or scarcely detectable staining of cortical epithelial cells (12). These findings are similar to observations on expression of class I antigens in murine (117) and human (27) thymuses. In sections of bovine lymph node and spleen stained with mAb P3 and P12, there is much weaker staining of germinal center cells than of other cellular components of these tissues, suggesting that germinal center cells have low levels of expression of class I antigens (12). This has not been observed in other species.

The functional relevance of MHC molecules has been demonstrated in blocking studies employing mAb W6/32. mAb W6/32 can inhibit cytolytic activity of some BoT8$^+$, class I-restricted alloreactive (17) or antigen-specific T-cell clones (66). mAb W6/32 can weakly block cytolytic activity of uncloned effectors generated

Table 14 Distribution of Cells Expressing MHC Class I and Class II Antigens in Bovine Lymphoid Tissues[a]

MHC class	Identifying mAb[b]	Percentage positive cells in each tissue		
		PBM	Thymus	Spleen
I	P3	98%	6%	95%
I	P12	100%	9%	96%
II	R1	30%	1%	20%
II	H4	22%	1%	nd[c]
II	TH21A	22%	4%	nd

[a]More than 3 cattle were tested for each tissue and mAb.
[b]Data for P3, P12, and R1 are from Lalor et al. (12), and for H4 and TH12A from Lewin et al. (9).
[c]nd = not done.

in MLC after one stimulation in vitro, but no blocking is measured after the second stimulation in vitro (Fig. 5). This may reflect differences in the epitopes recognized by different cytotoxic T-cell clones in the bulk populations, concurring with the variability of blocking by mAb W6/32 among alloreactive clones (17). mAb B1.1G6 did not block bovine BoT8$^+$ antigen-specific cytolytic clones, even when blocking by mAb W6/32 was greater than 90% (66). Other antibodies to β_2-microglobulin have been shown to block cytotoxicity of human T-cell clones, possibly as a result of conformational changes in the class I molecule induced by binding of the antibody (118). The discrepancies in these findings may be due to the mAb recognizing different epitopes on β_2-microglobulin.

C. Class II

Results of Lalor et al. (12) and Letesson et al. (19) indicate that BoLA class II molecules are expressed on all sIg$^+$ PBM and on some monocytes. Letesson et al. (19) have also found using mAb B2 Val 7C7 that bovine class II antigens are expressed by 20% of non-Ig-bearing lymphocytes and nearly all monocytes. These results are contrary to those of Lewin et al. (9) who found a very high correlation between the percentage of PBM expressing sIg and those reacting with mAb H4, a mAb reactive with murine Ia molecules, and TH21A, a mAb with similar reactivity to H4, suggesting that no cells in PBM other than sIg$^+$ cells express class II molecules.

All of these mAb show little or no reactivity with bovine thymocytes (Table 14; 19), although mAb R1 (12) and mAb B2Val7C7 (19) react with epithelial cells in the cortex and medulla as well as with interdigitating cells of the thymic medulla. In spleen and lymph node, mAb R1 reacts with lymphocytes in B-cell follicles and with large interdigitating cells in the T-dependent areas (12). Mammary gland macrophages express high concentrations of class II antigens, whereas only about 50% of pulmonary macrophages express class II antigens (Ellis, personal communication). Expression of class II antigens by mammary gland macrophages may prove useful for purifying macrophages from mammary gland inflammatory cells, since granulocytes do not express class II antigens but constitute a substantial proportion of mammary gland exudates.

It would appear from these results that bovine class II molecules generally are not expressed by resting T lymphocytes, as occurs in dogs and horses, but have the same distribution on lymphoid cells as class II molecules in mice and humans (see 91). There is some doubt, however, since Letesson et al. (19) showed some reactivity of mAb B2Val7C7 with non-sIg$^+$ lymphocytes. Lalor et al. (12) have shown the appearance of R1$^+$ cells in PBM which were depleted of R1$^+$ cells prior to being stimulated with Con A, indicating that blasting T cells express class II. Furthermore, T cells infected with the protozoan parasite *T. parva*, which induces continual replication of infected lymphocytes, have an apparently cell cycle-related expression of the R1 antigen (22). Expression of class II antigens by blasting sIg^- lymphocytes has been described in other species (see 12).

PBM expressing class II antigens have been shown to be required to generate mixed leukocyte reactions of cattle PBM (12), consistent with results in other species. Goddeeris (personal communication) has also shown that mAb J11 blocks proliferation of PBM in MLC. By FACS-separating PBM into $BoT8^+$ and $BoT4^+$ populations, we have shown that $BoT8^+$ lymphocytes, believed to respond to class I MHC antigens, also proliferate in mixed leukocyte reactions (Fig. 4), albeit to a lesser extent than $BoT4^+$ lymphocytes (1,2). However, $BoT8^+$ PBM require exogenous TCGF in order to proliferate (2) to alloantigens, whereas $BoT4^+$ cells do not (1). From this we can conclude that in unseparated PBM populations, $BoT4^+$ lymphocytes must be stimulated by class II alloantigens in order to produce the TCGF required by $BoT8^+$ lymphocytes to proliferate in response to the class I alloantigens.

Teale and colleagues at ILRAD have demonstrated the ability of mAb to HLA-DR to block cytolytic activity of some $BoT4^+$ alloreactive clones, but not $BoT8^+$ clones (17), further indicating that class II molecules are involved in the effector-target interaction of $BoT4^+$ cells (see Section II.C). mAb J11 was effective in blocking antigen-specific proliferation of PBM from some, but not all, cattle to stimulation by keyhole limpet hemocyanin presented on autologous monocytes (Table 15). This indicates that class II molecules are required for stimulation of bovine PBM by soluble antigens and, based on results with alloreactive clones, the responding PBM are probably $BoT4^+$ cells. However, other mAb reactive with bovine class II molecules, including R1 and a mAb which reacts with HLA-DR, did not block antigen-stimulated proliferation of PBM, suggesting they do not

Table 15 Effect of mAb J11 on Proliferation of Bovine PBM from Animals Primed to Keyhole Limpet Hemocyanin[a]

	Proliferative response[b]			
Animal	Medium background	Antigen	Antigen + mAb J11 Ig	% Inhibition by J11
D242	1500	132.5	11.6	91%
D247	3170	3.8	5.6	0%
D254	858	8.5	0.9	89%

[a]Assays were conducted essentially as described elsewhere (13).
[b]Medium background presented as counts per minute of [^{125}I]iododeoxyuridine uptake after 4 days of culture. Responses to antigen are indicated as stimulation indices.

react with the class II epitopes involved in presentation of the antigen (Emery, personal communication).

VI. CONCLUSIONS

Bovine cells of hemopoietic origin can be divided into various lineages and subsets by reactivity with a variety of monoclonal antibodies (mAb). Monoclonal antibodies are available which distinguish T and B lymphocytes from other cells of hemopoietic origin. Mature T lymphocytes may be identified by mAb which react with the bovine analogues of human T11 (CD2) and T3 (CD3), named BoT2 and BoT3, respectively. T lymphocytes may be further distinguished as belonging to two subsets which express BoT4 or BoT8, equivalent to CD4 and CD8 in humans, respectively. All four T-cell molecules, identified by precipitation or blotting, have biochemical characteristics similar to their proposed analogues in other species. The two major T-lymphocyte subsets display distinctive functional characteristics: $BoT4^+$ lymphocytes respond to stimulation by mitogens or alloantigens without requiring exogenous growth factors, whereas the majority of $BoT8^+$ lymphocytes do not; recognition of foreign antigen on cell surfaces by $BoT4^+$ lymphocytes is apparently restricted by class II MHC determinants, whereas $BoT8^+$ lymphocytes are restricted by class I molecules; moreover, within alloreactive and parasite-specific cytolytic T-cell populations, most of the cytolytic activity resides within the $BoT8^+$ population. Mature B lymphocytes may be distinguished from T lymphocytes by their expression of surface immunoglobulin. Monoclonal antibodies are available which react specifically with bovine IgM and IgG.

Several mAb have been produced which are specific for cells of the myelomonocytic lineage. Some of these mAb react with monocytes, macrophages, and granulocytes, whereas others react with subpopulations of monocytes and macrophages. Of particular interest is one mAb that is specific for pulmonary macrophages and another that is of importance in the accessory function of monocytes and precipitates molecules of 75 and 110 Kd.

A variety of mAb exist which react with bovine class I and class II major histocompatibility complex molecules. They have been employed to examine the expression of these molecules on cells of various lymphoid tissues and to demonstrate their functional relevance in recognition of antigens by cells of the two T-lymphocyte subsets.

Several other mAb react with antigens whose functional relevance have not been determined. The mAb have been useful in evaluating subpopulations of cells in functional assays and in assessing the state of activation of mononuclear cells. These include mAb which recognize T-lymphocyte blast antigens and those which react with differentiation markers shared by T lymphocytes, monocytes, and/or granulocytes.

ACKNOWLEDGMENTS

We would like to recognize and thank our colleagues at ILRAD who participated in generating and defining many of the mAb described herein: Albert Bensaid, Sam Black, John Ellis, Bruno Goddeeris, Paul Lalor, Kathleen Logan, Niall MacHugh, Janet Newson, Joseph Olobo, Stuart Shapiro, and Alan Teale; the FACS unit, including James Magondu and Dennis Wambuthi; and Peter Belsoi, Anita Kaushal and Chris Hinson for technical assistance.

We thank the following people for information quoted as personal communications: S. Black, W. Davis, J. Ellis, D. Emery, B. Goddeeris, D. Hurley, S. Kar, V. Lutje, N. MacHugh, A. Mastro, J. Newson, J. Olobo, M. Pinder, G. Roelants, A. Teale, and P. Wells.

This is ILRAD publication no. 457.

ABBREVIATIONS

AET	aminoethylisothioronium.
β_2-mgl	β 2-microglobulin.
BoT	prefix for bovine T-cell antigen.
BoLA	bovine leukocyte antigens.
CD	cluster differentiation antigen.
Con A	Concanavalin A.
CTL	cytotoxic T lymphocyte(s).
EAC	erythrocyte-antibody-complement.
FACS	fluorescence-activated cell sorter.
Fc	crystallizable fraction of immunoglobulin.
gp	glycoprotein.
HLA	human leukocyte antigen.
Kd	kilodalton.
nd	not done.
nk	not known.
mAb	monoclonal antibody(ies).
MHC	major histocompatibility complex.
MLC	mixed leukocyte culture(s).
PBM	peripheral blood mononuclear cells.
PHA	phytohemagglutinin.
RBC	red blood cells.
SD	standard deviation.
SDS-PAGE	sodium dodecylsulfate-polyacrylamide gel electrophoresis.
sIg	surface immunoglobulin.
TCGF	T-cell growth factor.

REFERENCES

1. C. L. Baldwin, A. J. Teale, J. Naessens, B. M. Goddeeris, N. D. MacHugh, and W. I. Morrison, Characterization of a subset of bovine T lymphocytes expressing BoT4 by monoclonal antibodies and function: Similarity to lymphocytes defined by human T4 and murine L3T4, *J. Immunol., 136*: 4385 (1986).
2. J. A. Ellis, C. L. Baldwin, N. D. MacHugh, A. Bensaid, A. J. Teale, B. M. Goddeeris, and W. I. Morrison, Characterization by a monoclonal antibody and functional analysis of a subset of bovine T lymphocytes that express BoT8, a molecule analogous to human CD8, *Immunology, 58*: 351 (1986).
3. J. A. Ledbetter, R. L. Evans, M. Lipinski, C. Cunningham-Rundles, R. A. Good, and L. A. Herzenberg, Evolutionary conservation of surface molecules that distinguish T lymphocyte helper/inducer and cytotoxic subpopulations in mouse and man, *J. Exp. Med., 153*: 310 (1981).
4. J. F. Maddox, C. R. Mackay, and M. R. Brandon, Surface antigens, SBU-T4 and SBU-T8 of sheep T lymphocyte subsets defined by monoclonal antibodies, *Immunology, 55*: 739 (1985).
5. A. Matsuura, Y. Ishii, H. Yuasa, H. Narita, S. Kon, T. Takami, and K. Kikuchi, Rat T lymphocyte antigens comparable with mouse Lyt-1 and Lyt-2, 3 antigenic systems: characterization by monoclonal antibodies, *J. Immunol., 132*: 316 (1984).
6. M. D. Pescovitz, J. K. Lunney, and D. H. Sachs, Murine anti-swine T4 and T8 monoclonal antibodies: Distribution and effects on proliferative and cytotoxic T cells, *J. Immunol., 134*: 37 (1985).
7. E. L. Reinherz, P. C. Kung, G. Goldstein, and S. F. Schlossman, Separation of functional subsets of human T cells by a monoclonal antibody, *Proc. Natl. Acad. Sci. USA, 76*: 4061 (1979).
8. E. L. Reinherz, P. C. Kung, G. Goldstein, and S. F. Schlossman, A monoclonal antibody reactive with the human cytotoxic/suppressor T cell subset previously defined by a heteroantiserum termed TH, *J. Immunol., 129*: 1301 (1980).
9. H. A. Lewin, W. C. Davis, and D. Bernoco, Monoclonal antibodies that distinguish bovine T and B lymphocytes, *Vet. Immunol. Immunopathol., 9*: 87 (1985).
10. J. Naessens, J. Newson, A. Bensaid, A. J. Teale, J. G. Magondu, and S. J. Black, *De novo* expression of T cell markers on *Theileria parva*-transformed lymphoblasts in cattle, *J. Immunol., 135*: 4183 (1985).
11. E. D. Rabinovsky and Tsu-Ju Yang, Production and characterization of a bovine T cell-specific monoclonal antibody identifying a mature differentiation antigen, *J. Immunol., 136*: 609 (1986).
12. P. A. Lalor, W. I. Morrison, B. M. Goddeeris, R. J. Jack, and S. J. Black, Monoclonal antibodies identify phenotypically and functionally distinct cell types in the bovine lymphoid system, *Vet. Immunol. Immunopathol., 13*: 121 (1986).
13. J. A. Ellis, W. C. Davis, N. D. MacHugh, D. L. Emergy, A. Kaushal, and W. I. Morrison, Differentiation antigens on bovine mononuclear phagocytes identified by monoclonal antibodies, submitted.

14. M. Pinder, A. J. Musoke, W. I. Morrison, and G. E. Roelants, The bovine lymphoid system III. A monoclonal antibody specific for bovine cell surface and serum IgM, *Immunology, 40*: 359 (1980).
15. M. Pinder, T. W. Pearson, and G. E. Roelants, The bovine lymphoid system: II. Derivation and partial characterization of monoclonal antibodies against bovine peripheral blood lymphocytes, *Vet. Immunol. Immunopathol., 1*: 303 (1980).
16. A. Bensaid, J. Naessens, S. J. Kemp, S. J. Black, S. Z. Shapiro, and A. J. Teale, An immunochemical analysis of class I (BoLA) molecules on the surface of bovine cells, *Immunogenetics,* in press.
17. A. J. Teale, C. L. Baldwin, J. A. Ellis, J. Newson, W. I. Morrison, and B. M. Goddeeris, Alloreactive bovine T cell clones: An analysis of function, phenotype and specificity, *J. Immunol., 136*: 4392 (1986).
18. M. Hoang-Xuan, D. J. Charron, M. T. Zilber, and D. Levy, Biochemical characterization of class II bovine major histocompatibility complex antigens using cross-species reactive antibodies, *Immunogenetics, 15*: 621 (1982).
19. J. J. Letesson, Ph. Coppe, N. Lostrie-Trussart, and A. Depelchin, A bovine 'Ia-like' antigen detected by a xenogeneic monoclonal antibody, *Anim. Blood Groups Biochem. Genet., 14*: 239 (1983).
20. C. L. Baldwin, N. D. MacHugh, J. A. Ellis, J. Naessens, J. Newson, and W. I. Morrison, Monoclonal antibodies which react with bovine T lymphocyte antigens and induce blastogenesis: Tissue distribution and functional characteristics, submitted.
21. W. Davis, J. A. Ellis, N. D. MacHugh, and C. L. Baldwin, Bovine pan T-cell monoclonal antibodies reactive with a molecule similar to CD2, *Immunology,* in press.
22. P. A. Lalor, W. I. Morrison, and S. J. Black, Monoclonal antibodies to bovine leukocytes define heterogeneity of target cells for *in vitro* parasitosis by *Theileria parva*, in *The Ruminant Immune System in Health and Disease* (W. I. Morrison, ed.), Cambridge University Press, Cambridge, 1986, p. 72.
23. M. Pinder and R. S. Hewett, Monoclonal antibodies detect antigenic diversity in *Theileria parva* parasites, *J. Immunol., 124*: 1000 (1980).
24. IUIS-WHO Nomenclature Subcommittees, Nomenclature for clusters of differentiation (CD) antigens defined by human leukocyte populations, *Bull. W.H.O., 62*: 809 (1984).
25. F. D. Howard, J. A. Ledbetter, J. Wong, C. P. Bieber, E. B. Stinson, and L. A. Herzenberg, A human T lymphocyte differentiation marker defined by monoclonal antibodies that block E rosette formation, *J. Immunol., 126*: 2117 (1981).
26. M. Kamoun, P. J. Martin, J. A. Hansen, M. A. Brown, A. W. Siadak, and R. C. Nowinski, Identification of a human T lymphocyte surface protein associated with the E-rosette receptor, *J. Exp. Med., 153*: 207 (1981).
27. A. K. Bhan, E. L. Reinherz, S. Poppema, R. T. McCluskey, and S. F. Schlossman, Location of T cell and major histocompatbility complex antigens in the human thymus, *J. Exp. Med., 152*: 771 (1980).
28. A van Agthoven, C. Terhorst, E. Reinherz, and S. Schlossman, Characterization of T cell surface glycoproteins T1 and T3 present on all human peripheral T lymphocytes and functionally mature thymocytes, *Eur. J. Immunol., 11*: 18 (1981).

29. E. L. Reinherz, P. C. Kung, G. Goldstein, and S. F. Schlossman, A monoclonal antibody with selective reactivity with functionally mature thymocytes and all peripheral human T cells, *J. Immunol., 123*: 1312 (1979).
30. P. J. Martin, J. A. Hansen, A. W. Siadak, and R. C. Nowinski, Monoclonal antibodies recognizing normal human T lymphocytes and malignant human B lymphocytes: A comparative study, *J. Immunol., 127*: 1920 (1981).
31. S. L. Swain, Significance of Lyt phenotype: Lyt-2 antibodies block antibodies of T cells that recognize class I major histocompatibility complex antigens regardless of their function, *Proc. Natl. Acad. Sci. USA, 78*: 7101 (1981).
32. S. L. Swain, T cell subsets and the recognition of MHC class, *Immunol. Rev., 74*: 129 (1983).
33. W. E. Biddison, P. E. Rao, M. A. Tale, G. Goldstein, and S. Shaw, Possible involvement of the OKT4 molecule in T cell recognition of class 2 HLA antigens. Evidence from cytotoxic T lymphocytes specific for S.B. antigens, *J. Exp. Med., 156*: 1065 (1982).
34. S. C. Meuer, S. F. Schlossman, and E. L. Reinherz, Clonal analysis of human cytotoxic T lymphocytes: $T4^+$ and $T8^+$ effector T cells recognize products of different major histocompatibility complex antigens, *Proc. Natl. Acad. Sci. USA, 79*: 4395 (1982).
35. Y. Thomas, L. Rogozinski, and L. Chess, Relationship between human T cell functional heterogeneity and human T cell surface molecules, *Immunol. Rev., 74*: 113 (1983).
36. E. L. Reinherz, S. C. Meuer, and S. F. Schlossman, The delineation of antigen receptor on human T lymphocytes, *Immunol. Today, 4*: 5 (1983).
37. H. Yamada, P. J. Martin, M. A. Bean, M. P. Braun, P. G. Beatty, K. Sadamoto, and J. A. Hansen, Monoclonal antibody 9.3 and anti-CD11 antibodies define reciprocal subsets of lymphocytes, *Eur. J. Immunol., 15*: 1164 (1985).
38. T. R. Malek, R. J. Robb, and E. M. Shevach, Identification and initial characterization of a rat monoclonal antibody reactive with the murine interleukin 2 receptor-ligand complex, *Proc. Natl. Acad. Sci. USA, 80*: 5694 (1983).
39. W. J. Leonard, J. M. Depper, T. Uchiyama, K. A. Smith, T. A. Waldmann, and W. C. Greene, A monoclonal antibody that appears to recognize the receptor for human T-cell growth factor: Partial characterization of the receptor, *Nature, 300*: 267 (1982).
40. I. S. Trowbridge and M. Bishr Omary, Human cell surface glycoprotein related to cell proliferation is the receptor for transferrin, *Proc. Natl. Acad. Sci. USA, 78*: 3039 (1981).
41. A. S. Grewal, B. T. Rouse, and L. A. Babiuk, Erythrocyte rosettes—a marker for bovine T cells, *Can. J. Comp. Med., 40*: 298 (1976).
42. D. A. Higgins and M. J. Stack, Bovine lymphocytes enhanced E-rosette formation after storage or gradient centrifugation, *Clin. Exp. Immunol., 29*: 304 (1977).
43. J. H. Reeves and H. W. Renshaw, Surface membrane markers on bovine peripheral blood lymphocytes, *Am. J. Vet. Res., 39*: 917 (1978).

44. P. S. Paul, D. R. Senogles, C. C. Muscoplat, and D. W. Johnson, Enumeration of T cells, B cells and monocytes in the peripheral blood of normal and lymphocytotic cattle, *Clin. Exp. Immunol., 35*: 306 (1979).
45. T. W. Pearson, G. E. Roelants, L. B. Lundin, and K. S. Mayor-Withey, The bovine lymphoid system: Binding and stimulation of peripheral blood lymphocytes by lectins, *J. Immunol. Methods, 26*: 271 (1979).
46. B. Morein, V. Hellstrom, L. G. Axelson, C. Johansson, and S. Hammerstrom, *Helix pomatia* A agglutinin, a surface marker for bovine T lymphocytes, *Vet. Immunol. Immunopathol., 1*: 27 (1979).
47. W. I. Morrison, C. L. Baldwin, N. D. MacHugh, A. J. Teale, B. M. Goddeeris, and J. Ellis, Phenotypic and functional characterisation of bovine lymphocytes, *Prog. Vet. Micro. Immunol.*, in press.
48. W. R. Usinger and G. A. Splitter, Two molecularly independent surface receptors identify bovine T lymphocytes, *J. Immunol. Methods, 45*: 209 (1981).
49. T. J. Yang, P. A. Jantzen, and L. J. Williams, Acid alpha-naphthyl acetate esterase: presence of activity in bovine and human T and B lymphocytes, *Immunology, 38*: 85 (1979).
50. S. C. Meuer, R. E. Hussey, M. Fabbi, D. Fox, D. Acuto, K. A. Fitzgerald, J. C. Hodgdon, J. P. Protentis, S. F. Schlossman, and E. L. Reinherz, An alternative pathway of T-cell activation: A functional role for the 50 kd T11 sheep erythrocyte receptor protein, *Cell, 36*: 897 (1984).
51. E. L. Reinherz, A molecular basis for thymic selection: Regulation of T11 induced thymocyte expansion by the T3-Ti antigen/MHC receptor pathway, *Immunol. Today, 6*: 75 (1985).
52. H. W. Renshaw, Non immune erythrocyte rosette formation of bovine peripheral blood and thymus lymphocytes, *Comp. Immunol. Microbiol. Infect. Dis., 4*: 75 (1981).
53. F. Emmrich and S. Meuer, Human T-cell clones find ever wider application, *Immunol. Today, 6*: 197 (1985).
54. J. Borst, M. A. Prendville, and C. Terhorst, Complexity of the human T lymphocyte-specific cell surface antigen T3, *J. Immunol., 128*: 1560 (1982).
55. L. E. Samelson, J. B. Harford, and R. D. Klausner, Identification of the components of the murine T cell antigen receptor complex, *Cell, 43*: 223 (1985).
56. J. P. Van Wauwe, J. R. De Mey, and J. G. Goossens, OKT3: A monoclonal anti-human T lymphocyte antibody with potent mitogen properties, *J. Immunol., 124*: 2708 (1980).
57. H. Spits, H. Yssel, J. Leeuwenberg, and J. E. deVries, Antigen-specific cytotoxic T cell and antigen-specific proliferating T cell clones can be induced to cytolytic activity by monoclonal antibodies against T3, *Eur. J. Immunol., 15*: 88 (1985).
58. E. L. Reinherz and S. F. Schlossman, The differentiation and function of human T lymphocytes, *Cell, 19*: 821 (1980).
59. E. L. Reinherz, P. C. Kung, G. Goldstein, R. H. Levey, and S. F. Schlossman, Discrete stages of intrathymic differentiation: Analysis of normal thymocytes and leukemic lymphoblasts of T-cell lineage, *Proc. Natl. Acad. Sci. USA, 77*: 1588 (1980).

60. B. M. Goddeeris, C. L. Baldwin, O. Ole-moiYoi, and W. I. Morrison, Improved methods for purification and depletion of monocytes from bovine peripheral blood mononuclear cells. Functional evaluation of monocytes in response to lectins, *J. Immunol. Methods, 89*: 165 (1986).
61. L. Andrus, S. J. Prowse, and K. J. Laferty, Interleukin 2 production by both Ly 2^+ and Ly 2^- T-cell subsets, *Scand. J. Immunol., 13*: 297 (1981).
62. A. J. Teale, W. I. Morrison, B. M. Goddeeris, C. M. Groocock, D. A. Stagg, and R. L. Spooner, Bovine alloreactive cytotoxic T cells generated *in vitro*: Target specificity in relation to BoLA phenotype, *Immunology, 55*: 355 (1985).
63. D. Vidovic, J. Klein, and Z. Nagy, The role of T cell subsets in the generation of secondary cytolytic responses *in vitro* against class I and class II major histocompatibility complex antigens, *J. Immunol., 132*: 1113 (1984).
64. H. Spits, H. Ijssel, A. Thompson, and J. E. deVries, Human $T4^+$ and $T8^+$ cytotoxic T lymphocyte clones directed at products of different class II major histocompatibility complex loci, *J. Immunol., 131*: 678 (1983).
65. R. L. Spooner et al., Analysis of alloantiserum against bovine lymphocytes. Joint report of the 1st international bovine lymphocyte antigen (BoLA) workshop, *Anim. Blood Groups Biochem. Genet., 10*: 63 (1979).
66. B. M. Goddeeris, W. I. Morrison, A. J. Teale, G. Bensaid, and C. L. Baldwin, Bovine cytotoxic T cell clones specific for cells infected with the protozoan parasite *Theileria parva*: Parasite strain specificity and class I MHC restriction, *Proc. Natl. Acad. Sci. USA, 83*: 5238 (1986).
67. D. B. Wilde, P. Marrack, J. Kappler, D. P. Dialynas, and F. W. Fitch, Evidence implicating L3T4 in class II MHC antigen reactivity; monoclonal antibody GK 1.5 (anti-L3T4a) blocks class II MHC antigen-specific proliferation, release of lymphokines and binding by cloned murine helper T lymphocyte lines, *J. Immunol., 131*: 2178 (1983).
68. A. Moretta, G. Pantaleo, M. C. Mingari, L. Moretta, and J. C. Cerottini, Clonal heterogeneity in the requirement for T3, T4, and T8 molecules in human cytolytic T lymphocyte function, *J. Exp. Med., 159*: 921 (1984).
69. H. R. MacDonald, N. Thiernesse, and J. C. Cerottini, Inhibition of T-cell mediated cytolysis by monoclonal antibodies directed against Lyt-2: Heterogeneity of inhibition at the clonal level, *J. Immunol., 126*: 1671 (1981).
70. P. H. Sayre and E. L. Reinherz, Structural invariance of T4 molecules from T cell clones of different antigens and major histocompatibility complex specificities, *Eur. J. Immunol., 15*: 291 (1985).
71. D. P. Dialynas, Z. S. Quan, K. A. Wall, A. Pierres, J. Quintans, M. R. Loken, M. Pierres, and F. W. Fitch, Characterization of the murine T cell surface molecule, designated L3T4, identified by monoclonal antibody GK 1.5: Similarity of L3T4 to the human Leu-3/T4 molecule, *J. Immunol., 131*: 2445 (1983).
72. S. Jonjic and U. H. Koszinowski, Monoclonal antibodies reactive with swine lymphocytes. I. Antibodies to membrane structures that define the cytolytic T lymphocyte subset in the swine, *J. Immunol., 133*: 647 (1984).
73. M. D. Pescovitz, J. K. Lunney, and D. H. Sachs, Preparation and characterization of monoclonal antibodies reactive with procine PBL, *J. Immunol., 133*: 368 (1984).

74. C. L. Baldwin, B. M. Goddeeris, and W. I. Morrison, Bovine BoT4+ T cell clones specific for lymphocytes infected with the protozoan parasite *Theileria parva, Parasite Immunol., 9*: 499 (1987).
75. J. A. Ledbetter, R. V. Rouse, H. S. Micklem, and L. A. Herzenberg, T cell subsets defined by expression of Lyt-1,2,3 and Thy-1 antigens. Two-parameter immunofluorescence and cytotoxicity analysis with monoclonal antibodies modifies current views, *J. Exp. Med., 152*: 280 (1980).
76. L. Lanier, N. L. Warner, J. A. Ledbetter, and L. A. Herzenberg, Expression of Lyt 1 antigen on certain murine B-cell lymphomas, *J. Exp. Med., 153*: 998 (1981).
77. V. Manohor, E. Brown, W. M. Leiserson, and T. M. Chused, Expression of Lyt-1 by a subset of B lymphocytes. *J. Immunol., 129*: 532 (1982).
78. S. P. Morzaria, P. L. Roeder, D. H. Roberts, D. Chasey, and T. W. Drew, Characteristics of a continuous suspension cell line derived from a calf with sporadic bovine leukosis, in *Eighth International Symposium of Bovine Leukosis* (A. C. Straub, ed.), Martinus Nijhoff, London, 1983.
79. A. S. Grewel, B. T. Rouse, and L. A. Babiuk, Characterization of surface receptors on bovine leukocytes, *Int. Archs Allergy Appl. Immunol., 56*: 289 (1978).
80. K. Nielsen, J. R. Duncan, and B. Stemshorn, Preparation of heavy chain specific antiserum to bovine IgA, IgM, IgG1 and IgG2, *Vet. Immunol. Immunopathol., 9*: 361 (1985).
81. W. R. Usinger, W. G. Smith, and G. A. Splitter, Bovine T cells do not require auxillary cells for response to selected mitogens, *Vet. Immunol. Immunopathol., 2*: 381 (1981).
82. W. I. Morrison, P. A. Lalor, A. K. Christensen, and P. Webster, Cellular organization and structural organization of the bovine thymus and lymph node, in *The Ruminant Immune System in Health and Disease* (W. I. Morrison, ed.), Cambridge University Press, Cambridge, 1986, p. 220.
83. M. L. Rose, R. J. Booth, J. A. Habeshaw, and D. Robertson, Separation and characterisation of tonsiller germinal centre lymphocytes using peanut lectin, in *In Vivo Immunology: Histophysiology of the Lymphoid System* (P. Nienovenhuis, A. A. van den Broek, and M. G. Hanna, eds.), *Adv. Exp. Med. Biol., 149*: 773 (1982).
84. S. P. Kumar, P. S. Paul, K. A. Pomeroy, D. W. Johnson, C. C. Muscoplat, M. J. van der Maaten, J. M. Miller, and D. K. Sorensen, Frequency of lymphocytes bearing Fc receptors and surface membrane immunoglobulins in normal, persistent lymphocytotic and leukemic cows, *Am. J. Vet. Res., 39*: 45 (1978).
85. R. Van Furth, Cells of the mononuclear phagocyte system. Nomenclature in terms of sites and conditions, in *Mononuclear Phagocytes Functional Aspects* (R. Van Furth, ed.), Martinus-Nijhoff Publishers, The Hague, 1980, p. 1.
86. J. V. Desiderio and S. G. Campbell, Bovine mammary gland macrophage: Isolation, morphologic features, and cytophilic immunoglobulins, *Am. J. Vet. Res., 41*: 1595 (1980).
87. R. C. Wardley, B. T. Rouse, and L. A. Babiuk, The mammary gland of the ox: a convenient source for the repeated collection of neutrophils and macrophages, *J. Reticuloendothel. Soc., 19*: 29 (1976).

88. J. R. Birmingham and E. L. Jeska, The isolation, longterm cultivation and characterization of bovine peripheral blood monocytes, *Immunology, 41*: 807 (1980).
89. N. V. Raff, L. J. Picker, and J. D. Stobo, Macrophage heterogeneity in man: A subpopulation of HLA-DR-bearing macrophages required for antigen-induced T cell activation also contains stimulator for autologous reactive T cell, *J. Exp. Med., 152*: 581 (1980).
90. R. F. Todd, L. M. Nadler, and S. F. Schlossman, Antigens on human monocytes identified by monoclonal antibodies, *J. Immunol., 126*: 1435 (1981).
91. R. Todd and S. F. Schlossman, Analysis of antigenic determinants on human monocytes and macrophages, *Blood, 59*: 775 (1982).
92. W. W. Hancock, H. Zola, and R. C. Atkins, Antigenic heterogeneity of human mononuclear phagocytes: Immunohistologic analysis using mononuclear antibodies, *Blood, 62*: 1271 (1983).
93. H. Rumpold, O. Forster, G. Bock, P. Swetly, and M. Riedl. Antigenic heterogeneity of rat macrophages. A monoclonal antibody reacting only with alveolar but not other types of macrophages, *Immunology, 45*: 637 (1982).
94. A. Biondi, T. H. Rossing, J. Bennett, and R. F. Todd, Surface membrane heterogeneity among human mononuclear phagocytes, *J. Immunol., 132*: 1237 (1984).
95. A. Dimitriu-Bona, G. R. Burmester, S. J. Waters, and R. J. Winchester, Human mononuclear phagocyte differentiation antigens. I. Patterns of antigenic expression on the surface of human monocytes and macrophages defined by monoclonal antibodies, *J. Immunol., 130*: 145 (1983).
96. U. Mauer-Gross, D. Von Steldern, U. Hadding, D. Bitter-Suermann, and R. Burger, Cell surface antigens on the guinea-pig macrophage: identification by monoclonal antibodies and association with activation state, *Immunology, 55*: 519 (1985).
97. T. Taniyama and T. Tokunaga, Monoclonal antibodies directed against mouse macrophages in different stages of activation for tumor cytotoxicity, *J. Immunol., 131*: 1032 (1983).
98. H. Wacker, H. Radzun, and M. Parwaresch, KI-M2R, a new specific monoclonal antibody, discriminates tissue macrophages from reticulum cells and monocytes *in vivo* and *in vitro, J. Leukocyte Biol., 38*: 509 (1985).
99. H. A. Lewin, J. W. Casey, and D. Bernoco, Lymphoblastoid cell lines derived from two cases of enzootic bovine lymphosarcoma express a T-cell phenotype, *Fed. Proc., 44*: 1717 (1985).
100. B. M. Goddeeris, P. A. Lalor, and W. I. Morrison, Bovine mixed leukocyte reactions and generation of cytotoxic cells *in vitro*, in *The Ruminant Immune System in Health and Disease* (W. I. Morrison, ed.), Cambridge University Press, Cambridge, 1986, p. 299.
101. Anon., Proceedings of the 2nd bovine lymphocyte antigen BoLA workshop, *Anim. Blood Groups Biochem. Genet., 13*: 33 (1982).
102. Anon., *European Workshop on Bovine Histocompatibility. Les Collogues de L'INRA No. 14,* Jouy-en-Josas, France, 1982.

103. M. J. Stear, M. J. Newman, and F. W. Nicholas, Two closely linked loci and one apparently independent locus code for bovine lymphocyte antigens, *Tissue Antigens, 20*: 289 (1982).
104. M. J. Newman, T. E. Adams, and M. R. Brandon, Serological and genetic identification of a bovine lymphocyte alloantigen system, *Animal Blood Groups Biochem. Genet., 13*: 123 (1982).
105. S. J. Black, R. Jack, P. Lalor, and J. Newson, Analyses of *Theileria*-infected cell surface antigens with monoclonal antibodies, in *Advances in the Control of Theileriosis* (A. D. Irvin, M. P. Cunningham, and A. S. Young, eds.), Martinus Nijhoff Publishers, The Hague, 1981, p. 327.
106. J. M. Brodsky, W. H. Stone, and P. Parham, Of cows and men: A comparative study of histocompatibility antigens, *Hum. Immunol., 3*: 143 (1981).
107. R. L. Spooner and I. Ferrone, Cross reaction of monoclonal antibodies to human MHC class I and class II products with bovine lymphocyte subpopulations, *Tissue Antigens, 24*: 270 (1984).
108. P. Chardon, J. Kalil, H. Leveziel, J. Colomboni, and M. Vaiman, Monoclonal antibodies to HLA recognize monomorphic and polymorphic epitopes on BoLA, *Tissue Antigens, 22*: 62 (1983).
109. C. J. Barnstable, W. J. Bodmer, G. Brown, G. Galfre, C. Milstein, A. F. Williams, and A. Ziegler, Production of monoclonal antibodies to group A erythrocytes, HLA and other human cell surface antigens: New tools for genetic analysis, *Cell, 14*: 9 (1978).
110. P. Parham, C. J. Barnstable, and W. F. Bodmer, Use of a monoclonal antibody (W6/32) in structural studies of HLA-A, B, C antigens, *J. Immunol., 123*: 342 (1979).
111. A. Liabeuf, C. Le Borgne de Kaouel, F. M. Kounlsky, B. Malissen, Y. Manuel, and A. R. Sanderson, An antigenic determinant of human beta 2-microglobulin masked by the association with HLA heavy chains at the cell surface: Analysis using monoclonal antibodies, *J. Immunol., 127*: 1542 (1981).
112. J. L. Teillaud, D. Crevat, P. Chardon, J. Kalil, C. Goujet-Zalc, G. Mahouy, M. Vaiman, M. Fellous, and D. Pious, Monoclonal antibodies as a tool for phylogenetic studies of major histocompatibility antigens and beta 2-microglobulin, *Immunogenetics, 15*: 377 (1982).
113. D. L. Emery, N. K. Puri, J. H. Dufty, M. D. Gorrell, and M. R. Brandon, A functional and biochemical analysis of bovine class II MHC antigens using monoclonal antibodies, submitted.
114. S. Chatterjee, D. Bernoco, and R. Billing, Treatment with anti-Ia and anti-blast/monocyte monoclonal antibodies, *Immunogenetics, 15*: 151 (1982).
115. D. Levy, M. Hoang-Xuan, and M. T. Zieber, Biochemical analysis of products of the bovine major histocompatibility complex, in *The Ruminant Immune System in Health and Disease* (W. I. Morrison, ed.), Cambridge University Press, Cambridge, 1986, p. 152.
116. N. D. MacHugh, A. Bensaid, W. C. Davis, C. J. Howard, K. R. Parsons, B. Jones, and A. Kaushal, Characterization of a bovine thymic differentiation antigen analogous to CD1 in the human system, submitted.

117. R. V. Rouse, W. van Ewijk, P. P. Jones, and I. l. Weissman, Expression of MHC antigens by mouse thymic dendritic cells, *J. Immunol., 122*: 2508 (1979).
118. D. W. Dongworth and A. J. McMichael, Inhibition of human T lymphocyte function with monoclonal antibodies, *Brit. Med. Bull., 40*: 254 (1984).

15

Differentiation Antigens in Lymphohemopoietic System of the Sheep

MASAYUKI MIYASAKA,* SUSAN McCLURE, WAYNE R. HEIN, and ZDENEK TRNKA
Basal Institute for Immunology, Basel, Switzerland

I. INTRODUCTION

Laboratory rodents possessing explicit genetic backgrounds have been the conventional experimental animals in immunology, and their immune systems have been extensively studied. Nevertheless, certain aspects of immunological phenomena cannot be investigated readily using murine species, either because of their size limitations or because of some important physiological differences between rodents and large animal species such as humans.

The sheep has often been used in the study of lymphocyte migration and has proved to be a useful animal model for understanding the cellular mechanisms underlying lymphocyte recirculation (1). In this species, the development of lymphatic cannulation techniques (2) made it possible to study separately the ingress and egress of different lymphocyte populations in different lymphoid organs (3). The epitome of this type of study is found in the investigation of migratory behavior of lymphocytes in the fetal lamb, where it was firmly established that lymphocyte recirculation commences during gestation in the absence of any exogenous antigenic stimuli (4). Other studies in which sheep have provided important knowledge in immunology are the ontogeny of immune responses in fetuses and the study of cell production in primary lymphoid organs. In sheep a peculiar placental structure completely separates the fetus from the mother so that the fetal immune system develops without maternal influence. By taking

**Present affiliation*: Tokyo Metropolitan Institute of Medical Science, Tokyo, Japan.

advantage of this physiological peculiarity, genuine primary immune responses to various antigens could be chronologically monitored following antigenic challenge to the fetal lamb (5,6). Another peculiarity of this animal that permits the detailed investigation of interesting immunological phenomena concerns the anatomy of primary lymphoid organs. The thymus of the sheep consists of cervical and thoracic portions, and the cervical thymus is readily accessible to surgical manipulations with minimal stress to the animal (7) because of its extrathoracic location. A major site of B-cell production in the sheep, the Peyer's patches in the ileum, also lie in a surgically accessible location. The ileal Peyer's patches develop in a fetal environment and acquire their histological maturity before birth. By the use of a sophisticated extracorporeal perfusion system (8), the ileal Peyer's patches have been demonstrated to generate and export enough B cells to maintain the peripheral pool of sIg^+ cells in the sheep, and it has been suggested that they may be homologous to the avian bursa (9).

While such studies in sheep have over the last two decades made many significant contributions to our knowledge of the immune system, the advent of hybridoma technology and the development of monoclonal antibodies to surface markers on sheep lymphocytes now permit a more precise definition of lymphocyte subpopulations in this animal and will help researchers to dissect the complexity of lymphocyte physiology in more detail.

In this review we will summarize what is currently known about differentiation antigens of the sheep lymphohemopoietic system and discuss the antigens in relation to nomenclature recently introduced for the human differentiation antigens (10).

II. CELL-SURFACE ANTIGENS IN THE LYMPHOHEMOPOIETIC SYSTEM OF THE SHEEP

A. Antigens Present on All Sheep T Cells

1. Antigens Homologous to Human CD5 (T1) Antigens

ST-1a/b Antigen. We have reported two mAb, ST-1a and ST-1b, that recognize antigens present on all sheep T cells (11-13). Flow cytometric analysis on thymocytes, and separated T and B lymphocytes from peripheral blood or lymph, revealed that the mAb ST-1a/b label all thymocytes and T cells but not B cells, and that the labeling intensity is relatively weak with thymocytes, intermediate with peripheral blood T cells, and strongest with efferent lymph T cells, suggesting that the expression of the ST-1a/b-reactive antigen on the T-cell surface increases along the course of T-cell differentiation. Lymphocytes responding to T-cell mitogens in vitro remain positive for the mAb binding, indicating that the ST-1a/b antigen is a stable T-cell marker.

The ontogeny of cells bearing ST-1a/b determinants in fetal lambs of various ages has been investigated by means of an immunoperoxidase staining on frozen

Table 1 Monoclonal Antibodies to Sheep Cell-surface Antigens

Cell populations defined	Identifying mAb	MW of antigen[a] recognized	Homologous antigens in other species	Refs.
All T cells	ST-1a/b	60-65K/67K	human CD5 (mouse Ly-1)	11-13
	25-91	67K	human CD5 (mouse Ly-1)	14
T-cell subsets				
Helper T cells	11.2 G11	57K	human CD4 (mouse L3T4)	15
	44-38	56K	human CD4 (mouse L3T4)	16,17
	T-80	?	?	18
CTL & CTLp[b]	ST-8	33-35K	human CD8 (mouse Ly-2)	19,20
	24-96 38-65	33K636K	human CD8 (mouse Ly-2)	16,17
Others	A1E1	12K/45K	human CD1 (mouse TL)	UP[c]
	20-27	12K/46K	human CD1 (mouse TL)	14
	19-19	215K	?	17
	197	220K	?	11
Pre-T cells?	E-79	?	?	UP
All B cells	E-53	?	?	11
B cells and activated T cells	28-1	24-26K/30-32K	MHC class II Ag	21
	SW73.2	24-26K/30-32K	MHC class II Ag	22
	SB-1	?	MHC class II Ag?	11
All cells	41-19	12K/44K	MHC class I Ag	23
	S064.6	12K/44K	MHC class I Ag	24
All leucocytes	151	190/200/220K	LCA (mouse T-200 & B-220)	11
	1-32	190/210/225K	LCA	25
Erythroid and myeloid cells	175	?	?	11

[a]Under reduced conditions.
[b]Cytotoxic T lymphocytes and their precursors.
[c]Unpublished.

sections of lymphoid organs and flow cytometric analysis of single-cell organ suspensions. In a 42-day-old fetus (gestation period of sheep = about 150 days), upon which immunoperoxidase staining of serial transverse sections of the whole body was performed, it was found that only the thymus contains demonstrable accumulations of the antigen-bearing cells. ST-1a/b$^+$ cells subsequently appear in the spleen, and the precapsular lymph node, followed by the mesenteric lymph node. The number of positive cells increases markedly in these secondary lymphoid organs after midgestation. These cells show nonrandom localization in secondary lymphoid organs in that they are found in accumulations around central arterioles in the white pulp of the spleen, paracortex of lymph nodes, and the interfollicular area of the jejunal Peyer's patches.

Biochemical analysis of the ST-1a/b-reactive antigens revealed that these T-cell-specific antigens are glycoproteins that consist of two noncovalently linked polypeptides of apparent molecular weight 67 Kd and 60-65 Kd. It is unclear whether the 67-Kd and 60-65-Kd subunits represent two different polypeptides, or whether they have the same polypeptide backbones but differ in the extent of glycosylation. Binding inhibition experiments showed that mAb ST-1a blocked the binding of mAb ST-1b on T cells in a dose-dependent manner and that saturating amounts of mAb ST-1a completely blocked subsequent binding of mAb ST-1b. In the reverse experiments mAb ST-1b blocked the binding of mAb ST-1a in an identical manner, indicating that ST-1a/b epitopes are either identical or topographically closely related. Sequential immunoprecipitation experiments showed that no immunoprecipitate could be obtained with mAb ST-1b if a cell lysate of T cells was immunoprecipitated extensively with mAb ST-1a. A cell lysate absorbed with ST-1b conversely yielded no immunoprecipitate with mAb ST-1a. In both cases, the absorbed cell lysates were successfully immunoprecipitated with an irrelevant monoclonal antibody, indicating the specific removal of the ST-1a-reactive antigen with mAb ST-1b, and of ST-1b antigen with mAb ST-1a. These results clearly indicate that determinants recognized by mAb ST-1a and ST-1b are identical.

The ST-1a/b antigen does not appear to mediate any important T-cell functions, since blocking of the cell-surface antigen with mAb ST-1a/b does not result in the inhibition of T-cell proliferation in response to lectins and alloantigens. Induction of cytotoxic T cells also cannot be inhibited by the treatment. However, both mAb ST-1a/b are cytotoxic antibodies and can lyse T cells in the presence of complement. Therefore, the mAb can be used as an effective means of removing contaminating T cells from non-T-cell preparations (26).

Characteristics of the ST-1a/b-reactive antigens with regard to the molecular mass and tissue distribution are very similar to those of pan-T-cell markers in other species, namely the CD 5 (T1/Leu 1) antigen in humans and the Ly-1 antigen in mice. Furthermore, the antigen is sensitive to trypsin and is expressed more abundantly by medullary thymocytes than by cortical thymocytes. These characteristics are identical to those of the human and mouse pan-T-cell markers and are compatible with the notion that the ST-1a/b-reactive antigen is the sheep homologue of the human CD 5 and the mouse Ly-1 antigens (12,13,19).

Both human CD 5 and mouse Ly-1 are known to be expressed by a very small subset of B cells and also by B-cell-type leukemia cells (27,28). However, there is no indication that a significant population of sheep B cells expresses the ST-1 defined antigen.

mAb ST-1a/b do not cross-react with T cells of any other species of animals so far examined (man, monkey, rat, mouse, guinea pig, chicken, frog, pig, horse, goat, and cattle), suggesting that the antigen appeared after the divergence of sheep and other ruminants from a common ancestor.

SBU-T1 Antigen. Mackay et al. (1985) have suggested that the SBU-1 antigen is the sheep homologue of the human CD 5 and mouse Lyt-1 antigens as has been suggested with ST-1a/b reactive antigens (19). The tissue distribution of antigen-bearing cells, the biochemistry (glycoprotein consisting of two polypeptide chains of 67 Kd and 62 Kd), and the ontogeny (17) are very similar to those of the ST-1a/b antigen. However, there are minor differences. The lower molecular weight form of the SBU-T1 antigen is claimed not to be expressed by lymph node T cells and possibly not by medullary thymocytes, whereas with the ST-1a/b-reactive antigen, the lower molecular weight form is more abundantly expressed by lymph node T cells and also by the medullary cell population in the thymus. Although the SBU-T1 antigen clearly resembles the human CD 5 and mouse Ly-1 antigens, functional significance of the SBU-T1 antigens has not been reported.

B. Antigens Present on T-cell Subsets

1. Antigens Homologous to Human CD 1 (T6) Antigen

SBU-T6 Antigen. SBU-T6 antigen recognized by mAb 20.27 has been suggested to be homologous to the human CD 1 (T6) antigen. The SBU-T6 antigen consists of two noncovalently associated polypeptides of 46 Kd and 12 Kd molecular weight and is expressed abundantly by cortical thymocytes of the sheep (14). Human CD 1 (T6) is detected on the surface of cortical thymocytes but not on medullary thymocytes or on peripheral T and B lymphocytes, and is called "thymocyte-restricted" antigen (29). The functional role of the molecule is not known, but its homology to the mouse TL antigens has been suggested on the basis of its association with β_2-microglobulin, the tissue distribution and molecular mass (29). Although the SBU-T6 antigen is similar to the human CD 1 (T6) and the mouse TL in molecular mass profile, its association with β_2-microglobulin has not been formally demonstrated. The tissue distribution is also different from that of the human CD 1 and of the mouse TL in that not only cortical thymocytes, but also B cells in peripheral blood, express detectable levels of the antigen.

A1E1. mAb A1E1 was generated against afferent lymph cells at the University of Edinburgh (J. Hopkins, unpublished). The tissue distribution of A1E1-reactive antigen is identical to that of human CD 1 (T6) antigen, in that it is detected on cortical thymocytes and interdigitating cells in lymph nodes. Unlike SBU-T6, the A1E1 antigen is not found on B cells.

The antigen consists of two polypeptide chains of 45 Kd and 12 Kd. Therefore, the A1E1 antigen is identical to the human CD 2 (T6) antigen in terms of the tissue distribution and molecular mass, and it can be said that the A1E1 antigen is more likely to be the sheep homologue of the human CD 1 than the aforementioned SBU-T6 antigen.

2. Antigens Homologous to Human CD 2 Antigens

CD 2 (T11) antigen, a single polypeptide of about 45 Kd molecular weight, is a human T-cell antigen associated with the receptor for sheep erythrocytes. The antigen is found on greater than 95% of thymocytes and peripheral T cells (30). mAb to the CD 2 blocks not only erythrocyte rosette formation (31) but also inhibits the mixed lymphocyte reaction (32). Anti-CD 2 mAb are also known to induce polyclonal activation of T cells (33). In the sheep some mAb show these characteristics but the biochemistry of the antigen is not clear (T. Hünig, personal communication). In this context, it is relevant to describe briefly a mAb L180/1 that has been reported to recognize the ligand of T11 (CD 2) or T11 target structure (T11-TS) (34,35). The mAb L180/1 was selected from a panel of mAb against sheep erythrocytes by its ability to block the rosette formation of human T cells with sheep erythrocytes. It also blocks the E-rosette formation of sheep activated T cells. The L180/1-reactive antigen, a presumptive T11-TS, is a glycoprotein of about 42 Kd molecular weight and is present not only on sheep erythrocytes but also on leukocytes. Since the L180/1 can block the mixed lymphocyte reaction but not the IL-2-driven antigen-independent phase of T-lymphocyte proliferation, the L180/1-reactive antigen or the presumptive T11-TS has been suggested to function as a cell-interaction molecule in antigen-specific immune responses.

3. Antigens Homologous to Human CD 3 Antigen

CD 3 (T3) antigen is noncovalently associated with the human T-cell receptor and is present on all mature T cells in humans (36). Anti-T3 mAb are able to block the induction and effector phase of cell-mediated lympholysis (36a,37), inhibit T-cell responses to soluble antigens, and are mitogenic for resting T cells (38). No homologous antigen to the human CD 3 has been reported in the sheep. Since mAb to the CD 3 has been a useful tool for examining the mechanism of antigen recognition and for studying the ontogeny of T lymphocytes, the generation of monoclonal reagents against the CD 3 homologue in the sheep is an urgent task.

4. Antigens Homologous to Human CD 4 (T4) Antigen

In humans it is believed that lymphocytes expressing CD 4 (T4) or CD 8 (T8) antigen belong to a mutually exclusive cell population and can exhibit different cellular functions. Lymphocytes bearing CD 4 recognize specific antigen in the context of MHC class II molecules and function as helper/inducer T cells, whereas cells bearing CD 8 recognize antigen in association with MHC class I molecules and function as cytotoxic/suppressor T cells. CD 4 and CD 8 are 55-Kd and 32-33-Kd glycoproteins, respectively.

In the sheep mAb that react to CD 4-like molecules or antibodies that recognize helper/inducer-type T cells have been reported.

SBU-T4 Antigen. SBU-T4 antigen is recognized by mAb 44-38 and 44-97 and consists of a major polypeptide of 56 Kd (14a) and minor polypeptides of 110-120 Kd (17,39) and 17 Kd (17) and has been suggested to be the structural homologue of the human CD 4 (T4) antigen. The antigen is expressed on about 80% of thymocytes, 20% of peripheral blood mononuclear cells, and 50% of efferent lymph lymphocytes. These SBU-T4$^+$ thymocytes co-express SBU-T8 antigen, whereas SBU-T4$^+$ peripheral T cells do not express the SBU-T8. The SBU-T8 has been claimed to be the sheep homologue of the human CD 8 antigen (25) as described later.

Although the functional role of SBU-T4 has still to be elucidated, the N-terminal sequence has been examined and the primary structure of the SBU-T4 has been shown to be highly homologous to that of the mouse CD 4-equivalent, L3T4 antigen (39). Therefore, despite the lack of information on the function of cells expressing the SBU-T4 antigen, it is perhaps valid to conclude, based on the tissue distribution, its molecular mass, and the N-terminal sequence homology, that the SBU-T4 is the sheep CD 4 molecule.

Antigen Recognized by mAb 11.2 G11. The mAb 11.2 G11 precipitates a single polypeptide chain of 57 Kd present on a T-cell subset (15). Approximately 40% of peripheral blood mononuclear cells express the 11.2 G11-defined antigen as determined by microcytotoxicity. Immunohistochemical studies show that the antigen-bearing cells are located mainly in the thymic cortex, the paracortex of lymph nodes, and the periarteriolar lymphoid sheath of the spleen. Treatment of sheep lymphocytes with this mAb and complement significantly inhibits mitogen- and antigen-induced lymphocyte proliferation. Therefore, the 11.2 G11-defined antigen is expressed on helper-type T cells, and its molecular mass and tissue distribution also correspond to those of the human CD4

5. Antigens Homologous to Human CD 8 (T8) Antigen

ST-8 Antigen. This antigen is defined by mAb ST-8 and expressed on a subset of T cells that can mediate cytotoxic function (19,20). The antigen molecule is a 35-Kd glycoprotein similar to the human CD 8 and mouse Ly-2 antigens.

The tissue distribution of cells bearing the ST-8 antigen is also highly similar to that of human CD 8 and mouse Ly-2. ST-8$^+$ cells were found mainly in the thymic cortex, T-dependent areas of the peripheral lymphoid organs, and the splenic red pulp and marginal zone, but not in B-dependent areas, such as germinal centers or lymph follicles of the Peyer's patches. Approximately 10% of peripheral blood mononuclear cells and 15% of efferent lymph lymphocytes are ST-8$^+$.

The elimination of ST-8$^+$ cells can result in the complete abrogation of the in vitro generation of CTL and their effector function, but does not interfere with the proliferative responses to the alloantigens and T-cell mitogens. Furthermore, the mAb ST-8 can block the CTL killing in the absence of complement, as has been demonstrated with antibodies against the human CD 8 (40) and mouse Ly-2 (41). These observations support the notion that the ST-8 antigen is the sheep homologue of the human CD 8 and mouse Ly-2. However, it is not clear whether the mAb ST-8 recognizes suppressor T-cell subpopulations.

SBU-T8 Antigen. This antigen is recognized by two mAb, 24.96 and 38.65, and is present on about 12% of peripheral blood mononuclear cells and 80% of thymocytes (17). Biochemical analysis suggests that the antigen consists of two polypeptides of 33 and 36 Kd, respectively (25). The 33-Kd molecule is expressed more abundantly than the 36-Kd molecule in thymocytes, but only the 36-Kd is detected in peripheral T cells. The antigen is trypsin-sensitive. Two-color immunofluorescence analysis employing mAb against SBU-T4, as presumptive sheep CD 4, and SBU-T8 revealed that the large majority of cortical thymocytes coexpress these two antigens but peripheral T cells express only one of them. These characteristics of SBU-T8 all correspond to those reported with the human CD 8, and the SBU-T8 antigen has been suggested to be the sheep homologue of the human CD 8. Nevertheless, no functional role of cells expressing the SBU-T8 has been reported.

6. Other Antigens Present on Sheep T-cell Subsets

Antigen Recognized by mAb T-80. mAb T-80 was the first mAb to be reported as a monoclonal reagent reactive with sheep T cells (18). Neither B cells nor other cells in the hemopoietic system show detectable levels of the surface binding of the mAb T-80. The tissue distribution of cells recognized by this antibody is similar to cells expressing SBU-T4 or the 11.2 G11-defined antigen. In the fetal environment, the antigen-bearing cells can be detected in the thymus as soon as the thymus becomes lymphoid. In postnatal animals T-80$^+$ cells are the major constituent of the thymic cortex and they are scattered in the thymic medulla. They are also abundant in the white pulp of the spleen, particularly around central arterioles. In lymph nodes the positive cells accumulate in the paracortex. The only notable difference in the tissue distribution between T-80$^+$ cells and SBU-T4$^+$ cells is that the former are absent in germinal centers, while the latter are frequently found in the B-cell follicles.

Although only about 50% of peripheral blood T cells are T-80$^+$, over 90% of T cells are T-80$^+$ in efferent lymph into which recirculating lymphocytes selectively enter by extravasation. These T-80$^+$ cells in efferent lymph have been shown to have very high membrane-associated actin activity compared to other lymphocyte populations (24) and appear to be better equipped for the extravasation and passage through labyrinthine lymph node parenchyme.

Various attempts to characterize the biochemical nature of the T-80 defined antigen have been unsuccessful. Nevertheless, functional results suggest that helper-type T cells are recognized by the mAb T-80. The mAb T-80 strongly inhibits the proliferative responses in the presence of complement to T-cell mitogens and alloantigens, and also the induction phase of cytotoxic T cells (CTL), but not CTL effector activity (19). The binding of the mAb alone does not affect any of the in vitro T-cell functions, suggesting that the T-80 defined antigen is not directly involved in the antigen recognition of helper-type T cells.

SBU-T19 Antigen. mAb 19-19 is reactive with a T-cell subset that expresses neither SBU-T4 nor SBU-T8 antigen (17). The 19-19 defined antigen has been designated as SBU-T19 antigen and has an apparent molecular mass of 215 Kd. Sequential immunoprecipitation analysis suggests that, although the molecular mass profile is similar to that of common leukocyte antigen (LCA) (16), the SBU-T19 is not antigenically related to the LCA. SBU-T19$^+$ cells represent about 1% of thymocytes and can be found as foci around blood vessels in the thymic medulla and scattered throughout the cortex. In the periphery the positive cells constitute about 15% of peripheral blood mononuclear cells, 7% of efferent lymph lymphocytes, and 1-3% of lymph node lymphocytes. SBU-T19$^+$ cells are found in the subcapsular region in nodes. The functional role of the SBU-T19 antigen is not known.

Antigen Recognized by mAb 197. Similar to the mAb 19-19, mAb 197 defines a minor subpopulation of T cells that are negative for the expression of aforementioned T-80 defined or ST-8 defined antigens (Beya and Miyasaka, unpublished). The antigen precipitated by the mAb 197 is a glycoprotein of an apparent molecular weight of approximately 220 Kd. The tissue distribution of 197$^+$ cells also bears a resemblance to that of SBU-T19$^+$ cells in that the positive cells are scattered throughout the thymus, and are localized in the subcapsular region in lymph nodes. In the spleen the positive cells are found in the peripheral region of the white pulp. Flow cytometric analysis showed that mAb 197 labels about 15% of peripheral blood mononuclear cells and 10% of efferent lymph lymphocytes. One interesting aspect of the cell population defined by the mAb 197 is that chronic lymphatic drainage of the animal results in the early disappearance of 197$^+$ cells, suggesting that this particular cell population is easily mobilizable. The functional significance of this high molecular weight molecule remains to be explored.

Antigen Recognized by mAb E-79–A Marker for Pre-T cells? mAb E-79 was prepared by Ezaki at our laboratory and labels a very small population of thymocytes in postnatal animals. Less than 1% of thymocytes are labeled and they are almost exclusively found in the cortex, particularly in the subcapsular region where pre-T cells are believed to be located in rodents (42). In the fetal environment, when the sheep thymus appears at about 35-40 days, all cells in the thymus appear to express the E-79-reactive antigen. After 45 days in gestation the proportion of antigen-bearing cells decreases rapidly and the cells are found to be localized predominantly in the subcapsular region of the thymus. This area is rich in dividing cells and is negative for the expression of ST-8-reactive antigen but weakly positive for ST-1 and T-80 defined antigens. No accumulation of E-79 cells is found in the liver and bone marrow throughout gestation. We are currently investigating the biochemistry of the antigen as well as the cell cycle status of the cells bearing the antigen in the hope that mAb 79 defines immature cells in the T lineage or pre-T cells of sheep.

C. Antigens Present on B Cells

1. Immunoglobulins

Detection of surface and cytoplasmic immunoglobulins in the sheep has depended on the use of heteroantisera. Heavy chain-specific anti-sheep immunoglobulin sera have been used successfully to detect surface immunoglobulins of the major isotypes, namely IgM, IgG, and IgA (43) and also to detect class-specific immunoglobulin-secreting cells (44,45). The immunoglobulin class detectable on the surface of sheep B cells in lymph and blood is predominantly IgM. Nothing is known about sheep IgD and IgE. IgG and IgA bearing cells are extremely rare in the circulation. Evidence has accumulated that the Peyer's patches in the ileum (IPP) are the major site of the surface IgM^+ cell production (46,47). The sheep IPP bear a close resemblance to the bursa of Fabricius in birds with regard to their morphology, cell composition, precocious development in gestation in the absence of external antigenic stimuli, extent of cell proliferation and subsequent export of cells into the periphery, and involution occurring at around the time the animal reaches its sexual maturity (reviewed in Ref. 9). Like the avian bursa, IPP consist of numerous follicles of B cells, whereas T cells account for less than 1% of total cells. The surgical resection of a large proportion of the IPP before birth or during the first week of postnatal life results in a severe reduction in the number of circulating B cells in lambs (43,46). Fetal IPP show lymphopoiesis in the absence of maternal or exogenous antigen (48). IPP undergo a significant degree of postnatal involution as seen in the bursa of Fabricius. The extent of emigration of newly formed B cells from the IPP of young lambs is sufficient to replace the B-cell pool in the peripheral blood within 2 to 5 days (49). Flow cytofluorometric analysis shows that the majority of IPP cells express small amounts of surface IgM (low sIgM$^+$) (11,50,65). These low-sIgM$^+$ cells are immature, in that they respond poorly to B-cell mitogens such as LPS and protein A, but they express receptors to peanut agglutinin (PNA) and proliferate rapidly in vitro. They can also be induced to express and secrete IgM upon stimulation with phorbol myristate acetate (50). Approximately 5% of IPP cells bear no sIgM. These cells do not bear detectable levels of cytoplasmic Ig and differ from pre-B cells reported in other species. However, these cells can also be induced into high-sIgM$^+$ cells upon exposure to phorbol myristate acetate, which may indicate the presence of precursors of sIgM$^+$ cells within the IPP. Examination of cells leaving IPP revealed that the level of sIgM expression was higher on IPP emigrant cells but not as high as that of peripheral B cells (26). Therefore, the level of sIgM expression of B cells can be related to the stage of cell differentiation in the sheep as follows: In IPP, where B cells are produced and expanded, there is a small population of sIg$^-$ cells that can be stimulated to become sIgM$^+$ cells, whereas the majority of IPP cells express low levels of sIgM. Cells leaving IPP express intermediate levels of sIgM, and circulating B cells express the highest levels of sIgM.

Attempts to produce monoclonal reagents against sheep Ig have been initiated, and mAb against IgA is becoming available (J. Hall, personal communication). Since differentiation and migration pathways of sheep B cells are becoming better defined, acquisition of more monoclonal reagents against sheep Ig is urgently needed.

2. Other Determinants on B Cells

Two mAb have been reported to discriminate B cells from T cells in the sheep. mAb E-53 (11,13) binds to cells of Peyer's patch follicles, splenic follicles, and germinal centers of lymph nodes on frozen sections. The thymus and T-dependent areas of peripheral lymphoid tissues are almost devoid of E-53$^+$ cells. No accumulations of the positive cells are found in the bone marrow and fetal liver. Although mAb E-53 shows specific reactivity towards B cells on fixed sections, it does not stain living B cells in suspensions, suggesting that the E-53-reactive antigen is cryptic on the B-cell membrane or present in the cytoplasm of B cells. Repeated attempts to immunoprecipitate the antigen have been unsuccessful (Beya and Miyasaka, unpublished). Although the biochemical nature of the antigen is unclear, the mAb E-53 is useful in determining the localization of B cells on frozen sections and can be a useful reagent to study the ontogeny of B cells.

mAb SB-1 has been shown to react to a non-Ig determinant on sheep B cells (11). The biochemistry of this antigen is unknown. Small T cells show no detectable binding of this mAb, whereas all B cells in efferent lymph and blood are positively labeled. The antigen defined by SB-1 increases its expression along the course of B-cell differentiation, as described above, with sIgM. However, a recent observation that the SB-1-reactive antigen can be induced on T cells by stimulation with lectins (Miyasaka and Beya, unpublished) indicates that the antigen is not a B-cell-specific marker.

Peanut agglutinin (PNA), a lectin with specificity for terminal galactose residues on cell-surface oligosaccharides has been shown to bind to germinal center cells in sheep lymph nodes (51). Peyer's patch cells also show high PNA binding, whereas circulating B cells have only meager binding. B cells in the circulation can exhibit high PNA binding if they are treated with neuraminidase, indicating that cells in the B lineage retain PNA receptors but that these become masked by sialic acid on mature B cells (26). PNA receptors are easily detectable on circulating T cells as well and thus, contrary to an earlier suggestion (52), they are not cell-lineage-specific markers.

D. Major Histocompatibility Antigens

The major histocompatibility complex is a chromosomal region that contains loci coding for molecules that are involved in recognition of non-self by T lymphocytes. There are two major loci, namely class I and class II. The class I gene products or MHC class I antigens (H-2 K,D,L in the mouse; HLA-A,B,C in the human) are found on every nucleated cell in varying amounts and function as targets for cytotoxic T lymphocytes. MHC class II antigens (I-A, I-E in the mouse; HLA-DR,DC,SB in the human) are present on B cells, antigen-presenting cells and a number of other cell types, and are recognized predominantly by helper/inducer T lymphocytes. The expression of these MHC antigens on lymphoid cells appears to be associated with the stage of cell differentiation.

mAb defining the MHC class I and II antigens are becoming available in the sheep. These antibodies appear to recognize nonpolymorphic determinants of the MHC antigens and are useful tools for the study of lymphocyte differentiation.

1. MHC Class I Antigens

Class I antigens are classical alloantigens consisting of a polymorphic glycoprotein heavy chain of 40-45 Kd noncovalently associated with an oligomorphic nonglycosylated light chain (β_2-microglobulin) of approximately 13 Kd. The heavy chain maps to the MHC, whereas the light chain is encoded by a gene not linked to the MHC.

Three mAb, SBU.I 41-17, SBU.I 41-19, and SBU.I 41-28, were generated at the University of Melbourne by immunizing mice with pokeweed mitogen-stimulated sheep lymphocytes (23). They all precipitate a 44-Kd heavy chain that is noncovalently associated with a 12-Kd light chain. The antigens recognized are detected on almost all lymphoid cells as well as on vascular endothelium. In nonlymphoid tissues cells show variable expression of the antigen. The molecular mass profile and tissue distribution of the antigen suggest that the mAb recognize the framework region of the MHC class I-like antigens of the sheep, and, hence, the antigens are designated OLA (ovine leukocyte antigen) class I antigens. Serological studies suggest that these mAb recognize different epitopes on the nonpolymorphic region of the OLA class I antigens. However, the MHC nature of the molecules, such as the polymorphism of the heavy chain and the oligomorphism of the presumptive β_2-microglobulin light chain, has not been reported, and genetic studies are required before the antigens recognized are qualified as the sheep MHC class I antigens.

Rat mAb SO64-6 was generated by J. Hopkins at the University of Edinburgh and recognizes 44 Kd/12 Kd glycoproteins that are ubiquitously present on nucleated cells in the blood (Beya and Miyasaka, unpublished). In the thymus the antigen is detected easily on cells in the medulla but is scarce or absent on the majority of cells located in the cortex. Similar to the antigen recognized by SBU.I antibodies, the SO64.6 reactive antigen also bears some important characteristics of MHC class I antigens, although it remains to be demonstrated that the antigen actually maps to the MHC.

2. MHC Class II Antigens

Class II antigens are heterodimeric transmembrane glycoproteins composed of α and β chains. The α chain is 30-33 Kd in size and has two N-linked glycans, whereas the β chain is 28-30 Kd and has one N-linked glycan in humans (53).

Some antibodies against class II antigens of the mouse (A.TH anti A.TL serum) (54) and of the human (65; J. Hopkins, personal communication) have been shown to recognize "Ia-like" molecules of the sheep.

Recently monoclonal reagents were produced which are believed to react to the sheep MHC class II antigens. SBU.II 28-1, 38-27, and 38-64 antibodies were generated by Puri and others (21). Antigens immunoprecipitated with these mAb all give typical two-chain patterns of 30-32 Kd/24-26 Kd by SDS-polyacrylamide gel electrophoresis. The antigen can be detected on the majority of B cells, a small proportion of sIg^- cells in the blood, macrophages in afferent lymph, and reticular epithelial cells in the thymic cortex and medulla. It remains to be demonstrated, however, whether these molecules are mapped to the MHC or whether they are associated with antigen recognition by helper/inducer T cells.

A rat mAb SW73.2 also recognizes 33-35-Kd/28-30-Kd glycoproteins present on a subpopulation of sheep lymphocytes (55). Immunofluorescence analysis shows that sIg^+ cells and veiled cells in afferent lymph express large amounts of the antigen. Small resting T cells in blood and efferent lymph show no detectable expression of the SW73.2 reactive antigen, but in vivo activated T cells (55) or lectin-stimulated T cells in vitro express the antigen abundantly (Miyasaka, unpublished). Histologically the antigen-positive cells are found mainly in germinal centers of lymphoid tissues. An observation that the mAb 73.2 can inhibit the antigen-specific proliferation of T cells against alloantigens and PPD (55), together with the biochemical nature and the tissue distribution of the antigen, strongly suggest that the antigen defined by the mAb 73.2 is the sheep MHC class II antigen. The formal proof will be obtained by genetic studies.

E. Antigens on Other Hemopoietic Cells

1. Leukocyte Common Antigen (LA)

Three mAb have been reported to react with the LCA of the sheep.

mAb 1.11.32 and 1.28.124, produced at the University of Melbourne, label all leukocytes by recognizing the LCA (16). The antigen consists of glycoproteins of 190, 215, and 220 Kd. The cross-reactive antigen is found on bovine cells but not on cells obtained from mouse, rat, man, or chicken.

mAb 151 produced at our laboratory also recognizes all myeloid and lymphoid cells but not erythroid cells (11). It precipitates glycoproteins of 190, 200, and 220 Kd. SDS-polyacrylamide gel electrophoresis analysis on various separated lymphoid cell populations suggest that different lineages of cells express different molecular forms of the antigen. Cell lysates obtained from the thymus or purified T cells yield immunoprecipitates of apparent molecular weight of 190 and 200 Kd, and lysates of ileal Peyer's patch cells and of circulating B cells provide the 220-Kd form. These 190-200-Kd molecules on T cells and 220-Kd molecules on B cells in the sheep probably correspond to the mouse T-200 (56) and B-220 (57) protein, respectively. The mouse T-200 protein appears as two closely electrophoresing bands of 190-200 Kd in precipitates obtained from splenic T cells, whereas the B-200 protein is a glycoprotein of 220 Kd expressed on cells in the B lineage of the mouse.

2. Antigen Present on Myeloid and Erythroid Cells

mAb 175 recognizes a biochemically unknown antigen present on nonlymphoid cells such as myeloid and erythroid cells (11). The antibody is useful to detect contamination of nonlymphoid cells in lymphoid cell preparations. For instance, proportions of monocytes in Percoll-separated mononuclear cell populations from the blood can be easily enumerated by immunofluorescence methods with mAb 175, and the results correspond well to those obtained by cytochemical methods such as nonspecific esterase staining (58) performed separately on fixed cells.

These two mAb, 151 and 175, have been shown to be very useful in performing differential counts on mixed populations of cells such as bone marrow cells or fetal blood cells which contain various lineages of cells that are not easily identified by their morphology (11). The phenotyping of mixed cell populations can be obtained by immunofluorescence staining and subsequent flow cytometric analysis, since these mAb show differential binding patterns to different lineages of hemopoietic cells. The mAb 151 recognizes myeloid and lymphoid but not erythroid cells, and the mAb 175 recognizes meyloid and erythroid but not lymphoid cells. Therefore, a proportion (%) of erythroid cells, for instance, is given by subtracting a percentage value of 151^+ cells (lymphoid + myeloid) determined by cytometric analysis from 100. Similarly, a proportion of lymphoid cells can be determined by subtracting a percentage value of 175^+ cells (myeloid + erythroid) from 100; a proportion of myeloid cells is given by subtracting a percentage value of erythroid cells obtained as above from a percentage of 175^+ (erythroid + myeloid) cells. Necessary assumptions to be made in this approach are 2-fold; first, any cells within a given cell lineage, be it erythroid, myeloid, or lymphoid, would express a lineage-specific marker to be identified as positive or negative by these mAb 151 and 175; second, any given hemopoietic cell population is composed of cells belonging to these three lineages. The former notion is supported by various biological precedents observed in the hemopoietic system in cell differentiation of various species of animals so far examined. The latter assumption is not unreasonable, since it is well established that the compartment of nonerythroid, nonmyeloid, nonlymphoid cells such as uncommitted stem cells and megakaryocytes in the hemopoietic system is extremely small.

Phenotyping of fetal mononuclear cells by the use of this method has been initiated in our laboratory and results show a good correlation with those separately obtained by more subjective analysis such as differential cell counting based on the May-Grunwald Giemsa morphology. The preliminary results have been reported (11).

3. Antigens Present on Follicular Dendritic Cells

Recently a mAb against follicular dendritic cells (FDC) was produced by Kennedy-Stoskopf at our laboratory. FDC are present only in lymph follicles and are known to retain antigens in the form of immune complexes on the surface of their membranes (59). The mAb V.5 is IgM.κ and stains cells with extremely slender processes in germinal centers in lymph nodes on frozen sections. Germinal centers in the spleen and lymph follicles in the Peyer's patches of the ileum and jejunum also contain cells with the same appearance, and they are intensively stained with the mAb V.5. No other cell types in lymphoid tissues so far examined are stained. Cells with similar dendritic processes such as interdigitating cells in the lymph node cortex or in the thymus are clearly negative for the staining when examined by an indirect immunoperoxidase technique.

mAb against FDC have been reported in other species. mAb OX-2 (60) reacts with FDC but also with endothelial cells of high endothelial venules in lymph nodes. mAb Ki-M4 (61) labels FDC in fixed lymphoid tissues in humans and also a very small population of mononuclear cells in the blood. Interestingly, $V.5^+$ cells can be found in afferent lymph, albeit as a minor cell constituent. Veiled cells in afferent lymph which are believed to be of similar origin with interdigitating cells in the lymph node cortex appear to be V.5. The $V.5^+$ cells are much smaller in size than veiled cells and some of them extend multiple short processes from the cytoplasm. The biochemistry of the FDC-specific antigen defined by the mAb V.5 is under investigation.

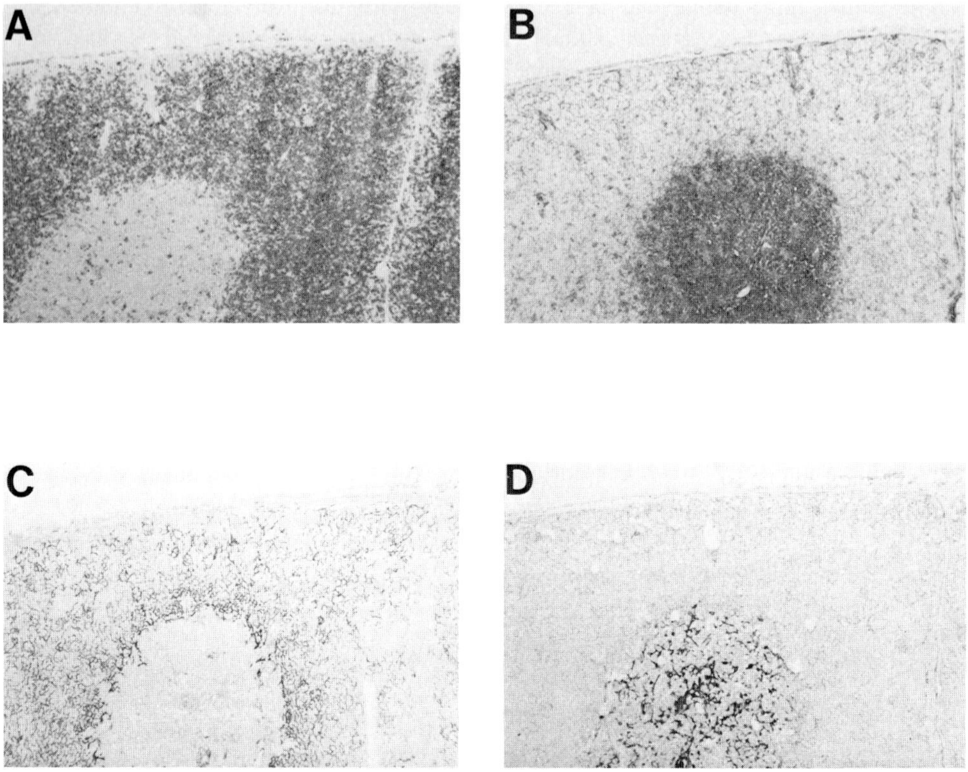

Figure 1 Immunoperoxidase staining pattern of serial frozen thymus sections. (A) mAb ST-8 (CD 8 equivalent) reacts predominantly with cortical lymphocytes. On the basis of the ST-8 staining pattern, the cortex and medulla can be clearly demarcated. (B) mAb SO64.6, in contrast, reacts predominantly with medullary lymphocytes. (C) mAb E-136 selectively stains reticular epithelial cells in the cortex, whereas mAb B43-42 (D) stains reticular epithelial cells in the medulla. (E) mAb 11 reacts with the capsule only. (F) mAb 175 reacts with

F. Antigens Present on the Thymic Microenvironment

Development of T cells initially takes place in the thymus, during which various antigenically definable subpopulations of lymphocytes differentiate in close contact with various types of stromal cells. These stromal components consist of epithelial cells, macrophages, and other types of nonlymphoid cells and are believed to influence the thymocyte maturation by providing a regulatory microenvironment for developing thymocytes. These various types of stromal cells are not only morphologically different but also antigenically distinct. In humans

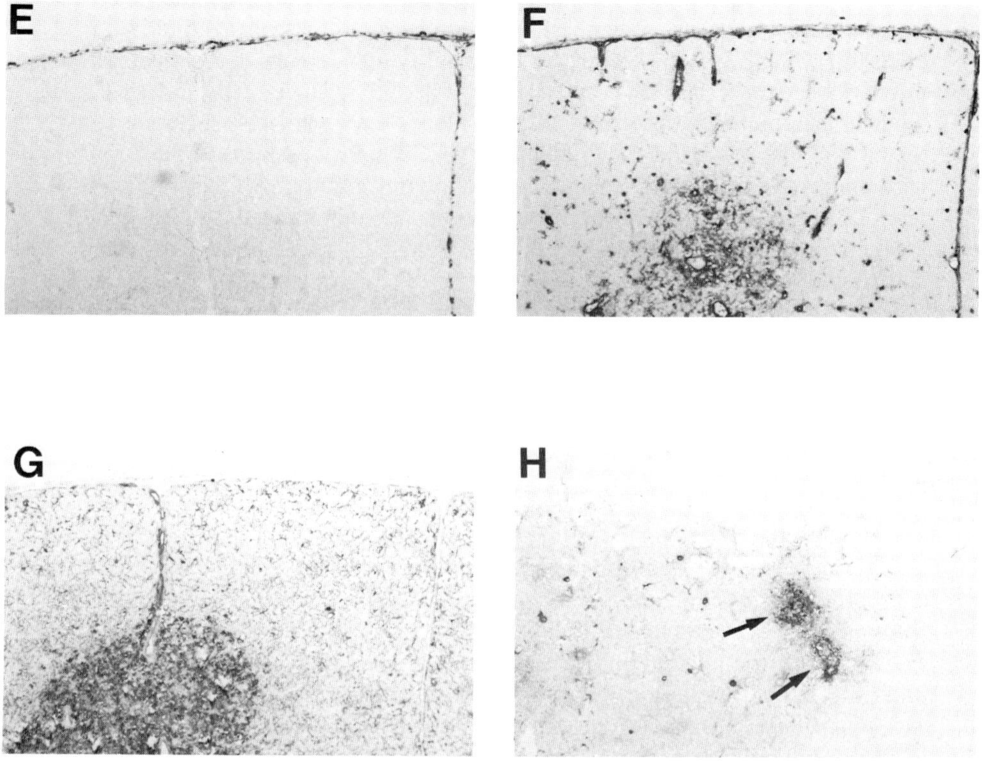

not only the capsule but also macrophages, reticular cells in the medulla, and blood vessel walls. (G) mAb SW73.2 recognizes a nonpolymorphic determinant of the MHC class II antigens and react with cortical reticular epithelial cells, medullary nonlymphoid cells and possibly medullary lymphocytes as well. (H) mAb B32-45 reacts with Hassall's corpuscles and some neighboring cells. Original magnification X 78.8. C = cortex, M = medulla, CA = capsule, Ha = Hassall's corpuscles.

and mice various mAb have been reported to show differential binding patterns to different components of the thymic microenvironment (62-64).

During the screening process of mAb that had been raised against thymocytes and fetal liver cells at our laboratory, we also found a few mAb that can selectively label various types of lymphoid cells and/or stromal cells in the thymus. Examination of serial sections of frozen thymic tissue stained by an immunoperoxidase method with various mAb show that some of these mAb are extremely selective in their binding to stromal cells (Fig. 1). mAb E-136 is reactive with cortical epithelial cells but not with medullary epithelial cells. Conversely, mAb B43-

42 labels medullary but not cortical epithelial cells. mAb SW73.2, which is believed to react with a nonpolymorphic determinant of MHC class II molecules, binds to epithelial cells of both types as well as lymphoid cells in the medulla. mAb B32-45 labels Hassall's corpuscles and adjacent epithelial cells. mAb 175 binds to macrophages, fibroblasts, and the blood vessel wall. mAb 11 binds to the interlobular septa and the thymic capsule. Reactivity patterns of these mAb with the thymic microenvironment, together with those of mAb that show differential binding to various lymphocyte subsets, are summarized in Table 2.

These observations clearly show that the thymic microenvironment is a complex tissue and that different types of stromal cells are in contact with different types of lymphocytes. The biochemical nature of these stromal antigens has yet to be determined, but a study of the ontogeny of antigen expression on thymic cells is under way and is hoped to provide some clue to the mechanism of generation and differentiation of various subsets of thymocytes.

III. SUMMARY

The hemopoietic system consists mainly of erythroid, myeloid, and lymphoid lineages and also their undifferentiated precursor cells. The widely used means of identifying the cellular lineage of hemopoietic cells has been morphological determination at the single-cell level. Although this can be done with relative ease on cells bearing mature morphology, the lineage assignment of cells with undifferentiated morphology has been difficult. Within the lymphoid cell lineage, in particular, although there exists functional heterogeneity that can easily be demonstrated by various in vivo and in vitro assays, the morphological heterogeneity is less obvious than in other cell lineages. It has been thus difficult to unravel the lymphocyte heterogeneity by depending on morphological investigation.

Recent development of hybridoma technology revealed that monoclonal antibodies (mAb) can have exquisite specificities and that they can selectively mark various cell populations in vitro. The cellular lineage of most cells in the lymphohemopoietic tissue of the sheep can now be identified without relying on morphological criteria by a panel of mAb that have been developed by various groups in the last several years.

mAb 151 labels myeloid and lymphoid cells by recognizing the common leukocyte antigen, and the 200-Kd form (T-200) and 220-Kd form (B-220) are detected on T and B lymphocytes, respectively. mAb 175 distinguishes erythroid and myeloid cells from lymphoid cells. Hence, by the use of these two mAb, sheep hemopoietic cells can be phenotyped into either the erythroid (175^+, 151^-), myeloid (175^+, 151^+), or lymphoid (175^-, 151^+) lineage.

Some mAb can distinguish T and B lymphocytes from other cells of hemopoietic origin. The sheep pan-T-cell marker is recognized by mAb ST-1a/b and 25-91 and is equivalent to the human CD 5. Functional markers on various

Table 2 Reactivity of mAb with Various Cellular Components of the Sheep Thymus

	Cortex				Medulla			
mAb	Capsule	Subcapsular blasts	Lymphocytes	Epithelial cells	Lymphocytes	Epithelial cells	Macrophages and fibroblasts	Hassall's corpuscles
11	+	–	–	–	–	–	–	–
E-136	–	–	–	+	–	–	–	–
B43-42	–	–	–	–	–	+	–	–
175	+	–	–	–	–	–	+	–
B32-45	–	–	–	–	–	–	–	+
SW73.2	–	–	–	+	+	+	–	–
SO64.6	–	–	–	±	+	+	–	–
E-79	–	+	–	–	–	–	–	–
ST-1	–	+	+	–	+	–	–	–
ST-8	–	–	+	–	– ~ +	–	–	–
A1E1	–	+	+	–	–	+[a]	–	–
T-80	–	+	+	–	– ~ +	–	–	–

[a]Cells with dendritic processes are positively stained.

lymphocyte subsets are also becoming available, although the picture hitherto obtained is not as complete as that which has been achieved in the man and mouse. Sheep cytotoxic T lymphocytes and their precursors are labeled by mAb ST-8 and the molecule recognized is equivalent to the human CD 8. The helper T-lymphocyte population is recognized by mAb T-80 but the biochemistry of the antigen is unclear. mAb 11 2 G11 also recognizes the helper T-cell population and its molecular mass and the tissue distribution suggest that the antibody recognizes the human CD 4. The SBU-T4 antigen recognized by mAb 44-38 and 44-97 is also likely to be the human CD-4 judging from its biochemistry, N-terminal amino acid sequence, and tissue distribution, although the functional role of the antigen-positive cell population remains to be elucidated.

mAb E-79 recognizes subcapsular blasts in the thymic cortex and the ontogeny of the cells reactive with the mAb E-79 suggests that the antibody labels the most immature cells in the thymus. A variety of mAb exist which react with various components of the thymic microenvironment. Cortical epithelial cells are positively labeled with mAb E-136 but negative with mAb 43-42. Conversely, medullary epithelial cells are positively marked with mAb 43-42 but negative with mAb E-136. Some mAb selectively bind to interlobular capsule, fibroblasts, or Hassall's corpuscles. These mAb should facilitate the investigation of the stromal cell function in relation to the T-cell development within the thymus.

Mature B lymphocytes are currently best identified in single-cell suspensions by polyclonal antisera. However, on frozen sections, mAb E-53 clearly distinguishes B cells from T cells and can be used as a useful anti-B-cell reagent. Monoclonal antibodies against sheep Ig are becoming available but more studies are required to expand the panel of anti-Ig mAb.

mAb against monomorphic determinants of the MHC class I and II antigens have been reported and used to study the expression of the MHC molecules in ontogenical development of lymphoid tissues. However, rigorous genetic studies are required to examine whether the molecules recognized by the mAb map to the MHC.

Obviously, more effort is to be made to expand the present library of monoclonal reagents against sheep hemopoietic cells, and it is hoped that the application of the mAb to the study of the lymphoid system of the sheep will help increase further the value of the sheep as a useful experimental animal to study immunology in vivo.

ACKNOWLEDGMENTS

We thank Ms. M.-F. Beya and Drs. S. Kennedy-Stoskopf and J. Hopkins for letting us use their unpublished materials. We would also like to thank Ms. L. Dudler and V. Stauffer for their excellent technical assistance, and Ms. C. Harley and Ms. C. Plattner for typing the manuscript.

REFERENCES

1. M. Miyasaka and Z. Trnka, Lymphocyte migration and differentiation in a large-animal model: The sheep, *Immunol. Rev., 91*: 87 (1986).
2. A. K. Lascelles and B. Morris, Surgical techniques for the collection of lymph from unanesthetized sheep, *Quart. J. Exp. Physiol., 46*: 199 (1961).
3. M. Miyasaka and Z. Trunka, Sheep as an experimental model for immunology: Immunological techniques *in vitro* and *in vivo*, in *Immunological Methods*, Vol. III (I. Lefkovits and B. Pernis, eds.), Academic Press, New York, 1985, p. 403.
4. L. D. Pearson, M. W. Simpson-Morgan, and B. Morris, Lymphopoiesis and lymphocyte recirculation in the sheep fetus, *J. Exp. Med., 143*: 167 (1976).
5. A. M. Silverstein and R. A. Prendergast, Lymphogenesis, immunogenesis and the generation of immunologic diversity, in *Developmental Aspects of Antibody Formation and Structure* (J. Sterzl and I. Riha, eds.), Academia, Prague, 1970, p. 69.
6. K. J. Fahey and B. Morris, Humoral immune responses in foetal sheep, *Immunology, 35*: 651 (1978).
7. A. Yamashita, M. Miyasaka, and Z. Trnka, Early postthymic T cells: Studies on lymphocytes in the lymph coming from the thymus of sheep, in *Immunology of the Sheep* (B. Morris and M. Miyasaka, eds.), Editiones Roche, Basel, 1985, p. 162.
8. R. Pabst and J. D. Reynolds, Evidence of extensive lymphocyte death in sheep Peyer's patches. II. The number and fate of newly-formed lymphocytes that emigrate from Peyer's patches, *J. Immunol., 136*: 2011 (1986).
9. J. D. Reynolds, Peyer's patches and the early development of B lymphocytes, *Contemp. Topics Microbiol. Immunol., 135*: 43.
10. A. Bernard, L. Boumsell, and C. Hill, Joint report of the first international workshop on human leukocyte differentiation antigens by the investigators of the participating laboratories, in *Leukocyte Typing: Human Leukocyte Differentiation Antigens Detected by Monoclonal Antibodies* (A. Bernard, L. Boumsell, J. Dausett, C. Milstein, and S. F. Schlossman, eds.), Springer-Verlag, New York, 1984.
11. M. Miyasaka, M.-F. Beya, L. Dudler, R. Parisot, T. Ezaki, and Z. Trnka, Studies on lymphocyte differentiation and migration in sheep by the use of monoclonal antibodies, in *Immunology of the Sheep* (B. Morris and M. Miyasaka, eds.), Editiones Roche, Basel, 1985, p. 68.
12. M.-F. Beya, M. Miyasaka, L. Dudler, T. Ezaki, and Z. Trnka, Studies on the differentiation of T lymphocytes in sheep. II. Two monoclonal antibodies that recognize all ovine T lymphocytes, *Immunology, 57*: 115 (1986).
13. M.-F. Beya and M. Miyasaka, Studies on the differentiation of T lymphocytes in sheep. III. Preliminary characterization of an antigen recognized by two pan T cell monoclonal antibodies, *Immunology, 58*: 71 (1986).
14. C. R. Mackay, F. J. Maddox, K. J. Gogolin-Ewens, and M. R. Brandon, Characterization of two sheep lymphocyte differentiation antigens, SBU-T1 and SBU-T6, *Immunology, 55*: 729 (1985).

14a. C. R. Mackay, J. F. Maddox, and M. R. Brandon, Three distinct subpopulations of sheep T lymphocytes, *Eur. J. Immunol., 16*: 19 (1985).
15. G. Lalonde, L. J. Gershwin, P. F. Moore, and D. Bernoco, Cytotoxic murine monoclonal antibody recognizing an ovine lymphocyte subpopulation similar to the human OKT-4-positive set, *J. Immunol., 136*: 2809 (1986).
16. J. F. Maddox, C. R. Mackay, and M. R. Brandon, The sheep analogue of leukocyte common antigen (LCA), *Immunology, 5*: 347 (1985).
17. C. R. Mackay, J. F. Maddox, and M. R. Brandon, Thymocyte subpopulations during early fetal development in sheep, *J. Immunol., 136*: 1592 (1986).
18. M. Miyasaka, I. Heron, L. Dudler, R. N. P. Cahill, L. Forni, T. Knaak, and Z. Trnka, Studies on the differentiation of T lymphocytes in sheep. I. Recognition of a sheep T-lymphocyte differentiation antigen by a monoclonal antibody T-80, *Immunology, 49*. 545 (1983).
19. T. Ezaki, R. Parisot, L. Dudler, M.-F. Beya, M. Miyasaka, and Z. Trnka, Monoclonal antibodies to surface markers which define functional subsets of sheep T lymphocytes, in *Immunology of the Sheep* (B. Morris and M. Miyasaka, eds.), Editiones Roche, Basel, 1985, p. 88.
20. T. Ezaki, M. Miyasaka, M.-F. Beya, L. Dudler, and Z. Trnka, A murine anti-sheep T8 monoclonal antibody, ST-8, that defines cytotoxic lymphocyte population, *Int. Arch. Allergy. Appl. Immunol., 82*: 168.
21. N. K. Puri, C. R. Mackay, and M. R. Brandon, Sheep lymphocyte antigens (OLA). II. Major histocompatibility complex class II molecules, *Immunology, 56*: 725 (1985).
22. J. Hopkins, I. McConnell, R. Bujdoso, and A. J. Munro, Studies of MHC class II products on sheep peripheral and efferent lymph cells, in *Immunology of the Sheep*, Editiones Roche, Basel, 1985, p. 441.
23. K. J. Gogolin-Ewens, C. R. Mackay, W. M. Mercer, and M. R. Brandon, Sheep lymphocyte antigens (OLA). I. Major histocompability complex class I molecules, *Immunology, 56*: 717 (1985).
24. M. Miyasaka, B. Mély-Goubert, W. M. Leiserson, L. Dudler, and Z. Trnka, Actin activity is high in the immunocompetent fraction of thymocytes, *Thymus, 6*: 57 (1984).
25. J. F. Maddox, C. R. Mackay, and M. R. Brandon, Surface antigens, SBU-T4 and SBU-T8, of sheep T lymphocyte subsets defined by monoclonal antibodies, *Immunology, 55*: 739 (1985).
26. M. Miyasaka, J. Reynolds, L. Dudler, M.-F. Beya, W. M. Leiserson, and Z. Trnka, Differentiation of B lymphocytes in sheep. II. Surface phenotype of B cells leaving the "Bursa-equivalent" lymphoid tissue of sheep, ileal Peyer's patches, in *Microenvironments in the Lymphoid System* (G. G. B. Klaus, ed.), Plenum Publ. Corp., New York, 1985, p. 119.
27. C. Y. Wang, R. A. Good, P. Ammirati, G. Dymbort, and R. L. Evans, Identification of a p69, 71 complex expressed on human T cells sharing determinants with B-type chronic lymphocytic leukemia cells, *J. Exp. Med., 151*: 1539 (1980).

28. K. Hayakawa, R. R. Hardy, D. R. Parks, and L. A. Herzenberg, The "Ly1 B" cell subpopulation in normal, immunodefective and autoimmune mice, *J. Exp. Med., 157*: 202 (1983).
29. C. Terhost, A. van Agthoven, K. LeClair, P. Snow, E. Reinherz, and S. Schlossman, Biochemical studies of the human thymocyte cell-surface antigens T6, T9 and T10, *Cell, 23*: 771 (1981).
30. F. D. Howard, J. A. Ledbetter, J. Wong, C. P. Bieber, E. B. Stinson, and L. A. Herzenberg, A human T lymphocyte differentiation marker defined by monoclonal antibodies that block E rosette formation, *J. Immunol., 126*: 2117 (1981).
31. W. Verbi, M. Greaves, D. Schneider, K. Konbek, H. Janossy, H. Stein, P. Kung, and G. Goldstein, Monoclonal antibodies OKT 11 and OKT11A have pan-T reactivity and block sheep erythrocyte "receptors," *Eur. J. Immunol., 12*: 81 (1982).
32. R. Palacios and O. Martinez-Maza, Is the E receptor on human T lymphocytes a "negative signal receptor"? *J. Immunol., 129*: 2479 (1982).
33. E. L. Larsson, J. Andersson, and A. Coutinho, Functional consequences of sheep red blood cell rosetting for human T-cells: gain of reactivity to mitogenic factors, *Eur. J. Immunol., 8*: 693 (1978).
34. T. Hünig, The cell surface molecule recognized by the erythrocyte receptor of T-lymphocytes. Identification and partial characterization using a monoclonal antibody, *J. Immunol., 162*: 890 (1985).
35. T. R. Hünig, The ligand of the erythrocyte receptor of T lymphocytes: Expression on white blood cells and possible involvement in T cell activation, *J. Immunol., 136*: 2103 (1986).
36. E. L. Reinherz, P. C. Kung, G. Goldstein, R. H. Levey, and S. F. Schlossman, Discrete stages of intrathymic differentiation: Analysis of normal thymocytes and leukemic lymphoblasts of T lineage, *Proc. Natl. Acad. Sci., 77*: 1588 (1980).
36a. E. L. Reinherz, R. E. Hussey, and S. F. Schlossman, A monoclonal antibody blocking human T cell function, *Eur. J. Immunol., 10*: 758 (1980).
37. G. F. Burns, A. W. Boyd, and P. C. Beverly, Two monoclonal anti-human T lymphocyte antigens have similar biologic effects and recognize the same cell surface antigen, *J. Immunol., 129*: 1451 (1982).
38. F. P. van Wauwe, J. R. De May, and J. G. Goossens, OKT3: A monoclonal anti-human T lymphocyte antibody with potent mitogenic properties, *J. Immunol., 124*: 2708 (1980).
39. B. J. Classon, J. Tsagaratos, L. Kirszbaum, J. Maddox, C. R. Mackay, M. Brandon, I. F. C. McKenzie, and I. D. Walker, The L3T4 antigen in mouse and the sheep equivalent are immunoglobulin-like, *Immunogenetics, 23*: 129 (1986).
40. S. C. Meuer, R. E. Hussey, J. C. Hussey, J. C. Hodgdon, T. Hercend, S. F. Schlossman, and E. L. Reinherz, Surface structures involved in target recognition by human cytotoxic T lymphocytes, *Science, 218*: 471 (1982).

41. E. Nakayama, H. Shiku, E. Stockert, H. F. Oettgen, and L. J. Old, Cytotoxic T cells: Lyt phenotype and blocking of killing activity by Lyt antisera, *Proc. Natl. Acad. Sci. USA, 76*: 1977 (1979).
42. S. L. Clark, Jr., The intrathymic environment, *Contemp. Topics Immunobiol., 2*: 77 (1973).
43. H. A. Gerber, B. Morris, and W. Trevella, Humoral immunity in B cell depleted sheep, in *Immunology of the Sheep* (B. Morris and M. Miyasaka, eds.), Editiones Roche, Basel, 1985, p. 187.
44. A. J. Husband, K. J. Beh, and A. K. Lascelles, IgA-containing cells in the ruminant intestine following intraperitoneal and local immunization, *Immunology, 37*: 597 (1979).
45. K. J. Beh, A. Husband, and A. K. Lascelles, Intestinal response of sheep to intraperitoneal immunization, *Immunology, 37*: 385 (1979).
46. H. A. Gerber, Functional studies on gut-associated lymphoid tissues, Ph.D. thesis, Australian National University, Canberra, 1979.
47. J. D. Reynolds and B. Morris, The evolution and involution of Peyer's patches in fetal and neonatal sheep, *Eur. J. Immunol., 13*: 627 (1983).
48. J. D. Reynolds and B. Morris, The effect of antigen on the development of Peyer's patches, *Eur. J. Immunol., 14*: 1 (1984).
49. J. D. Reynolds and R. Pabst, The emigration of lymphocytes from Peyer's patches in sheep, *Eur. J. Immunol., 14*: 7 (1984).
50. M. Miyasaka and L. Dudler, Differentiation of ovine immature B cells upon exposure to phorbol myristate acetate, *Int. Archs. Allergy Appl. Immunol., 74*: 281 (1984).
51. M. L. Rose and F. Malchiodi, Binding of peanut lectin to thymic cortex and germinal centres of lymphoid tissue, *Immunology, 42*: 583 (1981).
52. K. J. Fahey, The binding of lectins to sheep tissues and circulating cells: Peanut agglutinin, a marker for presumptive T-lymphocytes, *Aust. J. Exp. Med. Sci., 55*: 557 (198).
53. D. A. Schackelford and J. L. Strominger, Analysis of the oligosaccharides on the HLA-DR and DC1 B cell antigens, *J. Immunol., 130*: 274 (1983).
54. J. A. Falk, J. B. L. Addis, and M. Letarte, Species cross-reactive Ia determinants: Detection with a monoclonal antibody to human Ia of a murine Ia 7 epitope, *Human Immunol., 7*: 79 (1983).
55. J. Hopkins, B. M. Dutia, and I. McConnell, Monoclonal antibodies to sheep lymphocytes. I. Identification of MHC II molecules in lymphoid cells in resting lymph and after *in vivo* antigen inoculation, *Immunology, 59*: 433.
56. I. S. Trowbridge, Interspecies spleen-myeloma producing monoclonal antibodies against mouse lymphocyte surface glycoprotein T200, *J. Exp. Med., 148*: 313 (1978).
57. R. L. Coffman and I. L. Weissman, B220: A B cell-specific member of the T200 glycoprotein family, *Nature, 289*: 681 (1981).
58. L. T. Yam, C. Y. Li, and W. H. Crosby, Cytochemical identification of monocytes and granulocytes, *Am. J. Clin. Path., 55*: 283 (1971).

59. J. G. Tew, T. E. Mandel, R. P. Phipps, and A. K. Szakal, Tissue localization and retention of antigen in relation to the immune response, *Am. J. Anat.*, *170*: 420 (1984).
60. A. N. Barkley, Different reticular elements in rat lymphoid tissue identified by localization of Ia, Thy-1 and MRC OX2 antigens, *Immunology, 44*: 727 (1981).
61. M. R. Parwaresh, H. J. Radzun, M.-L. Hansmann, and K.-P. Peters, Monoclonal antibody Ki-M4 specifically recognizes human dendritic reticulum cells (follicular dendritic cells) and their possible precursor in blood, *Blood, 62*: 585 (1983).
62. B. F. Haynes, K. Shimuzu, and G. S. Eisenbarth, Identification of human and rodent thymic epithelium using tetanus toxin and monoclonal antibody A2B5, *J. Clin. Invest., 71*: 9 (1983).
63. B. F. Haynes, The human thymic microenvironment, *Adv. Immunol., 36*: 86 (1984).
64. E. van Vliet, M. Melis, and W. van Ewijk, Monoclonal antibodies of stromal cell types of the mouse thymus, *Eur. J. Immunol., 14*: 524 (1984).
65. M. Miyasaka, L. Dudler, G. Bordmann, W. M. Leiserson, H. A. Gerber, J. Reynolds, and Z. Trnka, Differentiation of B lymphocytes in sheep. I. Phenotypic analysis of ileal Peyer's patch cells and the demonstration of a precursor population for sIg^+ cells in the ileal Peyer's patches, *Immunology, 53*: 515 (1984).

Index